# Epstein-Barr Virus Protocols

# METHODS IN MOLECULAR BIOLOGY™

## *John M. Walker, Series Editor*

178. **Antibody Phage Display:** *Methods and Protocols,* edited by *Philippa M. O'Brien and Robert Aitken, 2001*
177. **Two-Hybrid Systems:** *Methods and Protocols,* edited by *Paul N. MacDonald, 2001*
176. **Steroid Receptor Methods:** *Protocols and Assays,* edited by *Benjamin A. Lieberman, 2001*
175. **Genomics Protocols**, edited by *Michael P. Starkey and Ramnath Elaswarapu, 2001*
174. **Epstein-Barr Virus Protocols,** edited by *Joanna B. Wilson and Gerhard H. W. May, 2001*
173. **Calcium-Binding Protein Protocols, Volume 2:** *Methods and Techniques,* edited by *Hans J. Vogel, 2001*
172. **Calcium-Binding Protein Protocols, Volume 1:** *Reviews and Case Histories,* edited by *Hans J. Vogel, 2001*
171. **Proteoglycan Protocols,** edited by *Renato V. Iozzo, 2001*
170. **DNA Arrays:** *Methods and Protocols,* edited by *Jang B. Rampal, 2001*
169. **Neurotrophin Protocols,** edited by *Robert A. Rush, 2001*
168. **Protein Structure, Stability, and Folding,** edited by *Kenneth P. Murphy, 2001*
167. **DNA Sequencing Protocols,** *Second Edition,* edited by *Colin A. Graham and Alison J. M. Hill, 2001*
166. **Immunotoxin Methods and Protocols**, edited by *Walter A. Hall, 2001*
165. **SV40 Protocols**, edited by *Leda Raptis, 2001*
164. **Kinesin Protocols,** edited by *Isabelle Vernos, 2001*
163. **Capillary Electrophoresis of Nucleic Acids, Volume 2:** *Practical Applications of Capillary Electrophoresis,* edited by *Keith R. Mitchelson and Jing Cheng, 2001*
162. **Capillary Electrophoresis of Nucleic Acids, Volume 1:** *Introduction to the Capillary Electrophoresis of Nucleic Acids,* edited by *Keith R. Mitchelson and Jing Cheng, 2001*
161. **Cytoskeleton Methods and Protocols**, edited by *Ray H. Gavin, 2001*
160. **Nuclease Methods and Protocols,** edited by *Catherine H. Schein, 2001*
159. **Amino Acid Analysis Protocols,** edited by *Catherine Cooper, Nicole Packer, and Keith Williams, 2001*
158. **Gene Knockout Protocols,** edited by *Martin J. Tymms and Ismail Kola, 2001*
157. **Mycotoxin Protocols,** edited by *Mary W. Trucksess and Albert E. Pohland, 2001*
156. **Antigen Processing and Presentation Protocols,** edited by *Joyce C. Solheim, 2001*
155. **Adipose Tissue Protocols,** edited by *Gérard Ailhaud, 2000*
154. **Connexin Methods and Protocols,** edited by *Roberto Bruzzone and Christian Giaume, 2001*
153. **Neuropeptide Y Protocols**, edited by *Ambikaipakan Balasubramaniam, 2000*
152. **DNA Repair Protocols:** *Prokaryotic Systems,* edited by *Patrick Vaughan, 2000*
151. **Matrix Metalloproteinase Protocols,** edited by *Ian M. Clark, 2001*
150. **Complement Methods and Protocols,** edited by *B. Paul Morgan, 2000*
149. **The ELISA Guidebook**, edited by *John R. Crowther, 2000*
148. **DNA–Protein Interactions:** *Principles and Protocols* **(2nd ed.)**, edited by *Tom Moss, 2001*
147. **Affinity Chromatography:** *Methods and Protocols*, edited by *Pascal Bailon, George K. Ehrlich, Wen-Jian Fung, and Wolfgang Berthold, 2000*
146. **Mass Spectrometry of Proteins and Peptides,** edited by *John R. Chapman, 2000*
145. **Bacterial Toxins:** ***Methods and Protocols***, edited by *Otto Holst, 2000*
144. **Calpain Methods and Protocols**, edited by *John S. Elce, 2000*
143. **Protein Structure Prediction:** *Methods and Protocols,* edited by *David Webster, 2000*
142. **Transforming Growth Factor-Beta Protocols**, edited by *Philip H. Howe, 2000*
141. **Plant Hormone Protocols**, edited by *Gregory A. Tucker and Jeremy A. Roberts, 2000*
140. **Chaperonin Protocols**, edited by *Christine Schneider, 2000*
139. **Extracellular Matrix Protocols**, edited by *Charles Streuli and Michael Grant, 2000*
138. **Chemokine Protocols**, edited by *Amanda E. I. Proudfoot, Timothy N. C. Wells, and Christine Power, 2000*
137. **Developmental Biology Protocols, Volume III**, edited by *Rocky S. Tuan and Cecilia W. Lo, 2000*
136. **Developmental Biology Protocols, Volume II,** edited by *Rocky S. Tuan and Cecilia W. Lo, 2000*
135. **Developmental Biology Protocols, Volume I,** edited by *Rocky S. Tuan and Cecilia W. Lo, 2000*
134. **T Cell Protocols:** *Development and Activation*, edited by *Kelly P. Kearse, 2000*
133. **Gene Targeting Protocols,** edited by *Eric B. Kmiec, 2000*
132. **Bioinformatics Methods and Protocols,** edited by *Stephen Misener and Stephen A. Krawetz, 2000*
131. **Flavoprotein Protocols,** edited by *S. K. Chapman and G. A. Reid, 1999*
130. **Transcription Factor Protocols,** edited by *Martin J. Tymms, 2000*
129. **Integrin Protocols,** edited by *Anthony Howlett, 1999*
128. **NMDA Protocols,** edited by *Min Li, 1999*
127. **Molecular Methods in Developmental Biology:** Xenopus *and Zebrafish*, edited by *Matthew Guille, 1999*
126. **Adrenergic Receptor Protocols,** edited by *Curtis A. Machida, 2000*
125. **Glycoprotein Methods and Protocols:** *The Mucins,* edited by *Anthony P. Corfield, 2000*
124. **Protein Kinase Protocols,** edited by *Alastair D. Reith, 2001*
123. ***In Situ* Hybridization Protocols (2nd ed.)**, edited by *Ian A. Darby, 2000*
122. **Confocal Microscopy Methods and Protocols,** edited by *Stephen W. Paddock, 1999*
121. **Natural Killer Cell Protocols:** *Cellular and Molecular Methods,* edited by *Kerry S. Campbell and Marco Colonna, 2000*
120. **Eicosanoid Protocols,** edited by *Elias A. Lianos, 1999*
119. **Chromatin Protocols,** edited by *Peter B. Becker, 1999*
118. **RNA–Protein Interaction Protocols,** edited by *Susan R. Haynes, 1999*
117. **Electron Microscopy Methods and Protocols,** edited by *M. A. Nasser Hajibagheri, 1999*
116. **Protein Lipidation Protocols,** edited by *Michael H. Gelb, 1999*
115. **Immunocytochemical Methods and Protocols (2nd ed.),** edited by *Lorette C. Javois, 1999*

METHODS IN MOLECULAR BIOLOGY™

# Epstein-Barr Virus Protocols

Edited by

**Joanna B. Wilson**

*I.B.L.S. Division of Molecular Genetics, University of Glasgow, United Kingdom*

and

**Gerhard H. W. May**

*I.B.L.S. Division of Biochemistry and Molecular Biology, University of Glasgow, United Kingdom*

**Humana Press** **Totowa, New Jersey**

Softcover reprint of the hardcover 1st edition 2001
999 Riverview Drive, Suite 208
Totowa, New Jersey 07512



This publication is printed on acid-free paper. ∞
ANSI Z39.48-1984 (American Standards Institute)
Permanence of Paper for Printed Library Materials.

Cover design by Patricia F. Cleary.
Cover illustration: Composition of the mini-EBV plasmid p1478A. See full caption on page 24.
Production Editors: Susan Giniger and John Morgan.

For additional copies, pricing for bulk purchases, and/or information about other Humana titles, contact Humana at the above address or at any of the following numbers: Tel.: 973-256-1699; Fax: 973-256-8341; E-mail: humana@humanapr.com; or visit our Website: http://humanapress.com.



10 9 8 7 6 5 4 3 2 1

Library of Congress Cataloging-in-Publication Data

Epstein-Barr virus protocols / edited by Joanna B. Wilson and Gerhard H.W. May.
p. cm. -- (Methods in molecular biology ; 174)
Includes bibliographical references.
ISBN 978-1-61737-137-0 e-ISBN 978-1-59259-227-2
1. Epstein-Barr virus--Laboratory manuals. I. Wilson, Joanna B. II. May, Gerhard H.W. III. Series.
QR400.2.E68 E654 2001
616'.0194--dc21

2001016991

# Preface

The discovery of Epstein-Barr virus (EBV) by Epstein, Achong, and Barr, reported in 1964 (*Lancet* **1**:702–703), was stimulated by Denis Burkitt's recognition of a novel African childhood lymphoma and his postulation that an infectious agent was involved in the tumor's etiology (*Nature* **194**:232–234, 1962). Since then, molecular and cellular biological and computational technologies have progressed by leaps and bounds. The advent of recombinant DNA technology opened the possibilities of genetic research more than most would have realized. Not only have the molecular tools permitted the analyses of viral mechanisms, but, importantly, they have formed the basis for discerning viral presence and, subsequently, viral involvement in an increasing number of diseases. Though in every field of science the search for further knowledge is likely to be a limitless phenomenon, the distinct goal in EBV research, namely, to gain sufficient insight into the viral–host interaction to be able to intercept the pathogenic process, is beginning to be realized.

Epstein-Barr virus research has effectively entered the postgenomic era that began with the sequencing of the first strains, cloned in the mid to late 1980s. Owing to the lack of a productive lytic system, for many years the difficulty in manipulating the viral genome virtually surpassed that of manipulating the mammalian genome. These difficulties have now largely been resolved and the use of recombinant and mini viral genomes demonstrate the continuing power of mutant analysis. Though a wealth of information on viral action has been amassed over the years, this has nevertheless been predictably dwarfed by the new questions it is possible to pose. This is evidenced by the number of laboratories working on EBV and reflected in the success of the International Association for Research on EBV and Associated Diseases and its biennial meetings (http://www.med.ic.ac.uk/ebv/home.htm). Information concerning viral infection, latency, immunogenicity, and immune evasion are being integrated into a holistic understanding of viral pathogenesis. Moreover, the decades of research on EBV provide by example a fast track for research work on newly identified, related viruses such as Kaposi's sarcoma–associated herpesvirus/human herpesvirus 8 (HHV8).

Seminal molecular techniques have opened avenues of research and several, such as Southern blotting, first described in 1975 (detailed in many variant forms in this volume), continue to yield highly informative data. With the advent of the polymerase chain reaction method in the late 1980s, assay sensitivity and detection of nucleic acids are no longer barriers to study, and new applications continue to emerge. The ability to harness homologous recombination and select for the desired products, which initiated the continuing explosion in analyzing genetic function in higher organisms by virtue of gene deletion or manipulation, has also been applied to EBV. Recently, sophisticated techniques for genomic, transcript, and proteomic comparative analyses are blooming, for which high-quality sample preparation is a prerequisite. Though these applications are not necessarily described herein, the underlying protocols for sample preparation are covered in several chapters.

All the protocols an EBV researcher could desire cannot possibly be covered in one single volume; however, we have endeavored to include many of the principal methods used and described by experts. Moreover, most of these protocols can be applied directly, or easily adapted, to address questions in fields of molecular biological research unrelated to EBV studies.

The editors would like to take this opportunity to thank John Walker, the series editor, and all the staff at Humana Press who were involved in producing this volume.

***Joanna Wilson***
***Gerhard May***

# Contents


Preface .......... *v*

Contributors .......... *xi*

I GENOME AND TRANSCRIPT ANALYSES

1 Epstein-Barr Virus: *The B95-8 Strain Map*
**Paul J. Farrell** .......... **3**

2 Analysis of Replication of oriP-Based Plasmids by Quantitative, Competitive PCR
**Ann L. Kirchmaier** .......... **13**

3 Genetic Analysis and Gene Expression with Mini-Epstein-Barr Virus Plasmids
**Ellen Kilger and Wolfgang Hammerschmidt** .......... **23**

4 Construction of cDNA Libraries for the Analysis of the Structure of Complementary Strand Transcripts (CSTs)
**Paul R. Smith** .......... **37**

5 Analysis of the Expression and Function of the EBV-Encoded Small RNAs, the EBERs, in Heterologous Cells
**Kenneth G. Laing, Volker Matys, and Michael J. Clemens** .......... **45**

6 Visualizing EBV Expression Patterns by FISH
**Anna Szeles** .......... **67**

II VIRAL DETECTION

7 *In Situ* Detection of Epstein-Barr Virus DNA and Viral Gene Products
**Gerald Niedobitek and Hermann Herbst** .......... **79**

8 Phenotype Determination of Epstein-Barr Virus-Infected Cells in Tissue Sections
**Hermann Herbst and Gerald Niedobitek** .......... **93**

9 Detection of EBV Infection at the Single-Cell Level: *Precise Quantitation of Virus-Infected Cells In Vivo*
**Gregory J. Babcock, Emily M. Miyashita-Lin, and David A. Thorley-Lawson** .......... **103**

10 Detection and Discrimination of Latent and Replicative Herpesvirus Infection at the Single Cell Level In Vivo
***Lisa L. Decker, Gregory J. Babcock, and David A. Thorley-Lawson*** ..... ***111***

III CULTURE METHODS

11 Virus Isolation
***Lindsey M. Hutt-Fletcher and Susan M. Turk*** ..... ***119***

12 Generation of Lymphoblastoid Cell Lines (LCLs)
***Teresa Frisan, Victor Levitsky, and Maria Masucci*** ..... ***125***

13 Cell Cycle Distribution of B-Lymphocytes and Cell Lines
***Alison J. Sinclair*** ..... ***129***

14 Introduction of Plasmid Vectors into Cells Via Electroporation
***Ann L. Kirchmaier*** ..... ***137***

15 Malignant Transformation and Immortalization Assays in Animal Cells Transfected with the BARF1 Gene
***Tadamasa Ooka*** ..... ***147***

16 Transient Gene Expression and MACS Enrichment
***Dieter Kube and Martina Vockerodt*** ..... ***155***

17 In Vitro Assays to Study Epithelial Cell Growth
***Christopher W. Dawson and Lawrence S. Young*** ..... ***165***

18 In Vitro Assays to Study Epithelial Cell Differentiation
***Christopher W. Dawson and Lawrence S. Young*** ..... ***173***

19 Cell Sensitivity Assays: *Quantitative Detection of Apoptotic Cells In Vitro Using the TUNEL Assay*
***Neil A. Jones and Caroline Dive*** ..... ***181***

20 Qualitative Detection of Apoptotic Cells Assessed by DNA Fragmentation
***Amanda J. McIlwrath*** ..... ***189***

IV IMMUNE ASSAYS

21 Regression Assay
***Teresa Frisan, Victor Levitsky, and Maria Masucci*** ..... ***199***

22 Generation of Polyclonal EBV-Specific CTL Cultures and Clones
***Victor Levitsky, Teresa Frisan, and Maria Masucci*** ..... ***203***

23 Determination of Antigen and Fine Peptide Specificity of EBV-Specific CTLs
***Victor Levitsky, Teresa Frisan, and Maria Masucci*** ..... ***209***

24 Limiting Dilution Assay
***Teresa Frisan, Victor Levitsky, and Maria Masucci*** ..... ***213***

## V VIRAL PROTEIN DETECTION

25 Antibodies for Detecting EBV Latent Proteins
*Martin Rowe and Anja Mehl* ........ 219
26 Detection of EBV Latent Proteins by Western Blotting
*Martin Rowe and Matthew Jones* ........ 229
27 Biosynthetic Radiolabeling of Virus Glycoproteins for Immunoprecipitation and Electrophoretic Analysis
*Lindsey M. Hutt-Fletcher and Susan M. Turk* ........ 243

## VI PROTEIN-PROTEIN, PROTEIN-DNA, AND PROTEIN-RNA INTERACTIONS

28 The Yeast Two-Hybrid Assay to Identify Interacting Proteins
*Kenneth M. Izumi* ........ 249
29 Identification of Transactivation, Repression, and Protein-Protein Interaction Domains Using GAL4-Fusion Proteins
*James J.-D. Hsieh and S. Diane Hayward* ........ 259
30 Magnetic DNA Affinity Purification of a Cellular Transcription Factor
*Lothar J. Strobl and Ursula Zimber-Strobl* ........ 271
31 Screening an Expression Library with a DNA Binding Site
*Qin Zhang and Eduardo A. Montalvo* ........ 279
32 Analysis of DNA Binding Proteins by Mobility Shift Assay
*Yi-Chun James Wang and Eduardo A. Montalvo* ........ 289
33 Analysis of RNA-Protein Interactions of the EBV-Encoded Small RNAs, the EBERs: *In Vitro Assays*
*Kenneth G. Laing, Androulla Elia, Ian W. Jeffrey, and Michael J. Clemens* ........ 297

## VII PROTEIN ACTIVITY ASSAYS

34 Chimeric and Mutated Variants of LMP1: *A Helpful Tool to Analyze the Structure-Function Relationship of a Pseudoreceptor*
*Olivier Gires, Marius Ueffing, and Wolfgang Hammerschmidt* ... 313
35 Assaying the Activity of Kinases Regulated by LMP1
*Arnd Kieser* ........ 325
36 In Vitro Assays for the Detection of Protein Tyrosine Phosphorylation and Protein Tyrosine Kinase Activities
*Sara Fruehling and Richard Longnecker* ........ 337

VIII TISSUE AND IN VIVO PROTOCOLS

37 Analysis of Apoptosis in Tissue Sections
*Vicki Save, Philip J. Coates, and Peter A. Hall* ............................ 347
38 Considerations in Generating Transgenic Mice: *DNA, RNA, and Protein Extractions from Tissues—Rapid and Effective Blotting*
*Joanna B. Wilson and Mark E. Drotar* ............................ 361
39 In Vivo Assay of Cellular Proliferation
*John Curran* ............................ 379
40 Topical Chemical Carcinogen Treatment in Mice
*John Curran* ............................ 391
41 Separation of Epidermal Tissue from Underlying Dermis and Primary Keratinocyte Culture
*Jennifer Macdiarmid and Joanna B. Wilson* ............................ 401
42 Selection and Enrichment of B Cells from Lymphoid Tissues
*Penelope Tsimbouri, Marie Anne O'Donnell, and Joanna B. Wilson* ............................ 411
43 Detection of Immunoglobulin Gene Rearrangements
*Robert G. Caldwell and Richard Longnecker* ............................ 423
Index ............................ 433

# Contributors

GREGORY J. BABCOCK • *Dana Farber Cancer Institute, Boston, MA*
ROBERT G. CALDWELL • *Microbiology and Immunology Department, Northwestern University Medical School, Chicago, IL*
MICHAEL J. CLEMENS • *Department of Biochemistry and Immunology, Cellular and Molecular Sciences Group, St. George's Hospital Medical School, University of London, London, United Kingdom*
PHILIP J. COATES • *Radiation and Genome Stability Unit, Medical Research Council Harwell, Didcot, Oxfordshire, United Kingdom*
JOHN CURRAN • *Athena Diagnostics, Inc., Division of Elar Pharmaceuticals, Worcester, MA*
CHRISTOPHER W. DAWSON • *CRC Institute for Cancer Studies, The University of Birmingham Medical School, Birmingham, United Kingdom*
LISA L. DECKER • *Department of Pathology, Harvard Medical School, Boston, MA*
CAROLINE DIVE • *Molecular and Cellular Pharmacology Group, School of Biological Sciences, University of Manchester, Manchester, United Kingdom*
MARK E. DROTAR • *I.B.L.S. Division of Molecular Genetics, University of Glasgow, Glasgow, United Kingdom*
ANDROULLA ELIA • *Department of Biochemistry and Immunology, Cellular and Molecular Sciences Group, St. George's Hospital Medical School, University of London, London, United Kingdom*
PAUL J. FARRELL • *Ludwig Institute for Cancer Research, Imperial College School of Medicine at St. Mary's, London, United Kingdom*
TERESA FRISAN • *Microbiology and Tumor Biology Center (MTC), Karolinska Institutet, Stockholm, Sweden*
SARA FRUEHLING • *Microbiology and Immunology Department, Northwestern University Medical School, Chicago, IL*
OLIVIER GIRES • *HNO-Forschung, Universitätsklinikum Grosshadern, München, Germany*
PETER A. HALL • *Department of Molecular and Cellular Pathology, University of Dundee, Dundee, United Kingdom*

WOLFGANG HAMMERSCHMIDT • *GSF, Institut für Klinische Molekularbiologie und Tumorgenetik, Abteilung Genvektoren, München, Germany*
S. DIANE HAYWARD • *Molecular Virology Laboratories, Department of Oncology, Johns Hopkins School of Medicine, Baltimore, MD*
HERMANN HERBST • *Gerhard-Domagk-Institut für Pathologie, Universität Münster, Münster, Germany*
JAMES J.-D. HSIEH • *Molecular Virology Laboratories, Department of Oncology, Johns Hopkins School of Medicine, Baltimore, MD*
LINDSEY M. HUTT-FLETCHER • *School of Biological Sciences, University of Missouri–Kansas City, Kansas City, MO*
KENNETH M. IZUMI • *Brigham and Women's Hospital, Boston, MA*
IAN W. JEFFREY • *Department of Biochemistry and Immunology, Cellular and Molecular Sciences Group, St. George's Hospital Medical School, University of London, London, United Kingdom*
MATTHEW JONES • *Section of Infection and Immunity, Department of Medicine, University of Wales College of Medicine, Cardiff, United Kingdom*
NEIL A. JONES • *Molecular and Cellular Pharmacology Group, School of Biological Sciences, University of Manchester, Manchester, United Kingdom*
ARND KIESER • *GSF, Institut für Klinische Molekularbiologie und Tumorgenetik, München, Germany*
ELLEN KILGER • *Boehringer Ingelheim Pharma KG, Ingelheim, Germany*
ANN L. KIRCHMAIER • *Department of Molecular and Cell Biology, Division of Genetics and Development, University of California, Berkeley, CA*
DIETER KUBE • *Sektion für Humanparasitologie, Institut für Tropenmedizin, Eberhard-Karls-Universität; Universitätsklinikum Tübingen, Tübingen, Germany*
KENNETH G. LAING • *Department of Medical Microbiology, St. George's Hospital Medical School, University of London, London, United Kingdom*
VICTOR LEVITSKY • *Department of Tumour Biology, Karolinska Institutet, Stockholm, Sweden*
RICHARD LONGNECKER • *Departments of Microbiology and Immunology, Northwestern University Medical School, Chicago, IL*
JENNIFER MACDIARMID • *I.B.L.S. Division of Molecular Genetics, University of Glasgow, Glasgow, United Kingdom*
MARIA MASUCCI • *Department of Tumour Biology, Karolinska Institutet, Stockholm, Sweden*

VOLKER MATYS • *BIOBASE—Biological Databases/Biologische Datenbanken GmbH, Braunschweig, Germany*
GERHARD H. W. MAY • *I.B.L.S. Division of Biochemistry and Molecular Biology, University of Glasgow, Glasgow, United Kingdom*
AMANDA J. MCILWRATH • *Technical and Customer Services United Kingdom, New England Biolabs (United Kingdom) Ltd, Hertfordshire, United Kingdom*
ANJA MEHL • *University of Wales College of Medicine, Department of Medicine, Section of Infection and Immunity, Cardiff, United Kingdom*
EMILY M. MIYASHITA-LIN • *Department of Psychiatry, University of California, San Francisco; Nina Ireland Laboratory of Developmental Neurobiology, San Francisco, CA*
EDUARDO A. MONTALVO • *Division of Infectious Diseases, Department of Pediatrics, University of Texas Health Science Center, San Antonio, TX*
GERALD NIEDOBITEK • *Pathologisches Institut, Friedrich-Alexander Universität, Erlangen, Germany*
MARIE ANNE O'DONNELL • *I.B.L.S. Division of Molecular Genetics, University of Glasgow, Glasgow, United Kingdom*
TADAMASA OOKA • *Laboratoire de Virologie Moléculaire, IVMC, CNRS, Faculté de Médecine R.T.H. Laënnec, Lyon, France*
MARTIN ROWE • *Section of Infection and Immunity, Department of Medicine, University of Wales College of Medicine, Cardiff, United Kingdom*
VICKI SAVE • *Directorate of Pathology, Ninewells Hospital and Medical School, Dundee, United Kingdom*
ALISON J. SINCLAIR • *School of Biological Sciences, University of Sussex, Falmer, Brighton, United Kingdom*
PAUL R. SMITH • *Section of Virology and Cell Biology, Division of Investigative Science, Imperial College School of Medicine at St. Mary's, London, United Kingdom*
LOTHAR J. STROBL • *Institut für Genetik der Universität zu Köln, Köln, Germany*
ANNA SZELES • *Microbiology and Tumor Biology Center, Karolinska Institute, Stockholm, Sweden*
DAVID A. THORLEY-LAWSON • *Department of Pathology, Tufts University School of Medicine, Boston, MA*
PENELOPE TSIMBOURI • *I.B.L.S. Division of Molecular Genetics, University of Glasgow, Glasgow, United Kingdom*
SUSAN M. TURK • *School of Biological Sciences, University of Missouri – Kansas City, Kansas City, MO*

MARIUS UEFFING • *GSF, Institut für Klinische Molekularbiologie und Tumorgenetik, München, Germany*
MARTINA VOCKERODT • *Universitätskliniken Köln, Zentrum für Molekulare Medizin, Klinik für Innere Medizin I, Köln, Germany*
YI-CHUN JAMES WANG • *Division of Infectious Diseases, Department of Pediatrics, University of Texas Health Science Center, San Antonio, TX*
JOANNA B. WILSON • *I.B.L.S. Division of Molecular Genetics, University of Glasgow, Glasgow, United Kingdom*
LAWRENCE S. YOUNG • *CRC Institute for Cancer Studies, The University of Birmingham Medical School, Birmingham, United Kingdom*
URSULA ZIMBER-STROBL • *Institut für Genetik der Universität zu Köln, Köln, Germany*
QIN ZHANG • *Division of Infectious Diseases, Department of Pediatrics, University of Texas Health Science Center, San Antonio, TX*

# I

# Genome and Transcript Analyses

# 1

# Epstein-Barr Virus

## *The B95-8 Strain Map*

**Paul J. Farrell**

## 1. Introduction

This chapter summarizes the genes and mRNAs that have been mapped on to the B95-8 EBV genome. The complete sequence of this strain of Epstein-Barr Virus (EBV) was established *(1,2)* and data from many publications has been integrated into the map, which is an update of that published previously *(3)*. The B95-8 strain grows well in laboratory culture and transforms human B lymphocytes efficiently, but B95-8 EBV has about 11.8 kb deleted relative to other strains of EBV. The sequence of that region has been determined in the Raji strain of EBV and a map has been published *(4)*. Detailed literature citations for most of the features have been published *(3)*. The map should be used in conjunction with the B95-8 EBV DNA sequence, which can be accessed in the European Molecular Biology Laboratory (EMBL; embl:ebv.seq) or Genbank databases. The feature tables shown in those database files have not yet been revised so the information shown in this map is considerably more up to date.

## 2. Repeat Sequences

There are several regions of the genome that contain tandem repeat sequences. Some of these are large repeat units (for example, the major internal repeat is 3072 bp and the terminal repeat is 538 bp) but some are much simpler repeats. In most virus preparations, there will be a distribution of copy number of these repeats, so it is important to appreciate that the viral map and coordinates are just one reference example of genome structure. Generally the repeat numbers in the B95-8 map are thought to be typical, although it now appears that the 11.5 copies of the major internal repeat inserted into the B95-8 sequence may be an over-estimate, about 8.5 being more usual in B95-8 EBV *(5)*.

The restriction maps for *Eco*RI and *Bam*HI are shown beneath the scale bar in kb. The restriction fragments are labeled according to size, A being the largest fragment

From: *Methods in Molecular Biology, Vol. 174: Epstein-Barr Virus Protocols*
Edited by: J. B. Wilson and G. H. W. May © Humana Press Inc., Totowa, NJ

**Table 1**
**EBV Gene Nomenclature**

| | |
|---|---|
| EBNA-3A | EBNA-3 |
| EBNA-3B | EBNA-4 |
| EBNA-3C | EBNA-6 |
| EBNA-LP | EBNA-5 |
| LMP-2A | TP-1 |
| LMP-2B | TP-2 |
| BZLF1 | ZEBRA, EB1, Zta |
| BRLF1 | Rta, R |
| BARF transcripts | BART, CST |

EBNA, Epstein-Barr virus nuclear antigen; LMP, latent membrane protein; TP, terminal protein; BART, *Bam* A rightward transcripts; CST, complementary strand transcripts.

and lower case letters being used for additional fragments when there are more than 26.

## 3. Open Reading Frames

The major open reading frames, presumed to correspond to the protein coding parts of genes are shown as boxes, pointed at one end to indicate the direction of translation. Coordinates shown below are generally from the presumed initiator methionine to the last translated amino acid. When there is no obvious initiator methionine or the RNA structure is uncertain, the coordinates of the reading frame are shown from the beginning of the open reading frame to the last translated amino acid; these reading frames are marked "orf" after the coordinates. Initiator methionine residues have generally not been confirmed by mutagenesis so it is important to appreciate that the map is an interpretation in this respect.

## 4. Nomenclature

Open reading frames of EBV are named systematically according to the *Bam*HI restriction fragment in which their transcription commences, designated L or R according to the direction and then marked F followed by a number. So BALF4 is the fourth leftward reading frame commencing in the *Bam*HI A restriction fragment. Many of the genes are also known by more common and useful names, which may describe their function. Abbreviations used here are EBNA, Epstein-Barr virus nuclear antigen, LMP, latent membrane protein, EBER, Epstein-Barr virus encoded RNA. There is unfortunately some variation in nomenclature for EBV genes in the published literature. A guide to equivalents is shown in Table 1; terms on the same horizontal line refer to the same gene that shown on the left, being the standard used in this map.

## 5. Gene Expression

The open reading frames are shaded according to their expression class. These classes are defined operationally in EBV. Latent cycle genes are expressed constitu-

*(text continued on p. 12)*

# Epstein-Barr virus
# B95-8 strain

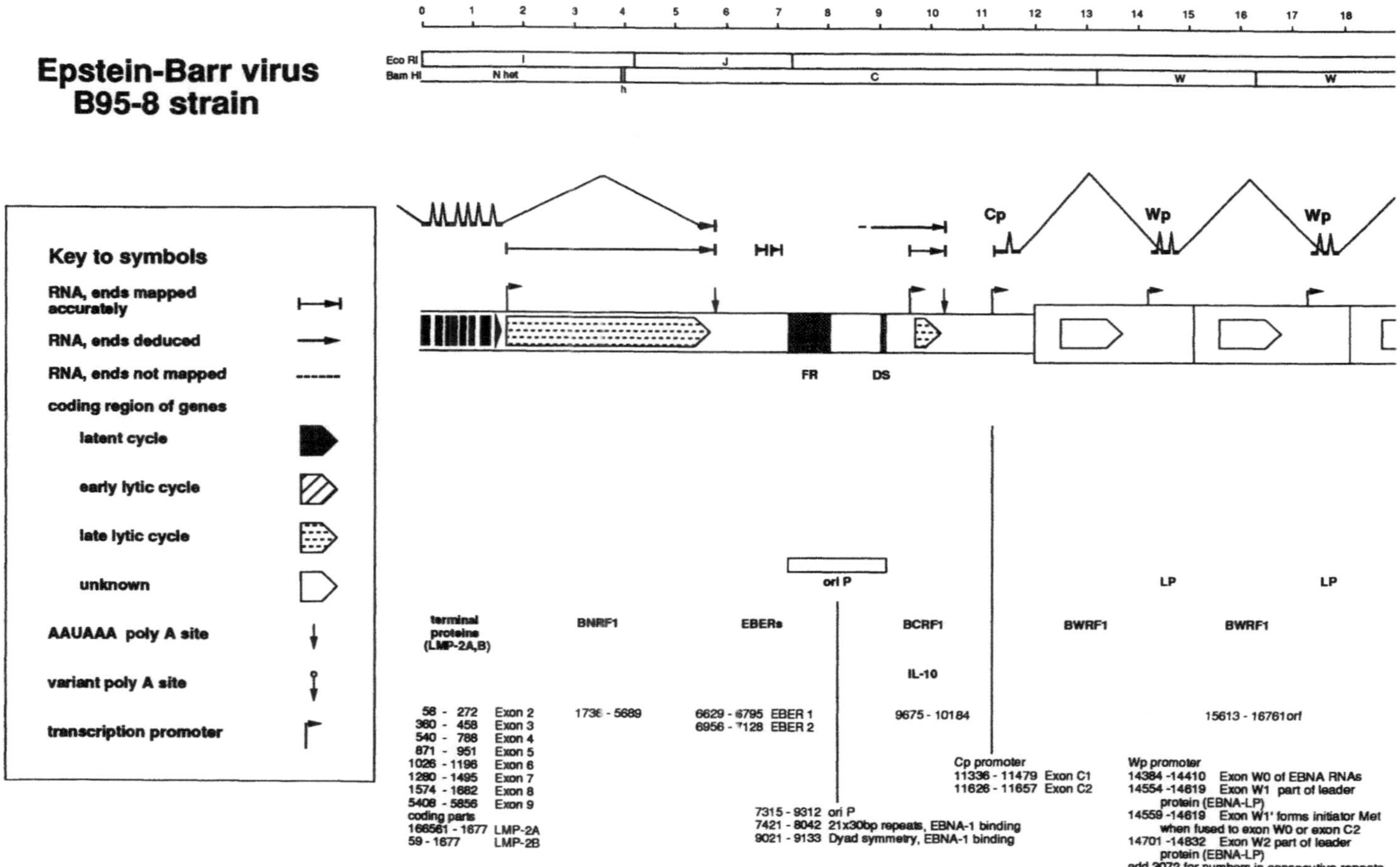

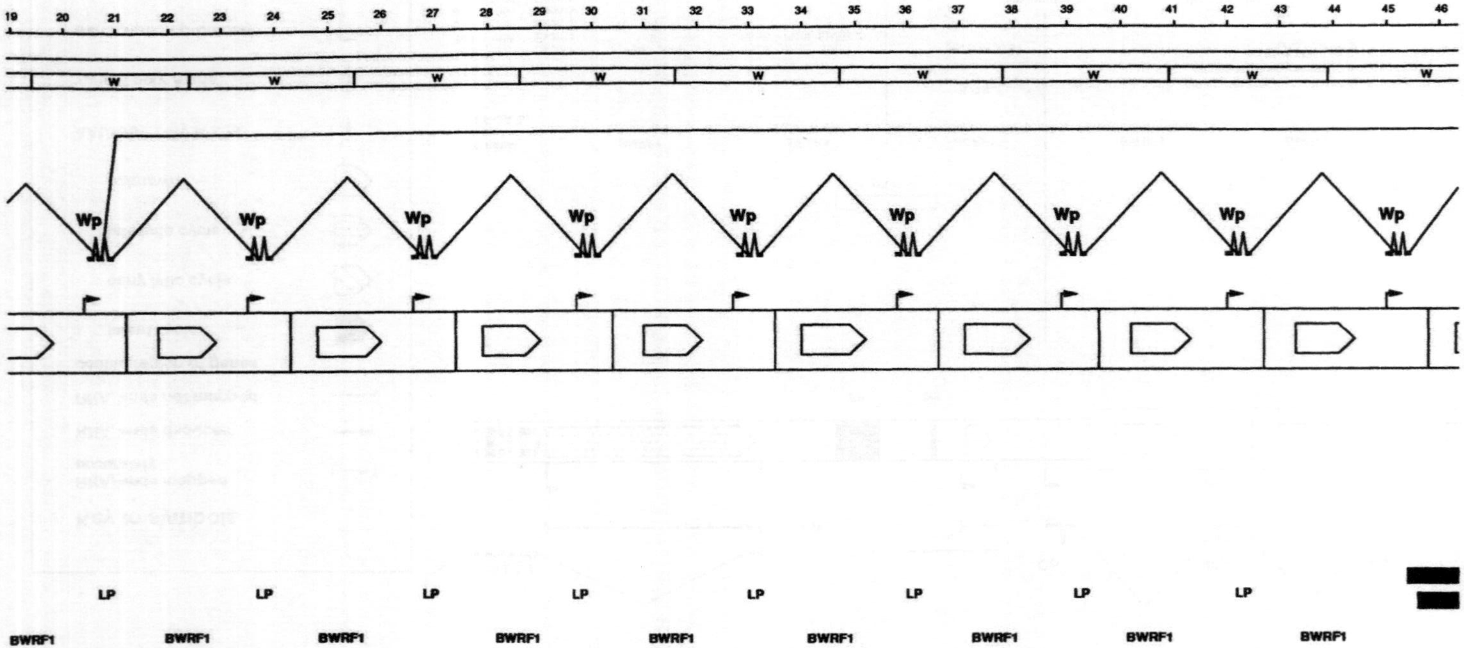

19
20
21
22
23
24
25
26
27
28
29
30
31
32
33
34
35
36
37
38
39
40
41
42
43
44
45
46
W
W
W
W
W
W
W
W
W
W
Wp
Wp
Wp
Wp
Wp
Wp
Wp
Wp
Wp
LP
LP
LP
LP
LP
LP
LP
LP
BWRF1
BWRF1
BWRF1
BWRF1
BWRF1
BWRF1
BWRF1
BWRF1
BWRF1

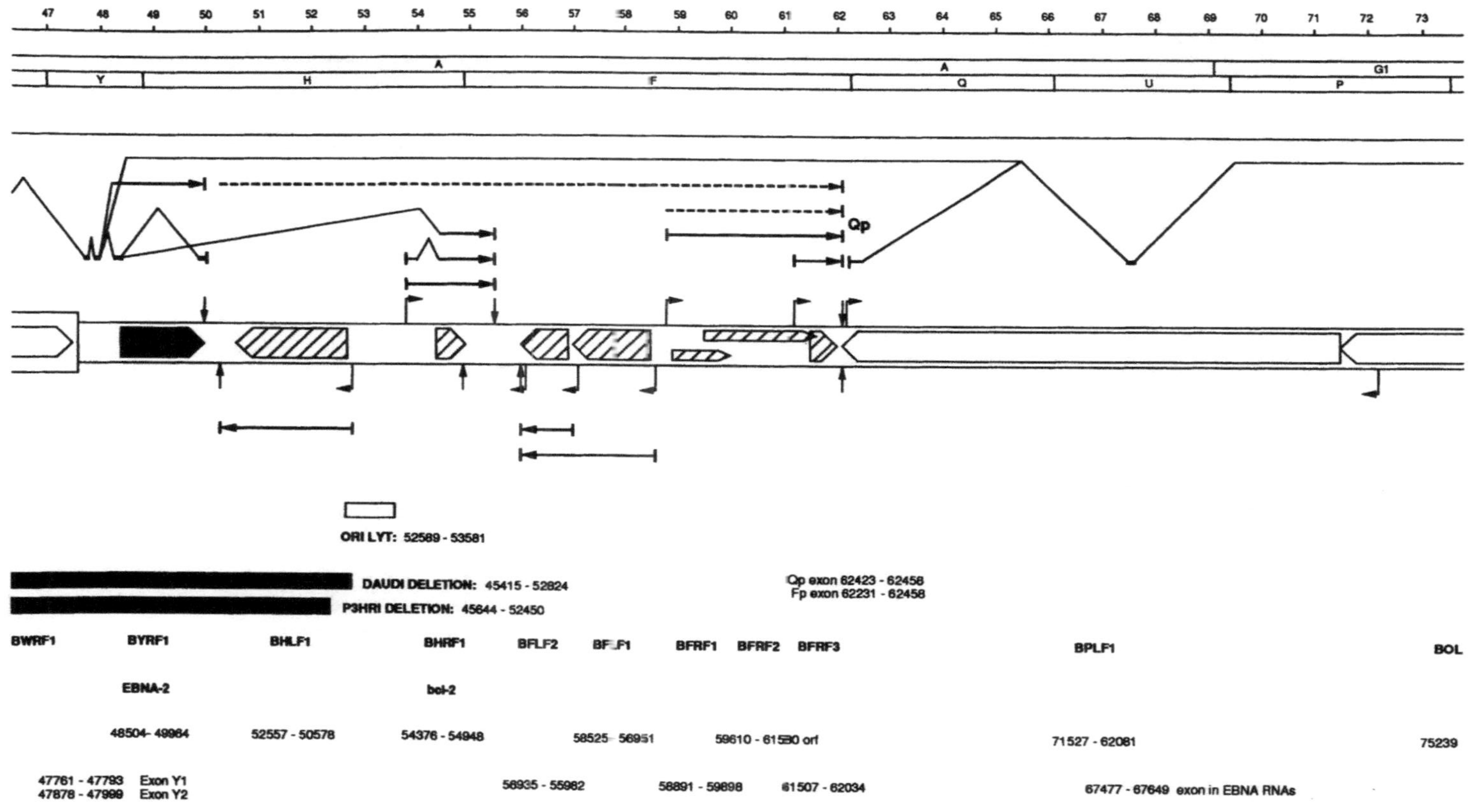

47 48 49 50 51 52 53 54 55 56 57 58 59 60 61 62 63 64 65 66 67 68 69 70 71 72 73
A
A
G1
Y
H
F
Q
U
P
Qp
ORI LYT: 52589 - 53581
DAUDI DELETION: 45415 - 52824
P3HRI DELETION: 45644 - 52450
Qp exon 62423 - 62458
Fp exon 62231 - 62458
BWRF1
BYRF1
BHLF1
BHRF1
BFLF2
BFRF1
BFRF2
BFRF3
BPLF1
BOL
EBNA-2
bcl-2
48504- 49964
52557 - 50578
54376 - 54948
59610 - 61530 orf
71527 - 62081
75239
47761 - 47793 Exon Y1
47878 - 47999 Exon Y2
56935 - 55982
58891 - 59898
61507 - 62034
67477 - 67649 exon in EBNA RNAs

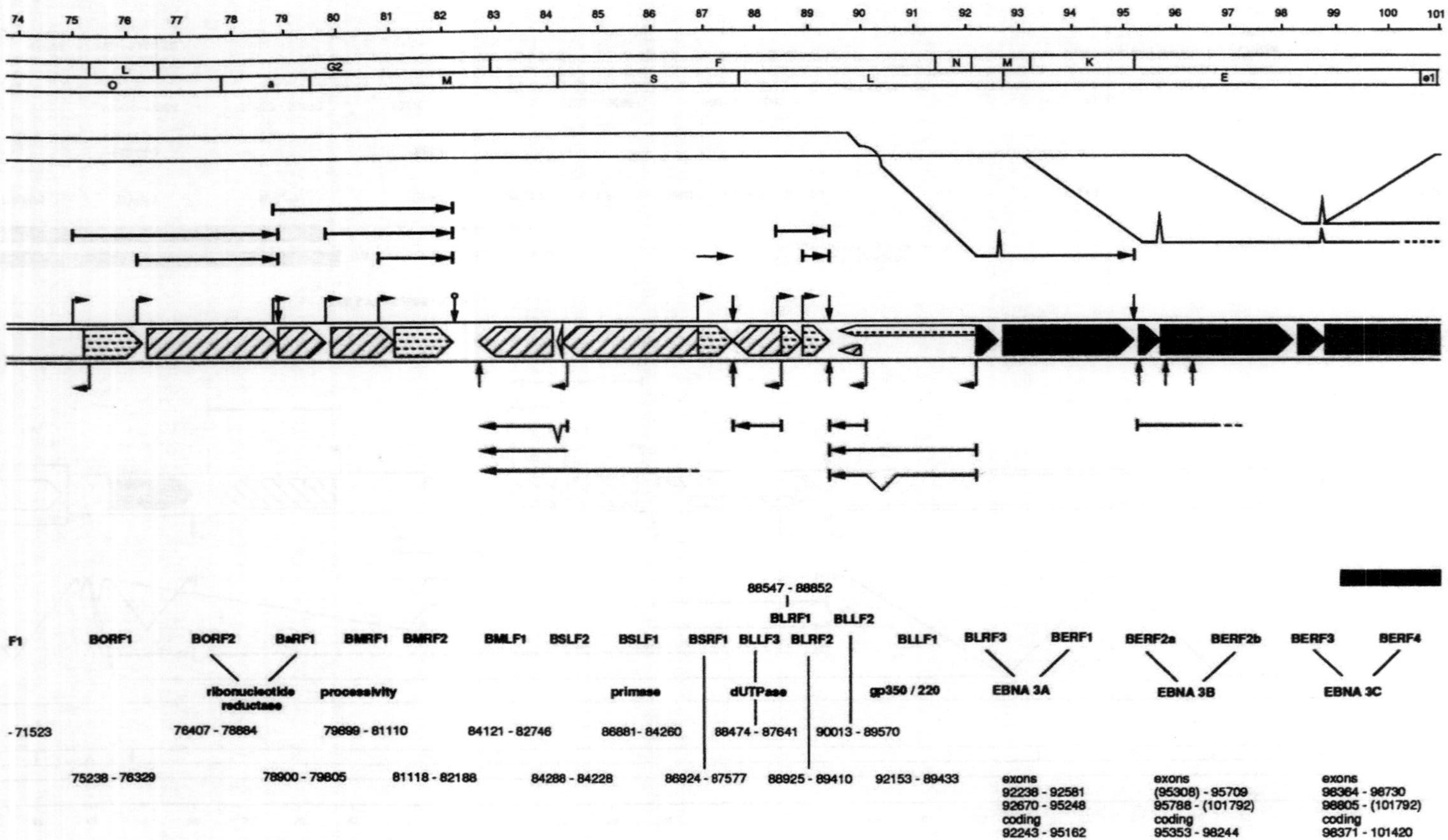
74
75
76
77
78
79
80
81
82
83
84
85
86
87
88
89
90
91
92
93
94
95
96
97
98
99
100
101
L
G2
F
N
M
K
O
a
M
S
L
E
e1
88547 - 88852
BLRF1
BLLF2
F1
BORF1
BORF2
BaRF1
BMRF1
BMRF2
BMLF1
BSLF2
BSLF1
BSRF1
BLLF3
BLRF2
BLLF1
BLRF3
BERF1
BERF2a
BERF2b
BERF3
BERF4
ribonucleotide reductase
processivity
primase
dUTPase
gp350 / 220
EBNA 3A
EBNA 3B
EBNA 3C
- 71523
76407 - 78884
79899 - 81110
84121 - 82746
86881 - 84260
88474 - 87641
90013 - 89570
75238 - 76329
78900 - 79805
81118 - 82188
84288 - 84228
86924 - 87577
88925 - 89410
92153 - 89433
exons
92238 - 92581
92670 - 95248
coding
92243 - 95162
exons
(95308) - 95709
95788 - (101792)
coding
95353 - 98244
exons
98364 - 98730
98805 - (101792)
coding
98371 - 101420

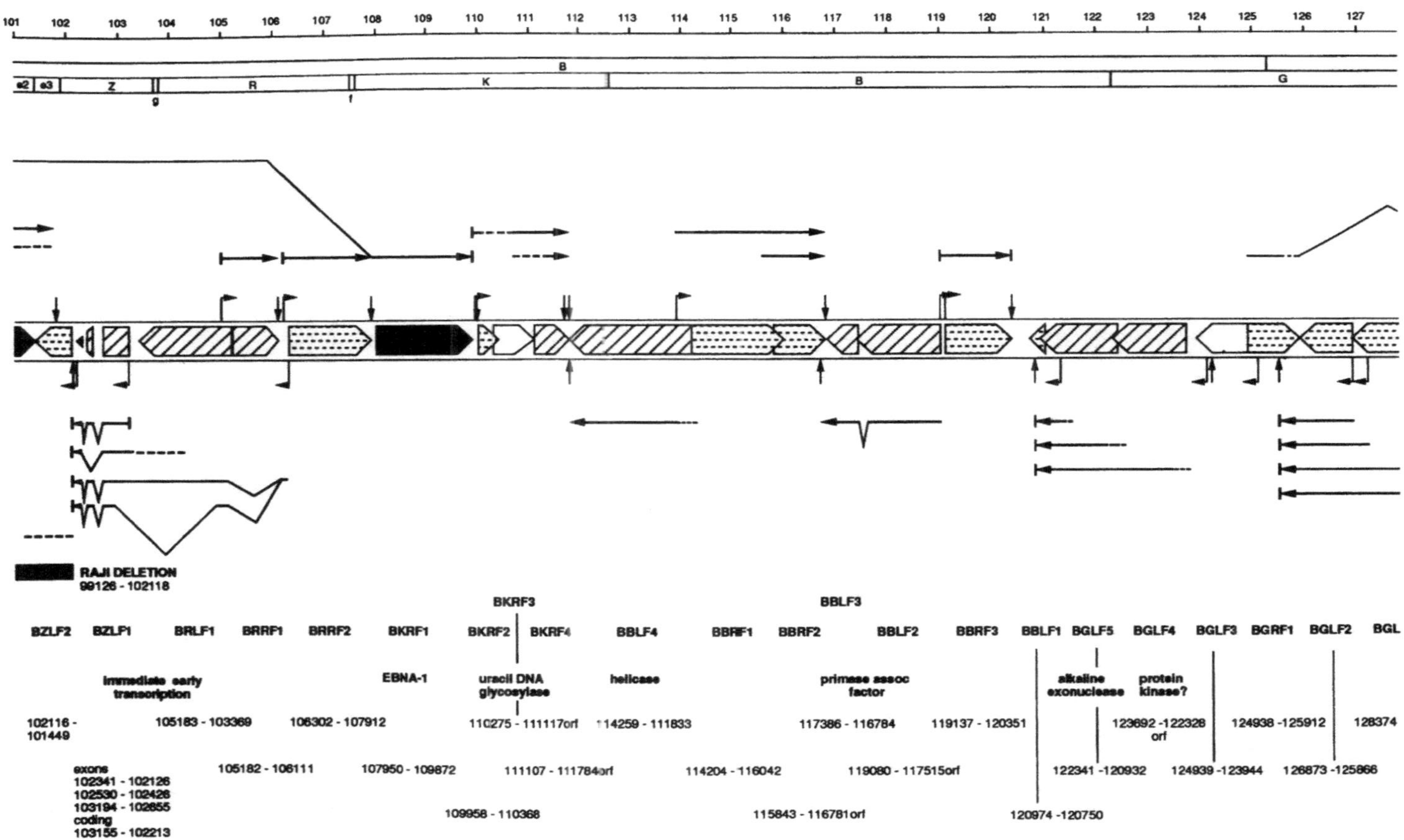

101 102 103 104 105 106 107 108 109 110 111 112 113 114 115 116 117 118 119 120 121 122 123 124 125 126 127
B
e2 e3 Z g R f K B G
RAJI DELETION
99126 - 102118
BKRF3
BBLF3
BZLF2 BZLF1 BRLF1 BRRF1 BRRF2 BKRF1 BKRF2 BKRF4 BBLF4 BBRF1 BBRF2 BBLF2 BBRF3 BBLF1 BGLF5 BGLF4 BGLF3 BGRF1 BGLF2 BGL
immediate early transcription
EBNA-1
uracil DNA glycosylase
helicase
primase assoc factor
alkaline exonuclease
protein kinase?
102116 - 101449
105183 - 103369
106302 - 107912
110275 - 111117orf
114259 - 111833
117386 - 116784
119137 - 120351
123692 -122328 orf
124938 -125912
128374
exons
102341 - 102126
102530 - 102426
103194 - 102855
coding
103155 - 102213
105182 - 106111
107950 - 109872
111107 - 111784orf
114204 - 116042
119080 - 117515orf
122341 -120932
124939 -123944
126873 -125866
109958 - 110368
115843 - 116781orf
120974 -120750

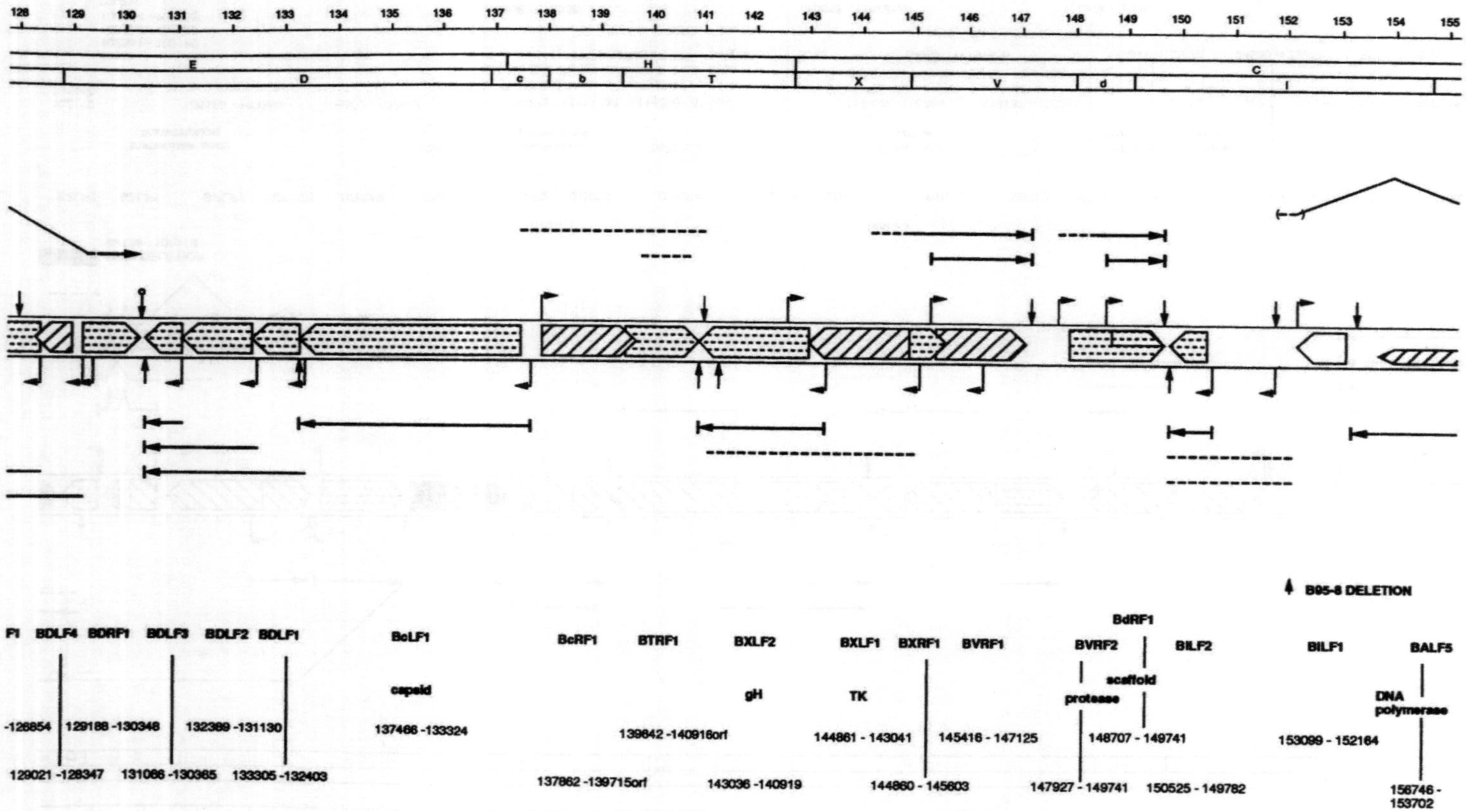
128
129
130
131
132
133
134
135
136
137
138
139
140
141
142
143
144
145
146
147
148
149
150
151
152
153
154
155
E
H
C
D
c
b
T
X
V
d
I
B95-8 DELETION
Fl
BDLF4
BDRF1
BDLF3
BDLF2
BDLF1
BcLF1
capsid
BcRF1
BTRF1
BXLF2
gH
BXLF1
TK
BXRF1
BVRF1
BdRF1
BVRF2
protease
scaffold
BILF2
BILF1
BALF5
DNA polymerase
-126854
129188 -130348
132389 -131130
137466 -133324
139642 -140916orf
144861 - 143041
145416 - 147125
148707 - 149741
153099 - 152164
129021 -128347
131066 -130365
133305 -132403
137862 -139715orf
143036 -140919
144860 - 145603
147927 - 149741
150525 - 149782
156746 - 153702

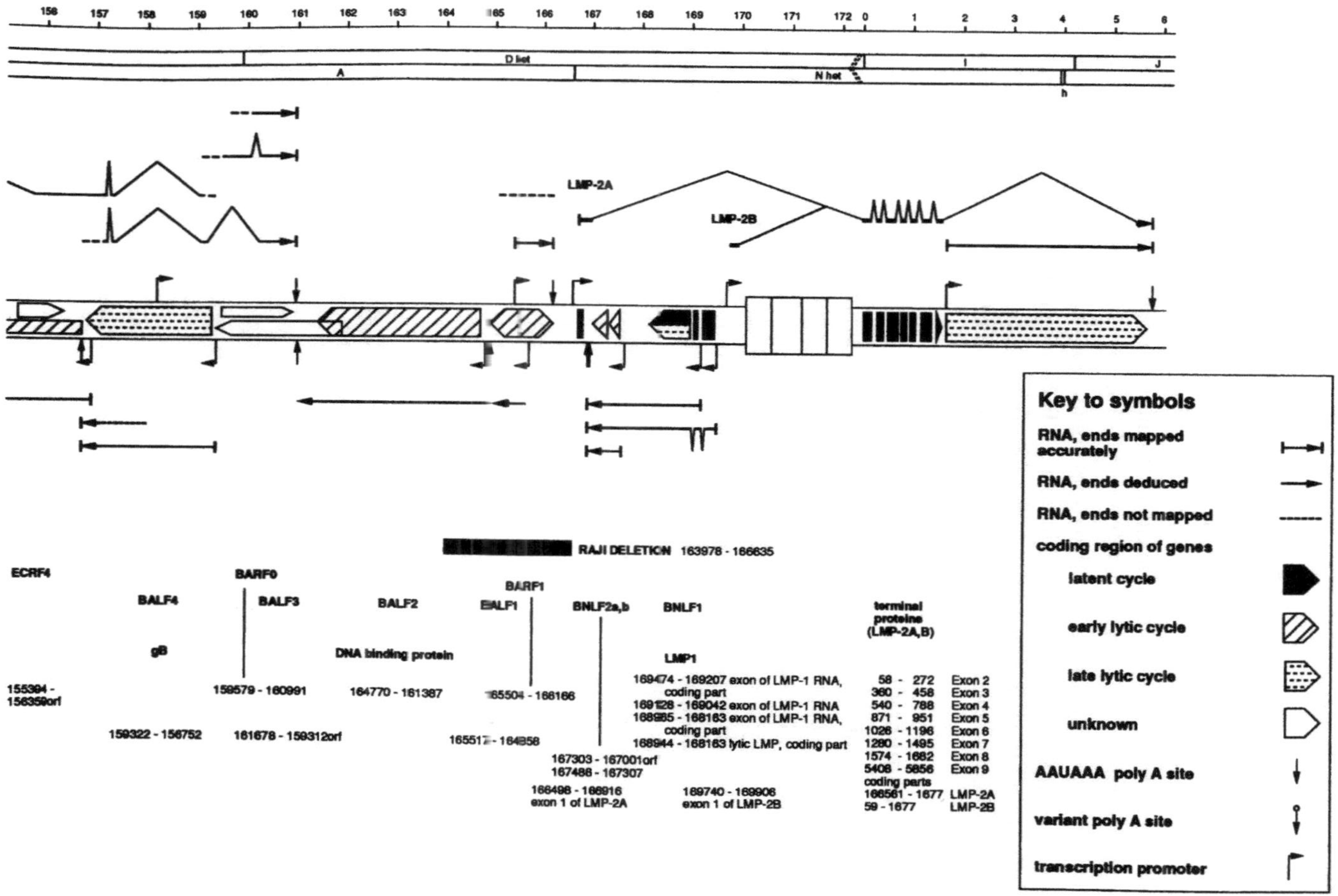
156
157
158
159
160
161
162
163
164
165
166
167
168
169
170
171
172
0
1
2
3
4
5
6
D het
A
I
J
N het
h
LMP-2A
LMP-2B
RAJI DELETION 163978 - 166635
ECRF4
BALF4
BARF0
BALF3
BALF2
BARF1
BALF1
BNLF2a,b
BNLF1
gB
DNA binding protein
LMP1
terminal proteins (LMP-2A,B)
155394 - 156359orf
159322 - 156752
159579 - 160991
161678 - 159312orf
164770 - 161387
165504 - 166166
167303 - 167001orf
167488 - 167307
166498 - 166916 exon 1 of LMP-2A
169474 - 169207 exon of LMP-1 RNA, coding part
169128 - 169042 exon of LMP-1 RNA
168944 - 168163 lytic LMP, coding part
169740 - 169906 exon 1 of LMP-2B
58 - 272 Exon 2
360 - 458 Exon 3
540 - 788 Exon 4
871 - 951 Exon 5
1026 - 1196 Exon 6
1280 - 1495 Exon 7
1574 - 1682 Exon 8
5408 - 5856 Exon 9
coding parts
166561 - 1677 LMP-2A
59 - 1677 LMP-2B
Key to symbols
RNA, ends mapped accurately
RNA, ends deduced
RNA, ends not mapped
coding region of genes
latent cycle
early lytic cycle
late lytic cycle
unknown
AAUAAA poly A site
variant poly A site
transcription promoter

tively in B cell lines immortalized by EBV and these genes are filled in black. Lytic cycle genes are induced by phorbol ester treatment of B95-8 cells (30 ng/mL for 3 d), induction of early genes being unaffected by the presence of phosphonoacetic acid, whereas induction of late genes is blocked by phosphonoacetic acid (125 μg/mL). Reading frames whose expression cannot readily be related to an mRNA or for which no mRNA has been detected are left unfilled. The likely expression class of some of these may be deduced by comparison with homologous genes in other herpes viruses. A recent summary of the relationship between EBV and genetic maps of other gamma herpesviruses (HHV8 and Herpesvirus Saimiri) has been published *(6)* and comparisons of EBV with the well characterized alpha and beta herpesviruses have been made earlier *(7)*.

## 6. Viral Transcription

RNAs transcribed from the EBV genome are shown as arrowed lines above and below the open reading frames with splices shown as narrow connections bridging between the exons. When the boundaries of an RNA have been determined accurately (within a few nucleotides), they are shown on the map with a small bar across the end of the RNA. Spliced exons whose boundaries are known precisely from cDNA sequence analysis are listed below. Other RNAs have not been mapped so precisely and RNAs whose structure is very uncertain are shown as dashed lines. RNA polymerase II promoters, which lead to the transcription of mRNA that have been mapped, are marked (see Key for symbol) and the positions of the sequence AATAAA in the DNA, which is part of the cleavage signal for generation of the 3' ends of mRNAs are marked by short vertical arrows. Some variant sites are also marked (see Key for symbol). Because the EBV genome is relatively GC rich (about 60% GC), the AATAAA sequence occurs only rarely by chance and has generally been a reliable indicator of the 3' ends of RNAs.

## References

1. Baer, R., Bankier, A. T., Biggin, M. D., Deininger, P. L., Farrell, P. J., Gibson, T. J., et al. (1984) DNA sequence and expression of the B95–8 Epstein-Barr virus genome. *Nature* **310,** 207–211.
2. Laux, G., Perricaudet, M., and Farrell, P. J. (1988) A spliced EBV gene expressed in immortalised lymphocytes is created by circularisation of the linear viral genome. *EMBO J.* **7,** 769–774.
3. Farrell. P. J. (1993) Epstein-Barr Virus, in *Genetic Maps,* 6th ed. (O'Brien, S. J., ed.), Cold Spring Harbor Laboratory Press, Cold Spring Harbor, New York, pp. 120–133.
4. Parker, B. D., Bankier, A., Satchwell, S., Barrell, B., and Farrell, P. J. (1990) Sequence and transcription of Raji Epstein-Barr virus DNA spanning the B95-8 deletion. *Virology* **179,** 339–346.
5. Allan, G. J. and Rowe, D. T. (1989) Size and stability of the Epstein-Barr virus major internal repeat (IR-1) in Burkitt's lymphoma and lymphoblastoid cell lines. *Virology* **173,** 489–498.
6. Ganem, D. (1997) KSHV and Kaposi's Sarcoma: the end of the beginning? *Cell* **91,** 157–160.
7. McGeoch, D. J. and Schaffer, P. A. (1993) Herpes Simplex Virus, in *Genetic Maps,* 6th ed. (O'Brien, S. J., ed.), Cold Spring Harbor Laboratory Press, Cold Spring Harbor, New York, pp. 147–156.

# 2

# Analysis of Replication of oriP-Based Plasmids by Quantitative, Competitive PCR

**Ann L. Kirchmaier**

## 1. Introduction

The quantitative, competitive polymerase chain reaction (PCR) assay outlined in this chapter was designed for the detection and quantitation of replicated DNAs in both short-term and long-term assays *(1)*. Quantitative, competitive PCR can be used to study both the contribution of proteins to the replication of oriP-based plasmids *(1)* as well as the requirements for specific DNA sequences to support replication of a plasmid *(2)*. Advantages of this assay include an increased sensitivity and a decreased time required to analyze samples relative to DNA blots, the traditional assay used to study replication of oriP-containing plasmids in the presence of EBNA-1 *(3–8)*.

In long-term experiments, quantitative, competitive PCR can be used to determine whether replicated DNAs are maintained as plasmids in cells under selection and to determine how many copies of those plasmids are present in those cells. However, this assay does not allow the determination of what type of rearrangement, if any, the input DNA may have undergone to be maintained as a plasmid in the host cells under drug selection. Instead, DNA blots are more useful to determine the nature of rearrangements that may occur in the input DNAs. Therefore, although quantitative, competitive PCR does have limitations, it is a sensitive and powerful experimental approach for studying the effects of proteins and the requirements for DNA sequences involved in replication.

For the quantitative, competitive PCR assay, primers are chosen that allow simultaneous amplification of up to three templates: the reporter DNA, the replication-defective DNA and the competitor DNA. Both the reporter DNA, and the replication defective DNA (generated in a *dam* + strain of *Escherichia coli* to incorporate the prokaryotic methylation signature) are introduced into the host cell. Subsequently, after culture, low molecular weight DNA is harvested from cells using a modified Hirt method *(9)* and digested with *Dpn*I to fragment any remaining DNA with a prokary-

From: *Methods in Molecular Biology, Vol. 174: Epstein-Barr Virus Protocols*
Edited by: J. B. Wilson and G. H. W. May © Humana Press Inc., Totowa, NJ

otic methylation pattern, which corresponds to the unreplicated, input DNA. The reporter DNA will be amplified during the PCR only if it has been replicated by the host cell and is therefore *Dpn*I-resistant. The replication defective DNA serves as an internal control and will be amplified during the PCR only if it too has been replicated, or if the *Dpn*I digestions have not gone to completion. Mammalian cells do support synthesis of prokaryotic vectors inefficiently for short times ***(1,2,10)***.

In order to quantitate the PCR products, known concentrations of the competitor DNA are added to a series of PCR assays. The use of $^{32}$P-end labeled oligonucleotide primers allows incorporation of $^{32}$P into the PCR products and facilitates the quantification. In a given PCR, the competitor DNA and the reporter DNA will be amplified with equal efficiency when the two templates are present in equal amounts, consequently, the amount of radioactive label incorporated for each template will be identical.

Oligonucleotide primers for use in competitive, quantitative PCR should be designed that will amplify a region of DNA on the reporter plasmid, the replication-defective plasmid and the competitor plasmid simultaneously. This region of DNA should be designed so that it varies in length between the three plasmids, so that amplification will yield products of three distinguishable sizes. For example, in previously reported experiments ***(1)*** the replication-competent reporter plasmid, *oriP-Bam*HI C-Luc, contains a wild-type gene encoding aminoglycoside phosphotransferase II. The replication-defective plasmid, *oriP*-minus (that serves as an internal control for digestion of nonreplicated DNA by *Dpn*I), lacks oriP and contains a 233 bp insertion at the *Msc*I site within the gene encoding aminoglycoside phosphotransferase II. The competitor DNA introduced into the PCR assay lacks oriP and contains a 222 bp deletion between the *Bsa*A1 and *Msc*I sites within the gene encoding aminoglycoside phosphotransferase II. One pair of primers will anneal to all three plasmids and amplify the corresponding fragment from each plasmid with equal efficiency. The sizes of amplified fragments generated for each of these constructs using one set of primers are 964, 742, and 1197 bp, respectively. Other primers and templates for this assay can be readily designed and used to monitor replication of oriP-based plasmids. However, these templates must be tested for their ability to be amplified with equal efficiency using the corresponding primers.

## 2. Materials

### 2.1. Cell Culture and DNA Transfection

1. Appropriate complete tissue culture medium (TCM): For example, for 143B cells ***(11)***, Dulbecco's Modified Eagle's medium (DMEM-HG), 10% calf serum, 0.2 mg/mL streptomycin sulfate, 200 U/mL penicillin G potassium. Store at 4°C.
2. Phosphate buffered saline (PBS): 0.137 *M* NaCl, 2.7 m*M* KCl, 5.4 m*M* $Na_2HPO_4$, 1.8 m*M* $KH_2PO_4$. Adjust pH to 7.4 and filter through a 0.2-µm filter.
3. 1X trypsin: Dilute 10X trypsin (Gibco BRL, containing 0.5% trypsin, 5.3 m*M* ethylenidiaminetetraacetic acid (EDTA)-4Na) in PBS. Filter through a 0.2-µm filter and store at 4°C.
4. 1X Eosin Y: 0.1% Eosin Y, 0.2% sodium azide in PBS. Filter through a 0.2-µm filter.
5. TCM-H: Add 1/20 vol of 1 *M* HEPES (N-2-hydroxyethylpiperazine-N'-2-ethanesulfonic acid, Gibco BRL cat no 15630–023 or equivalent), pH 7.4–7.6, to complete tissue culture medium, giving a final concentration of 50 m*M* HEPES. Store at 4°C.

6. Tissue culture flasks and dishes.
7. 50-mL conical tubes.
8. Hemocytometer.
9. 37°C $CO_2$ humidified incubator.
10. CsCl-gradient purified plasmid DNAs.

### 2.2. Isolation of Low Molecular Weight DNA

1. Cell resuspension buffer: 50 m*M* Tris-HCl, pH 7.6, 1 m*M* EDTA, 0.1 *M* NaCl.
2. Lysis buffer: 1.2% sodium dodecyl sulfate (SDS), 10 m*M* EDTA, 0.2 *M* Tris-HCl, pH 7.6.
3. 5 *M* NaCl.
4. RNAse A: 20 mg/mL, heat to >70°C for 20 min, store at –20°C.
5. Proteinase K: 20 mg/mL, store at –20°C.
6. Phenol:chloroform: 1:1 ratio, buffered to pH 8.0.
7. Chloroform.
8. Glycogen (20 mg/mL).
9. 100% ethanol.
10. 5 *M* ammonium acetate.
11. 70% ethanol in $H_2O$.
12. 1XTE7.5: 10 m*M* Tris-HCl, pH 7.5, 1 m*M* EDTA.
13. 0.1X TE7.5: 10-fold dilution of 1X TE7.5 with $H_2O$.
14. Microfuge tubes and microcentrifuge.

### 2.3. Competitive, Quantitative PCR

#### 2.3.1. Digestion of Sample DNA and Competitor DNA

1. *Dpn*I and other restriction enzymes and their buffers: store at –20°C.
2. 10X KGB: 1 *M* K-glutamate, 250 m*M* Tris-acetate, 100 m*M* Mg-acetate, 5 m*M* β-mercapto-ethanol, 0.5 mg/mL bovine serum albumin (BSA); Store at –20°C.
3. Phenol:chloroform: 1:1 ration, buffered to pH 8.0.
4. Chloroform.
5. 100% ethanol.
6. 5 *M* ammonium acetate.
7. 70% ethanol in $H_2O$.
8. 1XTE7.5 (as in **Subheading 2.2.**).
9. 0.1X TE7.5: 10 fold dilution of 1X TE7.5 with $H_2O$.
10. Microfuge tubes and microcentrifuge.

#### 2.3.2. Agarose Gel Electrophoresis

1. 1X TBE: 90 m*M* Tris, 80 m*M* boric acid, 2 m*M* EDTA.
2. 1.0% or 1.5% agarose (as indicated) in 1X TBE, microwaved to melt.
3. 5X Blue Juice: 0.05% Bromophenol Blue, 30% glycerol in $H_2O$.
4. Ethidium bromide (10 mg/mL).
5. Electrophoresis apparatus for slab agarose gels.
6. UV light transiluminator.

#### 2.3.3. End-Labeling Primers

1. T4 polynucleotide kinase (New England Biolabs), store at –20°C.
2. 10X T4 polynucleotide kinase buffer (New England Biolabs), store at –20°C.
3. $^{32}P$ γ-ATP (6000 Ci/mmol), e.g., Dupont NEN, store at –20°C.

4. QIAquick nucleotide removal kit (Qiagen) or equivalent kit.
5. 2-mL microfuge tubes.
6. 10 m*M* Tris-HCl, pH 8.0, heat to 60°C prior to use.

### 2.3.4. Competitive, Quantitative PCR

1. Microfuge tubes and microcentrifuge.
2. 0.1X TE7.5 (as in **Subheading 2.3.1.**).
3. 10X Taq buffer (Boehringer), store at –20°C.
4. 20 μ*M* dNTPs, store at –20°C.
5. 20 μ*M* 5' primer, store at –20°C.
6. 20 μ*M* 3' primer, store at –20°C.
7. Taq polymerase (5 U/μL, Boehringer), Store at –20°C.
8. 500 μL GeneAmp tubes (Perkin Elmer) or equivalent.
9. PCR thermocycler (e.g., Perkin Elmer thermocycler 480).
10. Mineral oil.
11. India ink.
12. 7.5% trichloroacetic acid (TCA), in $H_2O$.
13. Whatman 3MM paper.
14. DE81 paper (Fisher 05-717-A).
15. Saran wrap.
16. Vacuum gel dryer.
17. PhosphorImager with screens (e.g., Molecular Dynamics).

## 3. Methods

### 3.1. DNA Transfection into Cells and Subsequent Isolation of Low Molecular Weight DNA

1. Harvest cells and count viable cells as described in Chapter 12, **Subheading 3.1., step 1** and resuspend viable cells to $2 \times 10^7$ cells/mL in TCM-H.
2. Electroporate 10 μg of each plasmid DNA (oriP-containing DNA [the reporter], oriP-minus DNA [replication defective] and effector DNA encoding a derivative of EBNA-1) into 0.5 mL of cell suspension ($1 \times 10^7$ cells) as described in Chapter 12 (*see* **Note 1**).
3. Incubate one electroporated sample in 20 mL of complete tissue culture medium in a 15-cm dish at 37°C in 6% $CO_2$ for 94–98 h.
4. Harvest and count the viable cells as described in Chapter 12, **Subheading 3.1., steps 1–4**.
5. Resuspend the cells to $2 \times 10^7$ cells/mL in cell resuspension buffer and transfer the cells to microfuge tubes, filling the tubes to no more than one third (*see* **Note 2**).
6. To each sample, add an equal volume of lysis buffer. Rock gently for 10 min at room temperature. (Do not pipet or vortex the sample as this may shear the chromosomal DNA).
7. Add 0.5 mL of 5 *M* NaCl/1 mL sample (equivalent to $2 \times 10^7$ cells). Rock gently for 10 min at room temperature.
8. Incubate the samples at 4°C for 24–48 h to precipitate the high molecular weight DNA.
9. Pellet the high molecular weight DNA and cell debris by centrifugation at 9600*g* at 4°C for 45 min in a microfuge or other appropriate centrifuge (*see* **Note 2**).
10. Carefully transfer the supernatant, which contains the majority of the low molecular weight DNA to a fresh tube. Discard the pellet (*see* **Note 3**).
11. Incubate the supernatant for 2 hours at 42°C with RNAse A added to a final concentration of 0.1 mg/mL.

12. Incubate the supernatant for 2 h at 42°C with Proteinase K added to a final concentration of 0.2 mg/mL.
13. Extract the supernatant with an equal volume of phenol:chloroform, then an equal volume of chloroform by vortexing the sample with the organic solvent, centrifugation (10,000–16,000*g* for 30 s), and collection of the aqueous phase. Repeat if the samples contain a large amount of proteinaceous material.
14. Add 1 µL of glycogen (20 mg/mL) as carrier to each sample for precipitation. Add ammonium acetate to each sample to a final concentration of 0.3 *M*. Add 2 vol of 100% ethanol and mix well. Incubate the samples on dry ice for approx 20 min, or at –70°C for approx 1 h or at –20°C overnight, to precipitate the DNA.
15. Pellet the DNA by centrifugation at 9600*g* for 10 min in a microfuge, decant the ethanol. Wash the pellet with 70% ethanol and centrifuge at 9600*g* for 5 min, decant the ethanol. Dry the low molecular weight DNA in a Speed Vac or air dry.
16. Resuspend the samples in 300–500 µL of 1X TE7.5. Store the samples at –20°C.

## 3.2. Competitive, Quantitative PCR

### 3.2.1. Digestion of Low Molecular Weight Sample DNA

1. Incubate the samples overnight at 37°C with 100–160 U of *Dpn*I per 1 × $10^7$ cell equivalents of low molecular weight DNA (in the appropriate buffer) to digest any unreplicated DNA.
2. Add a further 80 U of *Dpn*I and 20–40 U of an appropriate restriction enzyme (to linearize the input plasmid DNA) and incubate at 37°C for one hour.
3. To determine whether the digestions with *Dpn*I have gone to completion, perform one nonradioactive, competitive PCR per sample using 0.1 pg or less of competitor DNA in the reaction (*see* **Subheading 3.2.4.**).
4. If the digestions have gone to completion, extract the sample with an equal volume of phenol:chloroform and then an equal volume of chloroform as described in **Subheading 3.1., step 13**.
5. Precipitate the DNAs as described in **Subheading 3.1., steps 14–15**.
6. Resuspend the samples in 0.1X TE7.5 to a concentration of 1 × $10^5$ cell equivalents/µL. Store the samples at –20°C (*see* **Note 4**).

### 3.2.2. Generation of Competitor DNA

1. Linearize 20 µg of competitor plasmid DNA with an appropriate restriction enzyme. To check that the digestion is complete, take an aliquot of competitor DNA and add loading buffer (to 1X Blue Juice). Electrophorese the aliquot in a 1.0% agarose gel (containing approx 0.5 µg/mL ethidium bromide) in 1X TBE.
2. Purify the competitor DNA sample by extraction with an equal volume of phenol:chloroform and then an equal volume of chloroform (*see* **Subheading 3.1., step 13**).
3. Precipitate the competitor DNA as described in **Subheading 3.1., steps 14–15**.
4. Resuspend the competitor DNA to an estimated concentration of 0.5–1 mg/mL in TE7.5.
5. Determine the concentration of the competitor DNA using a Hoescht dye assay ***(12)***, or by comparing the intensity under ultraviolet (UV) light of serial dilutions of agarose gel electrophoresed competitor DNA in the presence of ethidium bromide (0.5 µg/mL) to similar dilutions of known concentrations of a standard DNA ***(13)***.
6. Generate a working stock of competitor DNA at 1–10 ng/mL in 1XTE7.5 for PCR. Store at –20°C in a screw cap tube in a nonfrost free freezer.

### 3.2.3. End-Labeling Primers

1. Incubate (separately) 75 pmol of each primer with 10 U of T4 polynucleotide kinase, and 125 pmol of $^{32}$P γ-ATP (750 mCi) in 1X T4 polynucleotide kinase buffer in a 30 μL total reaction volume for 30 min at 30°C (*see* **Note 5**).
2. Add an additional 10 U of T4 polynucleotide kinase to each primer reaction and incubate for an additional 30 min at 30°C.
3. Separate the primers from unincorporated $^{32}$P γ-ATP by purification using the QIAquick nucleotide removal kit according to manufacturer's instructions as outlined below in **steps 4–8**.
4. Add 300 μL of buffer PN (Qiagen kit) to the $^{32}$P-end labeled primer and mix. Incubate for 1 min at room temperature. Transfer the sample mix to a QIAquick column placed in a 2 mL microfuge tube. Centrifuge the column at approx 4000*g* in a microfuge for 1 min. Discard the radioactive eluate.
5. Transfer the column to new microfuge tube. Add 300 mL of buffer PE (Qiagen kit) to the column. Centrifuge the column at approx 4000*g* in a microfuge for 1 min. Transfer the column to a new microfuge tube and discard the radioactive eluate.
6. Add 400 μL of buffer PE (Qiagen kit) to the column. Centrifuge the column at approx 4000*g* in a microfuge for 1 min. Transfer the column to a new microfuge tube and discard the radioactive eluate.
7. Centrifuge the column at approx 9600*g* in a microfuge for 30 s. Transfer the column to a new microfuge tube and discard the radioactive eluate.
8. Add 40 μL of 10 m*M* Tris, pH 8.0 (preheated to 60°C) to the column. Centrifuge the column at approx 9600*g* for 1 min to elute the $^{32}$P-end labeled primer. Transfer the $^{32}$P-labeled primer to a screw-cap tube. Store at –20°C.

### 3.2.4. Quantitative, Competitive PCR Assay

1. Generate the following master reaction mix containing a multiple of each reagent to equal the number of samples to be analyzed plus two extra (*see* **Note 6**). Vortex to mix. Master reaction mix (per one PCR) for a total reaction volume of 100 mL: 10 μL 10X Taq buffer (Boehringer), 1 μL 20 m*M* dNTPs, 1 μL 20 μ*M* 5' primer, 1 μL 20 μ*M* 3' primer, 0.1 μL $^{32}$P γ-ATP-labeled 5' primer, 0.1 μL $^{32}$P γ-ATP-labeled 3' primer, 75.3 mL $H_2O$, 0.5 μL 5 U/μL Taq polymerase (Boehringer).
2. Dilute the competitor DNA from the working stock (**Subheading 3.2.2.**) to known concentrations (e.g., 0.00025, 0.0010, 0.0040, 0.16, 0.64, and 2.5 pg/μL) in 0.1X TE7.5 in order to generate a standard curve (*see* **Note 7**).
3. To 500 μL tubes add 10 μL of one concentration of competitor DNA, and 1 μL of sample DNA (1 × $10^5$ cell equivalents/μL). Set up five reactions per sample, with an increasing amount of competitor DNA per reaction. Then aliquot 89 μL of the master reaction mix to each tube and mix to give a total volume of 100 μL/tube. Overlay with 70 μL of mineral oil.
4. Set up the PCR using the following conditions: initially denature the DNA templates at 94°C for 5 min once. Then set cycle: denature at 94°C for 30 s, anneal at 55°C for 30 s, and elongate at 72°C for 1 min. Repeat for 20-25 cycles. Finally, elongate at 72°C for 10 min, and transfer samples to 4°C. Store the samples at –20°C.
5. Take 15 μL of each PCR reaction, add 4 μL of 5X Blue Juice, and electrophorese the samples in a 1.5% agarose gel (containing approx 0.5 μg/mL ethidium bromide) in 1X TBE. When loading the gel, do not load the lane between the lowest amount of competitor of one sample and the highest amount of competitor in the next sample in order to avoid obscuring the signal of the lowest amount of competitor DNA and therefore compromising data analysis. Electrophorese overnight at 0.5–1 V/cm or for approx 4 h at 4 V/cm.

6. Examine the gel under UV light and mark the location of the molecular weight markers with a needle dipped in India Ink.
7. Precipitate the DNA in the gel by incubating the gel in 7.5% TCA for approx 30 min, until the dye front is yellow.
8. Optional: Place the gel on a stack of dry Whatman 3MM paper, cover with Saran wrap and place a book or equivalently weighted flat object on top for 15 min. This will facilitate wicking excess buffer out of the fixed gel, and reduce the amount of time required to dry the gel.
9. Transfer the gel onto a sheet of DE81 paper with two new sheets of Whatman 3MM paper underneath. Cover the gel with Saran wrap. Dry the gel in a gel dryer for 2–2.5 h. Remove the dried gel from the gel dryer and replace the Saran wrap with a new sheet.
10. Expose the dried gel to a PhosphorImager screen overnight. Collect data from the PhosphorImage (*see* **Fig. 1A**) and analyze as described in **Subheading 3.2.5.**

### 3.2.5. Data Analysis

1. To measure the amount of replicated reporter DNA in the sample, plot the graph log (molecules of competitor DNA) vs log (PhosphorImager Units of competitor DNA/ PhosphorImager Units of reporter DNA) (*see* **Fig. 1B**).
2. When the amount of the competitor DNA is equivalent to the amount of the reporter DNA in the sample, the two templates will be amplified with equal efficiency. Graphically, this represents the point on the x-axis where the log of 1/1 = 0. Therefore, the inverse log of the intercept equals the number of *Dpn*I-resistant molecules present in $1 \times 10^5$ cell equivalents of the sample, assuming all cells took up DNA upon transfection.
3. The average number of replicated molecules per transfected cell can be determined by correcting for the transfection efficiency of the cell line used in the experiment. To do this, divide the number of *Dpn*I-resistant molecules present in $1 \times 10^5$ cell equivalents of the sample by $1 \times 10^5$ cells and multiply that number by the transfection efficiency of the cell line tested. A method for determining the transfection efficiency of cell lines is described in Chapter 12.
4. To ensure that the *Dpn*I digestions have gone to completion, plot the graph log (molecules of competitor DNA) vs log (PhosphorImager Units of competitor DNA/PhosphorImager Units of *oriP*-minus DNA) and analyze the data as described earlier.

## 4. Notes

1. DNA may also be introduced by other means (e.g., calcium phosphate precipitation *[14]*) depending on the cell type.
2. Use larger tubes appropriate to the centrifugation in **Subheading 3.1., step 9** for larger sample volumes.
3. If desired, the high molecular weight, chromosomal DNA separated from the low molecular weight DNA can be analyzed as well. To do so, resuspend the pellet (containing primarily chromosomal DNA and cell membranes) in 1 m*M* EDTA, 0.1 *M* NaOH. This resuspension takes time and can be accelerated by incubating at 45°C and by gentle vortexing. Once resuspended, extract with phenol, phenol:chloroform, and chloroform. Precipitate the sample as described in **Subheading 3.1., steps 14–15**. However, do not dry the sample. Instead, immediately resuspend the high molecular weight DNA in 1X TE7.5. Continue to process high molecular weight DNA as described in **Subheading 3.1., steps 11–16.**

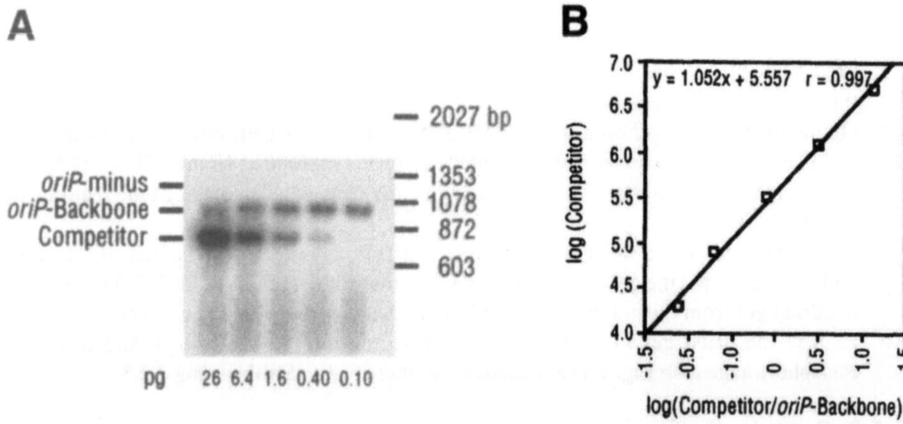


Fig. 1. Short-term replication of a reporter plasmid containing oriP in 143 cells that stably express wild-type EBNA-1 as measured by quantitative, competitive PCR. **(A)** Example of PhosphorImage of a sample analyzed by quantitative, competitive PCR. Ten µg each of reporter DNA (*oriP*-backbone) *(2)* and replication-defective DNA (*oriP*-minus) *(1)* were introduced into $1 \times 10^7$ 143/EBNA-1 cells *(15)* and analyzed as described in this chapter. Briefly, the low molecular weight DNA was harvested 12 d postelectroporation by Hirt extraction *(9)*, digested with *Dpn*I to fragment any unreplicated DNA, and *Acc*I to linearize the templates. Five quantitative, competitive PCRs with varying amounts of competitor DNA *(1)* were performed for the sample. 15 µL of each PCR were run on a 1.5% agarose gel in 1X TBE, and data were analyzed using a PhosphorImager. The migration patterns of molecular weight markers are noted to the right of the gel and the migration patterns of *oriP*-minus, o*oriP*-backbone, and competitor DNAs are shown to the left. The amount of competitor DNA in pg added to each PCR is noted below each lane. **(B)** Graph of the data from the sample shown in (A). Data from the PhosphorImage were analyzed as described in this chapter. Briefly, to measure the amount of replicated reporter DNA (in this case, *oriP*-backbone) in the sample, the graph log (molecules competitor) vs log (PhosphorImager units competitor/PhosphorImager units reporter) was plotted. r = correlation coefficient. The number of *Dpn*I-resistant molecules per $1 \times 10^5$ cell equivalents of sample was determined from the inverse log of the intercept. The number of replicated molecules per transfected cell was determined by dividing by the number of cell equivalents used in the competitive, quantitative PCR and multiplying by the transfection efficiency (approx 25% under the conditions used in this example) of the cell line. In this example, approx 14 copies of replicated *oriP*-backbone was present per transfected cell.

4. Prior to setting up a large experiment using radiolabeled primers, it is often useful to run a subset of samples in a nonradioactive competitive, quantitative PCR (*see* **Subheading 3.2.4.**) to ensure that the number of replicated plasmids detected are within the chosen range of concentrations of competitor DNA.
5. To increase the efficiency of the labelling reaction, the reaction samples can be incubated on ice overnight instead of 30 min at 30°C.
6. The quantitative, competitive PCR assay is linear over the range of at least $1 \times 10^4$–$1 \times 10^6$ cell equivalents of sample, and between at least 0.025 and 26 pg of competitor DNA. If

$1 \times 10^4$ cell equivalents of sample DNA are used in the PCR reaction, $1 \times 10^5$ cell equivalents of a low molecular weight DNA extracted from non-transfected cells, processed as described earlier, should be added to each PCR as a carrier DNA. If $1 \times 10^6$ cell equivalents of sample are used per point of standard curve, low molecular weight DNA from at least $5 \times 10^6$ cells must be harvested initially. The lower limit of detection in the assay can be adjusted by either starting with more sample DNA in each PCR or using less Competitor DNA and increasing the number of cycles used during the PCR analysis.

7. A new standard curve (even from the same competitor DNA stock) must be generated for each experiment.

## Acknowledgments

I thank Bill Sugden for his helpful discussions while developing the use of quantitative, competitive PCR to study EBV and for his suggestions for improving this manuscript. This was supported by Public Health Service grants CA-22443 and CA-07175 in the laboratory of Bill Snyder at the McArdle Laboratory for Cancer Research, University of Wisconsin, 1400 Wisconsin Ave., Madison, WI 53706.

## References

1. Kirchmaier, A. L. and Sugden, B. (1997) Dominant-negative inhibitors of EBNA-1 of Epstein-Barr virus. *J. Virol.* **71,** 1766–1775.
2. Kirchmaier, A. L. and Sugden, B. (1998) Rep*: a viral element that can partially replace the origin of plasmid DNA synthesis of EBV. *J. Virol.* **72,** 4657–4666.
3. Lupton, S. and Levine, A. J. (1985) Mapping genetic elements of Epstein-Barr virus that facilitate extrachromosomal persistence of Epstein-Barr virus-derived plasmids in human cells. *Mol. Cell. Biol.* **5,** 2533–2542.
4. Reisman, D., Yates, J., and Sugden, B. (1985) A putative origin of replication of plasmids derived from Epstein-Barr virus is composed of two *cis*-acting components. *Mol. Cell. Biol.* **5,** 1822–1832.
5. Sugden, B., Marsh, K., and Yates, J. (1985) A vector that replicates as a plasmid and can be efficiently selected in B-lymphocytes transformed by Epstein-Barr virus. *Mol. Cell. Biol.* **5,** 410–413.
6. Yates, J., Warren, N., Reisman, D., and Sugden, B. (1984) A *cis*-acting element from the Epstein-Barr viral genome that permits stable replication of recombinant plasmids in latently infected cells. *Proc. Natl. Acad. Sci. USA* **81,** 3806–3810.
7. Yates, J. L. (1996) Epstein-Barr virus DNA replication, in *DNA Replication in Eukaryotic Cells* (DePamphilis, M. L., ed.), Cold Spring Harbor Laboratory Press, Plainview, NY, pp. 751–773.
8. Yates, J. L., Warren, N., and Sugden, B. (1985) Stable replication of plasmids derived from Epstein-Barr virus in various mammalian cells. *Nature* **313,** 812–815.
9. Hirt, B. (1967) Selective extraction of polyoma DNA from infected mouse cell cultures. *J. Mol. Biol.* **26,** 365–369.
10. Aiyar, A., Tyree, C., and Sugden, B. (1998) The plasmid replicon of EBV consists of multiple cis-acting elements that facilitate DNA synthesis by the cell and a viral maintenance element. *EMBO J.* **17,** *6394–6403.*
11. Bacchetti, S. and Graham, F. L. (1977) Transfer of the gene for thymidine kinase to thymidine kinase-deficient human cells by purified herpes simplex viral DNA. *Proc. Natl. Acad. Sci. USA* **74,** 1590–1594.

12. Labarca, C. and Paigen, K. (1980) A simple, rapid, and sensitive DNA assay procedure. *Anal. Biochem.* **102,** 344–352.
13. Mackey, D. and Sugden, B. (1997) Studies on the mechanism of DNA linking by Epstein-Barr virus nuclear antigen 1. *J. Biol. Chem.* **272,** 29873–29879.
14. Graham, F. L. and Van der Eb, A. J. (1973) A new technique for the assay of infectivity of human adenovirus 5 DNA. *Virology* **52,** 456–467.
15. Middleton, T. and Sugden, B. (1992) A chimera of EBNA1 and the estrogen receptor activates transcription but not replication. *J. Virol.* **66,** 1795–1798.

# 3

## Genetic Analysis and Gene Expression with Mini-Epstein-Barr Virus Plasmids

**Ellen Kilger and Wolfgang Hammerschmidt**

### 1. Introduction

Upon infection with Epstein-Barr virus (EBV), primary human B-lymphocytes are efficiently immortalized and give rise to lymphoblastoid cell lines in vitro. Four of the 11 viral genes expressed in the immortalized B cells have been found to be essential genetically for the process of immortalization: the EBV nuclear antigens EBNA2, EBNA3a, and EBNA3c, and the latent membrane protein 1 (LMP1) *(1–5)*. Since EBNA1 maintains the status of the EBV genomes in the proliferating B cells, it might also be indispensable *(6)*.

To analyze the role of latent EBV genes in the process of immortalization in this way, it is necessary to generate recombinant viruses that carry a mutation in a certain gene. However, the genetic analysis of EBV genes is difficult owing to the fact that no permissive cell line is available that allows simple preparation of recombinant viruses. This problem can be overcome by the use of mini-EBV plasmids. Mini-EBV plasmids are constructed in *Escherichia coli* with the aid of an F-factor replicon such that they encompass all functional elements of EBV necessary for B-cell immortalization *(7,8)*. The mini-EBV p1478A is an example that is 82 kb in size and carries 71 kb of EBV sequences encompassing the latent EBV genes EBNA1, EBNA2, EBNA3a, -3b, -3c, EBNA-LP, LMP1, LMP2a, -2b, EBER1, and -2 and the *cis*-elements for replication: oriP and oriLyt, and the TR elements for packaging of the DNA into virions (**Fig. 1**). Upon transfection or infection of primary B-cells the mini-EBV p1478A immortalizes B-cells as efficiently as wild-type virus *(7,8)*. The advantage of this system is that a mini-EBV plasmid can be genetically altered and amplified in *E. coli*. This allows the mutation of latent EBV genes as well as the addition of new genes into the mini-EBV plasmid. The appropriately modified mini-EBV plasmid can then be packaged into virions in the helper cell line HH514, which carries the endogenous nonimmortalizing EBV strain P3HR1 *(9)*. These virus-stocks can be used to immortalize primary B-cells

From: *Methods in Molecular Biology, Vol. 174: Epstein-Barr Virus Protocols*
Edited by: J. B. Wilson and G. H. W. May © Humana Press Inc., Totowa, NJ

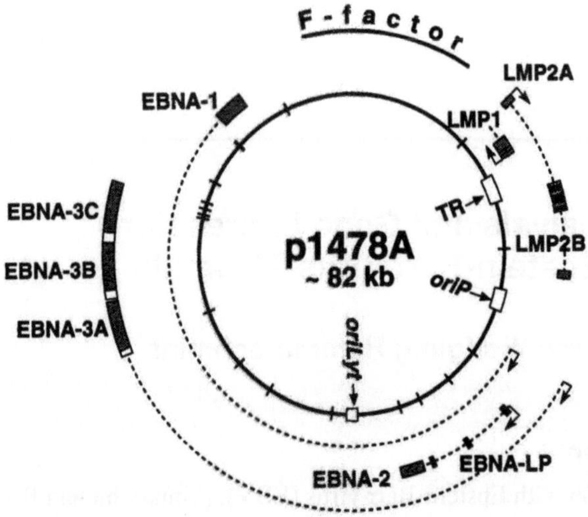


Fig. 1. Composition of the mini-EBV plasmid p1478A. The 11 viral genes (EBNA1, EBNA-LP, EBNA2, EBNA3a, -b, -c, LMP1, LMP2a, -b, EBER1, EBER2) generally expressed in the latent phase of the EBV life cycle are either denoted as gray boxes together with the extension of their primary RNA transcripts (dashed lines) and promoters (→) or are too small to be represented (EBER1 and EBER2). The map also shows the *cis*-acting elements (open boxes) *oriP*, *oriLyt*, and TR which constitute the plasmid origin, the lytic origin of replication, and the terminal repeats, respectively. *OriP* is involved in plasmid replication in latently infected cells whereas *oriLyt* is essential for viral DNA replication in the lytic phase of EBV infection. The terminal repeats TR are involved in packaging of the plasmid into virions. The prokaryotic plasmid backbone of the F-factor is annotated together with the location of *Bam*HI sites in the inner circle of the map.

to study the effect of the specific mutation. We have used this system to establish a B-cell line that expresses LMP1 in a conditional fashion and demonstrated that LMP1 expression is essential to maintain B-cell proliferation in EBV-infected B-cells in vitro ***(10)***.

Apart from the genetic analysis of latent EBV genes mini-EBV plasmids can also be used as vectors to express a foreign gene of interest in virus-free immortalized B-cells. For example, an expression cassette for a specific tumor antigen can be added into the mini-EBV plasmid and virus-free B-cell lines can be established that express this tumor antigen. Such B-cells supply an indefinite and safe source of antigen-presenting cells (APCs) that can be used to generate antigen specific T-cells for adoptive immune therapy trials. We have recently demonstrated that this approach is feasible by establishing B-cell lines expressing the human tumor antigen mucin (MUC-1) from a mini-EBV plasmid and generating a mucin specific cytotoxic T-cell response ***(11)***. In a different setting these B-cell lines could also be used as antitumor cell vaccines.

Here we describe the techniques needed to modify the original mini-EBV plasmid p1478A in *E. coli* and to establish B-cell lines with a newly constructed mini-EBV.

First, how to mutate an EBV gene on the mini-EBV plasmid is described (*see* **Subheading 3.1.**) and second, how to add a new gene (*see* **Subheading 3.2.**). Both methods use the chromosomal building technique *(12)*, which is based on recombination events in *E. coli*. We then describe how to amplify and purify these large plasmids (*see* **Subheading 3.3.**) and to establish B-cell lines immortalized by a newly constructed mini-EBV plasmid (*see* **Subheading 3.4.**).

## 2. Materials

### 2.1. Chromosomal Building

#### 2.1.1. Plasmids

1. p1478A is a mini-EBV plasmid that contains fragments of the B95.8 EBV genome (*13*, and *see* Chapter 1) with the nucleotide coordinates 163,477-19,359; 43,935-56,018 and 79,658-113,282 on an *E. coli* F-factor backbone encoding chloramphenicol resistance. p1478A is the direct precursor of p1495.4 *(7)* and has the same structure except for the last building step.
2. pMBO96: tet shuttle plasmid (**Fig. 2**) *(12)*.
3. p929.4: pMBO96 tet shuttle plasmid with different cloning sites, made by inserting the oligonucleotide NEB#1060 into *Sal*I-Klenow/*Bam*HI-Klenow treated pMBO96, contains single sites for *Hind*III, *Sal*I, *Nhe*I, *Bam*HI (**Fig. 2**).
4. p1242.1: derivative of pMBO96 tet shuttle plasmid with additional B95.8 EBV *(13)* fragment (coordinates 110,491-113,282) and hygromycin resistance gene (**Fig. 2**).
5. DCM111: plasmid-expressing resolvase (resD), obtained from M. O'Connor *(12)*.
6. pCMV-BZLF1: expression plasmid for BZLF1 *(14)*.

#### 2.1.2. Bacterial Strains

1. *E. coli* DH5α *(15)*.
2. *E. coli* CBTS: *recA* strain with a temperature-sensitive *recA* amber suppressor, which is $RecA^+$ at 30°C and $RecA^-$ at 42°C. Genotype: *leu*(am), *trp*(am), *lacZ2210*(am), *galK*(am), *galE?*, *sueC*, *rpsL*, *supD43,74*, *sueB*, *metB1*, *RecA99*(am).

#### 2.1.3. Media and Solutions

1. LB-medium: 1% tryptone, 0.5% yeast-extract, 0.5% NaCl.
2. LB-agar-plates: 15 g bacto-agar and 1 L LB-medium, supplemented with 30 µg/mL of tetracycline (LB-tet), 50 µg/mL chloramphenicol (LB-cam), or 100 µg/mL ampicillin (LB-amp).
3. TE8: 10 m*M* Tris-HCl, 1 m*M* ethylenediaminetetraacetic acid (EDTA), pH 8.0.
4. 1X TAE: 0.04 *M* Tris-acetate, 0.001 *M* EDTA.
5. Solution I: 50 m*M* glucose, 25 m*M* Tris-HCl, pH 8.0, 10 m*M* EDTA.
6. Solution II: 0.2 *M* NaOH, 1% SDS.
7. Solution III: Mix 600 mL of 5 *M* KAc with 115 mL of 100% glacial acetic acid and 285 mL of $H_2O$.
8. Sorval centrifuge with GS3 rotor or equivalent and 1000-mL bottles.
9. CsCl: solid and 1.55 $g/cm^3$ solution.
10. 13.5-mL Ultracrimp tubes (Kontron #9091-90387).
11. 38.5-mL Ultracrimp tubes (Kontron #9091-90389).
12. Ultracentrifuge and Centrikon TFT70.38 rotor or equivalent.
13. Syringes and needles (19 G).

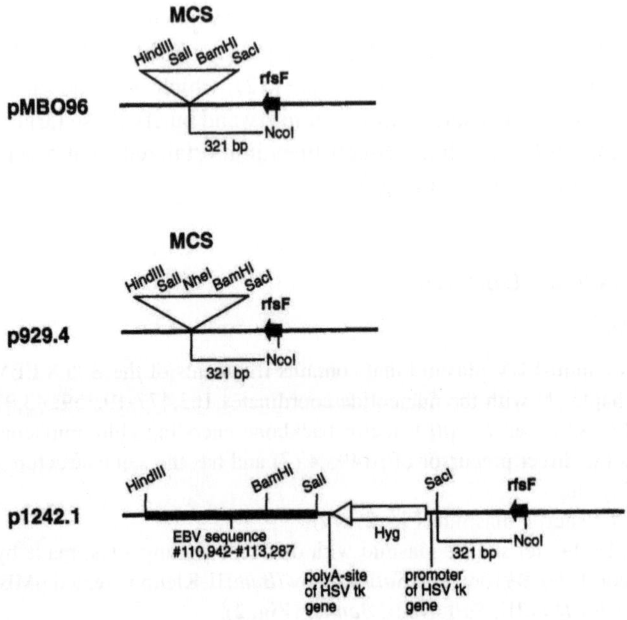


Fig. 2. Composition of pMBO96-derived tet shuttle plasmids. The figure shows a schematic representation of only that part of the tet shuttle plasmids that contains the multiple cloning site (MCS) adjacent to the *rfsF* site. pMBO96 contains single sites for *Hind*III, *Sal*I, *BamH*I, and *Sac*I, whereas p924.4 carries an additional single *Nhe*I site that can be used for cloning. The plasmid p1242.1 is derived from pMBO96 and contains an EBV fragment (coordinates 110,942-113,287 from B95.8 EBV *[13]*), which is homologous to the end of the EBV sequence on p1478A. In addition, the plasmid contains the hygromycin phosphotransferase gene (Hyg) with the HSV tk gene promoter and polyadenylation site. Both were cloned into the MCS of pMBO96 with the aim to transfer the Hyg gene into the mini-EBV p1478A. One can use the p1242.1 tet shuttle plasmid to transfer any gene of interest into p1478A. When the single *BamH*I or *Sal*I sites of p1242.1 are used for cloning, the desired gene will be transferred to p1478A together with the Hyg gene (*see* also Fig. 4). When a combination of *Sal*I and *Sac*I is used for cloning, the Hyg gene will be removed from the tet shuttle plasmid. In all three tet shuttle vectors, the *Sac*I site is 321 bp away from one of several *Nco*I sites present in the *rfsF*. The complete sequences of pMBO96 derived plasmids *(12)* will soon be available in international databases.

## 2.2. Generation of Mini-EBV Immortalized B-Cells

1. RPMI medium: RPMI 1640 (Gibco BRL) supplemented with 2 m*M* L-glutamine, 1 m*M* pyruvate, 50 µg/mL streptomycin, 50 IE/mL penicillin, 1.25 µg/mL amphotericin B and with or without 10% fetal calf serum (FCS).
2. HH514 *(16)* is a single cell clone of the Burkitt's lymphoma cell line P3HR1 *(9)*.
3. WI38 human fibroblast cells obtained from the American Type Culture Collection, (ATCC).
4. PBS: 0.8% NaCl, 0.02% KCl, 0.14% $Na_2HPO_4$, 0.02% $KH_2PO_4$, pH 7.0.
5. PBS/versene: dilute versene (Gibco BRL) 1:500 in PBS.

6. Lysis buffer: 0.1 *M* EDTA, pH 8.0, 0.1 *M* NaCl, 50 m*M* Tris-HCl pH 8.0, 1% SDS.
7. ΔB95.8 primer pair: 5'-GTCAGCCGCCAGGGTCCGTTTA-3'/5'-AAGTTTCC-TTG CCATCTAAAGC-3'.
8. CAM primer pair: 5'-TTCTGCCGACATGGAAGCCATC-3'/5'-GGAGTGAATA-CCA CGACGATTTCC-3'.
9. Whole sheep blood (Oxoid GmbH, Wesel, Germany).
10. Ficoll (Amersham Pharmacia Biotech).
11. Culture flasks and 96-well plates.
12. 37°C, 5% $CO_2$ humidified incubator.

## 3. Methods

### *3.1. Mutation of the Mini-EBV Plasmid p1478A by Allelic Exchange (Fig. 3)*

1. Flank the desired mutation of a latent EBV gene with 2–4 kb EBV sequences homologous to the mini-EBV plasmid p1478A. The mutation should be in the middle of the EBV sequence, so that the probability for homologous recombination is equal for both sides.
2. Ligate the EBV fragment containing the mutation and flanking regions into an appropriately prepared pMBO96 derived tet shuttle vector like p929.4 (**Fig. 2**) *(12)*. Transfect the new tet shuttle vector into competent bacteria of the DH5α strain *(15)* and select on tetracycline containing LB-plates (LB-tet) at 30°C.
3. To amplify bacteria for a plasmid mini-preparation streak single colonies onto the quarter of an LB-plate containing the appropriate antibiotic and cultivate overnight (*see* **Note 1**). For a plasmid mini-preparation, scratch the bacterial lawn from the plate with a toothpick, and resuspend the bacteria in 200 μL of TE containing 100 μg/mL RNase by vortexing. Add 200 μL of Solution II, vortex immediately for 1 s, and subsequently keep at room temperature for 5 min. Add 200 μL of Solution III, mix by shaking 2–3 times, and keep lysates on ice for 10 min. Centrifuge at 18,320*g* for 10 min at 4°C. Transfer the supernatant to a new tube and add 400 μL of isopropanol. After mixing centrifuge at 18,320*g* for 10 min at room temperature, wash the precipitated DNA with 70% ethanol. Aspirate the ethanol off completely, then dissolve the plasmid DNA in 20 μL of TE8 and keep on ice (*see* **Note 2**). Use 5–10 μL of the plasmid DNA for analysis with an appropriate restriction enzyme.
4. Transfect 5 μL of the tet shuttle plasmid DNA from the mini-preparation into competent bacteria of the CBTS strain *(12)*, containing the mini-EBV p1478A, and select on LB-tet-cam plates at 30°C overnight.
5. Restreak 5–10 bacterial colonies onto LB-tet-cam plates and incubate at 42°C overnight to derive cointegrates between the tet shuttle and the mini-EBV plasmid. Because of the perdurance of the tet proteins, one sees growth in the heavy portion of the streak and even some pinpoint colonies in the lighter portion. The desired clones, however, will form large colonies within 24 h (*see* **Note 3**).
6. Restreak several of these candidate colonies onto LB-tet-cam plates and incubate at 42°C and prepare plasmid DNA as described earlier (**Subheading 3.1., step 3**). Analyze the plasmid DNA with appropriate restriction enzymes, usually *Bam*HI and *Bgl*II to ensure the right composition of the co-integrate (*see* **Notes 4** and **6**).
7. For the second recombination step cultivate a clone containing the co-integrate in 5 mL of LB-cam at 30°C overnight, then plate aliquots of the culture onto an LB-cam plate and incubate at 30°C overnight to derive single colonies.

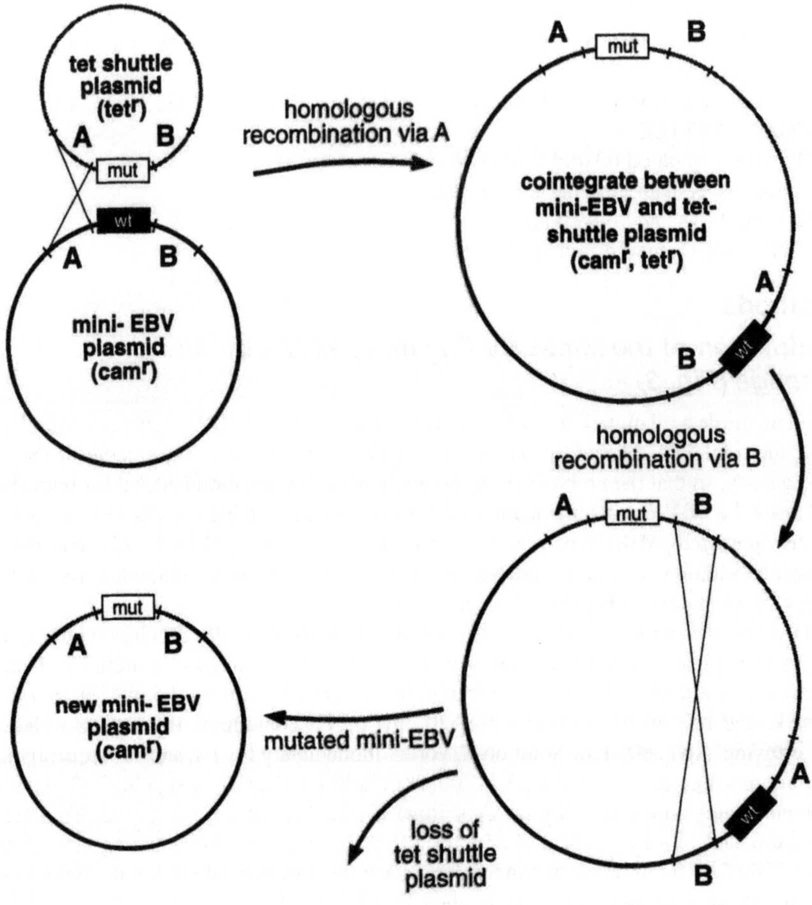


Fig. 3. Mutation of the mini-EBV plasmid p1478A by allelic exchange. The tet shuttle plasmid shown on the upper left side carries the modified allele of a latent EBV gene (mut) flanked by stretches of 2–4 kb EBV DNA on either side termed "A" and "B". The mini-EBV plasmid p1478A carries the wild-type form of the latent EBV (wt) within the identical EBV sequences "A" and "B". Homologous recombination via the "A" sequences of both plasmids leads to the formation of a co-integrate as is shown on the upper right side. The co-integrate is resolved by a second step of homologous recombination. Whereas recombination via the "A" sequences results in the original p1478A plasmid (not shown), recombination via the "B" sequences leads to a derivative of the original mini-EBV, which now carries the modified allele of the latent EBV gene (shown below on the left side).

8. Pick 50–100 single colonies and make short streaks onto LB-cam master plates and LB-tet plates and cultivate overnight at 42°C to test for cam-resistant clones that have lost the tet shuttle backbone and are now tet-sensitive (*see* **Note 5**).
9. Pick cam-resistent clones that are tet-sensitive and prepare plasmids as described in **Subheading 3.1., step 3.**

10. Analyze clones with appropriate restriction enzymes to ensure the composition of the resulting mini-EBV plasmid and the incorporation of the desired mutation (*see* **Notes 2** and **6**).
11. Freeze the new mini-EBV in CBTS bacteria for further chromosomal building. In parallel transfect mini-EBV DNA from the plasmid mini-preparation into competent DH5α bacteria for stable preservation and large scale plasmid amplification.
12. To amplify and purify the new mini-EBV plasmid follow the method described in **Subheading 3.3.**

### 3.2. Addition of a New Gene into the Mini-EBV Plasmid p1478A (Fig. 4)

1. Clone the desired gene into the polylinker of the tet shuttle plasmid p1242.1. The unique sites for *Sal*I or *BamH*I or the combination of *Sal*I and *Sac*I can be used for cloning (*see* **Fig. 2**). The new tet shuttle plasmid is amplified in DH5α on LB-tet plates at 30°C.
2. Follow **steps 4–6** from **Subheading 3.1.** to derive a cointegrate plasmid between p1478A and the new tet shuttle plasmid carrying the desired gene.
3. To resolve the cointegrate via the *rfsF* sites prepare competent bacteria from the clone carrying the correct cointegrate and transfect 100 ng of the plasmid DCM111 *(12)*, which encodes the resolvase enzyme (resD) and ampicillin resistance. Select on LB-amp-cam plates at 42°C.
4. Pick and select clones that are cam-resistant and tet-sensitive as in **Subheading 3.1., steps 8** and **9** (*see* **Note 7**).
5. Transfect 5 μL of plasmid mini-preparations from several tet-sensitive clones into competent DH5α and select on LB-cam plates at 37°C. In the majority of the clones the DCM111 plasmid will be lost by retransfection of *E. coli.*
6. Pick several colonies (20–30) and make short streaks onto an LB-cam master plate and an LB-amp plate at 37°C to test for amp-sensitive clones that have lost the DCM111 plasmid.
7. Prepare plasmid DNA from amp sensitive clones as described in **Subheading 3.1., step 3**.
8. Analyze the plasmid DNA with appropriate restriction enzymes to ensure the composition of the new mini-EBV plasmid (*see* **Notes 2** and **6**).
9. To amplify and purify the new mini-EBV plasmid follow the method described in **Subheading 3.3.**

### 3.3. CsCl Purification of Mini-EBV Plasmids

1. Prepare an overnight culture of DH5α containing the mini-EBV plasmid in 800 mL LB-cam with added 0.3 *M* NaCl.
2. Transfer bacteria to a fermenter and grow them in 5 L of LB-cam with 0.3 *M* NaCl and 100 mL of glycerol until they have reached an $OD_{600}$ of 5.
3. Spin down bacteria in five 1000 mL-centrifuge bottles for 15 min at 4000*g*, 20°C and discard the supernatant.
4. To prepare plasmid-DNA resuspend each pellet in 50 mL of solution I and transfer the suspension to 500 mL-centrifuge tubes that fit in a Sorvall-GS3 rotor. Add 100 mL of solution II to each tube and mix gently. Keep on ice for 10 min. Add 74 mL of ice-cold solution III to each tube and mix well by shaking. Keep on ice for at least 10 min then centrifuge in a GS3 rotor for 20 min at 4200*g*, 4°C. Transfer the supernatant to a new 500 mL-centrifuge tube and add 1 volume of isopropanol to precipitate the DNA. Mix well and keep on ice for 20 min. Centrifuge for 20 min at 4200*g*, 4°C. Dilute all five pellets in a total volume of 100 mL of TE8.
5. Dissolve 110 g of CsCl in the 100 mL DNA solution. Fill 800 μL of ethidium bromide (10 mg/mL) and then 25 mL of the plasmid/CsCl solution into each of four 38.5-mL

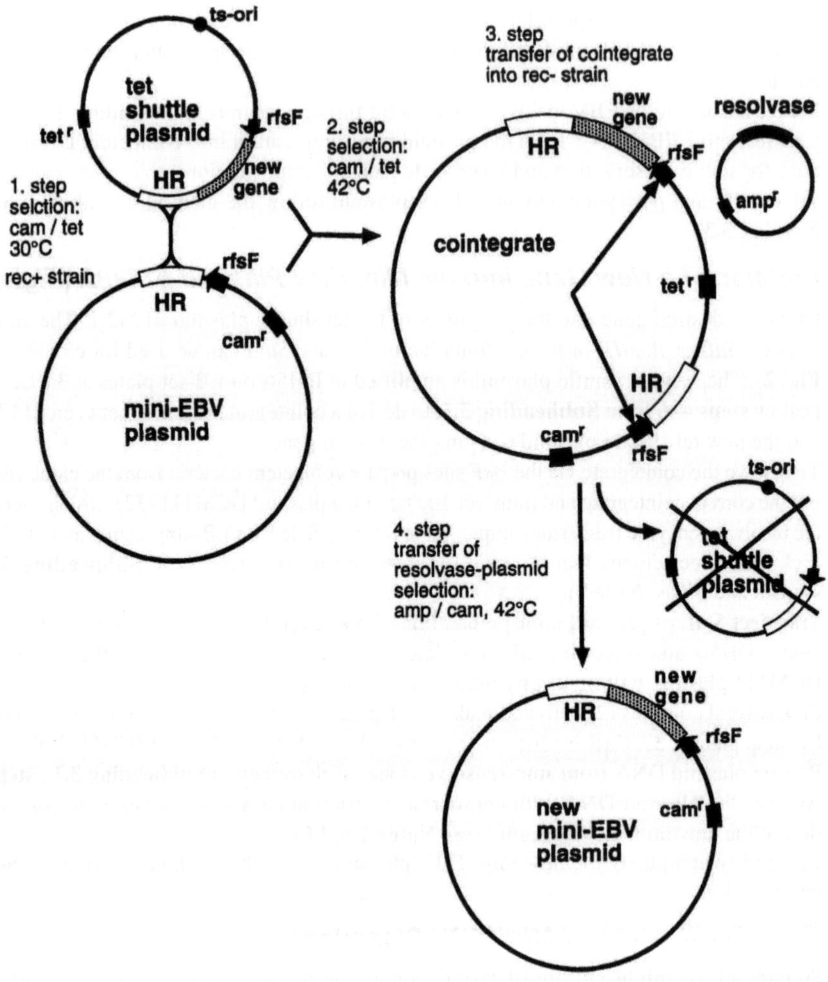


Fig. 4. Addition of a new gene onto the mini-EBV plasmid p1478A. The tet shuttle plasmid shown on the upper left side carries the desired gene flanked by 3–4 kb of EBV DNA (HR) and a *rfsF* site. The mini-EBV plasmid p1478A carries at the end of its EBV insert a homologous region (HR) to the EBV DNA of the tet shuttle plasmid and a second *rfsF* site. Homologous recombination between the HR regions of both plasmids leads to the formation of a co-integrate as shown on the upper right side. The enzyme resolvase encoded by the DCM111 plasmid carries out recombination between the two *rfsF* sites of the cointegrate leading to loss of the tet shuttle backbone. The resulting new mini-EBV plasmid has the same structure as p1478A but carries the new gene adjacent to the HR region (shown on the lower left side). The tet shuttle plasmid is lost through selection.

ultracentrifuge tubes (Kontron Ultracrimp) and fill the tube up with a 1.55 g/cm$^3$ CsCl solution.

6. Seal the tubes and run in an ultracentrifuge (Centrikon TFT70.38 rotor) for 3 d at 92,000*g* and 20°C. Two clearly visible bands should be apparent under 300 nm UV light. Collect

the lower band of the gradient from each of the four centrifuge tubes using syringes and needles.

7. Combine the content of the four syringes into two 13.5-mL ultracentrifuge tubes (Kontron Ultracrimp), top off with a 1.55g/cm$^3$ CsCl solution, and centrifuge at 84,000*g* (Beckman 70.ITi rotor) and 20°C for 2 d.
8. Two bands should be clearly visible without UV light. Both can be collected separately. The upper band contains circular DNA in excellent quality for mapping. The lower band contains supercoiled, high quality mini-EBV plasmid DNA, which can be used for transfections of eukaryotic cells.
9. Add 3 mL of isopropanol (saturated with $H_2O$ and CsCl). Mix well, centrifuge at 5000*g* for 1 min. Discard the upper phase containing ethidium bromide. Repeat this procedure at least three times until no more ethidium bromide is visible in the upper phase. Mix with three volumes of TE8 and precipitate DNA with 0.7 vol of isopropanol, wash with 70% ethanol, and resuspend the pellet in 200–300 µL of TE8. Store mini-EBV plasmid DNA at 4°C because freezing and thawing will damage the large plasmids. Always pipet the DNA with a tip with its end clipped off such that the opening is wider than usual to avoid shearing.

### 3.4. Infection of Primary B-cells with Mini-EBV (Fig. 5)

1. Centrifuge $10^7$ HH514 cells for 5 min at 1000*g* and room temperature. Wash cells in serum-free RPMI medium and resuspend the cells in 250 µL of serum-free RPMI medium at room temperature.
2. Mix 250 µL of HH514 cells with 20 µg of CsCl-purified mini-EBV plasmid DNA (*see* **Subheading 3.3.**) and 10 µg of pCMV-BZLF1 *(14)* plasmid DNA in an electroporation cuvet with 4-mm gap.
3. Electroporate the cells with 250 V, 960 µF in a Bio-Rad Gene Pulser™ and add 500 µL of FCS immediately afterwards (for further details on electroporation parameters, *see* Chapter 14). Then transfer the cells to 10 mL of RPMI medium containing 10% FCS and incubate them for 5 d at 37°C. During that time DNA replication, encapsidation into virions and lysis of the cells occurs.
4. Centrifuge the 10 mL supernatant of the cells containing released virus particles for 5 min at 1000*g* and room temperature to remove cells and cellular debris. Subsequently filter the virus-stock through a 0.45-µm filter. The virus-stock can be kept at 4°C for up to 1 wk.
5. To isolate primary human B-lymphocytes from tonsillectomies or adenectomies generate a single cell suspension in a small volume of PBS containing versene in a 1:500 dilution (PBS/versene). Wash the cells three times with PBS/versene then add 2 mL of whole sheep blood to 100 mL of cells in PBS/versene to rosette T-cells. Carefully pipet 30 mL of the cell suspension on top of 15 mL of ficoll in a 50-mL Falcon tube so that the phases do not mix. Centrifuge at 740*g*, 4°C for 30 min. Collect the interphase of the gradient containing the B-cells, mix with at least 1 volume of PBS/versene, and pellet the B-cells at 700*g* at room temperature for 5 min. Wash the cells two times with PBS/versene by pelleting the cells first at 550*g* and then at 430*g*, each at room temperature for 5 min. Resuspend the primary B-cells in RPMI medium with 10% FCS. It is best to use the cells immediately but they can also be stored at RT for short time periods or in a cell-culture flask at 37°C overnight.
6. Mix 2–3.5 × $10^7$ primary B-cells with 2.5–5 mL of virus stock in a final volume of 11 mL RPMI medium with 10% FCS. Plate the cells in a 96 well plate with 100 µL of the culture per well on a lethally irradiated (50 Gy) human fibroblast feeder-cell layer (Wi38) (*see*

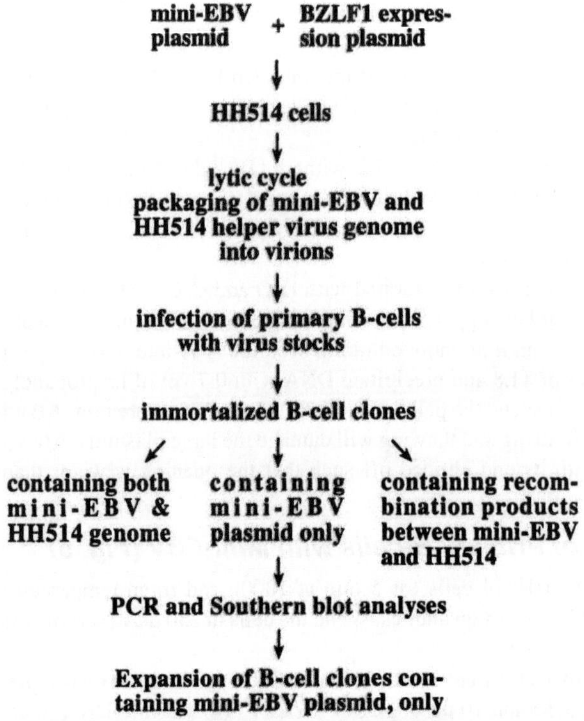


Fig. 5. Schematic representation of the consecutive steps involved in generation of virus-free B-cell clones by infection with helper-virus packaged mini-EBV plamids.

**Notes 8** and **9**). Incubate the cells at 37°C and replace 50 μL of the culture medium with 50 μL of fresh RPMI medium with 10% FCS every week. Outgrowing clones should be visible after 3–5 wk of cell culture.

### *3.5. Cell Culture and Analyses of B-cell Clones*

1. When B-cell clones become clearly visible by light microscopy, transfer, and expand them sequentially to higher culture volumes. In the beginning the cells should be diluted 1:2 until a culture volume of 1 mL has been reached. Dense cultures can then be diluted 1:3 or 1:4.
2. Prepare cellular DNA from an aliquot of 2.5–5 × $10^6$ cells: Pellet the cells for 5 min at 1000*g* and room temperature and wash with PBS. Lyse the cells in 1 mL of lysis buffer, add 50 μL of proteinase K (10 mg/mL), and incubate the lysate at 50°C for 2–3 h. Extract the DNA with buffered phenol and precipitate with 1 vol of isopropanol (further details on high molecular weight DNA preparation are given in **ref. *20***).
3. Use 1 μg of total cellular DNA for PCR analyses to detect helper virus or wild-type EBV with the primer pair ΔB95.8. Use cellular DNA from an EBV-infected cell line (e.g., HH514) as a positive control. PCR is carried out with 1 pmol of each primer under standard conditions for 30 cycles (94°C for 45 s, 58°C for 1 min, 72°C for 1 min). The ΔB95.8 primer pair amplifies a 434 bp fragment from nucleotide position 33 to 466 of the Raji strain sequence ***(17)***, which is absent in the prototype EBV strain B95.8 ***(13)*** and the mini-EBV plasmid.

4. Carry out a second PCR analyses with all clones that were negative for HH514 helper virus or wild-type EBV. Use the CAM primer pair to detect the presence of mini-EBV plasmid. A 294 bp product is amplified from the chloramphenicol resistance gene of the mini-EBV.
5. Carry out Southern blot analysis (***18,20***) with an appropriate probe ***(19)*** to ensure that no structural changes of the mini-EBV plasmid have occurred and that no helper virus DNA is present.
6. Expand (*see* **Subheading 3.5., step 1**) and freeze B-cell clones that contain the mini-EBV plasmid but no helper virus or wild-type EBV.

## 4. Notes

1. Bacteria transfected with a tet shuttle plasmid grow only at 30°C on LB-tet because of the temperature sensitive replication origin of the plasmid. Bacteria will grow slowly and sometimes need more than 1 d to grow to clearly visible colonies. It is obligatory to purify tet shuttle plasmids by CsCl gradient centrifugation (*see* **Subheading 3.3.** and **ref.** ***20***) when the DNA is used for cloning purposes. To make plasmid DNA mini-preparations, it is better to spread the cells on thick LB-tet-plates and let them grow to a dense lawn than to make a liquid culture because the bacteria will grow faster on a plate. We normally use one quarter of a plate to spread one clone.
2. DNA from plasmid mini-preparations should always be kept on ice and stored at –20°C to avoid degradation. Not all restriction enzymes will work with these preparations. For tet shuttle plasmids, one can also purify them with commercially available ion exchange columns to test with other restriction enzymes if necessary. Mini-EBV and co-integrate plasmid-DNA from mini-preparations can be analyzed with *BamH*I, *Bgl*II, *Xho*I, and some other commercially available enzymes.
3. Streaks to derive cointegrates are carried out as dilution streaks. First pick the colony and streak it on a small part of the plate. Then make long streaks out of this patch with a new sterile loop. This can be done on one half of a plate for restreaking one colony. The number of colonies chosen here depends on the efficiency of the process. Five to ten are usually enough.
4. Usually the analysis of 10 clones is enough to find an intact co-integrate.
5. The resolution of the co-integrate by homologous recombination is a spontaneous process that can not be selected for. Therefore only a few tet-sensitive clones will be found in 50–100 clones.
6. Analyses of cointegrate or mini-EBV plasmid DNA with restriction enzymes should always be compared to the original mini-EBV to ensure the overall structure of the plasmid. One should use long gels with 0.8% agarose in TAE-buffer, run them without ethidium bromide, and stain the gels afterwards. In the recombination process, unwanted nonhomologous recombination can occur and the structure of the plasmid can be found altered or copy numbers of repetitive sequences can vary considerably. Therefore, a careful analysis with several restriction enzymes is mandatory.
7. Resolution of the cointegrate via the *rfsF* sites is catalyzed by the resolvase enzyme usually with an efficiency of about 10%.
8. How much of the virus-stock is needed to yield good infection results depends on the efficiency of the packaging procedure. It is helpful to plate at least two dilutions of the virus-stock (1:2 and 1:4 dilution). B-cell clones should then be expanded from wells with the highest dilution, because here the probability of doubly infected clones is lowest.

9. WI38 feeder cells can be irradiated and plated 1–2 d in advance or irradiated feeder cells can be immediately mixed with primary B-cells and virus-stock.

## References


1. Cohen, J. I., Wang, F., Mannick, J., and Kieff, E. (1989) Epstein-Barr virus nuclear protein 2 is a key determinant of lymphocyte transformation. *Proc. Natl. Acad. Sci. USA* **86,** 9558–9562.
2. Kaye, K. M., Izumi, K. M., and Kieff, E. (1993) Epstein-Barr virus latent membrane protein 1 is essential for B-lymphocyte growth transformation. *Proc. Natl. Acad. Sci. USA* **90,** 9150–9154.
3. Tomkinson, B., Robertson, E., and Kieff, E. (1993) Epstein-Barr virus nuclear proteins EBNA-3A and EBNA-3C are essential for B-lymphocyte growth transformation. *J. Virol.* **67,** 2014–2025.
4. Hammerschmidt, W. and Sugden, B. (1989) Genetic analysis of immortalizing functions of Epstein-Barr virus in human B lymphocytes. *Nature* **340,** 393–397.
5. Kempkes, B., Spitkovsky, D., Jansen-Dürr, P., Ellwart, J. W., Delecluse, H.-J., Rottenberger, C., et al. (1995) B-cell proliferation and induction of early G1-regulating proteins by Epstein-Barr virus mutants conditional for EBNA2. *EMBO J.* **14,** 88–96.
6. Yates, J. L. (1996) Epstein-Barr virus DNA replication, in *DNA Replication in Eukaryotic Cells,* (DePamphilis, M. L., ed.), Cold Spring Harbor Laboratory Press, Cold Spring Harbor, NY, pp. 751–773.
7. Kempkes, B., Pich, D., Zeidler, R., and Hammerschmidt, W. (1995) Immortalization of human primary B-lymphocytes *in vitro* with DNA. *Proc. Natl. Acad. Sci. USA* **92,** 5875–5879.
8. Kempkes, B., Pich, D., Zeidler, R., Sugden, B., and Hammerschmidt, W. (1995) Immortalization of human B-lymphocytes by a plasmid containing 71 kpb of Epstein-Barr viral DNA. *J. Virol.* **69,** 231–238.
9. Rabson, M., Gradoville, L., Heston, L., and Miller, G. (1982) Non-immortalizing P3J-HR-1 Epstein-Barr virus: a deletion mutant of its transforming parent, Jijoye. *J. Virol.* **44,** 834–844.
10. Kilger, E., Kieser, A., Baumann, M., and Hammerschmidt, W. (1998) Epstein-Barr virus-mediated B-cell proliferation is dependent upon latent membrane protein 1, which simulates an activated CD40 receptor. *EMBO J.* **17,** 1700–1709.
11. Kilger, E., Pecher, G., Schwenk, A., and Hammerschmidt, W. (1998) Expression of mucin (MUC-1) from a mini-Epstein-Barr virus in immortalized B-cells to generate tumor antigen specific cytotoxic T-cells. *submitted for publication*
12. O'Connor, M., Peifer, M., and Bender, W. (1989) Construction of large DNA segments in Escherichia coli. *Science* **244,** 1307–1312.
13. Baer, R., Bankier, A. T., Biggin, M. D., Deininger, P. L., Farrell, P. J., Gibson, T. J., et al. (1984) DNA sequence and expression of the B95–8 Epstein-Barr virus genome. *Nature* **310,** 207–211.
14. Hammerschmidt, W. and Sugden, B. (1988) Identification and characterization of *oriLyt,* a lytic origin of DNA replication of Epstein-Barr virus. *Cell* **55,** 427–433.
15. Hanahan, D. (1985) Techniques for transformation of *E. coli,* in *DNA Cloning: A Practical Approach, vol. 1,* (Glover, D.M., ed.) IRL Press, Oxford, pp. 109–135.
16. Heston, L., Rabson, M., Brown, N., and Miller, G. (1982) New Epstein-Barr virus variants from cellular subclones of P3J-HR-1 Burkitt lymphoma. *Nature* **295,** 160–163.

17. Parker, B. D., Bankier, A., Satchwell, S., Barrell, B., and Farrell, P. J. (1990) Sequence and transcription of Raji Epstein-Barr virus DNA spanning the B95-8 deletion region. *Virology* **179,** 339–346.
18. Southern, E. M. (1975) Detection of specific sequences among DNA fragments separated by gel electrophoresis. *J. Mol. Biol.* **98,** 503–517.
19. Kempkes, B., Zimber-Strobl, U., Eissner, G., Pawlita, M., Falk, M., Hammerschmidt, W., and Bornkamm, G. W. (1996) Epstein-Barr virus nuclear antigen 2 (EBNA2)-oestrogen receptor fusion proteins complement the EBNA2–deficient Epstein-Barr virus strain P3HR1 in transformation of primary B cells but suppress growth of human B cell lymphoma lines. *J. Gen. Virol.* **77,** 227–237.
20. Maniatis, T., Fritsch, E. F., and Sambrook, J. (1989) *Molecular Cloning: A Laboratory Manual.*Cold Spring Harbor Laboratory Press, Cold Spring Harbor, New York.

# 4

# Construction of cDNA Libraries for the Analysis of the Structure of Complementary Strand Transcripts (CSTs)

**Paul R. Smith**

## 1. Introduction

The Epstein-Bar virus (EBV)-encoded complementary strand transcripts (CSTs) are a recently described *(1,2)* group of related transcripts initiating from a common promoter that exhibit a complex splicing pattern and contain a number of small open reading frames with the potential to encode a number of proteins *(3)*. The CSTs have been detected in most types of EBV infection, including nasopharyngeal carcinoma (NPC) *(4)*, oral hairy leukoplakia *(5)*, EBV-positive gastric carcinoma *(6)*, and latently infected lymphoblastoid cell lines *(7,8)*. The function of these transcripts is still unclear.

The requirement for the production of a complementary strand DNA library is today in many cases unnecessary, because in most instances, a ready-made library can be purchased from a number of suppliers, or, alternatively, isolation of cDNA clones can be accomplished by use of polymerase chin reaction (PCR)-based methods. For the study of the EBV CSTs, these approaches have limitations. First, commercially available libraries containing EBV are largely restricted to those constructed from B-lymphoblastoid cell lines. In these particular cell lines, however, the levels of the CSTs are low *(7)*. Secondly, studies of the CSTs suggest that the splicing pattern of the CSTs is complex *(3,9)*, making PCR amplification of large, full-length, or less abundant clones more difficult. Because many of the clones isolated to date do not contain large open reading frames, the identification of potential proteins encoded by CSTs is facilitated by the isolation of large or full-length cDNA clones, which can be sequenced and possible open reading frames identified.

Most groups that have analyzed CST structure have, therefore, chosen to construct cDNA libraries from cells which contain CSTs expressed to a high level. These are usually derived from human NPC, either a xenograft, such as C15, a human NPC tumor passaged in nude mice *(10)*, or directly from NPC biopsy material *(4)*.

From: *Methods in Molecular Biology, Vol. 174: Epstein-Barr Virus Protocols*
Edited by: J. B. Wilson and G. H. W. May © Humana Press Inc., Totowa, NJ

There are many different cloning vectors on the market for the construction of cDNA libraries. For the analysis of CST structure, most groups have utilized a basic λgt10-based vector. The remainder of this chapter will therefore concentrate on the use of this type of library.

## 2. Materials

### 2.1. Library Construction

1. Tissue source. Construction of libraries from C15 tumor will require at least 0.5 g of tissue. Freshly isolated tumor generally gives a greater yield of RNA than that isolated from frozen material.
2. Dounce homogenizer.
3. Method for purification of poly(A)+ RNA.
4. Method for construction of cDNA. Most reagents for these kits will be supplied by the manufactures, however some basic materials will be required.
5. DEPC-treated water. Add diethyl pyrocarbonate to 0.1% (v/v), stand overnight and then autoclave.
6. Phenol/Chloroform/Isoamyl alcohol (25:24:1). Phenol is saturated with Tris-HCl, pH 8.0, and an equal volume of chloroform containing isoamyl alcohol is added.
7. Absolute ethanol (–20°C).
8. Packaging kits.
9. Materials for plating libraries (*see* **Subheading 2.2.**).

### 2.2. Plating the Library

1. LB broth: 10 g tryptone, 5 g yeast extract, 5 g sodium chloride in 1 L of water. Autoclave.
2. LBM broth: LB broth containing 20 m*M* magnesium chloride and 2% maltose.
3. LBM agar plates: LBM broth containing 1.5% agar. Autoclave.
4. Top agarose: LBM broth containing 0.7% agarose.
5. 20% maltose: Filter-sterilized.
6. 2 *M* magnesium sulfate. Autoclaved.
7. 37°C Incubator.
8. 10-cm diameter Petri dishes.
9. SM buffer: 50 m*M* Tris-HCl, pH 7.4, 0.1 *M* NaCl, 10 m*M* $MgSO_4$, 0.01% gelatin. Autoclaved.

### 2.3. Screening the Library

1. Materials for plating the library (*see* **Subheading 2.2.**).
2. Nitrocellulose filters (Schleicher and Schüll, 137-mm diameter, 0.45-μm pore size).
3. 3 MM paper.
4. Hybridization buffer: 1.5 m*M* sodium pyrophosphate, 20 m*M* sodium dihydrogen orthophosphate, 0.1% sodium dodecyl sulfate (SDS), 6X SSC, 0.25% Ficoll, 0.25% bovine serum albumin (SA), 0.25% poly vinyl pyrrolidine.
5. Radiolabeled DNA.
6. 20X SSC: 3 *M* sodium chloride, 0.3 *M* sodium citrate, pH 7.0.
7. 10% SDS.
8. Saran wrap.
9. Hybridization oven.
10. Chloroform.

### 2.4. Phage Isolation

1. Materials for plating the library (*see* **Subheading 2.2.**).
2. LBM agarose plates: LBM broth containing 1.5% agarose. Autoclave.
3. DNaseI, 10 mg/mL.
4. RNaseA, 10 mg/mL.
5. 20% PEG/2 *M* NaCl solution in $H_2O$, using PEG 8000.
6. 0.5 *M* ethylenediaminetetraacetic acid (EDTA), pH 8.0.
7. 10% SDS.
8. Proteinase K, 10 mg/mL.
9. Phenol/Chloroform/Isoamyl alcohol, (25:24:1).
10. 3 *M* sodium acetate, adjusted to pH 5.5.
11. Absolute ethanol (–20°C).
12. 80% ethanol.
13. TE8: 10 m*M* Tris-HCl, pH 8.0, 1 m*M* EDTA.

## 3. Methods

### 3.1. Library Construction

1. Isolation of mRNA from the chosen tissue source will depend on the choice of RNA isolation method (*see* **Note 1**). For isolation from C15 tumor, homogenize tissue in a chilled Dounce homogenizer using 10–15 strokes on ice, being careful to avoid excess heat or froth generation. Subsequent steps should follow the manufacturers instructions to obtain high-purity poly(A)+ RNA. From 0.5 g of C15 tumor, it should be possible to obtain up to 10 mg of mRNA.
2. Production of cDNA. There are many kits for the construction of cDNA; the choice of kit will be determined in many cases by the availability of the required cloning vector. Construct the cDNA from the mRNA according to the manufacturers instructions (*see* **Note 2**).
3. Ligation of the cDNA into λgt10 vectors. It is best to buy predigested, phosphorylated vectors to maximize ligation efficiency. In some cases it may be necessary to perform several test ligations before a satisfactory cDNA library is produced. Ligation conditions will depend on the methods used to construct the library and will be supplied by the providers of the construction kits or the lambda vectors (*see* **Note 3**).
4. Packaging and amplification. It is necessary first to test the ligations to check the number of recombinants and also the size and number of inserts before proceeding to amplify the library (*see* **Note 4**). Ligations should be packaged into phage particles using commercially available packaging kits, there are again a variety of these. Plate packaged ligations using a suitable strain of plating bacteria (usually supplied with the packaging kit) and analyze resulting phage plaques for number of recombinants and size and frequency of inserts. In the case of λgt10 libraries, all plaques will contain inserts; for λgt11-based libraries it is necessary to confirm that at least 80% of plaques contain inserts. If the library is satisfactory, containing at least $10^6$ individual recombinants with an average size of at least 1 kb, then the library can be amplified. For amplification, enough LBM agar plates will be required to plate the entire library at a density of 50,000 plaques/plate. Plate the entire library as described in **Subheading 3.2.** Following plating and incubation, add 10–15 mL of SM buffer to each plate and incubate at 4°C for at least 1 h and preferably overnight, to allow the phage to leach out. Remove SM buffer containing phage into sterile containers. The amplified library can be kept at 4°C, but some loss in titer will

result with time. For long-term storage, glycerol should be added to a concentration of 40% and the library divided into aliquots and stored at –70°C

### 3.2. Plating the Library

1. Following amplification, determine the titer of the amplified library. About 106 clones can be easily screened with approx $5 \times 10^4$ plaques plated on each 10-cm LBM agar plate.
2. Dilute the library with SM buffer to 50,000 plaques/100 µL (for each plate).
3. Prepare competent bacteria. For the analysis of a λgt10 library grow 50 mL of an appropriate *Escherichia coli* strain (usually Hfl c600) overnight in LBM broth, pellet at 1500*g* for 10 min, and resuspend the bacteria in 10 mL of 0.2% maltose/20 m*M* magnesium sulfate and maintain at 4°C until required (up to 1 wk).
4. For each plate, add 100 µL of library dilution to 900 µL of competent bacteria and incubate at 37°C for 30 min. Add to 9 mL of melted top agarose (kept at 55°C; *see* **Note 5**) and pour onto prewarmed LBM agar plates. Once set, incubate inverted at 37°C for 3–4 h or until plaques appear. Store plates at 4°C, wrapped to prevent dehydration

### 3.3. Screening

1. Probing of $10^6$ plaques will require 20 LBM agar plates; duplicate lifts are taken from each plate. First, label the nitrocellulose filters (*see* **Note 6**). Place carefully on the top agarose. Leave the first filter on the plate for 30 s, during which time orientation holes can be marked by punching needle holes through the filter and into the agar (*see* **Note 6**). Remove the filter using blunt forceps and air dry for 15 min. The duplicate lift is allowed to remain on the agarose for 1 min, using the same orientation holes to mark the filter. If other lifts are to be taken from the same plate, then place the plates at 4°C for at least 1 h prior to taking subsequent lifts.
2. An easy way to denature the DNA on the filter prior to probing is to place the filters in a 3 MM paper wallet and wrap in aluminum foil. Then place the wallets containing the filters in a pressure cooker and heat for 2 min under medium pressure. Immediately remove the pressure and dry at 60°C for 2 h ***(11)***.
3. Prior to probing pre-incubate the dried filters in hybridization buffer for 2–3 h at 68°C. During this time it is possible to radiolabel the purified DNA fragments using standard protocols (*see* **Note 7**). 2.5 µg of purified DNA is sufficient to screen 20 filters (*see* **Note 8**).
4. Following pre-hybridization place the filters in 1 mL fresh hybridization buffer/filter, and add the denatured, labeled probe(s). Incubate the filters overnight at 68°C (*see* **Note 9**).
5. Following hybridization, wash the filters for 15 minutes in 2X SSC/0.5% SDS, followed by 2 × 60 min washes in 0.3X SSC/0.1% SDS, 2 × 60 min washes in 0.1X SSC/0.1% SDS, and finally 2 × 60 min with 0.1X SSC/0.5% SDS; all washes at 68°C. Place the damp filters between two sheets of Saran wrap and set up for autoradiography. Expose the films at –70°C for 7–10 d (*see* **Note 10**).
6. Develop the films and check for plaques positive on both sets of filters. Remove plugs of agar containing the positive plaques with a small diameter cork borer or Pasteur pipet. Store the plugs in 500 µL of SM buffer and add a small drop of chloroform to lyse any bacteria, until required for secondary screening.
7. Owing to the high density of plaques on the primary plates, it is necessary to re-screen the phage from the positive plaques at a lower density in order to isolate individual positive plaques. Firstly determine the titer of the phage from the plugs necessary to give a density allowing separation of individual plaques and then plate and probe using the protocols

described earlier for primary screening. Once individual, positive plaques have been identified, use toothpicks to harvest phage into 200 μL of SM buffer.

### 3.4. Isolation of Lambda Phage

Isolation of phage particles follows standard protocols, we generally find that plate purification gives better yields than liquid purification.

1. Add 50–100 μL of phage in SM buffer to 300 μL of competent *E. coli* cells (prepared as described in **Subheading 3.2.**) and incubate for 15 min at 37°C.
2. Add 3 mL of top agarose and pour onto an LBM agarose plate (*see* **Note 11**) and incubate for about 6 h at 37°C until plaques form.
3. Place the plates at 4°C for 30–60 min, then add 5 mL cold SM buffer and leave the plates overnight at 4°C.
4. Remove the SM buffer and clarify by centrifugation at 2500*g* for 15 min.
5. Add DNaseI to 10 μg/μL and RNaseA to 10 μg/μL and incubate for 30 min at 37°C.
6. Add an equal volume of 20% PEG/2 *M* NaCl, mix well, and place on ice for 2 h. Spin at 2500*g* for 20 min, discard supernatant, and re-spin briefly. Discard remainder of supernatant.
7. Add 500 μL of SM buffer to resuspend the phage and leave for at least 60 min at 4°C (preferably overnight), add SDS (final concentration, 0.5%), EDTA (final concentration, 20 m*M*), and Proteinase K (final concentration, 100 μg/μL), and incubate for 30 min at 37°C.
8. Extract twice with an equal volume of phenol/chloroform/isoamyl alcohol, remove upper phase, add 1/10th vol of 3 *M* sodium acetate and two volumes of cold ethanol, and precipitate at –20°C overnight.
9. Wash pellet with 80% ethanol, and briefly air-dry the pellet.
10. Resuspend the precipitate in 100 μL of TE8. Digest 10 μL and characterize the insert by digestion with relevant restriction enzymes (*see* **Note 12**).

## 4. Notes

1. The starting point for the construction of cDNA libraries requires isolation of high-quality mRNA. There are many commercially available kits for the purification of RNA from tissue or tissue culture cells, and several kits for selection of poly(A)+ RNA from total RNA.
2. Production of libraries is aided by the availability of many kits for cDNA synthesis. Choice of kit depends mainly on the use of the final library. Construction of expression based libraries will be aided by the use of randomly priming oligonucleotides, whereas the isolation of full-length cDNAs will require oligonucleotides that prime from the 3'-polyadenylated sequence. For the construction of libraries for a specific purpose, as for analyzing the structure of CSTs, it is possible to prime the first-strand synthesis with a specific oligonucleotide. For example, use of an oligonucleotide complementary to the 3 region common to all CST transcripts described to date should result in synthesis of a library enriched for CST cDNA clones.
3. There are many kits available for maximizing the efficiency of ligation for libraries. We have found that the methods described in the cDNA kits are adequate if the cDNA synthesis has been efficient.
4. Amplification provides a stock of the library for several screenings. If the library is needed for one specific analysis, then amplification may not be necessary and the whole library can be screened at once. This has the advantage that all cDNA clones will be screened, including slower-growing or rare clones. However, repeat screenings are not possible.

5. The use of agarose in the top layer provides a better base when nitrocellulose lifts are taken. It is not advisable to use agar in the top layer as the filters have a greater tendency to stick to the agar. Avoid creating air bubbles when pouring the phage/agarose mix because these will impair the screening process.
6. There are many methods for marking filters, we use a soft pencil to label the filters and a broad-gauge needle to mark the holes. We do not use ink or a weak radio-isotope solution to mark orientation.
7. Complete plasmid DNA can be used to screen λgt10 libraries, but it is preferable to digest and purify a specific insert to remove vector sequences prior to labeling.
8. To isolate full-length clones, one set of filters should be screened with DNA from the 3'-end of the transcripts; for example, between EBV co-ordinates 160250 and 160990. A duplicate set of filters should be screened from the 5' region of the CSTs, preferably covering exon I *(3)*. The complex splicing patterns of the isolated clones described to date make it difficult to describe a probe from the "middle" of the CSTs common to all clones; however, a probe from exon V *(3)*, between EBV co-ordinates 155730 and 156000, will cover most of the clones described so far.
9. Incubation of the filters will depend on how many are being screened. Any commercially available hybridization oven with large incubation chambers will be satisfactory; alternatively, the filters can be placed in a plastic box and incubated in a shaking water bath.
10. The length of time taken for the spots to develop will depend on several factors. To ensure that the background is not too high, it is sensible to monitor the filters with a Geiger counter prior to setting up for autoradiography, alternatively develop one sheet of film after an overnight exposure.
11. The use of agarose rather than agar in the base of the plates as well as the top aids isolation of good quality phage DNA.
12. Initial analysis of the isolated clones will rely on restriction digestion to identify the size of the insert present in the clone. This will depend on the restriction enzyme sites present in the linkers used in the initial library construction. A useful reference is the presence of a single *Eco*RI site in the CST clones. Because many λgt10-based vectors use *Eco*RI in the linkers, digestion of the isolated phage DNA with this enzyme can give an initial idea of the structure of the clone, as two separately spliced CST clones have been identified at the 3'-end. *Eco*RI digestion will produce a fragment of approx 1140 bp or 972 bp depending on the splicing pattern present in the clones, in addition to the (usually) larger band containing the 5' sequences.

## References


1. Hitt, M. M., Allday, M. J., Hara, T., Karran, L., Jones, M. D., Busson, P., et al. (1989) EBV gene expression in an NPC related tumor. *EMBO J.* **8,** 2639–2651.
2. Gilligan, K., Sato, H., Rajadurai, P., Busson, P., Young, L., Rickinson, A., et al. (1990) Novel transcription from the Epstein-Barr virus terminal EcoRI fragment, DIJhet, in a nasopharyngeal carcinoma. *Virology* **64,** 4948–4956.
3. Smith, P. R., Gao, Y., Karran, L., Jones, M. D., Snudden, D., and Griffin, B. E. (1993) Complex nature of the major viral polyadenylated transcripts in Epstein-Barr virus associated tumors. *J. Virol.* **67,** 3217–3225.
4. Chen, H.-L., Lung, M. M. L., Sham, J. S. T., Choy, D. T. K., Griffin, B. E., and Ng, M. H. (1992). Transcription of BamHI-A region of the EBV genome in NPC tissues and B cells. *Virology* **191,** 193–201.

5. Lau, R., Middledorp, J., and Farrell, P. J. (1993). Epstein Barr virus gene expression in oral hairy leukoplakia. *Virology* **195,** 463–474.
6. Sugiura, M., Imai, S., Tokunga, M., Koizumi, S., Uchizawa, M., Okamoto, K., and Osato, T. (1996). Transcriptional analysis of Epstein-Barr virus gene expression in EBV-positive gastric carcinoma: unique viral latency in the tumor cells. *Br. J. Cancer* **74,** 625–631.
7. Karran, L., Gao, Y., Smith, P. R., and Griffin, B. E. (1992) Expression of a family of EB virus complementary strand transcripts in latently infected cells. *Proc. Natl. Acad. Sci. USA* **89,** 8058–8062.
8. Brooks, L. A., Lear, A. L., Young, L. S., and Rickinson, A. B. (1993). Transcripts from the Epstein-Barr virus BamHI A fragment are detectable in all three forms of virus latency. *J. Virol.* **67,** 3182–3190.
9. Sadler, R. H. and Raab-Traub, N. (1995). Structural analyses of the Epstein-Barr virus BamHI A transcripts. *J. Virol.* **69,** 1132–1141.
10. Busson, P., Ganem, G., Flores, P., Mugneret, B., Clauss, B., Caillou, K., et al. (1988). Establishment and characterization of three transplantable EBV-containing nasopharyngeal carcinomas. *Int. J. Cancer* **42,** 599–606.
11. Allday, M. J. and Jones, M. D. (1987) Rapid processing of nitrocellulose filter lifts of bacteriophage lambda libraries. *Nucleic Acids Res.* **15,** 10592.



5

# Analysis of the Expression and Function of the EBV-Encoded Small RNAs, the EBERs, in Heterologous Cells

**Kenneth G. Laing, Volker Matys, and Michael J. Clemens**

## 1. Introduction

The two small virally encoded RNA species, EBER-1 and EBER-2, are abundantly expressed in almost all Epstein-Barr virus (EBV)-infected cell types. Their functions in relation to the physiology of the virus remain enigmatic. In recent years, the main interest in the EBERs has been in connection with the use of these RNAs as targets for identification of EBV infection using *in situ* hybridization. However evidence for a possible function for the EBERs is now emerging and it seems likely that these small RNAs constitute another weapon in the armory used by EBV to infect and immortalize the host cell. EBER-1 and EBER-2 are uncapped, nonpolyadenylated, untranslated RNAs of 167 and 172 nucleotides, respectively. Even in cells with the most restricted range of EBV gene expression (e.g., most Burkitt's lymphomas), where EBNA-1 is the only viral protein synthesized, the EBERs are always present. The two RNAs are also found in cells in which EBV replication is actively occurring. In this chapter we describe techniques for the expression of the EBERs in EBV-negative cells, and for the analysis of the functions of these small RNAs in the control of cellular protein synthesis.

### *1.1. Requirements for In Vivo Expression of the EBERs in Heterologous Cells*

Jat and Arrand *(1)* showed that the transcription of EBER-1 and -2 from the *Eco*RI J fragment of EBV in whole cell extracts was sensitive to inhibition by high concentrations of α-amanitin, thus indicating that the synthesis of these nontranslated RNAs is carried out by RNA polymerase III. In order to construct and manipulate competent expression vectors containing the EBER genes, it is essential to understand something of the polymerase III promoter structure. These promoters fall into four main categories, sometimes referred to as type I, II, III, and IV *(2,3)*, and contain various essential elements that are internal and/or proximal to the gene itself. Type I promoters (e.g.,

From: *Methods in Molecular Biology, Vol. 174: Epstein-Barr Virus Protocols*
Edited by: J. B. Wilson and G. H. W. May © Humana Press Inc., Totowa, NJ

those of 5S rRNA genes) have the classical polymerase III promoter structure. They contain internal A and C box consensus sequences associated with an intermediate (I) domain. All the elements of the type I promoter have a fixed spatial organization. The type II promoters, which include those of the tRNAs *(4)* and the adenovirus VA RNA genes *(5)*, are more varied in their spatial organization. Although they also have the classical A box consensus sequence, which is important in selection of the transcriptional start site, they lack a C box element. Instead this type of promoter contains a B box element, which has a major role in determining the level of gene activity and is usually located at a variable distance downstream of the A box. Both type I and II promoters have a 5' proximal TATA-box. The third class of promoters comprises those containing only proximal elements with an organization more recognizable to those familiar with polymerase II promoters. Examples are the promoters of the vertebrate U6 small-nuclear RNA genes *(6)*. The fourth arrangement of elements is a hybrid of the type II and III promoters, with both internal elements such as the A and B boxes and the proximal elements common to both RNA polymerases II and III. This class of polymerase III promoters is found in several viral genes, including those for the small RNAs of EBV. Jat and Arrand *(1)* showed that the truncation of the EBER-2 gene to a position adjacent to a B box consensus sequence led to a loss of synthesis of the RNA in their whole cell extract system, suggesting that such internal gene sequences are necessary for efficient transcription. However, surprisingly, truncation 3' to this sequence also gave a reduced level of activity from the gene, suggesting the region influencing transcription may extend 3' to the proposed intragenic element. Deletion of the A box element from the EBER-2 gene has been shown to result in a product of heterogeneous length, suggesting that the A box is important in positioning the transcriptional start site, whereas deletion of the B box led to a reduction in transcription to 3% *(7)*. Surprisingly, the positions of the A and B boxes of EBER-1 have not been experimentally determined and their identities are still defined by homology to the consensus sequences. The proposed elements of both genes show some divergence from the classical consensus sequences but this is common amongst polymerase III-transcribed viral genes.

Howe and Shu *(7)* described the proximal sequences of EBER-1 and -2 as including Sp1, ATF, and TATA-like elements. By making sequential deletions and mutations proximal to the gene, they showed that these elements make a significant contribution to the activity of the promoter in both transfected BJAB and HeLa cells and in nuclear extracts in vitro. Howe and Shu *(8)* later showed that the TATA-like sequence of EBER-2 is important for the exclusive transcription of EBER-2 by RNA polymerase III.

Calcium phosphate transfection of 293 cells, as a means of obtaining high level expression of genes such as the EBERs, is a useful technique, given the absence of EBV genes in this cell line. 293 cells are a human embryonic kidney line transformed by the introduction of sheared adenovirus DNA *(9)*. They are highly transfectable by the calcium phosphate method and under optimal conditions, greater than 90% of the cells will show high levels of expression of a transfected reporter gene such as β-galactosidase, using an *in situ* assay.

Calcium phosphate precipitation, as described by Graham and van der Eb *(10)*, essentially utilizes the formation of a calcium phosphate-DNA co-precipitate upon the mixing of $CaCl_2$ and a phosphate-containing buffer (HEPES Buffered Saline) at a neutral pH. The uptake of the DNA is an active process requiring endocytosis and differs from that occurring after electroporation or liposome-mediated transfection in this respect. The processing and transportation of DNA taken up by the phagosome results in the vast proportion of DNA being rapidly degraded or simply lost from the nucleoplasm with time and only transient expression of genes introduced by this means is therefore observed. Various modifications of the basic protocol have been introduced, directed at improving the transfection efficiency in cell lines that yield poor results with the standard technique. Such modifications usually entail the treatment of cells post-transfection with various reagents such as glycerol *(11)*, dimethyl sulfoxide (DMSO) *(12)*, tubulin *(13)*, or lysosomal inhibitors *(14)*. Because these modifications are unnecessary for 293 cells and efficient alternatives such as liposome-mediated transfection *(15)* and electroporation *(16)* have subsequently become available for other cell types, only the basic protocol is described in **Subheadings 2.1.** and **3.1.**

### 1.2. Small-Scale RNA Isolation from Transfected Cells

Small scale isolation of RNA is often required in transfection experiments and necessitates a rapid and simple extraction protocol designed to minimize handling errors and the losses of material these incur. Although there are many differing protocols that have been used for the recovery of cellular RNA *(17)*, very few are appropriate to the small-scale isolation required in these types of analyses.

One of the major difficulties in dealing with small numbers of cells and the consequent small volumes of cellular extract that result is the need to remove the nuclear DNA during the procedure. In many protocols the release of this material into solution inevitably leads to RNA losses, owing in part to the increase in viscosity of the lysate and the inability to remove the DNA from solution easily and consistently. The two methods described below avoid this problem in one of two ways. The first is by the exclusion of the nuclei, following gentle lysis with a nonionic detergent (NP40), and is a modification of the method described by Bodescot et al. *(18)*. The second is by a modification of a technique first described by Chomczynski and Sacchi *(19)*, which dissolves the DNA using a mixture of guanidinium thiocyanate and acid phenol. This is followed by selective precipitation of the DNA during the procedure. However, the protocol described differs from that of Chomczynski and Sacchi by the inclusion of both guanidinium thiocyanate and acid phenol in the lysis buffer in place of guanidinium thiocyanate alone. This necessitates the addition of chloroform separately at a later stage in order to partition the aqueous and phenolic phases, allowing the separation of the RNA from both the protein and genomic DNA.

The differences in the two approaches described later have the consequence that the first method (proteinase K/SDS) selectively recovers cytoplasmic RNA, whereas the second (phenol/guanidinium thiocyanate) recovers total cellular RNA. This difference should therefore be borne in mind, particularly if the species of interest predominates in one or other cellular fraction. Although the subcellular partitioning of the EBERs is still subject to some controversy *(20–22)*, both methods yield significant amounts of RNA, although a proportion of RNA is retained in the nuclear fraction using the former method and is therefore lost if the nuclei are discarded.

### 1.3. Northern Blotting of the EBV-Encoded Small RNAs

The small RNAs of EBV, EBER-1 and -2, the VA RNAs of adenovirus, and many small cellular RNAs such as the Y or U RNAs have complex and highly stable secondary structures. As a result they are difficult to resolve, even under denaturing conditions, by gel electrophoresis through agarose and often have a mobility differing from that expected for their size. However, it is sometimes necessary to carry out Northern blots whereby both these small RNAs and the larger mRNAs are to be probed for simultaneously. To this end, it is preferable to use a denaturing agarose system and capillary blotting similar to that originally described by Southern *(23)*. Such a technique necessitates the acceptance of a loss of resolution at the lower range of molecular weights in order to be able to resolve species larger than one kilobase. Where a high resolution is required below 0.5 kilobases or the sole species to be identified is a small RNA such as EBER-1 or -2, the system of choice is denaturing polyacrylamide gel electrophoresis followed by electroblotting.

Denaturing agarose gel electrophoresis can be carried out using various different denaturants such as formaldehyde, both formaldehyde and formamide *(24–26)*, glyoxal/DMSO *(27)*, or methyl-mercury hydroxide *(28)*. Although the latter is by far the best denaturant, it is highly toxic and presents numerous problems in handling. The other denaturants have little to choose between them. Northerns of glyoxal/DMSO gels tend to give sharper banding, but they present difficulties if unacceptable $H^+$ gradients are generated during electrophoresis. Therefore the most common and consistent approach to Northern blotting uses the combination of formaldehyde and formamide and is the method described. Although the gel conditions are in reality only semi-denaturing, this matters very little for the small RNAs such as EBER-1 and -2 owing to the poor resolving power of agarose.

As with agarose, polyacrylamide gel electrophoresis can also utilize a number of different denaturants including formamide, glyoxal/DMSO *(27)* and urea. By far the easiest and safest method is the use of urea as a denaturant and anyone familiar with DNA or RNA sequencing or RNA mapping will immediately recognize the gel system described.

Capillary blotting of denaturing agarose gels differs very little from that of Southern blotting *(23)*, with the exception of one or two important details. Fewer people will, however, be familiar with electroblotting of nucleic acids. In principle the technique does not differ from Western blotting of proteins, in that a charged molecule is transferred from the gel on to a membrane by creating a potential across two electrodes. A protocol for electroblotting agarose gels is described in Chapter 37. Electrotransfer of RNA from polyacrylamide gels can be carried out using either a semi-dry or wet blotting apparatus, although the method described uses the more traditional wet system and yields consistent and extremely good results.

### 1.4. The Use of Radiolabeled Probes in Northern Blotting for the EBV-Encoded Small RNAs

The detection of immobilized RNA by hybridization is a technique dating back to the late 1970s, using diazobenzyloxymethyl-cellulose paper *(29)* or nitrocellulose paper to immobilize the RNA following denaturation. Using such techniques, relatively low abundance RNA species can be detected with high efficiency with radioactive DNA or RNA probes. Many different types of membrane are now available for use in Northern blotting and although nitrocellulose is still commonly used, the greater durability and versatility of nylon membranes means they are generally more popular. However, nylon membranes are prone to give high background signals if care is not taken. Since the inception of hybridization as a means of detecting nucleic acids, a large number of variants on the standard protocol have arisen. When using DNA probes, the inclusion of formamide as a denaturant in the Northern hybridization is desirable because it favors the greater stability of DNA/RNA hybrids over DNA/DNA hybrids formed from self-hybridization of a double-stranded probe. This means that a reduction in the temperature is necessary with a concomitant decrease in the rate of hybridization, leading to longer hybridization times. A phosphate-buffered solution with a greater buffering capacity is also necessary instead of the standard citrate buffer generally used. The choice to include formamide when using RNA probes (riboprobes) falls more to one of personal preference than having any real advantage. Several different blocking agents are used in combination with fragmented DNA, including Denhardt's solution *(30)* and nonfat powdered milk *(31)*. Denhardt's solution tends to be used more commonly and gives a better signal-to-noise ratio, whereas nonfat milk powder also has the risk that it may contain RNases, which may present problems particularly when using riboprobes. Other compounds frequently included in hybridization protocols include dextran sulfate and polyethylene glycol (PEG). These increase the rate of association between the probe and target sequence, but are not further considered here as only very short hybridization times are necessary with probes to the small RNAs like the EBERs. There are few other factors specifically influencing Northern hybridization protocols with riboprobes to the small RNAs such as EBER-1 and -2. However, the high G/C content of these RNAs means that sense/antisense hybrids of these molecules are highly stable and allow higher stringency washes than would often be used.

### *1.5. Protein Synthesis Measurements In Vivo*

One of the characteristic features of the EBERs is their ability in vitro to associate with and inhibit the activity of the double-stranded RNA activated protein kinase (PKR), one of the principle regulators of protein synthesis initiation *(32–35)*. PKR regulates protein synthesis by phosphorylating the alpha subunit of the eukaryotic initiation factor eIF2 *(36)*. This prevents the recycling of this factor between successive rounds of initiation of protein synthesis *(37–39)*. Thus protein synthesis measurements in vivo can be indicative of PKR activity, although activation of this protein kinase is not of course the only means by which translation can be downregulated. Inhibition of protein synthesis has been demonstrated following the treatment of cells with known activators of PKR such as the calcium ionophores, A23187, ionomycin, or thapsigargin *(40–42)*, or with inducers of the glucose-regulated stress protein (GRP) chaperones, such as sodium arsenite *(42)*.

Treatment with A23187 results in the phosphorylation of eIF2α *(40–43)* and can be prevented by the expression of catalytically inactive dominant negative mutants of PKR or a nonphosphorylatable serine to alanine mutant of eIF2α. Protection against the effects of A23187 has been extended to other inhibitors of PKR such as the HIV TAR RNA binding protein *(40)* and RNAs such as the EBERs (our unpublished data). It is therefore in this context that we describe a simple but useful protocol for the in vivo measurement of protein synthesis with $^{35}$S-labeled methionine.

Many different circumstances arise in cell biology where it is advantageous to be able to measure the quantity of protein in an extract following treatment of cells. This is particularly so with treatments that may be expected to affect protein synthesis or cell growth, such as reduced serum concentrations or the prolonged treatment of cells with calcium ionophores. Although this would rarely be the only or even the principal measurement undertaken, it may be an important factor in understanding the effect of a treatment. With this in mind, a microtiter assay modified from that described by Bradford *(44)*, allowing the measurement of total cellular protein simultaneously in a large number of extracts, is described. The Bradford assay has a number of advantages over many of the previous assays used for proteins, not least of which is its speed and simplicity. The assay measures the intercalation of Coomassie Brilliant Blue G250 with protein and the resultant shift in its absorption spectrum from a $\lambda_{max}$ of 465 nm to 595 nm. An adaptation of this assay to a microtiter format is described later and allows the assay to be read in an automated plate reader. This adaptation allows the reading of 96 samples in a matter of seconds with the obvious benefit to those who have spent long hours changing cuvets and noting down readings from a conventional spectrophotometer. For those without access to an appropriate reader, the protocol can be scaled up to 1 mL and read in the conventional way.

## 2. Materials

### 2.1. Calcium Phosphate-Mediated Transfection of the EBER Genes

1. Supercoiled DNA in TE (10 m*M* Tris-HCl, pH 8.0, 1 m*M* ethylenediaminetetraacetic acid [EDTA]) at 1 mg/mL (*see* **Note 1**).
2. 2.5 *M* $CaCl_2$, filter-sterilized and stored at 4°C.
3. 2X HBS: 50 m*M* HEPES, pH 7.1 (HEPES: N-2-Hydroxyethylpiperazine-N-2-ethane-sulphonic acid), 280 m*M* NaCl, 1.5 m*M* $Na_2HPO_4$. Adjust pH using 1 *M* NaOH and filter-sterilize. Store at 4°C.
4. $H_2O$, filter-sterilized.
5. 5 mL or similar sterile polystyrene or glass tubes (*see* **Note 2**).
6. 293 cells (human embryonic kidney cell line).
7. Medium: Dulbecco's modified Eagle's medium (DMEM) with 10% (v/v) fetal calf serum (FCS).

### 2.2. RNA Isolation

#### 2.2.1. RNA Isolation: Proteinase K/Sodium Dodecyl Sulfate (SDS) Method

1. PBS/EDTA: 0.137 *M* NaCl, 2.7 m*M* KCl, 5.4 m*M* $Na_2HPO_4$, 1.8 m*M* $KH_2PO_4$, 5 m*M* EDTA. Adjust pH to 7.4 and filter through a 0.2-μm filter.

2. Lysis buffer: 140 m*M* NaCl, 10 m*M* Tris-HCl, pH 8.6, 0.5% (v/v) NP40, 1 m*M* dithiothreitol (DTT) (*see* **Note 3**).
3. 200 m*M* vanadyl ribonucleoside complex (VRC). VRC should be stored at –20°C in aliquots and freeze-thawing should be avoided.
4. Protease buffer: 200 m*M* Tris-HCl, pH 8.0, 25 m*M* EDTA, 0.3 *M* NaCl, 2% (w/v) SDS.
5. 20 mg/mL proteinase K in 100 m*M* Tris-HCl, pH 8.0, 100 m*M* NaCl, 50% (v/v) glycerol.
6. Phenol/chloroform/isoamyl alcohol (25:24:1), equilibrated in 10 m*M* Tris-HCl, pH 8.0, 1 m*M* EDTA.
7. Chloroform/isoamyl alcohol (24:1).
8. 20 mg/mL glycogen.
9. Isopropanol
10. 70% (v/v) ethanol.
11. Diethyl pyrocarbonate (DEPC)-treated $H_2O$ (*see* **Note 3**).

#### 2.2.2. RNA Isolation: Phenol/Guanidinium Thiocyanate Method

1. Acidic phenol/guanidinium thiocyanate: phenol (water saturated) (1 vol); 4 *M* guanidinium thiocyanate, 25 m*M* sodium citrate, 0.5% (w/v) sodium sarcosyl, 0.1 *M* 2-mercaptoethanol (1 vol); 2 *M* sodium acetate, pH 4.0 (0.1 vol) (*see* **Note 4**).
2. Chloroform.
3. Isopropanol.
4. 70% (v/v) ethanol.
5. DEPC-treated $H_2O$ (*see* **Note 3**).

### 2.3. Electrophoresis and Blotting

#### 2.3.1. Formaldehyde/Formamide Agarose Gel Electrophoresis and Capillary Blotting

1. Agarose (ultra-pure or molecular biology grade).
2. Formaldehyde (*see* **Note 5**).
3. De-ionized formamide (*see* **Note 6**).
4. 5X running buffer: 40 m*M* sodium acetate, 5 m*M* EDTA, 20.6 g/L MOPS (0.1 *M*), pH 7.4 (*see* **Note 7**).
5. 10X loading buffer: 50% (v/v) glycerol, 1 m*M* EDTA, pH 8.0, 0.25% (w/v) bromophenol blue, 0.25% (w/v) xylene cyanol.
6. 20X SSC: 3 *M* NaCl, 300 m*M* tri-sodium citrate.
7. Whatman 3MM paper.
8. Glass tray (e.g., Pyrex dish).
9. Parafilm or equivalent.
10. Tissue paper.
11. Plastic food wrap film.
12. Blotting membrane, e.g., Hybond-N™ (Amersham; *see* **Note 8**).

#### 2.3.2. Urea/Acrylamide Gel Electrophoresis and Electroblotting

1. 10X TBE: 0.89 *M* Tris, pH 8.0, 0.89 *M* boric acid, 20 m*M* EDTA.
2. 30% (w/v) acrylamide.
3. 2% (w/v) bis-acrylamide.
4. Urea.
5. Whatman no. 1 filter paper or equivalent.
6. 10% (w/v) ammonium persulphate.

7. N,N,N',N'-tetramethyl-ethylenediamine (TEMED).
8. Loading buffer: 98% (v/v) de-ionized formamide (*see* **Note 6**), 10 m*M* Tris-HCl, pH 8.0, 1 m*M* EDTA.
9. Whatman 3 MM paper.
10. Transfer buffer: 0.025 *M* phosphate, pH 6.5. Dissolve 11.86 g $Na_2HPO_4 \cdot 12H_2O$ and 12.67 g $NaH_2PO_4 \cdot H_2O$ in 5 L of sterile $H_2O$ (*see* **Note 9**).
11. Wet blotting apparatus.
12. Blotting membrane (*see* **Note 8**).

## 2.4. Probing of Northern Blots for the EBV-Encoded Small RNAs

1. 20X SSC: 3 *M* NaCl, 300 m*M* tri-sodium citrate or 20X SSPE: 3.6 *M* NaCl, 200 m*M* $NaH_2PO_4$, 20 m*M* EDTA.
2. 10% SDS.
3. 100X Denhardts solution: 2% (w/v) Ficoll™, 2% (w/v) BSA, 2% (w/v) polyvinylpyrrolidone.
4. Blocking DNA: salmon sperm/calf thymus DNA (10 mg/mL) sheared by passing through a 19 gauge hypodermic needle, denatured by heating to 95°C for 5 min.
5. Wash buffers: A: 2X SSC, 0.1% (w/v) SDS; B: 1X SSC, 0.1% (w/v) SDS; C: 0.1X SSC, 0.1% (w/v) SDS.
6. Radiolabeled probe (*see* **Subheading 3.1.2.** in Chapter 31).
7. Plastic wrap, e.g., Saran wrap.

## 2.5. Protein Synthesis Measurements In Vivo

### 2.5.1. Treatment of Cells with Calcium Ionophore A23187 and $^{35}S$ Methionine Labeling

1. $^{35}S$-methionine, 10 mCi/mL, 1000 Ci/mmol.
2. 0.5 m*M* A23187 dissolved in DMSO.
3. Cell culture medium.
4. PBS: 0.137 *M* NaCl, 2.7 m*M* KCl, 5.4 m*M* $Na_2HPO_4$, 1.8 m*M* $KH_2PO_4$. Adjust pH to 7.4 and filter through a 0.2-μ filter.
5. 0.3 *M* NaOH.
6. 10% (w/v) trichloroacetic acid (TCA) containing 0.5% (w/v) sodium pyrophosphate.
7. Methanol.
8. Acetone.
9. Scintillation vials.
10. Beckman Ready Organic™ or equivalent organic scintillation fluid.
11. Scintillation counter.

### 2.5.2. Microtiter Bradford Protein Assay

1. PBS/EDTA: 0.137 *M* NaCl, 2.7 m*M* KCl, 5.4 m*M* $Na_2HPO_4$, 1.8 m*M* $KH_2PO_4$, 5 m*M* EDTA. Adjust pH to 7.4 and filter through a 0.2-μm filter.
2. 0.1 *M* Tris-HCl, pH 7.8.
3. 0.15 *M* NaCl.
4. 1 mg/mL BSA in 0.15 *M* NaCl.
5. Bradford solution: 100 mg Coomassie Brilliant Blue G250, dissolved in 50 mL 95% (v/v) ethanol; add 100 mL 85% (w/v) phosphoric acid (phosphoric acid is normally supplied at this concentration), make up to 1 L with $H_2O$.
6. Microtiter plates, microtiter plate reader (capable of reading 595 nm).

## 3. Methods

### 3.1. Calcium Phosphate-Mediated Transfection of the EBER Genes

1. Cells should either be seeded the same day as the transfection is to be carried out at a density of 2.5–3 × $10^4$ cells per $cm^2$ or the previous evening at a slightly lower density of 2 × $10^4$ cells per $cm^2$ and allowed to attach for a minimum period of 6 h (*see* **Note 10**). If the cells are seeded in the morning then the transfection may be carried out in the late afternoon.
2. To a microcentrifuge tube add 20 µg of DNA (equivalent to 0.5 µg/$cm^2$, *see* **Note 11**), 40 µL of 2.5 *M* $CaCl_2$ (1 µL/$cm^2$) and $H_2O$ to a final volume of 400 µL.
3. Add 100 µL of the DNA mix to a 5 mL or similar sterile polystyrene or glass tube, add 100 µL of 2X HBS dropwise while gently vortexing and allow to stand at room temperature for 10–15 min (*see* **Note 12**). Repeat this process for each replicate treatment.
4. The precipitate may have a slightly milky appearance at this stage. Gently mix the suspension as the precipitate tends to settle. Add 200 µL of precipitated calcium phosphate-DNA suspension to each 10 $cm^2$ well or dish containing approx 5 mL of medium.
5. Allow the cells to take up the DNA for 8–16 h (may be conveniently done overnight).
6. Carefully change the media on the cells. Because 293 cells are easily detached extreme care is required not to remove cells that have become detached or loosened by the treatment.
7. Cells should be harvested 48–60 h post-transfection (*see* **Note 13**).

### 3.2. RNA Isolation

#### 3.2.1. RNA Isolation: Proteinase K/SDS Method

1. Cells that are not strongly adherent, such as 293 cells, can be dislodged and collected by pipetting ice-cold PBS/EDTA on to the cell monolayer (*see* **Note 14**). For a 10 $cm^2$ dish (containing up to 10 × $10^6$ cells), 0.8 mL should be used. Add this to the dish and allow to stand on ice for 3–5 min and then repeatedly pipet it on to the monolayer until the cells have detached. The cells are then removed to a microcentrifuge tube and the dish rinsed out with a further 0.2 mL of ice-cold PBS/EDTA.
2. Pellet the cells in a pre-chilled bench top centrifuge at 1000*g* at 4°C for 5 min.
3. On ice, remove as much of the supernatant as possible (care is necessary as the cell pellet is relatively loose and can be easily lost at this stage).
4. Loosen the cell pellet, by carefully flicking the tube (*see* **Note 15**).
5. Add 180 µL of lysis buffer and immediately add 20 µL of vanadyl ribonucleoside complex.
6. Allow lysis to take place on ice for 5 min.
7. Pellet the nuclei, organelles and cell debris in a bench top centrifuge at 12,000*g* for 5 min, at 4°C.
8. Remove and retain the supernatant, add 200 µL of protease buffer and proteinase K to 50 µg/mL. Incubate at 37°C for 30 min.
9. Extract once with phenol/chloroform/isoamyl alcohol and once with chloroform/isoamyl alcohol, retaining the aqueous phase each time.
10. Add 1 µL of 20 mg/mL glycogen as a carrier, 400 µL of isopropanol and incubate on ice for 30 min.
11. Pellet the precipitated RNA (*see* **Note 16**) at 15000*g* for 20 min at 4°C and wash the pellet with ice-cold 70% (v/v) ethanol. Allow the pellet to dry and resuspend in 5 µL of DEPC-treated water or 15 µL of formamide loading buffer if the entire sample is to be loaded on a urea polyacrylamide gel (*see* **Subheadings 2.3.1.** and **2.3.2.**).

### 3.2.2. RNA isolation: Acidic Phenol/Guanidinium Thiocyanate Method

1. Follow the method for harvesting cells above (**Subheading 3.2.1., steps 1–4**). Then add 100 µL of phenol/guanidinium thiocyanate mixture per $1–10 \times 10^5$ cells in a microcentrifuge tube (*see* **Note 17**).
2. Mix by inversion or if necessary to disrupt poorly dispersed cell pellets, by gentle pipetting (*see* **Note 18**). Allow samples to stand for 5 min at room temperature.
3. Add 20 µL of chloroform per 100 µL of phenol/guanidinium thiocyanate mixture. It is important that the chloroform used should not contain isoamyl alcohol. Mix vigorously by inversion until a uniform emulsion is obtained and allow to stand for 2 min at room temperature.
4. Centrifuge at 15,000*g* for 15 min at 4°C and remove the aqueous phase containing the RNA to a fresh tube, being careful not to contaminate this material with DNA and protein contained within the inter- and phenolic phases.
5. Add 50 µL of isopropanol per 100 µL of phenol/guanidinium thiocyanate mixture used and allow the samples to stand for 5 min at room temperature.
6. Pellet the precipitated RNA at 15000*g* for 20 min at 4°C and wash the pellet with ice cold 70% (v/v) ethanol. Allow the pellet to dry and resuspend in 5 µL of DEPC treated water or 15 µL of formamide loading buffer if the entire sample is to be loaded on a urea polyacrylamide gel (*see* **Subheadings 2.3.1.** and **2.3.2.**).

## 3.3. Electrophoresis and Blotting

### 3.3.1. Agarose Gel Electrophoresis and Capillary Blotting

1. To make 100 mL of a 1% (w/v) gel, add 1 g of agarose to 60 mL of water, melt it and allow it to cool to 60°C. In a fume hood add 20 mL of 5X running buffer while mixing (this can be achieved by gently swirling the gel mix, being careful not to introduce bubbles into the gel). Add 18 mL of formaldehyde (*see* **Note 5**), mixing as before, immediately check and adjust the volume if necessary and cast the gel. Leave the gel to set for 30 min in the fume hood.
2. Prepare the samples (containing up to 30 µg of RNA [*see* **Note 19**] in 4.5 µL of DEPC-treated water [*see* **Note 3**]) by adding 2 µL of 5X running buffer, 3.5 µL of formaldehyde and 10 µL of formamide.
3. Heat the samples at 65°C for 3–5 min and then snap cool on ice. Briefly centrifuge to collect the liquid in the bottom of the tube and add 2 µL of 10X loading buffer.
4. Pre-run the gel submerged in 1X running buffer for 5 min at 5 V/cm.
5. Load the gel (*see* **Note 20**).
6. Run the gel at 3 V/cm (*see* **Note 21**) until the bromophenol blue reaches two thirds of the way down the gel. RNAs such as the EBERs will run with or near the bromophenol blue running dye.
7. Remove the marker lane if it is to be stained (*see* **Note 22**). Rinse the gel in DEPC treated water in a clean oven-baked glass dish (previously baked at 200°C for 1 h) for 5 min to remove the formaldehyde.
8. Place a support (we normally use the inverted gel tray used to form and support the gel during electrophoresis) in a glass dish. Cut an appropriate-sized piece of 3MM paper to act as a wick and place it over the support such that the paper is the same width as the support and approx one and a half to two times its length, with equal lengths trailing over the ends. Place the transfer buffer (20X SSC) in the tray to a depth of 1–1.5 cm. Soak the wick with transfer buffer and remove any air bubbles by rolling with a sterile pipet.

9. Invert the gel on the support removing any air bubbles trapped below as before. Cut a corner of the gel to allow subsequent orientation of the membrane.
10. Wet the gel with transfer buffer. Place a piece of Hybond-N™ (Amersham) or equivalent membrane the same size as the gel on to its surface (*see* **Note 23**) cutting the corner corresponding to the cut corner of the gel. Roll the membrane to exclude air bubbles caught between the membrane and the gel.
11. Place a piece of parafilm around the gel where the wick is exposed (*see* **Note 24**).
12. Place several pieces of 3MM paper the same size as the gel on to the membrane. Pre-wet with 20X SSC buffer on top of the membrane, making sure again that there are no air bubbles between the layers.
13. Place a 5–10 cm stack of paper towels cut to the exact size of the gel on the 3MM paper and then place a weight on these such that the weight is evenly distributed over the gel (use a glass plate to spread the weight if necessary). A weight of approx 5 g/cm$^2$ is sufficient to compress the stack and allow the capillary action.
14. Cover the whole tray and stack with plastic film wrap to prevent evaporation of the buffer and leave overnight.
15. Transfer will be complete when the paper towels are wet to two thirds of the way to the top of the stack. The stack can then be dismantled, the membrane rinsed in 20X SSC buffer to remove adhering agarose and the RNA fixed to the membrane by the appropriate means. In the case of Hybond-N™ this may be done with UV light (*see* **Note 25**).

### *3.3.2. Urea/Polyacrylamide Gel Electrophoresis and Electroblotting*

1. Make gel mix (20:1 acrylamide to bis crosslinker): 2.5 mL of 10X TBE, 8.3 mL of 30% (w/v) acrylamide, 6.25 mL of 2% (w/v) bis-acrylamide, 10.5 g of urea, $H_2O$ to 25 mL and filter through Whatman no.1 filter paper or equivalent.
2. While slowly mixing add 125 µL of 10% (w/v) ammonium persulphate and 25 µL of TEMED and immediately pour the gel mix into pre-cleaned glass plates (*see* **Note 26**).
3. Allow to polymerize for 30 min (*see* **Note 27**).
4. Set up the vertical gel apparatus, containing 1X TBE running buffer in both the upper and lower reservoirs, load the wells of the gel with 7 *M* urea in 1X TBE and pre-run for 30 min at 30 V/cm.
5. Samples that are not already resuspended in loading buffer should be mixed with three volumes of loading buffer and heated for 3–5 min at 65°C (*see* **Note 28**). Samples that are not immediately loaded should be placed on ice to prevent renaturation until they are loaded on to the gel.
6. After the pre-run, carefully wash the wells out with 1X TBE and then load the gel (*see* **Note 29**). Run the gel at 30 V/cm until the xylene cyanol has reached within 1–2 cm of the bottom of the gel. In a 10% (w/v) polyacrylamide gel bromophenol blue runs at a position corresponding to 10–15 bases and xylene cyanol runs above at 50–60 bases.
7. Remove the gel from the apparatus and separate the plates. It is usually better to pull the spacers slightly away from the gel, remove one of the spacers completely and use a single-edged razor blade to separate the plates, by lifting the uppermost plate clear of the gel. Remove a corner of the gel in order to help determine the orientation. The gel is now ready for electroblotting.
8. Place a dry piece of Whatman 3MM paper on the gel and lift the gel from the separated electrophoresis plate (*see* **Note 30**).
9. First submerge the electroblot clamp in transfer buffer and then lay it open on a clean flat tray. Soak pieces of 3MM paper slightly larger than the gel in transfer buffer and lay one

on each of the open faces of the apparatus. Place the gel with the 3MM paper used to support it on to the wet paper on one side of the transfer apparatus with the gel uppermost. In order for the 3MM supporting the gel to wet evenly, pipet transfer buffer under the supporting 3MM. Once the paper is evenly wet, air bubbles must be removed by gently rolling a sterile pipet over the gel. Place the membrane (*see* **Note 23**), cut to the same size as the gel, carefully on the gel and wet with transfer buffer. Roll the membrane with a sterile pipet to exclude air bubbles before a last piece of soaked 3MM paper is placed on to the membrane. Close the clamp and place it into the transfer chamber containing transfer buffer with the membrane positioned between the gel and the positive electrode.

10. Transfer the RNA to the membrane at 0.5 A for 1–1.5 h (*see* **Note 31**). The chamber should be cooled if possible, especially if a blotting apparatus is used that contains a relatively small volume of buffer and/or longer transfer times are used. If the chamber does not incorporate a cooling coil, the transfer may be carried out in a cold room. The buffer should be slowly mixed by placing a magnetic flea in the chamber and positioning the apparatus on a magnetic stirrer.
11. After the transfer is complete, carefully disassemble the apparatus. If the membrane has any acrylamide adhering to it, rinse it briefly in transfer buffer, then blot the membrane dry and fix the RNA by an appropriate means (*see* **Note 25**).

## 3.4. Probing of Northern Blots for the EBV-Encoded Small RNAs

### 3.4.1. Pre-Hybridization

1. Both the prehybridization and hybridization can be conveniently and safely carried out in a glass bottle rotated in a hybridization oven (*see* **Note 32**). Mix 30 mL of prehybridization buffer (18 mL of $H_2O$, 9 mL of 20X SSC, 1.5 mL of 10% SDS, 1.5 mL of 100X Denhardt's solution) (*see* **Note 33**) and warm it to 68°C.
2. Insert the membrane, wrapped in a similar sized nylon mesh, into the hybridization bottle (*see* **Note 34**). Add 10 mL of the prehybridization buffer and 50 µL of blocking DNA.
3. Seal the bottle and rotate it in the hybridization oven at 68°C for 3–5 h (*see* **Note 35**).

### 3.4.2. Hybridization

1. Carry out the hybridization of the probe to the target RNA as for the prehybridization, by substituting 10 mL of fresh prehybridization buffer (*see* **Note 36**) containing 50 µL of 10 mg/mL heat-denatured, sheared DNA and the labeled probe. Hybridization can be conveniently carried out overnight (*see* **Note 37**).

### 3.4.3. Washing

1. Mix the wash solutions and warm to 70°C.
2. Remove the blot from the hybridization bottle to a plastic or glass tray (*see* **Note 38**) and rinse with 50 mL of wash buffer A.
3. Add 200–300 mL of wash buffer A and gently shake the blot in a shaking water bath for 15 min at 70°C (*see* **Note 39**).
4. Change the wash buffer to buffer B and gently shake as above for 10 min at 70°C.
5. Change the wash buffer to buffer C and again gently shake for 10 min at 70°C. Check the membrane for a high background signal and if necessary repeat the last high stringency wash.
6. Remove the excess liquid, wrap the damp membrane (*see* **Note 40**) in Saran Wrap or equivalent plastic film wrap and place in a light-tight cassette with X-ray film or a phosphorscreen to carry out autoradiography or phosphorimaging respectively.

### 3.5. Protein Synthesis Measurements In Vivo

#### 3.5.1. Treatment of Cells with Calcium Ionophore A23187 and $^{35}$S-Methionine Labelling

1. Pre-treat cells in mid to late exponential growth for 15 min by replacing the medium with fresh medium containing 0–0.5 µ*M* A23187 (*see* **Note 41**). Although the protocol describes the treatment and labeling of monolayers such as NIH 3T3 cells, it can be simply adapted for suspension cultures by substituting a centrifugation step where a medium change is required and carrying out the labeling in a tissue culture tube instead of a plate.
2. Add 10 µCi of $^{35}$S-labeled methionine to a 2 cm$^2$ well containing 1 mL of medium, giving a final concentration of 10 µCi/mL (*see* **Note 42**).
3. Incubate in the presence of A23187 for a further 30 min to 1 h (*see* **Note 43**).
4. Remove the medium and wash the cells with PBS.
5. Carefully remove all the PBS from the wells and add 100 µL of 0.3 *M* NaOH to each well (*see* **Note 44**).
6. Incubate at room temperature for 1 h.
7. Remove the lysate to a labeled microcentrifuge tube (*see* **Note 45**) and centrifuge at 10,000*g* for 10 min at 4°C, after which 25 µL of the supernatant should be spotted on to a marked piece of 3MM paper (*see* **Note 46**).
8. Allow the paper to dry, then soak in chilled 10% (w/v) trichloroacetic acid containing 0.5% (w/v) sodium pyrophosphate for 30 min.
9. Wash the 3MM paper by gently shaking in a cold methanol bath for 5 min, then wash in 1:1 methanol/acetone followed by acetone alone, gently shaking as before for 5 min in each bath.
10. Place the pieces of 3MM paper in scintillation vials, add an appropriate organic scintillation fluid such as Beckman Ready Organic™ and count the radioactive emissions in a beta counter.

#### 3.5.2. Microtiter Bradford Protein Assay

1. Cells such as 293s (*see* **Note 47**) that are not strongly adherent can be harvested in ice-cold PBS/EDTA. For a 2-cm$^2$ well (containing up to $1 \times 10^6$ cells) add 0.8 mL, allow to stand on ice for 3–5 min and then repeatedly pipet on to the monolayer until the cells have detached. Remove the suspension to a microcentrifuge tube and then rinse the dish out with a further 0.2 mL of ice-cold PBS/EDTA.
2. Pellet the cells in a pre-chilled bench top centrifuge at 1000*g* for 5 min at 4°C.
3. On ice, remove as much of the supernatant as possible (care is necessary as the cell pellet is loosely packed and can be easily lost at this stage).
4. Disperse the pellet by vortexing the tube.
5. Add 200 µL of 0.1 *M* Tris-HCl, pH 7.8, rapidly freeze-thaw three times by placing the tubes in dry ice until frozen, then in a 37°C water bath until fully thawed, and vortex between each cycle.
6. Take 5–10 µL of cell lysate and make up to 50 µL with 0.15 *M* NaCl.
7. Make a series of dilutions of bovine serum albumin (BSA) standards containing 0–10 µL of 1 mg/mL BSA in a final volume of 50 µL 0.15 *M* NaCl. Add 20 µL of each to a microtiter plate in duplicate.
8. Add 20 µL of the cell lysate in duplicate to the microtiter plate.
9. Add 180 µL of Bradford solution to the wells of the plate. Place in a plate reader and measure optical density (OD) at 595 nm. Construct and read off standard curve for protein concentration (*see* **Note 48**).

## 4. Notes

1. The topology of DNA is not of importance for the transfection *per se* and DNA is usually linearized for stable transfections, as this increases the frequency with which extra-chromosomal DNA is integrated. However, promoters are more active when supercoiled DNA is used and therefore transient transfections should be carried out using DNA that contains little or no relaxed DNA forms. The purity and topology of the donor DNA is therefore important when transiently transfecting eukaryotic cells. Most laboratory manuals covering the introduction of plasmid-borne genes into cells will suggest a variety of methods for purifying high-quality DNA. These include the more common Triton lysis/CsCl double-banding method described by Gorman ***(45)*** or a combination of the alkaline lysis method described by Birnboim ***(46)*** with CsCl double-banding or acidic phenol extraction such as that described by Zasloff et al. ***(47)***. For further reading, *see* Aubin et al. ***(48)*** and Sambrook et al. ***(17)***. In practice CsCl double-banding is not always necessary and the proportion of supercoiled DNA from a single gradient is often, although not always, sufficient. Although many of the molecular biological suppliers now provide convenient columns on which supercoiled plasmid DNA can be isolated, few such columns yield DNA of adequate purity for this purpose. If a column method is used, it is necessary to remove bacterial endotoxins during the preparation of the DNA as these are often carried over in the preparation and are extremely toxic to most cells. The carryover of such toxins can also be a problem with CsCl-purified DNA, especially where single banding is used.
2. Polystyrene or glass tubes should be used for the formation of the calcium phosphate precipitates.
3. DEPC treatment of buffers can be carried out by the addition of DEPC to 0.1% (v/v). However Tris-HCl buffers and heat labile compounds cannot be treated with DEPC and solutions should be made with treated water. DEPC-treated solutions should be allowed to stand at room temperature for 12 h and autoclaved to destroy any traces of DEPC. Although it is often appropriate to use DEPC-treated solutions, in practice only a few stock solutions need to be treated in this way, provided that common sense and care are taken to prevent solutions becoming contaminated with RNases when handling RNA. This means that all equipment must be kept clean and dust-free.
4. Several manufacturers supply RNA extraction kits based on the phenol/guanidinium thiocyanate method originally described by Chomczynski and Sacchi ***(19)*** as well as variants on several other methods; these are often little more than the reagents packaged in an attractive format at an inflated price. However, in deference to some manufacturers who simply supply the reagents, we use Tri-reagent™ (Sigma), although other suppliers do provide similar products in convenient quantities. This saves unnecessary handling of toxic reagents such as guanidinium thiocyanate and phenol when making up solutions. The stock solution of guanidinium thiocyanate (4 *M* guanidinium thiocyanate, 25 m*M* sodium citrate, pH 7.0, 0.5% (w/v) sodium sarcosyl, 0.1 *M* 2-mercaptoethanol) is stable at 4°C for 1 mo or more, although the solution may need to be heated to dissolve components prior to the addition of the 2-mercaptoethanol. Water-saturated phenol can be made by the addition of double-distilled or de-ionized water to solid phenol until saturated, or it can be purchased directly. Acidic phenol/guanidinium thiocyanate/sodium acetate should be made shortly prior to use by mixing the stock guanidinium thiocyanate solution, 2 *M* sodium acetate, pH 4.0, and water-saturated phenol in a ratio of 1:0.1:1 by volume respectively.

5. Formaldehyde has a molecular mass of 30.03 and is usually available as a 37% (w/v) solution in water (12.3 *M*). Caution should be used when handling formaldehyde as vapors are toxic and solutions should be prepared in a fume cupboard. Gel tanks containing formaldehyde should remain covered wherever possible and the electrophoresis should be run in a ventilated area.
6. Formamide should be de-ionized by the addition of 10% (w/v) Amberlite (AG-50f-x8) or Dowex (XG8) mixed bed resin and stirred for 30 min. The formamide can be separated from the resin by filtration. It should be aliquoted and stored at –20°C.
7. 950 mL 5X running buffer containing 40 mmoles sodium acetate and 5 mmoles EDTA can be made up without the addition of MOPS, autoclaved, then 20.6 g MOPS added and the pH adjusted to 7.4 with NaOH. This avoids the discoloration or decomposition of the buffer that occurs during autoclaving. Solutions containing MOPS should be stored at room temperature in the dark. Long-term storage will similarly result in slight discoloration and if the solution becomes discernibly yellow it should not be used.
8. A wide choice of appropriate membranes is available for Northern blotting. We routinely use a nylon membrane such as Hybond-N™ (Amersham).
9. Many wet-blotting apparatuses require the use of large volumes of transfer buffer as with the example described. We therefore recommend the addition of solid $Na_2HPO_4$ and $NaH_2PO_4$ to sterile water, as this saves on making large volumes of buffer in advance. In our experience the quality of the water used in most laboratories is adequate for the purpose and it is unnecessary to go to the extent of DEPC treatment of the transfer buffer or water used to make the buffer. We therefore recommend that sterile water or pre-made buffer is used. However, DEPC treatment of buffers can be carried out by the addition of DEPC to 0.1% (v/v). Tris-containing buffers are not compatible with DEPC, nor are heat-labile compounds, because it is necessary subsequently to autoclave a solution following the addition of DEPC. Such solutions should be made with treated water. The treated solution should be vigorously mixed, allowed to stand at room temperature for longer than 12 h and autoclaved to destroy any traces of DEPC.
10. Care should be taken to distribute the cells evenly over the surface of the dish as unevenly distributed cells may lead to differences in the local confluency of cells and potentially introduce an additional source of variation in the transfection efficiency and behavior of the cells.
11. The concentration of DNA suggested is an approximate guide to the optimal amount that should be expected to give maximal expression of a transfected gene. However, it is advisable with any transfection method and cells used that a series of experiments should be carried out using a reporter gene to establish the optimal conditions for transfection. In our experience the optimal amounts of DNA/$cm^2$ of cells at the stated density, required for maximal expression, tend to give a wide plateau over which no additional effect is seen on the level of expression of the transfected gene.
12. The exact length of time used has little noticeable effect on the transfection per se and various protocols suggest that different lengths of time should be allowed for the formation of calcium phosphate precipitates. However it is preferable to standardize the procedure to give as near identical conditions as possible during the formation of the precipitate and the transfection itself. The more appropriate type of replication in any experiment is that including the formation of precipitates, since a larger variation in the expression of transfected genes is attributable to use of different co-precipitates than to well-to-well variation using the same precipitate.
13. The expression of EBER-1 from the EBV transcription unit described earlier in a transient transfection into 293 cells reaches a maximum at about 48 h post-transfection and

declines thereafter, but is still clearly detectable by Northern blotting up to 60 h post-transfection. The EBV promoter described in the Introduction can be used also to express the EBERs in a wide range of heterologous cells including human EBV-negative Burkitt lymphoma lines such as DG-75 and mouse fibroblasts such as NIH 3T3.

14. Cells should be harvested by means appropriate to the individual cell line. Monolayers that are not strongly adherent (like the readily transfectable 293 cells) can be harvested as described earlier. However, most monolayer cells are more strongly adherent and can usually only be harvested by means of a cell scraper. This is often laborious in experiments with multiple treatments or large numbers of replicates and an alternative may be to release the cells from the dish by the use of trypsin/EDTA. However, following this procedure the trypsin should be neutralized by the addition of serum-containing media during the harvesting and the cells should be washed with ice-cold PBS/EDTA to remove the residual trypsin and serum components. Suspension cells are the simplest to harvest in that they only require pelleting followed by washing with PBS/EDTA. The force and time used is dependent on the individual cell lines but would normally be 800–1000*g* for 5–10 min, preferably but not necessarily in a chilled centrifuge. The protocol should then be followed as described earlier.
15. Inadequate dispersion of the cell pellet results in incomplete lysis and ultimately a proportionate reduction in yield.
16. Expected yields for total RNA from mammalian cells are in the range of 3–50 μg/$10^6$ cells. However, both methods are roughly equivalent with slightly lower yields obtained with the Proteinase K/SDS method.
17. Alternatively cells that are strongly adherent can be lysed *in situ* after washing with PBS. *In situ* lysis necessarily requires the use of 1 mL phenol/guanidinium thiocyanate mixture per 10 $cm^2$ of cells and proportionate increases in the volumes used in the subsequent steps.
18. The addition of the reagent to even a well-dispersed pellet at this stage can result in the formation of an insoluble aggregate. Where this is clearly a result of the compacted cell pellet not having been adequately dispersed (*see* **Note 10**) and gives rise to a large single aggregate, the latter may be broken up by gentle pipetting without substantial loss of yield and is more an inconvenience than a real problem. However, excessive pipetting will result in shearing of high molecular weight DNA and can lead to contamination of the RNA with fragmented DNA.
19. Abundant mRNAs constitute around 0.1% of the mRNA population and can normally be detected from 10–20 μg of total cellular RNA using this method. The relative abundance of the EBERs even in transfected cells (dependent on the transfection efficiency and cell type; *see* **Subheading 1.1.**) also allows their detection under these conditions.
20. If markers are to be run simultaneously, it is a good idea to leave an empty lane, especially if the markers are to be cut off before transfer. Alternatively, if transcripts of known RNAs such as the EBERs are to be probed for as a standard, it is also useful to leave an empty lane between these and the samples as overloading can easily lead to leaching from one lane into the adjacent one during transfer.
21. The voltage can be increased to 5 V/cm without adverse effects, although heating and the more rapid exhaustion of the buffer may occur at higher voltages. If prolonged runs or higher voltages are used, it will be necessary to mix the buffer after 1–2 h to prevent a pH gradient forming. This can be done by simply pipetting buffer between the two reservoirs.
22. Staining of gels that are to be transferred should be avoided as this can reduce the efficiency of subsequent hybridization. Greater care in handling agarose gels containing form-

aldehyde is necessary not only because formaldehyde is hazardous in itself but also because it makes the gel more brittle.

23. Membranes such as Hybond-N™ are hydrophilic in nature and do not require pre-wetting; however, other materials such as nitrocellulose are not and do require pre-soaking. Reference should therefore be made to individual suppliers' instructions with regard to pretreatment of membranes.
24. One of the common errors made particularly by inexperienced workers is either to cut the stack of paper towels or the 3MM paper placed on the gel too large or to place excessive weight on the stack so that, as the stack wets, it comes into contact with the wick. This short-cuts the capillary flow through the gel giving poor or uneven transfer and can be avoided by taking care in cutting the stack to the correct size, using an appropriate weight and placing Saran wrap or parafilm around the gel as a barrier to such contact.
25. UV cross-linking as a means of fixing RNA transferred to a membrane is only applicable to the nylon type membranes such as Hybond-N™ and it is therefore recommended that the supplier guidelines are followed in fixing any membranes used. However, it is our experience that membranes such as Hybond-N™ can be easily fixed by exposure to 0.3 J/cm$^2$ on the side of the membrane exposed to the gel. In practice, we tend to fix the membrane on both sides without loss of signal.
26. The gel system we routinely use has glass plates of approx 12 × 15 cm, 0.75 or 1 mm spacers and a comb with 0.5–1 cm wide wells. Because very narrow wells tend to give more uneven bands owing to the difficulty in removing residual urea left in the wells prior to loading the gel, particular care needs to be taken if these are to be used. The glass electrophoresis plates are cleaned with detergent, rinsed in distilled water, and then again cleaned alternately with methanol and distilled water to ensure they are sufficiently clean. One of the two plates can be siliconized with dimethyldichlorosilane solution to aid the separation of the plates on completion of the electrophoresis. This can be carried out by evenly wetting the surface of the clean plate with dimethyldichlorosilane, using towelling wetted with the siliconizing fluid, allowing the plate to dry in a fume cupboard and finally cleaning it with distilled water to remove any acid residue.
27. Gels can be prepared the previous day, if they are wrapped in plastic food wrap to prevent drying out and shrinkage. However, it takes little time to prepare gels such as those described and it is therefore preferable to prepare them immediately prior to use.
28. Exposure to excessive temperature, repeated or prolonged heating in the presence of high concentrations of formamide should be avoided as this can lead to hydrolysis of RNA.
29. If residual urea is allowed to remain in the well prior to loading the gel, the sample may not load evenly, and the resulting bands may appear uneven or form a trailing tail, giving less than satisfactory results.
30. It is essential that the 3MM paper is placed on the gel correctly the first time as it can only be removed by wetting the gel and repeating the process with a fresh piece of 3MM once the gel has had any excess liquid removed from the surface. If the gel fails to lift off with the 3MM, this is usually owing to excess liquid lying on the surface of the gel but may also be indicative of plates that have been poorly cleaned or are badly scratched.
31. Because transfer is complete in a relatively short time there is little need to have alternative transfer times or conditions; however, it is also possible to carry out effective transfers overnight using 0.25 A.
32. Prehybridization and hybridization are usually carried out in a sealed hybridization bottle rotated within a purpose-made oven. Where this type of equipment is available its use is

recommended as it reduces personal exposure to radioactive probes. However, this procedure can also be carried out in sealed plastic bags or containers.

33. With the addition of SDS to salt solutions or vice versa, the SDS can sometimes precipitate; this is easily remedied by adding the SDS lastly to the diluted salt solution and ensuring the prehybridization solution is at working temperature prior to addition to the blot.
34. The nylon mesh prevents uneven exposure of overlapping areas of membrane to either the pre-hybridization or hybridization solution, reducing the occurrence of uneven or high background signal. The membrane should be laid on a piece of mesh of equivalent size and tightly rolled up in such a way that the membrane is contained within the roll. It can then be inserted into the bottle and allowed to unroll.
35. Prehybridization should be carried out for a minimum of 1–2 h; however, it is often timely and convenient to set up the prehybridization in the morning, change the buffers 3–5 h later and add the probe for hybridization overnight.
36. Blocking agents such as Denhardts solution are sometimes left out of the hybridization solution, especially when nylon membranes are used, as they can interfere with the annealing of probe to the target sequence. However, this is not recommended as it can lead to a higher background signal. With the relative stability of RNA/RNA hybrids and the abundance of the small RNAs like EBER-1, quenching of the hybridization signal is not normally a problem.
37. The hybridization temperature used is determined by factors affecting the melting temperature ($T_m$) of the hybrid, such as composition (DNA:RNA or RNA:RNA), G/C content, salt concentration and the presence or absence of formamide. Although denaturants such as formamide are sometimes included in the hybridization in order to utilize lower temperatures ***(17)*** and maximize the formation of a DNA:RNA duplex when DNA is being used as the probe, they result in a decrease in the rate of hybridization ***(49)***. The hybridization should be carried out for approx one to three times the $C_o t_{1/2}$, that is one to three times the time required for 50% renaturation of the probe. This value is determined by the complexity of the probe (usually approximated to its length in kilobases), the mass of the probe added and the volume of the hybridization reaction. For 50 ng of a probe of the complexity of EBER-1, in a 10 mL hybridization volume as suggested, the required duration of hybridization is approx 4 h. In practice, however, hybridization can be conveniently carried out overnight.
38. Washing of blots can be carried out in the hybridization bottle if preferred; however, cleaner backgrounds are often obtained by removing the blot from the bottle, separating the nylon mesh and carrying out the washes in a larger volume of wash buffer using a shaking water bath.
39. In order to obtain low background and therefore a high signal-to-noise ratio, it is necessary to take care in maintaining the temperature of the wash solutions. This is especially important to remember while changing the washes, because removing the lid from water baths or opening the door of a hybridization oven in order to change the washes can cause a significant drop in the temperature of the bath or oven. It is therefore useful to monitor the temperature of the wash buffer within the tray itself during the washes if a water bath is used. Doing so allows for a greater degree of control over the wash conditions than if a hybridization bottle and oven are used. If the temperature falls more than 1°C below the wash temperature, the duration of the wash should be extended until the temperature has been regained. The wash temperature used is determined mainly by factors affecting the melting temperature ($T_m$) of the hybrid, such as the G/C content and the nature of the hybrid itself (DNA:RNA or RNA:RNA) (*see* **Note 37**). The temperature used should be around 10°C below the $T_m$ of the duplex.

40. If the blot is to be stripped and reprobed then it is essential that the blot is not allowed to dry.
41. The measurement of protein synthesis in cells such as NIH 3T3s upon exposure to increasing concentrations of calcium ionophores such as A23187 reveals a sigmoidal dose-response curve. The protective effect of the expression of dominant negative mutants of PKR or other inhibitors such as the EBERs results in a shift in the dose curve, thus requiring higher concentrations of A23187 to inhibit protein synthesis to a similar extent. However, the range of concentrations over which a response can be seen is cell type-dependent and although it is normally between 0–0.5 μ*M* for NIH 3T3 cells, it should be determined empirically. A23187 has low solubility in aqueous solutions and it is necessary to dissolve the stock solution in DMSO. It is therefore essential that all treatments contain similar concentrations of DMSO irrespective of the concentration of the ionophore, since DMSO itself can affect methionine incorporation. Pre-treatment need only last 15 min as the effect on protein synthesis is very rapid.
42. It is not necessary to use methionine-free medium as sufficient incorporation can be obtained under these conditions to measure the relative inhibition of protein synthesis. It is also necessary to maintain exposure to the ionophore for the duration of the labeling.
43. Methionine incorporation can be carried out for a shorter duration (e.g., 15 min); however, in such a case it may be necessary to use methionine-free medium in order to maximize the amount of incorporation.
44. NaOH conveniently lyses the cells and also prevents the inclusion of labeled Met-tRNA from the measurement by hydrolysing the charged tRNA.
45. If the cell number is high upon lysis the lysate may become viscous and difficult to pipet leading to significant pipetting errors. This can be remedied by increasing the NaOH volume proportionately to the cell number.
46. When carrying out labeling such as described earlier without special equipment, it is advantageous to spot the cell lysate on a grided piece of 3MM paper such that the layout and positioning of the treatments resemble that in the tissue culture plates used. The grid can be drawn with a soft leaded pencil and accordingly marked. Each piece of 3MM corresponding to a single plate can then be washed and the individual treatments or replicates can be more easily and rapidly identified than if individual pieces or filter circles are used.
47. Cells should be harvested by means appropriate to the individual cell line (*see* **Note 14**).
48. Since the amount of BSA added to the microtiter plate will be 0, 1, 2, 3, . . . 10 μg, the unit of concentration from the standard curve is therefore micrograms of BSA/50 μL and as the volume of the sample added to the microtiter plate is known, the concentration read off the scale is therefore equivalent to μg of BSA/ volume of lysate added; in the earlier instance 5–10 μL.

## Acknowledgments

Research in our laboratory that has led to the development of the methods described here was funded by grants from the Cancer Research Campaign, the Leukaemia Research Fund, the Wellcome Trust, and the Sylvia Reed Fund. V. Matys was supported by a Scholarship from the State of Baden-Wurttemberg, Germany.

## References

1. Jat, P. and Arrand, J. R. (1982) *In vitro* transcription of two Epstein-Barr virus specified small RNA molecules. *Nucleic Acids Res.* **10,** 3407–3425.
2. Willis, I. M. (1993) RNA polymerase III: Genes, factors and transcriptional specificity. *Eur. J. Biochem.* **212,** 1–11.

3. Kunkel, G. R. (1991) RNA polymerase III transcription of genes that lack internal control regions. *Biochem. Biophys. Acta* **1088,** 1–9.
4. Sprinzl, M., Dank N., Nock, S., and Schon, A. (1991) Compilation of tRNA sequences and tRNA genes. *Nucleic Acids Res.* **19(Suppl.),** 2127–2171.
5. Fowlkes, D. M. and Shenk, T. (1980) Transcriptional control regions of the adenovirus VAI RNA gene. *Cell* **22,** 405–413.
6. Gupta, S. and Reddy, R. (1991) Compilation of small RNA sequences. *Nucleic Acids Res.* **19(Suppl.),** 2073–2075.
7. Howe, J. G. and Shu, M. D. (1989) Epstein-Barr virus small RNA (EBER) genes: unique transcription units that combine RNA polymerase II and III promoter elements. *Cell* **57,** 825–834.
8. Howe, J. G. and Shu, M. D. (1993) Upstream basal promoter element important for exclusive RNA polymerase III transcription of EBER 2 gene. *Mol. Cell. Biol.* **13,** 2655–2665.
9. Graham, F. L., Smiley, J., Russell, W. C., and Nairn, R. (1977) Characteristics of a human cell line transformed by DNA from human adenovirus type 5. *J. Gen. Virol.* **36,** 59–74
10. Graham, F. L. and van der Eb, A. (1973) A new technique for the assay of infectivity of human adenovirus 5. *Virology* **52,** 456–467.
11. Parker, B. A. and Strak, G. R. (1979) Regulation of simian virus 40 transcription: Sensitive analysis of the RNA species present early in infections by virus or viral DNA. *J. Virol.* **31,** 360–369.
12. Lewis, W. H., Strinivasan, P. R., Stokoe, N., and Siminovitch, L. (1980) Parameters governing the transfer of the genes for thymidine kinase and dihydrofolate reductase into mouse cells using metaphase chromosomes or DNA. *Somatic Cell Genet.* **6,** 333–348.
13. Faber, F. E. and Eberle, R. (1976) Effect of cytochalasin and alkaloid drugs on the biological expression of herpes simplex virus. *Exp. Cell Res.* **103,** 15–22.
14. Luthman, H. and Magnusson, G. (1983) High efficiency polyoma DNA transfection of chloroquine treated cells. *Nucleic Acids Res.* **11,** 1295–1307.
15. Felgner, P. L. (1991) Cationic liposome-mediated transfection with lipofectin™, in *Methods in Molecular Biology, vol. 7: Gene Transfer and Expression Protocols* (Murry E. J., ed.), Humana Press, Clifton, NJ, pp. 81–90.
16. Spencer, S. C. (1991) Electroporation technique of DNA transfection, in *Methods in Molecular Biology, vol. 7: Gene Transfer and Expression Protocols* (Murry E. J., ed.), Humana Press, Clifton, NJ, pp. 45–52.
17. Sambrook, J., Fritsch, E. F., and Maniatis, T. (1989) *Molecular Cloning: A Laboratory Manual,* 2nd ed., vol. 2. Cold Spring Harbor Laboratory Press, Cold Spring Harbor, NY.
18. Bodescot, M., Chamberaud, B., Farrel, P., and Perricaudet, M. (1984). Spliced RNA from the IR1-U2 region of Epstein-Barr virus: presence of an open reading frame for a repetitive polypeptide. *EMBO J.* **3,** 1913–1917.
19. Chomczynski, P. and Sacchi, N. (1987) Single-step method of RNA isolation by acid guanidinium thiocyanate-phenol-chloroform extraction. *Anal. Biochem.* **162,** 156–159.
20. Howe, J. G. and Steitz, J. A. (1986) Localization of Epstein-Barr virus small RNAs by *in situ* hybridization. *Proc. Natl. Acad. Sci. USA* **83,** 9006–9010.
21. Wu, T.-C., Mann, R. B., Epstein, J. I., MacMahon, E., Lee, W. A., Charache, P., et al. (1991) Abundant expression of EBER1 small nuclear RNA in nasopharyngeal carcinoma. A morphologically distinctive target for detection of Epstein-Barr virus in formalin-fixed paraffin-embedded carcinoma species. *Am. J. Pathol.* **138,** 1461–1469.
22. Schwemmle, M., Clemens, M. J., Hilse, K., Pfeifer, K., Troster, H., Muller, W. E. G., and Bachmann, M. (1992) Localization of Epstein-Barr virus-encoded RNAs EBER1 and

EBER2 in interphase and mitotic Burkitt lymphoma cells. *Proc. Natl. Acad. Sci. USA* **89,** 10,292–10,296.

23. Southern, E. M. (1975) Detection of specific sequences among DNA fragments separated by gel electrophoresis. *J. Mol. Biol.* **98,** 503–517.
24. Lehrach, H., Diamond, D., Wozney, J. M., and Boedtker, H. (1977) RNA molecular weight determinations by gel electrophoresis under denaturing conditions, a critical re-examination. *Biochemistry* **16,** 4743–4751.
25. Goldberg, D. A. (1980) Isolation and partial characterisation of the *Drosophila* alcohol dehydrogenase gene. *Proc. Natl. Acad. Sci. USA* **77,** 5794–5798.
26. Seed, B. (1982) Attachment of nucleic acids to nitro-cellulose and diazonium substituted supports, in *Genetic Engineering: Principles and Methods,* vol. 4 (Setlow, J. K. and Hollaender, A., eds.), Plenum Publishing, New York, NY, p. 91.
27. McMaster, G. K. and Carmichael, G.G (1977) Analysis of double and single stranded nucleic acids on polyacrylamide and agarose gels by using glyoxal and acridine orange. *Proc. Natl. Acad. Sci. USA* **74,** 4835–4838.
28. Thomas, P. S. (1980) Hybridisation of denatured RNA and small DNA fragments transferred to nitro-cellulose. *Proc. Natl. Acad. Sci. USA* **77,** 5201–5205.
29. Alwine, J. C., Kemp, D. J., and Stark, G. R. (1977) Method for detection of specific RNAs in agarose gels by transfer to diazobenzyloxymethyl-paper and hybridisation with DNA probes. *Proc. Natl. Acad. Sci. USA* **74,** 5350–5354.
30. Denhardt, D. T. (1966) A membrane-filter technique for the detection of complementary DNA. *Biochem. Biophys. Res. Commun.* **23,** 641–646.
31. Johnson, D. A., Gautsch, J. W., Sportsman, J. R., and Elder, J. H. (1984) Improved technique utilising non-fat dry milk for analysis of proteins and nucleic acids transferred to nitro-cellulose. *Gene Anal. Tech.* **1,** 3.
32. Clarke, P. A., Schwemmle, M., Shickinger, J., Hilse, K., and Clemens, M. J. (1991) Binding of Epstein-Barr virus small RNA EBER-1 to the double-stranded RNA activated protein kinase DAI. *Nucleic Acids Res.*19, 243–248.
33. Sharpe, T. V. , Schwemmle, M., Jeffrey, I., Laing, K., Mellor, H., Proud, C., et al. (1993) Comparative analysis of the regulation of the interferon inducible protein kinase PKR by Epstein-Barr virus RNAs EBER1 and EBER2 and adenovirus $VA_I$ RNA. *Nucleic Acids Res.* **21,** 4483–4490.
34. Clemens, M. J. (1993) The small RNAs of Epstein-Barr virus. *Mol. Biol. Rep.* **17,** 81–92.
35. Clemens, M. J., Laing, K. G., Jeffrey, I. W., Schofield, A., Sharp, T. V., Elia, A., et al. (1994) Regulation of the interferon-inducible eIF-2α protein kinase by small RNAs. *Biochimie* **76,** 770–778.
36. Clemens, M. J. and Elia, A. (1997) The double-stranded RNA-dependent protein kinase PKR-structure and function. *J. Interferon Cytokine Res.* **17,** 503–524.
37. Pain, V. (1986) Initiation of protein synthesis in mammalian cells. *Biochem. J.* **235,** 625–637.
38. Pain, V. (1997) Initiation of protein synthesis in eukaryotic cells. *Eur. J. Biochem.* **236,** 747–771.
39. Clemens, M. J. (1994) Regulation of eukaryotic protein synthesis by protein kinases that phosphorylate initiation factor eIF-2. *Mol. Biol. Rep.* **19,** 201–210.
40. Srivastava, S. P., Davis, M., and Kaufman, R. (1996) Calcium depletion from the endoplasmic reticulum activates the double stranded RNA dependent protein kinase (PKR) to inhibit protein synthesis. *J. Biol. Chem.* **270,** 16,619–16,624.
41. Prostko, C. R., Dholakia, J. N., Brostrom, M. A., and Brostrom, C. O. (1996) Activation of the double stranded RNA-regulated protein kinase by depletion of endoplasmic reticular calcium stores. *J. Biol. Chem.* **270,** 6211–6215.

42. Brostrom, C. O., Prostko, C. R., Kaufman, R. J., and Brostrom, M. A. (1996) Inhibition of translational initiation by activators of the glucose-regulated stress protein and heat shock protein stress response systems. *J. Biol. Chem.* **271,** 24,995–25,002.
43. Alcazar, A., Bazan, E., Rivera, J., and Salinas, M. (1995) Phosphorylation of initiation factor 2 α subunit and apoptosis in $Ca^{2+}$ ionophore-treated cultured neuronal cells. *Neurosci. Lett.* **201,** 215–218.
44. Bradford, M. (1976) A rapid and sensitive method for the quantitation of microgram quantities of protein utilizing the principle of protein-dye binding. *Anal. Biochem.* 72, 248–254.
45. Gorman, C. (1985) High efficiency gene transfer into mammalian cells, in *DNA Cloning*: vol. II (Glover D. M., ed.), IRL, Oxford, pp.143–190.
46. Birnboim, H. C. (1983) A rapid alkaline extraction method for the isolation of plasmid DNA. *Methods Enzymol.* **100,** 243–255.
47. Zasloff, M., Ginder, G. D., and Felsenfeld, G. (1978) A new method for the purification and identification of covalently closed circular DNA molecules. *Nucleic Acids Res.* **5,** 1139–1152.
48. Aubin, R., Weinfeld, M., and Paterson, M. C. (1991) Preparation of recombinant plasmid DNA for DNA-mediated gene transfer, in *Methods in Molecular Biology, vol. 7: Gene Transfer and Expression Protocols* (Murry E. J., ed.), Humana Press, Clifton, NJ, pp. 3–14.
49. Casey, J. and Davidson, N. (1977) Rates of formation and thermal stabilities of RNA:DNA and DNA:DNA duplexes at high concentrations of formamide. *Nucleic Acids Res.* **4,** 1539–1552.

# 6

# Visualizing EBV Expression Patterns by FISH

**Anna Szeles**

## 1. Introduction

Fluorescence *in situ* hybridization (FISH) is the method of choice for visualization of viral nucleotide sequences in the infected cells. FISH methodology has been previously used for localization of Epstein-Barr virus (EBV) DNA sequences within interphase nuclei or on chromosomes *(1–4)*. The FISH technique has also been applied to visualization of specific viral RNAs within the nuclei of cells latently infected with EBV *(5,6)*. *In situ* two-color detection of EBV-specific nuclear RNA allows the study of different viral expression programs at the cellular level *(7)*.

In FISH, nucleotides of the probe DNA are replaced with modified (labeled) nucleotides. The probes are labeled either with haptens, such as biotin or digoxigenin, and detected subsequently by immunofluorescence, or are labeled directly with fluorochromes. After hybridization of the labeled probes with target DNA or RNA their intracellular location can be determined from fluorescence microscopy images. FISH is a technique that, in contrast to the other methods, allows the visualization of specific RNA sequences at the single cell level in a heterogeneous cell population.

The basic FISH technique involves preparation of cytological material, incorporation of labeled nucleotides into the DNA probes by standard labeling techniques, denaturation of the target chromosomes or nuclei and probe DNA (when the target cells or tissues are not denatured, only RNA will hybridize), followed by the hybridization of the single-stranded probe DNA to target DNA or RNA. Stable DNA-DNA or DNA-RNA hybrids are then viewed with epifluorescence optics.

The original protocols for FISH were developed by a number of research groups (for reviews, see refs. *8–10*). Optimization of technical variables has resulted in simplified but highly sensitive hybridization protocols. Various parameters are important to the overall process: (1) reagent quality is a critical factor, (2) fixation of the biological material for the retention of the target DNA or RNA, (3) labeling efficiency, (4) optimal probe length to allow penetration, and (5) hybridization conditions.

From: *Methods in Molecular Biology, Vol. 174: Epstein-Barr Virus Protocols*
Edited by: J. B. Wilson and G. H. W. May © Humana Press Inc., Totowa, NJ

The methodology presented below was originally developed by Lawrence et al. *(5)* for fluorescence detection of specific transcripts of integrated EBV within interphase nuclei using hapten-labeled DNA probes. It was later modified by Szeles et al. *(7)* for two-color FISH in order to visualize individual cells that use different EBV expression programs. Our approach utilizes fluorochrome labeling of EBV-specific DNA sequences so that antibody incubation is no longer required after the post-hybridization washes. This method is quick, simple, and yields no background signal.

In order to achieve simultaneous visualization for each FISH probe, different fluorochrome-conjugated nucleotides (e.g., FITC-dUTP, rhodamine-dUTP) are selected to identify the sites of hybridization. Each fluorochrome yields different colors (e.g., green or red), thereby permitting two-color FISH *(11–14)*. Fluorochrome-labeled probes can be hybridized together with biotin- or digoxigenin-labeled probes, increasing the number of simultaneously detected probes *(15)*.

In this chapter, a detailed description is given for: (1) cell preparation, (2) probe DNA labeling using nick translation, (3) probe preparation, (4) *in situ* hybridization, (5) posthybridization washing, (6) DNA counterstaining and embedding, and (7) digital-imaging microscopy.

**Figure 1 A–H** illustrates the DNA- and RNA-specific hybridization using EBV-specific DNA probes in EBV-transformed lymphoblastoid cell lines (LCLs) and EBV-carrying Burkitt lymphoma (BL) cells, visualized by this method.

---

Fig. 1. *(opposite page)* DNA and RNA FISH to EBV-carrying B-cell-derived cells using EBV-specific DNA probes. Interphase nuclei and metaphase chromosomes were analysed on standard cytogenetic preparations. **(A and E)** Hybridization to viral (EBV *Bam*HI W) DNA. RNase A treatment followed by DNA denaturation and hybridization with FITC-labeled *Bam*HI W DNA sequence detected the viral genomes (green) in interphase nuclei prepared from LCL IB4-D cell lines with integrated EBV DNA (A) and LCL970402 cell line with multiple episomal EBV DNA copies (E). The nuclei were counterstained with DAPI (blue). **(B)** Simultaneous hybridization of the *Bam*HI W probe and the chromosome 4 specific probe in denatured samples (the RNase treatment was omitted) indicate the two chromosome 4 domains (red) and the *Bam*HI W nuclear RNA track (green) in a DAPI stained nucleus of IB-4 cell. The chromosome 4 painting probe was labeled with (Cy3) and the EBV *Bam*HI W DNA with FITC. **(C)** Simultaneous hybridization to both viral (EBV *Bam*HI W) DNA and chromosome 4 in denatured and RNase A-treated samples from LCL IB4-D. Yellow signals on each sister chromatid on q25 of one chromosome 4 (red) indicate the localization of integrated EBV genomes. The chromosome 4 painting probe was labeled with (Cy3) and the EBV *Bam*HI W DNA with FITC. Chromosomes were counterstained with DAPI. **(D, and F–H)** Nuclear EBV specific RNA detection in LCLs and in type I BL cell. Two viral programs designated as type I and type III are used alternatively in EBV-carrying B cell lines and tumor biopsies. In type III, all six Epstein-Barr nuclear antigen (EBNA) messages are spliced from a polycistronic message. In type I, only EBNA1 is expressed from a monocistronic message *(7)*. A FITC-labeled EBV *Bam*HI K DNA probe that can hybridise to both the monocistronic and the polycistronic message and a rhodamine labeled *Bam*HI W DNA probe that can hybridize with the polycistronic but not with the monocistronic message were used to distinguish between cells that use a type III and type I program in two-color FISH. The nuclei were counterstained with DAPI. **(D)** Simultaneous detection of EBV *Bam*HI K (green) and *Bam*HI W (red) RNA tracks on a nondenatured prepa-

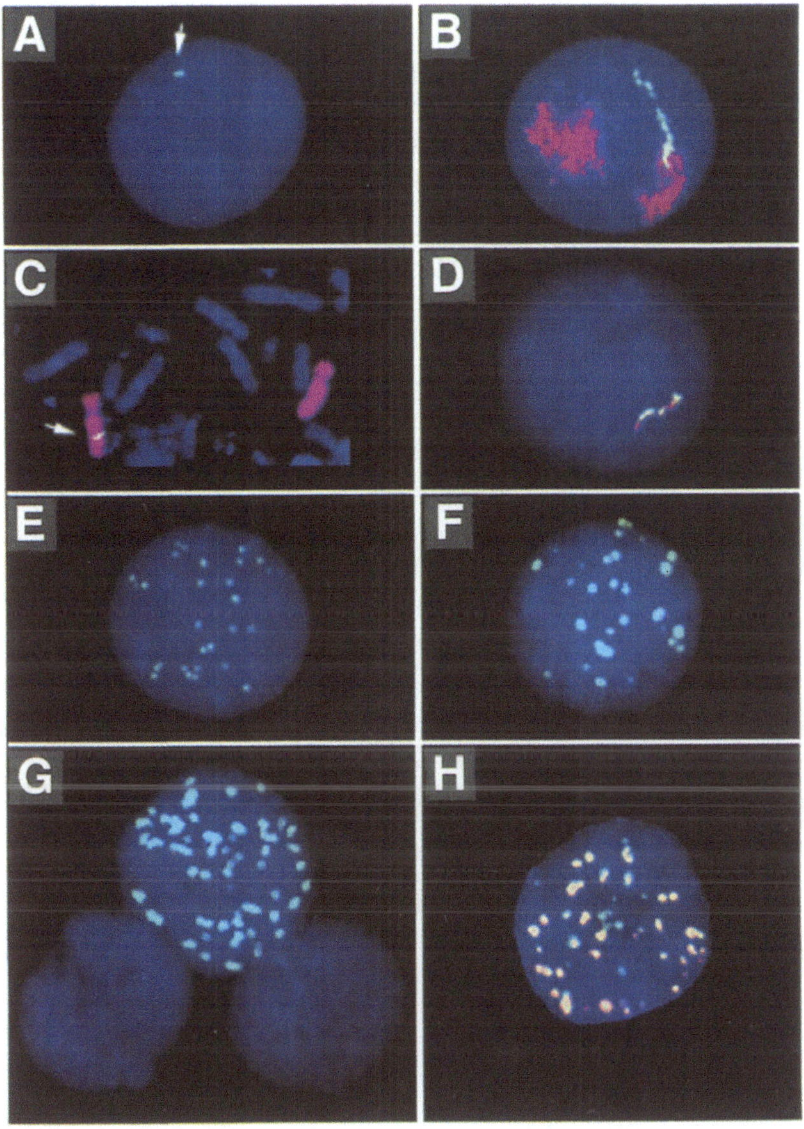


ration from the LCL line IB4-D. Both probes hybridized to the same nuclear foci. **(F)** Detection of *Bam*HI K (green) but not *Bam*HI W RNA in type I BL line Rael in two color experiments. **(G** and **H)** Two-color FISH shows heterogeneous EBV RNA expression in LCL IARC-171 cells that carry numerous episomal genomes. The *Bam*HI W probe was labeled with rhodamine and the *Bam*HI K with FITC. FISH shows many double-colored (green and red) RNA foci or tracks on one nucleus (H). Only green (BamHI K RNA) but not red (BamHI W RNA) signal was detected on the other nucleus (G) suggesting that a proportion of the cells may shift from a type III to a type I program. Two nuclei failed to hybridize with either one of the two probes (G) suggesting that the latency 0 program may exist.

## 2. Materials

### 2.1. Cytogenetic Preparations of Metaphase and Interphase Cells from EBV-Carrying B-Cell-Derived Human Cell Lines

1. Cell culture medium: RPMI 1640 containing 10% heat-inactivated fetal calf serum (FCS) and 200 µg/mL of Penicillin/Streptomycin.
2. Colcemid, stock 10 µg/mL (Gibco BRL, cat # 15210-040). Store at 4°C.
3. Centrifuge tubes, approx 15 mL.
4. Bench centrifuge for speeds up to 300*g*.
5. Hypotonic solution (0.075 *M* KCl).
6. Fixative: 3 parts of 100% methanol to 1 part of glacial acetic acid). Prepare fresh; do not store for more than 1–2 h before use.
7. Pasteur pipets.
8. Microscope slides.
9. Microscope with phase contrast condenser, and phase contrast 63× objective.
10. Diamond-tipped pencil.
11. 70, 90, and 100% ethanol.

### 2.2. Labeling DNA Sequence Probes by Nick Translation

1. Probes: Different fragments of the EBV genome (*Bam*HI W and *Bam*HI K DNA probes, *see* also **Note 1**) *(7)*.
2. dNTPs (Boehringer-Mannheim). Prepare an unlabeled stock nucleotide mixture of 0.5 m*M* dATP, dCTP, dGTP, 0.1 m*M* dTTP. Store at –20°C.
3. 10X Nick translation buffer: 0.5 *M* Tris-HCl, pH 7.8, 50 m*M* $MgCl_2$, 0.5 mg/mL BSA (nuclease-free). Store at –20°C.
4. Dithiothreitol (DTT): 100 m*M*.
5. Fluorescein-12-dUTP (Boehringer-Mannheim, cat. #1 373 242).
6. Tetramethyl-rhodamine-6-dUTP (Boehringer-Mannheim, cat. #1 534 378).
7. Enzymes: DNA polymerase I and DNase I (Boehringer-Mannheim, Mannheim, Germany).
8. 3 *M* sodium acetate (filter-sterilized and stored at room temperature).
9. 100% ethanol at –20°C.
10. 70% ethanol at –20°C.
11. TE: 10 m*M* Tris-HCl, pH 7.5, 1 m*M* EDTA.

### 2.3. RNA In Situ Hybridization

#### 2.3.1. Probe Preparation

1. Salmon sperm DNA (ssDNA) sheared or DNase digested to a size of approx 500 bp (Sigma, St. Louis, MO): 1 mg/mL in TE. Freeze in 20 µL aliquots.
2. *Escherichia coli* tRNA (Sigma or Calbiochem): 1 mg/mL in TE.
3. 3 *M* Sodium acetate.
4. Ethanol.
5. Deionized formamide (BDH AnalR). Store at 4°C for use within 3 mo and at –20°C for longer-term storage. Formamide is a potential carcinogen, therefore, wear gloves and handle in a fume hood.
6. 50% (w/v) solution of dextran sulfate in water, autoclaved. Store in 1 mL aliquots at –20°C.
7. 20X SSC: 3 *M* NaCl, 300 m*M* Na citrate adjusted with HCl to pH 7.0.
8. Programmable temperature-controlled heating block or water bath.

### *2.3.2. Hybridization*

1. Cytogenetic preparation.
2. Plastic coverslips: approximately 22 × 22 $mm^2$, cut from autoclavable waste disposal bags or Parafilm.
3. Moist chamber (*see* **Note 2**).
4. Incubator, set at 37°C.

### *2.3.3. Post-hybridization Washing*

1. Coplin jars.
2. Forceps.
3. Washing solution A: 50% formamide/2X SSC, pH 7.0. Heated to 42°C. Prepare freshly.
4. Washing solution B: 2X SSC (1 part 20X SSC, 9 parts distilled $H_2O$, pH 7.0). Heated to 42°C. Prepare fresh.
5. Washing solution C: 4X SSC (1 part 20X SSC, 4 parts distilled $H_2O$, pH 7.0).
6. Water bath at 42°C. (Preferably with variable temperature and shaking option for post-hybridization washes at 35–50°C).

### *2.3.4. DNA Counterstaining and Embedding*

1. DAPI (4,6-Diamidino-2-phenylindole, Sigma). Store stock solution of 10 µg/mL at –20°C.
2. Vectashield embedding medium (Vector Labs, Burlingame, CA).

### *2.3.5. Microscopy*

Modern epifluorescence microscope, appropriate filter sets, cooled-CCD (charge coupled device) camera, computer-assisted image analysis system.

## 3. Methods

### *3.1. Cytogenetic Preparations of Metaphase and Interphase Cells from EBV-Carrying B-Cell-Derived Human Cell Lines*

The technique outlined here is similar to that used in most cytogenetic laboratories.

1. Dilute cell cultures to 2 × $10^5$ cells/mL into fresh medium 2 d before harvest to obtain actively growing cultures.
2. Treat 10 mL of culture with colcemid (final concentration 0.02 µg/mL) for 1 h at 37°C to accumulate metaphases.
3. Transfer cells into a 15-mL glass or polypropylene centrifuge tube.
4. Centrifuge in a bench centrifuge at 300*g* for 10 min.
5. Pour the supernatant off carefully.
6. Re-suspend the cell pellet with the last drop of supernatant by shaking. Do not use a pipet.
7. Add about 10 mL of hypotonic solution, which has been pre-warmed to 37°C and pipet the cells gently in and out of a Pasteur pipet.
8. Incubate at 37°C for 20 min (*see* **Note 3**).
9. Centrifuge 300*g* for 10 min.
10. Pour off the supernatant, leaving about 0.5 mL of fluid above the cell pellet.
11. Re-suspend the cell pellet in this fluid by pipetting the cells gently in and out of a Pasteur pipet until a fine cell suspension with no large clumps of cells remains.
12. Draw the re-suspended cells into the Pasteur pipet and expel the suspension slowly into a fresh 15 mL centrifuge tube containing 10 mL of freshly prepared ice cold fixative (*see* **Note 4**).

13. Leave at room temperature for 30 min.
14. Centrifuge for 10 min at 300*g*.
15. Carefully discard the supernatant and gradually add 10 mL of fixative.
16. Repeat **steps 14** and **15** twice (*see* **Note 5**).
17. Centrifuge at 300*g* for 10 min after the last fixation.
18. Re-suspend the cells in a small volume of fixative, e.g., 0.5 mL.
19. Drop one drop of cell suspension out of a Pasteur pipet onto a cleaned, pre-chilled (stand on ice for 15 min) microscope slide from a height of a few centimeters (*see* **Note 6**).
20. Dry by blowing or shaking.
21. Check cell density, and quality of spreads under the microscope before making any further preparation using phase contrast optics (*see* **Note 7**).
22. Select top-quality preparations. Locate the best area on slide using a diamond tipped pencil.
23. Dehydrate slides in 70, 90, and 100% ethanol, 5 min each time.
24. Air-dry slides at room temperature.
25. Store slides at –20°C in an airtight slides box containing desiccant, and seal with tape (*see* **Note 8**).

### 3.2. Labeling DNA Sequence Probes by Nick Translation

1. Pipet the following components into a dark microcentrifuge tube on ice: X µL (1 µg) probe, 4 µL of dNTPs mix, 5 µL of 10X nick translation buffer, 5 µL of DTT (100 m*M*), 2 µL of 1 m*M* Fluorescein-12-dUTP, 2 µL of DNA polymerase I, 5 µL of DNase I. Immediately before use dilute 1 µL of stock DNase I (1 mg/mL) in 1 mL of ice cold distilled water, mix thoroughly, and add 5 µL to the reaction mixture. Sterile-distilled water to 50 µL. For labeling with rhodamine, replace the fluorescein-12-dUTP with 2 µL of tetramethyl-rhodamine-6-dUTP (*see* **Note 9**).
2. Close the lid of the tube, mix well by tapping the tube sharply with a finger several times and centrifuge briefly (16,000*g* for 5 s).
3. Incubate the mixture at 15°C for 2 h in a water bath or use a cooled PCR machine.
4. Keep the mixture at 4°C until verified by gel.
5. Run a 10 µL aliquot of labeled probe on a 1% agarose minigel together with molecular weight standards, to check fragment sizes. If the probe size is correct, go to **step 6** (*see* **Note 10**).
6. Precipitate the labeled DNA as follows: Add to the tube 5 µL (0.1 vol) of 3 *M* Sodium acetate, pH 5.6 and 150 µL (3 vol) of cold (–20°C) 100% ethanol. Vortex for 30 s. Place the tube in a –80°C freezer for 15 min. Centrifuge tube for 15 min at 16,000*g* and 4°C. Discard the supernatant and then wash the pellet by carefully adding 0.5 mL of ice cold 70% ethanol. Spin the tube for 5 min at 16,000*g*. Discard the supernatant and dry the pellet under vacuum or air dry.
7. Dissolve the pellet in 20 µL water or TE and store probe solution at –20°C.

### 3.3. RNA *In Situ* Hybridization

#### 3.3.1. Probe Preparation

1. Prepare DNA mix: Pool 50 ng of each labeled probe in a microcentrifuge tube. Precipitate labeled probes with 10 µg each of sonicated ssDNA and *E. coli* tRNA, 0.1 vol of 3 *M* sodium acetate and 3 vol of cold (–20°C) 100% ethanol. Leave at –80°C for 15 min to precipitate, centrifuge and wash once in 70% ethanol. Dry under vacuum.
2. Prepare hybridization mix for 10 µL: mix 5 µL of 100% formamide (deionized), 2 µL of 50% dextran sulfate, 2 µL of sterile double-distilled $H_2O$, and 1 µL of 20X SSC.
3. Re-suspend the pellet in 10 µL of hybridization mix (for 22 × 22 $mm^2$ Parafilm).

4. Denature the DNA mix at 80°C for 10 min.
5. Centrifuge briefly to collect vapors.
6. Place on ice until use.

### 3.3.2. Hybridization

1. Apply 10 µL of denatured probe mix to the slide. (The target cells are not denatured) (*see* **Notes 11** and **12**).
2. Lay a small piece (approx 22 × 22 mm$^2$) of Parafilm over the hybridization solution. Gently tap out air bubbles. They can be easily removed by lifting the Parafilm carefully.
3. Cover the sample with a large sheet of Parafilm and seal it completely around the edges.
4. Incubate slide in a moist chamber at 37°C overnight (*see* **Note 2**).

### 3.3.3. Post-hybridization Washing

Remove unhybridized probe by washing. Make sure slides do not dry out between washing steps and pour solution gently.

1. Remove Parafilm with forceps.
2. Wash slide in a Coplin jar with washing solution A for 3 min at 42°C.
3. Pour off solution and replace with fresh solution A. Leave for further 3 min at 42°C.
4. Repeat **step 3**.
5. Pour off solution and replace with solution B and incubate slides three times for 2 min at 42°C.
6. Place slides in solution C at room temperature for 5 min.

### 3.3.4. DNA Counterstaining and Embedding

1. Mount the slide with 10 µL of Vectashield antifade solution containing 75 ng/µL DAPI (*see* **Note 13** for procedure variation).
2. Cover with a 22 × 40 mm$^2$ glass coverslip.
3. Apply gentle downward pressure to flatten coverslip before examining slide.
4. Store preparations at 4°C in dark.

### 3.3.5. Microscopy

Visualize fluorescent probes with a fluorescent microscope with the appropriate filters. The following optical filters will visualize the fluorochromes used in the hybridization: a filter set specific for DAPI (pale-blue emission under UV, FITC (green emission under blue excitation), and rhodamine (red emission under green excitation) to view the counterstain and the hybridization signals, respectively. Double- or triple-band pass filter sets combine into one cube an excitation filter, a barrier filter, and a dichroic mirror. This permits the simultaneous detection of multiple fluorochromes. The best results are obtained using a digital imaging system. We use a gray scale cooled-CCD camera (Hamamatsu 4800). Color-specific images are collected (i.e., one image for DAPI, one image for FITC, and one image for rhodamine); these images are then pseudocolored and merged. *See* **Note 14** for a discussion on types of controls for FISH experiments.

## 4. Notes

1. EBV-specific probes can be derived from cloned *Bam*HI-digested fragments (*Bam*HI W and *Bam*HI K) of the B95-8 strain of EBV DNA ***(16)***. The 3.1 kilobases (kb) *Bam*HI W

fragment and the 5.1 kb *Bam*HI K fragment should be purified from the gels before using for FISH.

2. Moist chamber: Any airtight dark box to hold glass slides horizontally with a sheet of Whatman filter paper moistened with water or 2X SSC. It is best if the lid is gently sloping to prevent condensing water to drop onto the incubating slides. The slides must be placed on glass rods or bottle tops to raise them above the moist surface. Cover the box and seal with Parafilm.
3. Hypotonic treatment swells the cells and nucleus. It is important to achieve optimal conditions of hypotonic swelling. Time and temperature are critical and vary for each cell type. Extended treatment and higher temperatures increase swelling of cells. Undertreated cells do not spread well; over-treated cells burst too early and chromosomes may be lost.
4. Fixation: As previously described *(5,6)* EBV-specific nuclear RNAs can also be detected on paraformaldehyde-fixed cells. We are using methanol/acetic acid fixation for analysis of interphase nuclei and metaphase chromosomes on standard cytogenetic preparations. This method allows coupling the detection of the EBV genomes (*see* **Fig. 1A**, **C**, and **E**) with visualization of EBV-specific nuclear RNAs (*see* **Fig. 1B**, **D**, **F**, **G**, and **H**). One of the most important functions of the fixation step is the removal of much of the cell debris and proteinaceous material from the cell suspension, to produce a much cleaner preparation of chromosomes and to improve the quality of the spread.
5. Cells can be stored in the refrigerator at this point for several days. Cells that have been stored in fixative must be washed in fresh fixative. For spreading, centrifuge the suspension (as in **step 17**) and re-suspend in 0.5–1 mL of fresh fixative (as in **step 18**).
6. Use quality slides. Microscope slides that are frosted on one side are convenient for marking with pencil. Wash slides in acid-alcohol (99% ethanol: 1% concentrated HCl) and air-dry. Remove any particles of dust or tissue before use.
7. Cell density: Check that the concentration of cells is suitable; if it is too high, dilute the cell suspension with a little more fixative; if there are too few cells, spin at 200*g* for 5 min and re-suspend in a smaller volume of fresh fixative. An ideal cell suspension gives a single layer of cells. There should be little or no contact between nuclei. If only bright field optics are available, stain the slides in a 2% solution of Giemsa (Gurrs R66), in 0.01 *M* phosphate buffer ($Na_2HPO_4$ : $KH_2PO_4$), pH 6.8 for 10 min at room temperature and examine using bright field optics and a 63× objective.
8. Proper slide storage is important to ensure strong FISH signal and low background. If slides are kept at room temperature, the chromosomes and nuclei may dry out after a few weeks, resulting in abnormal morphology.
9. Probe labeling can be performed using other fluorochromes (e.g., SpectrumGreen, SpectrumOrange, SpectrumRed, or Texas red direct-labeled dUTP). Fluorochromes are easily photobleached by exposure to light. Handle all solutions and slides containing fluorochromes in reduced light.
10. Estimate the size range of the probe from the gel. The majority of the DNA smear should be around the 300 bp range. Probe fragments that are larger than 700 bp may produce bright fluorescent speckles across the hybridization areas. To produce smaller probe fragments incubate the reaction tube further at 15°C or adjust the optimal DNase concentration in the nick translation reaction.
11. For hybridization to EBV DNA sequences, we treat the target cells with RNase A (100 μg/mL in 2X SSC) at 37°C for 1 h, denature for 2–3 min in 70% formamide, 2X SSC at 70°C, and dehydrate through cold 70, 95, and 100% EtOH for 5 min each and air-dry. These

steps were followed by hybridization with the *Bam*HI W sequences for the detection of the viral genome (**Fig. 1A**, **C**, and **E**).

12. For simultaneous detection of chromosome-specific nuclear domains containing EBV integration sites and *Bam*HI W RNA, we omit the RNase A treatment. Cells were denatured and hybridized with chromosome 4-specific and *Bam*HI-W probes (*see* **Fig. 1B**).
13. Antifade mounting medium: 0.233 g DABCO (1,4-diazabicyclo-(2.2.2) octane, Sigma) in 800 μL distilled water, 200 μL of 1 *M* Tris-HCl, pH 8.0, 9 mL of glycerol; vortex and store in dark at –20°C. Add DAPI (0.5 μg/mL) to antifade working solution and store at –20°C.
14. Controls: Positive and negative cell lines will provide evidence that the FISH reaction has the expected pattern of reactivity. Pre-treatment of samples with RNase or DNase will prove that the hybridization depends on the presence of RNA or DNA in the cells (**Fig. 1A**, **C**, and **E**). Other controls include integrated EBV-carrying cell lines, in which the viral integration sites on both sister chromatids are only visible when denatured prior to hybridization (**Fig. 1C**) and no signals are observed on metaphase chromosomes (which do not transcribe RNA) when the denaturation step is omitted. Finally, probes specific for EBV sequences that are not being expressed in cells may also be used as controls for RNA hybridization (**Fig. 1F**).

## References


1. Teo, C. G. and Griffin, B. E. (1987) Epstein Barr virus genomes in lymphoid cells: activation in mitosis and chromosomal location. *Proc Natl Acad Sci USA* **84,** 8473–8477.
2. Lawrence, J. B., Villnave, C. A., and Singer, R. H. (1988) Sensitive high-resolution chromatin and chromosome mapping *in situ:* presence and orientation of two closely integrated copies of EBV in a lymphoma line. *Cell* **52,** 51–61.
3. Gargano, S., Caporossi, D., Gualandi, G., and Calef, E. (1992) Different localization of Epstein-Barr Virus genome in two subclones of the Burkitt lymphoma cell line Namalwa. *Genes Chromosomes Cancer* **4,** 205–210.
4. Hurley, E. A., Klaman, L. D., Agger, S., Lawrence, J. B., and Thorley-Lawson, D. A. (1991) The prototypical Epstein-Barr virus-transformed lymphoblastoid cell line IB4 is an unusual variant containing integrated but not episomal viral DNA. *J. Virol.* **65,** 3958–3963.
5. Lawrence, J. B., Singer, R. H., and Marselle, L. M. (1989) Highly localized tracks of specific transcripts within interphase nuclei visualized by *in situ* hybridization. *Cell* **57,** 493–502.
6. Xing, Y. and Lawrence, J. B. (1991) Preservation of specific RNA distribution within the chromatin-depleted nuclear substructure demonstrated by in situ hybridization coupled with biochemical fractionation. *J. Cell Biol.* **112,** 1055–1063.
7. Szeles, A., Falk, K. I., Imreh, I., and Klein, G. (1999) Visualization of alternative EBV expression programs by FISH at the cell level. *J. Virol.* **73,** 5064–5069.
8. Lichter, P., Boyle, A. L., Cremer, T., and Ward, D. C. (1991) Analysis of genes and chromosomes by non-isotopic *in situ* hybridization. *Genet. Anal. Techn. Appl.* **8,** 24–35.
9. McNeil, J. A., Johnson, C. V., Carter, K. C., Singer, R. H., and Lawrence, J. B. (1991) Localizing DNA and RNA within nuclei and chromosomes by fluorescence *in situ* hybridization. *Genet. Anal. Techn. Appl.* **8,** 41–58.
10. Raap, A. K., Nederlof, P. M., Dirks, R. W., Wiegant, J. C. A. G., and Van der Ploeg, M. (1990) Use of haptenized nucleic acid probes in fluorescent *in situ* hybridization, in *In Situ Hybridization*: *Application to Developmental Biology and Medicine* (Harris, N. and Williams, D. G., eds.), Cambridge University Press, Cambridge, pp. 33–41.
11. Nederlof, P. M., Robinson, D., Abuknesha, R., Wiegant, J., Hopman, A. H., Tanke, H. J., and Raap, A. K. (1989) Three color fluorescence *in situ* hybridization for the simultaneous detection of multiple nucleic acid sequences. *Cytometry* **10,** 20–27.

12. Nederlof, P. M., Van der Flier, S., Wiegant, J., Raap, A. K., Tanke, H. J., Ploem, J. S., and Van der Ploeg, M. (1990) Multiple fuorescence in situ hybridization procedures. *Cytometry* **11,** 126–131.
13. Ried, T., Baldini, A., Rand, T. C., and Ward, D. C. (1992) Simultaneous visualization of seven different DNA probes by *in situ* hybridization using combinatorial fluorescence and digital imaging microscopy. *Proc Natl Acad Sci USA* **89,** 1388–1392.
14. Wiegant, J., Wiesmeijer, C. C., Hoovers, J. M., Schuuring, E., d'Azzo, A., Vrolijk, J., et al. (1993) Multiple and sensitive *in situ* hybridization with rhodamine-, fluorescein- and coumarin-labeled DNAs. *Cytogenet Cell Genet.* **63,** 73–76.
15. Wiegant, J., Ried, T., Nederlof, P. M., Van der Ploeg, M., Tanke, H. J., and Raap, A. K. (1991) *In situ* hybridization with fluoresceinated DNA. *Nucleic Acids Res.* **19,** 3237–3241.
16. Arrand, J. R., Rymo, L., Walsh, J. L., Bjorck, E., Lindhal, T., and Griffin, B. E. (1981) Molecular cloning of the complete Epstein-Barr virus genome as a set of overlapping restriction endonuclease fragments. *Nucleic Acids Res.* **9,** 2999–3014.

# II

# Viral Detection

# 7

# *In Situ* Detection of Epstein-Barr Virus DNA and Viral Gene Products

**Gerald Niedobitek and Hermann Herbst**

## 1. Introduction

Primary Epstein-Barr virus (EBV) infection is followed by a life-long persistence of the virus in the B-cell compartment of the host *(1,2)*. Small numbers of EBV-carrying B cells have been identified in the peripheral blood as well as in lymphoid and nonlymphoid tissues of chronic virus carriers *(3,4)*. This is relevant to the study of human tumors. The detection of EBV DNA in a tumor by polymerase chain reaction (PCR) usually does not permit conclusions as to whether this is due to the presence of the virus in the tumor cell population or to the presence of EBV-carrying "by-stander" B cells in the tissue. For a meaningful analysis of EBV infection, it is therefore necessary in many instances to establish the cellular location of the virus using morphology-based techniques.

The methods described in this chapter can be broadly divided into those that are appropriate for the detection of the virus and those that can be used to characterize the prevalent form of EBV infection. In general, the *in situ* hybridization techniques fall into the former category whereas immunohistochemistry is useful for distinguishing latent from replicative infection and for identifying the prevailing form of EBV latency (*see* **Table 1**).

### *1.1. In Situ Hybridization*

The first reproducibly successful attempts to localize the virus in tissue sections were carried out using *in situ* hybridization for the detection of EBV DNA *(5)*. Most workers used the cloned *Bam*HI W fragment of the EBV genome (*see* Chapter 1) as a probe for this purpose. Because this fragment is repeated up to 10–15 times in the viral genome, this approach promised greater sensitivity than the use of single-copy gene probes. These probes can be labeled with a variety of radioactive (e.g., $^{35}S$, $^{33}P$, $^{3}H$) and nonradioactive (e.g., biotin, digoxigenin, bromodeoxyuridine, fluorescein-isothiocyanate [FITC]) reporter molecules *(5)*. In our hands, $^{35}S$-labeled probes have

From: *Methods in Molecular Biology, Vol. 174: Epstein-Barr Virus Protocols*
Edited by: J. B. Wilson and G. H. W. May © Humana Press Inc., Totowa, NJ

proved to be consistently more sensitive than nonradioactive probes. For practical purposes, this means that if latent EBV infection is to be detected by DNA *in situ* hybridization, $^{35}S$-labeled probes should be employed. Nonradioactive DNA probes are sufficient for the detection of replicative EBV infection, e.g., in oral hairy leukoplakia. However, virus replication is more appropriately and more conveniently demonstrated by simpler immunohistological assays.

In recent years *in situ* hybridization for the detection of the small EBV-encoded RNAs (EBER-1 and -2) has become the standard method for the detection of the latent EBV infection *(6)*. The EBERs are small (ca. 170 bases) nonpolyadenylated nuclear RNAs of unknown function that are expressed in all known forms of EBV latency at very high copy numbers (up to $10^7$ copies per cell) *(7)*. Owing to their abundance and their relative stability compared to mRNA, they represent ideal targets for *in situ* hybridization studies. *In situ* hybridization for the detection of the EBERs is applicable to frozen sections as well as formalin-fixed, paraffin-embedded tissue sections and has even been used successfully on *post mortem* tissues. Several types of probes are available for the detection of the EBERs. Oligonucleotides labeled with nonradioactive tags are available from several commercial sources. These probes are adequate for most routine applications. Alternatively, RNA probes derived from transcription vectors can be employed, and this approach is described here *(8)*. These probes can be labeled with radioactive nucleotides or with nonradioactive compounds. In most circumstances, e.g., the analysis of tumors, use of nonradioactive probes yields satisfactory results. However, for the detection of rare latently infected B-cells in chronic virus carriers, we prefer radioactive probes because of their higher sensitivity. In most laboratories, EBER *in situ* hybridization has replaced DNA *in situ* hybridization as the standard method for detecting latent EBV infection. It has to be kept in mind, however, that the use of EBER *in situ* hybridization relies on the active expression of the viral genome. Although expression of the EBERs has been demonstrated in all known forms of EBV latency, an EBER-negative viral latency remains at least a theoretical possibility.

### 1.2. Immunohistochemistry

Based on the variable patterns of EBV protein expression, at least three different forms of latent infection have been defined *(9)*. In EBV-immortalized lymphoblastoid cell lines (LCL) and in post-transplant lymphoproliferative disorders (PTLD), viral gene expression is usually restricted to a set of so-called latent genes, including six nuclear antigens (EBNA-1, -2, -3A, -3B, -3C, -LP), three latent membrane proteins (LMP-1, -2A, -2B), and the EBERs (latency III) *(7)*. The expression of these viral latent gene products is limited to the EBERs and EBNA-1 in Burkitt's lymphoma (BL, latency I), and to the EBERs, EBNA-1, and the LMPs in Hodgkin's disease (HD) and nasopharyngeal carcinoma (NPC, latency II) *(7,10-13)*. Thus, the only viral protein that is consistently expressed in all known forms of EBV latency is EBNA-1. Although monoclonal antibodies (MAbs) for the detection of EBNA-1 in paraffin sections have been described, staining results are usually weak and EBNA-1 staining cannot substitute for EBER *in situ* hybridization *(12)*. Expression of the other latent proteins is

**Table 1**
**Characterization of EBV Latency**

| Form of latency | Example | EBERs | LMP-1 | EBNA-2 |
|---|---|---|---|---|
| Latency I | BL | + | – | – |
| Latency II | HD, NPC | + | + | – |
| Latency III | LCL, PTLD | + | + | + |

EBERs, small nuclear EBV-encoded RNAs; EBNA-2, EBV-encoded nuclear antigen 2; LMP-1, latent membrane protein 1; BL, Burkitt's lymphoma; HD, Hodgkin's disease; NPC, nasopharyngeal carcinoma; LCL, lymphoblastoid cell line; PTLD, post-transplant lymphoproliferative disorder.

variable. Therefore, immunohistochemistry (IH) cannot be used for the detection of the virus *per se*. A possible exception to this rule is the detection of LMP-1 in HD because it is expressed in the neoplastic Hodgkin and Reed-Sternberg cells of practically all EBV-positive HD cases ***(11,14)***.

The immunohistochemical characterization of EBV gene expression can be used to assess the form of EBV infection, i.e., latent or lytic. Expression of the BZLF1 protein of EBV induces the switch from latent to replicative infection and precedes the expression of early and late genes ***(15)***. Antibodies against the BZLF1 protein and other EBV lytic cycle proteins have proved to be a useful marker for identifying viral replication *in situ* and can be applied to paraffin sections ***(16,17)***.

An important application of immunohistochemistry is the characterization of the prevalent form of EBV latency in virus-associated diseases. This has been greatly aided by an increasing number of antibodies applicable to routinely processed tissues (*see* Chapter 24). Thus, it is now possible to detect EBNA-1, EBNA-2, LMP-1, and LMP-2A in paraffin sections (*see* **Subheading 3.4.**). However, for practical purposes, antibodies directed against EBNA-2 and LMP-1 are sufficient to define the form of virus latency prevalent in EBV-associated diseases (*see* **Table 1**).

## 2. Materials

### 2.1. Slides, Coverslips, Tissue Sections and Cytospin Preparations (*see* Note 1)

1. Glass slides and coverslips.
2. Decon 90 (Prochem, Wesel, Germany).
3. Acetone.
4. APES: 3-aminopropyltriethoxysilane (Sigma, St. Louis, MO).
5. 0.2 *N* HCl.
6. Ethanol: 50, 70, 96, 100%.
7. Silicon solution (Serva, Heidelberg, Germany).
8. Physiological saline solution: 0.9% NaCl in $H_2O$.
9. 10X PBS: 2.07 g $NaH_2PO_4 \cdot H_2O$, 6.22 g $Na_2 PO_4 \cdot 2H_2O$, 38.0 g NaCl, 0.5 mL DEPC, made up to 500 mL with distilled $H_2O$, incubate for at least 1 h at room temperature, autoclave, allow to cool, adjust pH to 7.2 with 1*N* NaOH.

10. 4% paraformaldehyde: dissolve 4 g of paraformaldehyde in 80 mL of water with gentle heating and addition of 1 *M* NaOH until the powder dissolves. Make up to 90 mL with distilled water and add 10 mL of 10X PBS.
11. Oven.

### 2.2. Probe Labeling

1. Appropriate restriction enzymes with 10X buffer.
2. 3 *M* sodium acetate.
3. Ethanol.
4. DEPC: Diethylpyrocarbonate (Sigma).
5. Depc$H_2O$ (*see* **Note 1**): add 1 mL of depc/L of water, shake well, incubate for at least 1 h at room temperature and autoclave.
6. α-$^{35}$S-UTP (>1250Ci/mmol; 12.5 Ci/mL) or α-$^{35}$S-dCTP (>1250Ci/mmol; 12.5 Ci/mL).
7. RNase inhibitor (40 U/μL).
8. RNA polymerases (SP6, T3, or T7, 20U/μL) and appropriate buffer.
9. DTT: 100 m*M* dithiothreitol.
10. NTP mix (10 m*M* ATP, 10 m*M* CTP, 10 m*M* GTP).
11. Yeast tRNA solution: 50 mg/mL.
12. DNase I (RNase-free, 10 U/μL).
13. Phenol/chloroform/isoamylalcohol (25/24/1 v/v).
14. Deionized formamide, pH 7.0.
15. Nick translation kit (e.g., Amersham Pharmacia, Uppsala, Sweden).
16. Nick columns (Amersham Pharmacia).

### 2.3. In Situ *Hybridization*

1. Xylene.
2. Ethanol.
3. Depc$H_2O$.
4. 0.2 *N* HCl.
5. 20X SSC (Standard saline citrate): 0.15 *M* sodium chloride, 0.015 *M* sodium citrate, pH 7.0.
6. Triton X-100.
7. Pronase: Prepare stock solutions of pronase by dissolving commercially available freeze-dried pronase (Boehringer, Mannheim, Germany) in depc$H_2O$. Incubate the solution at 37°C for 4 h to digest contaminating enzymes such as nucleases.
8. PBS: Dilute 10X PBS in water.
9. Triethanolamine/acetic anhydride: 0.1% triethanolamine, pH 8.0, 0.25% acetic anhydride.
10. Deionized formamide: Make up a 50% stock solution by dissolving 25 g of dextran sulphate in 25 mL depc$H_2O$ at 80°C. Make up to 50 mL with depc$H_2O$, aliquot, and store at –20°C.
11. Dextrane sulphate.
12. 100 m*M* DTT.
13. Carrier DNA (1 mg/mL, e.g., calf thymus or herring sperm DNA).
14. 90°C heating block with plane surface.
15. Yeast tRNA (50 mg/mL).
16. Parafilm.
17. RNase A (10 mg/mL).
18. TBS (Tris-buffered saline): 0.05 *M* Tris-HCl, 0.15 *M* NaCl, pH 7.6.
19. Photographic emulsion (e.g., Ilford G5).
20. Kodak D19 developer.

**Table 2**
**Monoclonal Antibodies for the Immunohistochemical Detection of EBV-Encoded Proteins and Digoxigenin-Labeled EBER-Specific Probes**

| Clone | Species | Specificity | Source | Reference |
|---|---|---|---|---|
| 1H4 | Rat | EBNA-1 | E. Kremmer | *(12)* |
| 2B4 | Rat | EBNA-1 | E. Kremmer | *(12)* |
| PE-2 | Mouse | EBNA-2 | Dako | *(18)* |
| CS1-4 | Mouse | LMP-1 | Dako | *(19)* |
| 4E11 | Rat | LMP2A | E. Kremmer | *(20)* |
| 15F9 | Rat | LMP2A | E. Kremmer | *(20)* |
| BZ-1 | Mouse | BZLF1 | Dako | *(16)* |
| 1.71.256 | Mouse | Digoxigenin | Boehringer | |

21. Sodium thiosulphate.
22. Hematoxilin and eosin.

### 2.4. Immunohistochemistry

1. Acetone.
2. Xylene.
3. Ethanol.
4. 0.1 *M* citrate buffer, pH 6.0.
5. Domestic microwave oven.
6. TBS (Tris-buffered saline): 0.05 *M* Tris-HCl, 0.15 *M* NaCl, pH 7.6.
7. Primary antibodies (*see* **Table 2**).
8. Bovine serum albumin (BSA).
9. Biotinylated rabbit antiserum against rat immunoglobulins (Dako, Glostrup, Denmark).
10. Biotinylated rabbit antiserum against mouse immunoglobulins (Dako).
11. Streptavidin-biotinylated alkaline phosphatase complex (StreptABC-AP, Dako).
12. Naphthol AS-MX phosphate.
13. N,N-dimethylformamide.
14. 0.1 *M* Tris-HCl, pH 8.2.
15. 1 *M* levamisole.
16. Fast Red TR salt.
17. Filter paper.
18. Hematoxilin.
19. Aqueous mounting medium.

## 3. Methods

### 3.1. Preparation of Glassware, Slides, Coverslips, Sections, and Cytospins (*see* **Note 1**)

#### 3.1.1. Glassware

1. For RNA *in situ* hybridization, glassware has to be RNase-free. To achieve this, wrap clean glassware in tin foil and bake at 250°C for 6 h.
2. To improve adhesion of cells and sections glass slides should be coated with 3-aminopropyltriethoxysilane (APES). To do this, first wash glass slides in 2% Decon 90.

3. Rinse thoroughly in tap water, then briefly rinse in deionized water and air dry for about 15 min.
4. Place into acetone for 3 min at room temperature (RT), followed by 2% APES/acetone for 3 min at RT.
5. Briefly rinse in distilled water and air dry.
6. Glass coverslips should be siliconized to avoid sticking of probe DNA or RNA to the glass and to allow easy removal after hybridization. To do this, first clean cover slips in 0.2 N HCl for 20 min.
7. Rinse coverslips in deionized water and then briefly dip into 100% ethanol.
8. Air-dry for 15 min at RT and then bake at 250°C for 5 h. Allow to cool.
9. Dip coverslips into silicon solution.
10. Bake at 100–115°C for 2 h.

### *3.1.2. Paraffin Sections*

1. Fix tissues in neutral buffered formalin and embed in paraffin wax using routine histological procedures.
2. Cut approx 5 µm thick sections (3–5 µm for immunohistochemistry, 5–8 µm for *in situ* hybridization) from paraffin blocks and mount onto APES-coated slides.
3. Dry at 60°C for 1 h.

### *3.1.3. Frozen Sections*

1. Place fresh tissue samples into plastic vessels, cover with physiological saline solution, snap-freeze in liquid nitrogen, and store at –70°C.
2. Cut 6-µm frozen sections on a cryostat and mount them onto APES-coated slides.
3. For use in immunohistochemistry, air dry sections overnight. If the slides are not used for immunohistochemistry immediately, store unfixed at –70°C.
4. For use in *in situ* hybridization, dry sections on a 60°C hot plate for 3 min and fix immediately in 4% paraformaldehyde for 20 min at RT.
5. Wash slides twice in 3X PBS and twice in 1X PBS for 1 min each at RT.
6. Dehydrate sections through a series of graded ethanol dilutions, air-dry briefly and store at –70°C.

### *3.1.4. Cytospin Preparations*

1. Wash cells and resuspend in PBS.
2. Adjust cell concentration so that approx $5 \times 10^4$ to $1 \times 10^5$ cells are added per slide.
3. Following centrifugation, treat cytospins as described for frozen sections.

## *3.2. Probe Labeling*

### *3.2.1. RNA Probes* (*see* **Notes 2** and **3**)

Single-stranded RNA probes are generated from plasmids with the specific insert located between two bacteriophage-derived DNA-dependent RNA polymerase promoter sites to allow the transcription of probes in sense and anti-sense direction. To ensure transcription of the insert only, linearized plasmid template is used.

1. In order to linearize plasmids, mix 10 µg of plasmid DNA, 40 U of restriction enzyme and 4 µL of appropriate 10X restriction enzyme buffer, make up to 40 µL with $ddH_2O$. Incubate at 37°C overnight.

2. Precipitate linearized plasmid DNA by adding 4 µL of 3 *M* sodium acetate and 80 µL of ethanol to the linearization mix. Incubate at –70°C for 30 min and centrifuge at 16,000*g* in a micro-centrifuge for 30 min at 4°C. Air-dry pellet and resuspend in 12.5 µL of depc$H_2O$.
3. Verify linearization by running a 0.5 µL aliquot of the digestion mixture on a 0.5% agarose gel.
4. To generate $^{35}S$-labeled probes, carry out a transcription reaction as follows (*see* **Notes 2** and **3**): Mix 50 µCi α-$^{35}S$-UTP, 0.5 µL RNase inhibitor, 2 µL 5X transcription buffer, 1 µL 100 m*M* DTT, 0.5 µL NTP mix, 1 µL linearized plasmid, 1 µL RNA polymerase (SP6, T3, or T7). Make up to 10 µL with depc$H_2O$ and mix.
5. Incubate at RT for 60 min.
6. Add another 0.5 µL of RNA polymerase and incubate for another 30 min.
7. DNase digest plasmid DNA by adding 5 µL of yeast tRNA solution, 0.5 µL of RNase inhibitor, 0.5 µL of DNase I (RNase-free) to the reaction mix and incubating at 37°C for 8 min.
8. Extract proteins by adding 10 µL of 3 *M* sodium acetate, 74 µL of depc$H_2O$ and 100 µL of phenol/chloroform/isoamylacohol (25/24/1 [v/v]). Mix well and centrifuge at 16,000*g* for 2 min in a microcentrifuge and save the upper phase (ca. 100 µL).
9. Precipitation: Ethanol precipitate RNA by adding 1/10 vol of 3 *M* sodium acetate and 2 vol of ethanol as described in **step 2**, centrifuge and air dry the pellet. Resuspend in 100 µL of depc$H_2O$ and repeat ethanol precipitation with 1/10 vol of sodium acetate and 2 vol of ethanol. Resuspend pellet in 12.5 µL of depc$H_2O$. Take a 0.5 µL aliquot for scintillation counting (*see* **Note 4**). To the remaining 12 µL add 3 µL of 100 m*M* DTT and 15 µL of deionized formamide. Store at –20°C.

### *3.2.2. DNA Probes*

For the detection of EBV DNA, use a plasmid harboring the *Bam*HI W internal repetitive fragment of the EBV genome. Label total plasmid DNA with $^{35}S$-labeled dCTP using nick translation. Nick translation requires a balanced mixture of DNase I and DNA polymerase. Particularly if this reaction is not carried out frequently, use of kits is advised, which are available from several suppliers. Following the nick translation reaction, separate labeled DNA from unincorporated nucleotides using Sephadex columns (e.g., Nick columns, Pharmacia) according to the supplier's instructions. Alternatively, label DNA probes using random primer labeling kits (e.g., Boehringer).

## **3.3. In Situ *Hybridization***

### *3.3.1. Prehybridization*

1. Prehybridization treatment is essentially the same for DNA and RNA *in situ* hybridization. Dewax paraffin sections in xylene (two changes, 10 min each) and rehydrate them through a series of graded ethanols (e.g., 100, 96, 70, 50% depc$H_2O$). Take frozen sections or cytospin preparations out of the –70°C freezer and thaw for at least 1 h (keep wrapped to avoid condensation).
2. Incubate in 0.2 *N* HCl for 10 min at room temperature (RT), then rinse in 1X PBS.
3. Incubate in 0.01% Triton X-100 for 90 s at RT (*see* **Note 5**), rinse in 1X PBS.
4. Digest with Pronase (0.125–1 mg/mL) in 1X PBS (*see* **Note 6**), rinse thoroughly with 1X PBS.
5. Fix in 4% paraformaldehyde for 20 min at room temperature.
6. Acetylate sections with triethanolamine/acetic anhydride for 10 min at RT (*see* **Note 7**), rinse in 1X PBS.
7. Dehydrate sections through graded ethanols.

### 3.3.2. EBV DNA In Situ Hybridization

1. Make up the hybridization mix to give the following end concentrations: 50% deionized formamide, 2X SSC, 10% dextran sulphate (*see* **Note 9**), 10 m*M* DTT (*see* **Note 10**), 30 µg/mL herring sperm DNA, 20–40 ng/mL labeled probe.
2. Add 25 µL of hybridization mix to each slide.
3. Cover sections with siliconized coverslips (*see* **Note 11**).
4. Denature probe and cellular DNA by placing slides onto a 90°C heating block for 3 min.
5. Hybridize overnight at 37°C in an atmosphere of 50% formamide (*see* **Note 12**).
6. Remove coverslips and wash in 50% formamide, 1X SSC, 10 m*M* DTT at 37°C for 4 h with hourly changes of the wash solution.
7. Rinse in 2X SSC, 10 m*M* DTT for 30 min at RT.
8. Rinse in 0.1X SSC, 10 m*M* DTT for 30 min at RT.
9. Dehydrate sections through graded ethanols and air-dry.

### 3.3.3. EBER In Situ Hybridization

1. Make up the hybridization mix to give the following end concentrations (*see* **Note 8**): 50% deionized formamide, 2X SSC, 10% dextran sulphate (*see* **Note 9**), 10 m*M* DTT (*see* **Note 10**), 250 µg/mL yeast tRNA, 50,000–200,000 cpm $^{35}$S-labeled probe per section or digoxigenin-labeled probes to a final dilution of between 1:25 to 1:200 (*see* **Note 8**), depc$H_2O$ to final volume.
2. Place approx 25 µL of hybridization mix on each section.
3. Cover sections with a piece of parafilm cut to size (*see* **Note 11**).
4. Hybridize overnight at 50°C in an atmosphere of 50% formamide (*see* **Note 12**).
5. Remove parafilm and wash slides in 50% formamide, 1X SSC, 10 m*M* DTT at 52°C for 4 h with hourly changes of the wash solution.
6. Wash in 2X SSC, 10 m*M* DTT at 37°C for 30 min.
7. Incubate in 20 µg/mL RNase A, 2X SSC, 10 m*M* DTT at 37°C for 30 min.
8. Wash in 2X SSC, 10 m*M* DTT at RT for 10 min.
9. Wash in 0.1X SSC, 10 m*M* DTT at RT for 10 min.
10. Dehydrate sections subjected to *in situ* hybridization with $^{35}$S-labeled probes through graded ethanols and air dry. Autoradiographic detection of bound probes is described in **Subheading 3.3.4.**
11. Transfer sections exposed to digoxigenin-labeled probes to TBS. Bound probes are detected using immunohistochemistry as described in **Subheading 3.4.2.**

### 3.3.4. Dark Room Procedure (*see* **Note 13**)

1. Melt Ilford G5 photographic emulsion at 42°C and prepare a 1:2 dilution of the emulsion in dd$H_2O$. Before entering the dark room, fill 10 mL of dd$H_2O$ into a 50-mL plastic vial and highlight the 20 mL mark with a marker pen so that it can be seen using only a dim red light. Pour 10 mL of the melted emulsion carefully into the water and mix so as to avoid formation of froth.
2. Dip slides into the emulsion (*see* **Notes 14** and **15**).
3. Place coated slides onto an absorbent paper towel in an upright position to allow draining off of excess emulsion and air-dry for 1 h in complete darkness.
4. Still in complete darkness, place the slides into a light-proof box together with a drying agent, wrap in tin foil, and place into a 4°C refrigerator.
5. Expose slides at 4°C for 3–20 d (*see* **Note 16**).

6. Remove slide box from refrigerator and allow to adjust to room temperature for at least 30 min.
7. Prepare a 1:2 dilution of Kodak D19 developer in cold tap water.
8. Prepare a 25% (w/v) solution of sodium thiosulphate in cold tap water.
9. In complete darkness remove slides from the box and place into the developer for 3 min.
10. Wash in cold tap water.
11. Fix in 25% sodium thiosulphate for 3 min. Now switch on light.
12. Rinse thoroughly under running cold tap water.
13. Counterstain with hematoxylin and eosin (filter before use and mount using an aqueous mounting medium).

## 3.4. Immunohistochemistry

### 3.4.1. Fixation and Antigen Retrieval

#### 3.4.1.1. Frozen Sections and Cytospin Preparations

1. Remove from the –70°C freezer and allow to adjust to room temperature for at least 1 h.
2. Fix in acetone for 20 min and air-dry.

#### 3.4.1.2. Paraffin Sections

1. Dewax in xylene for 30 min at RT.
2. Rehydrate through graded ethanols (5 min each in 100, 96, 70% ethanol and water).
3. Place sections into a beaker with 1 L of 0.1 *M* citrate buffer, pH 6.0.
4. Irradiate in a domestic microwave oven (750 W) at maximum power for up to 60 min (*see* **Note 17**).
5. Allow to cool down and transfer into TBS.

### 3.4.2. Immunohistochemical Staining (see **Note 18**)

The primary antibodies regularly used in our laboratories for the detection of EBV-encoded proteins and of digoxigenin-labeled EBER probes are listed in **Table 2**. For the detection of LMP-1, BZLF1, and digoxigenin-labeled EBER probes, the following staining protocol is used.

1. Apply primary antibody diluted in TBS, 1% BSA and incubate for 60 min at RT.
2. Rinse with TBS.
3. Apply appropriate secondary antibody diluted in TBS and incubate for 30 min at RT. For the detection of bound primary mouse antibodies, we use a biotinylated rabbit antiserum against mouse immunoglobulins (Dako). Primary antibodies from the rat are detected using a biotinylated rabbit antiserum specific for rat immunoglobulins (Dako).
4. Whilst incubating, prepare streptavidin-biotinylated alkaline phosphatase complex (StreptABC-AP, Dako) according to the manufacturer's instructions. Note that the complex should be prepared 30 min before use.
5. Rinse with TBS.
6. Incubate with StreptABC-AP for 30 min at RT.
7. While incubation takes place, prepare substrate/chromogen solution (*see* **Note 19**): dissolve 2 mg Napthol AS-MX phosphate in 0.2 mL of N,N-dimethylformamide, add 9.8 mL of 0.1 *M* Tris-HCl, pH 8.2, and 10 µL of 1 *M* levamisole. Just before use dissolve 10 mg Fast-Red TR salt in the solution and filter through ordinary filter paper.
8. Rinse sections in TBS.

9. Apply chromogen/substrate solution for 30 min at RT.
10. Rinse with TBS.
11. Counterstain with hematoxylin and mount using an aqueous mounting medium.

## 4. Notes

1. Glassware and solutions used for RNA *in situ* hybridization have to be treated in order to inactivate RNases that are ubiquitous. For glassware, this is achieved by baking at 250°C for 6 h. All solutions which can be autoclaved are treated with diethylpyrocarbonate (DEPC). Add 1 mL of depc/L, shake well, incubate for at least 1 h to overnight, and autoclave. Autoclaving leads to the decomposition of DEPC into ethanol and $CO_2$. Therefore, pH has to be adjusted after autoclaving. Prepare solutions which cannot be autoclaved using DEPC-treated water (e.g., Tris-containing solutions, dextran sulfate).
2. For the generation of radiolabeled probes with high specific activity, no unlabeled UTP is added to the transcription reaction. In our hands, probes generated using a mixture of $^{35}$S-labeled and unlabeled UTP result in weaker *in situ* hybridization signals. To obtain probes of even higher specific activity, a second labeled nucleotide (e.g., $^{35}$S-CTP) can be added to the transcription reaction. If the volume of the radioactive nucleotide is too large, use a speed-vac or a similar centrifuge to freeze-dry the labeled NTP solution.
3. Generate digoxigenin-labeled probes using a commercially available labeling mix (DIG RNA labeling mix, Boehringer, Mannheim, Germany) according to the manufacturer's instructions.
4. Only use probes if scintillation counting of a 0.5 µL aliquot yields an activity of at least $5 \times 10^5$ cpm.
5. Treatment with Triton X-100 is optional and in our laboratories is used only for DNA *in situ* hybridization.
6. A variety of proteases have been recommended for *in situ* hybridization. In our hands, pronase has given reliable and reproducible results over many years. The concentrations given are meant as a guideline only. It is important to titrate the pronase to establish the conditions that will give the best signal without disrupting tissue morphology. It is possible to vary the pronase concentration, the duration of the digestion, and the temperature. In particular, when the ambient temperature in the laboratory may be variable, it is advisable to use an incubator, e.g., at 37°C. Factors which may effect the outcome of the pronase digestion are type of fixative, length of fixation, and other variables of the embedding procedure.

   Nevertheless, once the optimal pronase digestion conditions have been established, there is very little variation necessary for blocks from the same institution. Currently used concentrations in our laboratories are 0.5 mg/mL for paraffin sections and 0.125 mg/mL for frozen sections and cytospins. Higher concentrations may be required for DNA *in situ* hybridization. To identify an appropriate pronase concentration, digest tissue sections with different pronase concentrations, keeping temperature and incubation time constant. Counterstain sections and identify the pronase concentration, which visibly starts to damage the tissue. Then use half that concentration.
7. The mixture of triethanolamine and acetic anhydrid must be prepared fresh immediately before adding it to the sections. Acetylation is believed to reduce background by decreasing nonspecific probe binding to glass. Whether this actually works is uncertain. However, it is included in our protocol for *in situ* hybridization with $^{35}$S-labeled probes. We usually omit this step when working with nonradioactive probes.

8. Calculations are based on the assumption that 25 µL of hybridization mix are required for the average slide. Radioactive probe is included in the mix so that between 50,000 and 250,000 cpm are added per slide. The amount of radioactive probe necessary may vary depending on the abundance of the target, the individual probe and the labeling reaction. For the EBERs, usually between 50,000 and 100,000 cpm per slide suffice. Note that if the EBER1 and EBER2 probes are used as a mixture, 50,000–100,000 cpm per slide are added for each probe. Dilutions of digoxigenin-labeled probes have to be titrated using appropriate positive control sections. Note that before adding to the hybridization mix, RNA probes have to be heated at 80°C for 30 s and put on ice to remove secondary and tertiary structures.
9. The dextran sulphate solution is viscous and difficult to pipet. This may be facilitated by warming the solution. The following procedure has also proved useful. Set the pipet to the required volume and fit appropriate tip. Draw the required volume of water into the pipet tip and mark the level. Eject the water again, increase the volume setting of the pipet and draw dextran sulphate solution into the tip up to the marked level.
10. Add DTT to hybridization mix and washing solutions only when using $^{35}S$-labeled probes.
11. Siliconized glass cover slips may be used and this may be more appropriate for DNA *in situ* hybridization which requires heating the slides to denature the target DNA. However, for RNA *in situ* hybridization, use of parafilm is perfectly adequate.
12. We add a 50% formamide solution to the incubation chamber. In our experience, making a humid chamber just by adding water will lead to probe dilution.
13. Before entering the dark room, sort slides into a rack to facilitate dipping and to make sure that the slides are put into the correct light proof boxes in complete darkness. Dilute photographic emulsion in the dark room using a low-energy red light only.
14. For dipping the sections, plastic slide containers for mailing glass slides have proved useful. These hold a volume of approx 20 mL. Pour the diluted emulsion carefully into the slide container and dip the slides into the emulsion. If a larger number of slides is to be coated with emulsion, it is advisable to keep the emulsion in a 42°C water bath.
15. In our experience, it is safe to reuse diluted emulsion once. For this purpose, wrap the container with the emulsion tightly with tin foil and store at 4°C. To reuse the emulsion, place the container into a 42°C water bath and proceed as described.
16. Exposure times will vary depending on the abundance of the target. Three to seven days are usually sufficient for the EBERs, while detection of viral DNA and of low-copy mRNAs may require longer exposure. For every experiment it is advisable to prepare at least two or three sets of slides to allow development after different exposure times. Place each set of slides into a separate light-proof box.
17. Irradiation of formalin-fixed paraffin sections in citrate buffer using a microwave oven has proved useful for the detection of a variety of antigens ***(21)***. A variety of microwaveing conditions have been described including variations in energy, time, or buffer used. Alternatively, domestic pressure cookers may be used. Optimum conditions have to be determined individually in every laboratory. In our hands, use of a large volume of citrate buffer (1 L) has proved useful. It requires longer microwave irradiation time than smaller quantities but makes substitution of volume lost through evaporation unnecessary. When placing slides into a beaker for microwave irradiation, make sure they are not stacked too tightly to ensure even distribution of heat.
18. For enhancing weak immunohistochemical stains (for example when detecting EBNA-1, EBNA-2, and LMP-2A) amplification systems using biotinylated tyramide have proved useful. This method is based on the horseradish peroxidase-catalysed precipitation of

numerous biotin molecules at the site of primary antibody binding *(22,23)*. The precipitated biotin can then be detected using a variety of methods. In our laboratory, this is done by applying the StreptABC-AP reagent as described earlier followed by development of the alkaline phosphatase as described. Methods have been described for the preparation of biotinylated tyramide but if this reaction is not employed frequently, use of commercially available kits may be advantageous (Renaissance® TSA™ kits, NEN Life Science, Boston, MA).

19. The solution consisting of Napthol AS-MX phosphate, dimethylformamide, and Tris buffer can be stored at 4°C for several weeks. Fast Red TR salt is added immediately before use. To make sure that the substrate/chromogen solution is working before adding it to the slides, a small aliquot of the StreptABC-AP reagent can be mixed with an aliquot of the substrate/chromogen solution in a reaction tube. The solution should turn red quickly.

## Acknowledgment

We gratefully acknowledge the cooperation of A. Agathanggelou, T. Finn, R. Lisner, K. von Ostau, U. Tank, and D. Ung in developing and adapting these methods.

## References

1. Niedobitek, G. and Young, L. S. (1994) Epstein-Barr virus persistence and virus-associated tumours. *Lancet* **343,** 333–335.
2. Thorley-Lawson, D. A., Miyashita, E. M., and Khan, G. (1996) Epstein-Barr virus and the B cell: that's all it takes. *Trends Microbiol.* **4,** 204–208.
3. Niedobitek, G., Herbst, H., Young, L. S., Brooks, L., Masucci, M. G., Crocker, J., Rickinson, A. B., and Stein, H. (1992) Patterns of Epstein-Barr virus infection in non-neoplastic lymphoid tissue. *Blood* **79,** 2520–2526.
4. Hubscher, S. G., Williams, A., Davison, S. M., Young, L. S., and Niedobitek, G. (1994) Epstein-Barr virus in inflammatory diseases of the liver and liver allografts: an in situ hybridization study. *Hepatology* **20,** 899–907.
5. Niedobitek, G. and Herbst, H. (1991) Applications of in situ hybridization. *Int. Rev. Exp. Pathol.* **32,** 1–56.
6. Hamilton-Dutoit, S. J. and Pallesen, G. (1994) Detection of Epstein-Barr virus small RNAs in routine paraffin sections using non-isotopic RNA/RNA in situ hybridization. *Histopathology* **25,** 101–111.
7. Rickinson, A. B. and Kieff, E. (1996) Epstein-Barr virus, in *Fields Virology,* vol. 2 (Fields, B. N., Knipe, D. M., and Howley, P. M., eds.), Lippincott-Raven, Philadelphia, pp. 2397–2446.
8. Niedobitek, G., Young, L. S., Lau, R., Brooks, L., Greenspan, D., Greenspan, J. S., and Rickinson, A. B. (1991) Epstein-Barr virus infection in oral hairy leukoplakia: virus replication in the absence of a detectable latent phase. *J. Gen. Virol.* **72,** 3035–3046.
9. Rowe, M., Lear, A., Croom-Carter, D., Davies, A. H., and Rickinson, A. B. (1992) Three pathways of Epstein-Barr virus (EBV) gene activation from EBNA1-positive latency in B lymphocytes. *J. Virol.* **66,** 122–131.
10. Niedobitek, G., Herbst, H., Young, L. S., Rowe, M., Dienemann, D., Germer, C., and Stein, H. (1992) Epstein-Barr virus and carcinomas. Expression of the viral genome in an undifferentiated gastric carcinoma. *Diagn. Mol. Pathol.* **1,** 103–108.
11. Herbst, H., Dallenbach, F., Hummel, M., Niedobitek, G., Pileri, S., Müller-Lantzsch, N., and Stein, H. (1991) Epstein-Barr virus latent membrane protein expression in Hodgkin and Reed-Sternberg cells. *Proc. Natl. Acad. Sci. USA* **88,** 4766–4770.

12. Grässer, F. A., Murray, P. G., Kremmer, E., Klein, K., Remberger, K., Feiden, W., et al. (1994) Monoclonal antibodies directed against the Epstein-Barr virus-encoded nuclear antigen 1 (EBNA1): immunohistologic detection of EBNA1 in the malignant cells of Hodgkin's disease. *Blood* **84,** 3792–3798.
13. Murray, P. G., Niedobitek, G., Kremmer, E., Grasser, F., Reynolds, G. M., Cruchley, A., et al. (1996) In situ detection of the Epstein-Barr virus-encoded nuclear antigen 1 in oral hairy leukoplakia and virus-associated carcinomas. *J. Pathol.* **178,** 44–47.
14. Pallesen, G., Hamilton-Dutoit, S. J., Rowe, M., and Young, L. S. (1991) Expression of Epstein-Barr virus latent gene products in tumour cells of Hodgkin's disease. *Lancet* **337,** 320–322.
15. Miller, G. (1990) The switch between latency and replication of Epstein-Barr virus. *J. Infect. Dis.* **161,** 833–844.
16. Young, L. S., Lau, R., Rowe, M., Niedobitek, G., Packham, G., Shanaham, F., et al. (1991) Differentiation-associated expression of the Epstein-Barr virus BZLF1 transactivator protein in oral "hairy" leukoplakia. *J. Virol.* **65,** 2868–2874.
17. Niedobitek, G., Agathanggelou, A., Herbst, H., Whitehead, L., Wright, D. H., and Young, L. S. (1997) Epstein-Barr virus (EBV) infection in infectious mononucleosis: virus latency, replication and phenotype of EBV-infected cells. *J. Pathol.* **182,** 151–159.
18. Young, L., Alfieri, C., Hennessey, K., Evans, H., O'Hara, C., Anderson, K. C., et al. (1989) Expression of Epstein-Barr virus transformation-associated genes in tissues of patients with EBV lymphoproliferative disease. *N. Engl. J. Med.* **321,** 1080–1085.
19. Rowe, M., Evans, H. S., Young, L. S., Hennessy, K., Kieff, E., and Rickinson, A. B. (1987) Monoclonal antibodies to the latent membrane protein of Epstein-Barr virus reveal heterogeneity of the protein and inducible expression in virus-transformed cells. *J. Gen. Virol.* **68,** 1575–1586.
20. Niedobitek, G., Kremmer, E., Herbst, H., Whitehead, L., Dawson, C. W., Niedobitek, E., et al. (1997) Immunohistochemical detection of the Epstein-Barr virus-encoded latent membrane protein 2A (LMP2A) in Hodgkin's disease and infectious mononucleosis. *Blood* **90,** 1664–1672.
21. Shi, S.-R., Cote, R. J., and Taylor, C. R. (1997) Antigen retrieval immunohistochemistry: past, present, and future. *J. Histochem. Cytochem.* **45,** 327–343.
22. Bobrow, M. N., Harris, T. D., Shaughnessy, K. J., and Litt, G. J. (1989) Catalyzed reporter deposition, a novel method of signal amplification. *J. Immunol. Methods* **125,** 279–285.
23. Bobrow, M. N., Shaughnessy, K. J., and Litt, G. J. (1991) Catalyzed reporter deposition, a novel method of signal amplification. II. Application to membrane immunoassays. *J. Immunol. Methods* **137,** 103–112.

# 8

# Phenotype Determination of Epstein-Barr Virus-Infected Cells in Tissue Sections

**Hermann Herbst and Gerald Niedobitek**

## 1. Introduction

Epstein-Barr virus (EBV) has been found in a plethora of lesions phenotypically as diverse as malignant lymphomas of B- and T-cell type, Hodgkin's disease, infectious mononucleosis, carcinomas, neoplasms of follicular dendritic cells, and leiomyosarcomas. On the other hand, there are examples of cell types that were suspected to harbor EBV but were not found to be infected when applying appropriate methodology, examples comprising seminoma cells or macrophages in EBV-associated hemophagocytic syndrome. Confident assignment of EBV infection to a specific cell type may require the application of double-labeling techniques for the simultaneous detection of viral DNA or viral gene products on the one hand and cellular gene products on the other hand. Depending on the type of latency, EBV inflicts changes on infected cells such as morphological alterations as well as disturbances in the phenotypic make-up of the cell surface, in the cytokine expression profile, and in the signal transduction pathways. Because of the heterogeneous composition of many EBV-associated lesions, gene expression analysis of EBV-infected cells in tissue sections is, again, best achieved with double-labeling techniques. Moreover, simultaneous detection of EBV and immunoglobulin light-chain gene transcripts of kappa or lambda types, not only provides a phenotypic marker but also yields information as to the clonal composition of these cells by their display of an either monotypic or polytypic expression pattern.

Various combinations of immunohistology (IH) and *in situ* hybridization (ISH) with either radioactive or nonradioactive probes (IH/ISH), *in situ* hybridization with a *gemisch* of radioactive and nonradioactive probes (ISH-ISH), and even triple-labeling procedures (IH/ISH-ISH) have been used with success ***(1–5)***. For nonradioactive procedures, two major approaches are possible, double immunofluorescence and double immunoenzymatic techniques. Because of the considerable drawbacks of immunofluorescence, particularly when applied to formalin-fixed tissue sections, only immu-

From: *Methods in Molecular Biology, Vol. 174: Epstein-Barr Virus Protocols*
Edited by: J. B. Wilson and G. H. W. May © Humana Press Inc., Totowa, NJ

noenzymatic procedures are described here. To achieve proper signal discrimination, the choice of visualization systems and chromogens is important. For immunoenzymatic double labeling, various different color combinations based on the use of different marker enzymes have been described, and numerous reviews and application handbooks exist for those techniques (*see* **Note 1**). In this chapter, we will restrict ourselves to the following procedures: 1) sequential IH/ISH for the detection of differentiation antigens by IH and cellular or viral nucleic acids by radioactive or nonradioactive ISH, and 2) simultaneous radioactive ISH for the detection of cellular RNA (e.g., cytokine or immunoglobulin transcripts) with nonradioactive visualization of EBER transcripts (ISH-ISH).

The sequential procedure has previously been adapted to combinations of ISH with classical enzyme histochemistry, such as visualization of acid phosphatase or esterase activities ***(6,7)***.

## 2. Materials

1. 4% paraformaldehyde: dissolve 4 g of paraformaldehye in 80 mL of water with gentle heating and addition of 1 *M* NaOH until the powder dissolves. Make up to 90 mL with distilled water and add 10 mL of 10X PBS.
2. Xylene.
3. Acetone.
4. Ethanol: 50, 70, 96, 100%.
5. Tris-buffered saline (TBS): 0.05 *M* Tris-HCl, 0.15 *M* NaCl, pH 7.6.
6. 10X PBS: 80 g NaCl, 2 g KCl, 2 g $KH_2PO_4$, 11.5 g $Na_2HPO_4 \cdot 7H_2O$, made up to 1 L with distilled $H_2O$.
7. Pronase: 0.01 mg/mL in $H_2O$.
8. Glycin.
9. IH/ISH dilution buffer: RPMI-1640, 1% BSA (w:v), 5000 U/mL Heparin, 2.5 mg/mL yeast-tRNA, pH 7.5 (*see* **Note 2**).
10. Normal human serum, heat inactivated at 56°C for 30 min.
11. APAAP (alkaline phosphatase anti-alkaline phosphatase) complex.
12. 5% New fuchsin: dissolve 5 g in 100 mL of 2 *N* HCl, keep in a dark bottle at 4°C.
13. Propandiole: 0.2 *M* 2-Amino-2,2-methyl-propan-1,3-diole, store at 4°C in a dark bottle.
14. Levamisole.
15. Naphtol-AS-BI-phosphate.
16. Sodium nitrite.
17. DMF: N-N-Dimethylformamide.
18. 2 *N* HCl.
19. Diethylpyrocarbonate-treated water (depc$H_2O$; *see* Note 7, Chapter 7).
20. Triton X-100.
21. Triethanolamine/acetic anhydride: 0.1 *M* triethanolamine, pH 8.0, 0.25% acetic anhydride (v:v).
22. Hydrolysis buffer: 80 m*M* $NaHCO_3$, 120 m*M* $Na_2CO_3$, pH 10.2, 10 m*M* DTT.
23. Stop solution: 0.2 *M* sodium acetate, 1% Acetic acid, 10 m*M* dithiothreitol (DTT).
24. 10 m*M* DTT.
25. Glycerol gelatin.
26. Hematoxylin (Meyer's).
27. DAB: 3,3-Diaminobenzidine tetrahydrochloride.

28. 30% Hydrogen peroxide ($H_2O_2$).
29. Peroxidase-conjugated anti-digoxigenin-Fab fragment.
30. 0.05 *M* Tris-HCl, pH 7.6.
31. 100X Denhardt's solution: 2% bovine serum albumin (BSA), 2% Ficoll 400, 2% polyvinyl-pyrrolidone, freeze-dried.
32. Probe mix: 50% formamide, 10 m*M* Tris-HCl, pH 7.5, 10 m*M* sodium phosphate, 1X Denhardt's solution, 1 mg/mL yeast tRNA, 5 m*M* ethylenidiaminetetraaceticacid (EDTA), 10 m*M* DTT, 10% dextrane sulfate.
33. Alkaline phosphatase-conjugated anti-digoxigenin-Fab fragment.

## 3. Methods

The pretreatment of glass ware, slides, and cover slips is detailed in Chapter 7 as is DNA and RNA probe labeling.

### 3.1. Sequential IH/ISH Labeling (*see* Notes 3 and 4)

#### 3.1.1. Sectioning, Fixation, and Antigen Retrieval

Frozen sections, cytological preparations:

1. Kryostat sections of 6-µm thickness and cytocentrifuge slides are prepared immediately prior to use. Air-dry; do not use a hot plate.
2. Fix in ice-cold 4% paraformaldehyde for 20 min (*see* **Notes 5** and **6**).

Paraffin sections:

1. Dewax in xylene (2 changes) for a minimum of 30 min and in acetone for 10 min, all at room temperature (RT). Rehydrate through graded ethanols (5 min each in 100, 96, 70% ethanol and TBS) at RT.
2. Depending on the antibody, predigest the section with pronase (approx 0.01 mg/mL in PBS, *see* **Note 7**).
3. Use 0.1 *M* glycin in TBS for 30 s to inactivate pronase. Transfer to TBS.
4. Alternatively or additionally, some antibodies require epitope unmasking by heat-treatment: place sections into a beaker with 1000 mL of 0.1 *M* citrate buffer, pH 6.0, made up with $DEPCH_2O$. Irradiate in a domestic microwave oven (750 W) at maximum power for up to 60 min (*see* **Note 8**). Allow to cool down and transfer to TBS.

#### 3.1.2. Antibody Reactions

1. Apply the appropriately diluted primary antibody in IH/ISH dilution buffer and incubate for 20 min at RT (*8*; *see* **Notes 9** and **10**).
2. Flush the slides with 1X TBS. Take care to remove buffer as completely as possible to avoid diluting subsequently applied reagents, but do not let the section dry out.
3. Apply appropriate bridging antibody (e.g., rabbit anti-mouse immunoglobulin) diluted in IH/ISH dilution buffer including 1/8 vol of heat-inactivated normal serum for 20 min at RT (*see* **Note 10**).
4. Flush the slides with 1X TBS.
5. Apply secondary bridging antibody, if appropriate (*see* **Note 10**).
6. Flush the slides with 1X TBS.
7. Apply APAAP complex *(8)*, diluted 1:20 in IH/ISH dilution buffer for 20 min at RT. Save a few drops of the reagent to control the substrate solutions.
8. **Steps 2–7** may be repeated for increased sensitivity (*see* **Note 11**).

**Table 1**
**Solution A**

| Final volume | 50 | 100 | 150 | 200 | 250 | 300 | 350 | 400 | 450 | 500 | mL |
|---|---|---|---|---|---|---|---|---|---|---|---|
| TBS, pH 9.7 | 35 | 70 | 105 | 140 | 175 | 210 | 245 | 280 | 315 | 350 | mL |
| Propandiole | 12.5 | 25 | 37.5 | 50 | 62.5 | 75 | 87.5 | 100 | 112.5 | 125 | mL |
| Levamisole | 20 | 40 | 60 | 80 | 100 | 120 | 140 | 160 | 180 | 200 | mg |

**Table 2**
**Solution B**

| Final volume | 50 | 100 | 150 | 200 | 250 | 300 | 350 | 400 | 450 | 500 | mL |
|---|---|---|---|---|---|---|---|---|---|---|---|
| Na-AS-Bi-P | 25 | 50 | 75 | 100 | 125 | 150 | 175 | 200 | 225 | 250 | mg |
| DMF | 0.3 | 0.6 | 0.9 | 1.2 | 1.5 | 1.8 | 2.1 | 2.4 | 2.7 | 3.0 | mL |

**Table 3**
**Solution C**

| Final volume | 50 | 100 | 150 | 200 | 250 | 300 | 350 | 400 | 450 | 500 | mL |
|---|---|---|---|---|---|---|---|---|---|---|---|
| $NaNO_3$ | 10 | 20 | 30 | 40 | 50 | 60 | 70 | 80 | 90 | 100 | mg |
| $H_2O$ | 0.25 | 0.5 | 0.75 | 1.0 | 1.25 | 1.5 | 1.75 | 2.0 | 2.25 | 2.5 | mL |
| 5% New fuchsin | 0.1 | 0.2 | 0.3 | 0.4 | 0.5 | 0.6 | 0.7 | 0.8 | 0.9 | 1.0 | mL |

### *3.1.3. Alkaline Phosphatase Development*

The new fuchsin alkaline phosphatase (AP)-substrate solution (*9*; *see* **Note 12**) is prepared from the solutions A, B, and C, which are made up prior to use in the following order:

Solution A:

1. Mix APAAP development buffer consisting of TBS and 0.2 *M* propandiole in a baked glass beaker.
2. Dissolve the appropriate amount of levamisole in the APAAP development buffer according to **Table 1**.

Solution B:

3. In a fume hood, dissolve naphtol-AS-Bi-phosphate in DMF in a baked glass beaker according to **Table 2**.

Solution C:

4. Immediately before use, prepare a solution of the appropriate amount of sodium nitrite by dissolving the substance in bidistilled water.

5. Add the appropriate volume of 5% new fuchsin solution according to **Table 3** and allow to react under vigorous agitation for exactly 1 min (use a stopwatch!).
6. Combine the appropriate amounts of solutions A and B, mix well.
7. Add solution C, mix well, adjust to pH 8.8 by dropwise addition of 2 N HCl, filter, control the pH and, if necessary, adjust again to pH 8.8 and add $H_2O$ to the final volume (*see* **Note 12**).
8. Control the AP-substrate solution by mixing an aliquot with a minute amount of APAAP complex solution saved from **Subheading 3.1.2., step 7**.
9. Use the solution immediately, within 5 min, for developing of sections under constant agitation.
10. Wash 3 times with 1X TBS, examine the staining result by microscopy, and proceed with prehybridization.

### 3.1.4. Hybridization Pretreatment for In Situ Hybridization

1. Incubate sections in 0.2 *N* HCl for 10 min at RT.
2. Rinse with depc$H_2O$ and 1X PBS for 30 s each.
3. Incubate in 0.01% Triton X-100 for 90 s at RT (for DNA probes, *see* **Note 13**).
4. Rinse in 1X PBS.
5. Digest with pronase (approx 0.125 mg/mL in 1X PBS, pH 7.2) at RT (*see* **Note 7**).
6. Block pronase with 0.1 *M* glycin in 1X PBS for 30 s at RT.
7. Rinse with 1X PBS for 30 s.
8. Postfix in ice-cold 4% paraformaldehyde for 20 min.
9. Rinse with 1X PBS for 3 min.
10. Acetylate sections with freshly prepared triethanolamine/acetic anhydride for 10 min at RT (*see* **Note 14**).
11. Rinse with 1X PBS.
12. Dehydrate sections through graded ethanols with less than 10 s for each step (*see* **Note 15**).
13. Continue with application of the appropriate probe mixture.

### 3.1.5. DNA/RNA In Situ Hybridization

EBV DNA and RNA *in situ* hybridization protocols are detailed in Chapter 7. To increase probe penetration into tissues, the fragment size should be adjusted to 20–30 bases as follows:

1. Add an equal volume of hydrolysis buffer.
2. Incubate the mixture at 60°C. The hydrolysis time is calculated according to the formula *(10)*
$$t = (L_0 - L_f) / (k \cdot L_0 \cdot L_f),$$
with t = hydrolysis time in min, $L_0$ = initial transcript length, $L_f$ = final transcript length, and the constant $k = 0.11\ kb^{-1} \cdot min^{-1}$.
3. Terminate the reaction by adding an equal volume of stop solution.
4. Precipitate in 70% ethanol for more than 1 h at –70°C, centrifuge, re-dissolve in 10 m*M* DTT and determine the incorporation of [$^{35}$S] by scintillation counting.

Dehydrate sections subjected to *in situ* hybridization with [$^{35}$S]-labeled probes through graded ethanols and air-dry. Autoradiographic detection of bound probes is described in Chapter 7. If desired, use Meyer's hematoxilin for nuclear counterstaining and mount in glycerol gelatin. Transfer sections exposed to digoxigenin-labeled probes to TBS for immunohistology with digoxigenin-specific antibody.

### 3.1.6. Detection of Immobilized Digoxigenated Probe

Typically, this procedure applies to the detection of highly abundant transcripts such as EBER or BHLF1 RNA which are virtually exclusive to the nucleus except for mitotic figures. When alkaline phosphatase has been employed as a tag for the antibody used in the preceding steps of the IH/ISH procedure, peroxidase and 3,3-diaminobenzidine tetrahydrochloride (DAB) chromogen-substrate are a good choice to visualize the bound digoxigenated probe.

1. Block endogenous peroxidase using 3% hydrogen peroxide ($H_2O_2$) in distilled water for 5 min at RT (*see* **Note 16**).
2. Rinse 3 times for 2 min each with 1X TBS.
3. Apply peroxidase-conjugated anti-digoxigenin-$F_{ab}$ fragments in a dilution of up to 1:1000 and incubate for 20 min at RT.
4. Rinse 3 times for 2 min each with 1X TBS.
5. Dissolve 6 mg of DAB in 10 mL of 0.05 *M* Tris-HCl, pH 7.6, add 0.1 mL of 3% $H_2O_2$, filter, apply to the section, and incubate for 5 min at RT (*see* **Note 17**).
6. Rinse with TBS.
7. Counterstain nuclei with Meyer's hematoxilin, if desired, and mount with glycerol gelatin.

## 3.2. Combined ISH-ISH Labeling

For this procedure, sectioning, fixation, labeling of RNA probes, pre-hybridization and hybridization are carried out as described for simple ISH. However, the preparation of the hybridization mixture and the washing sequence differ *(1–3)*.

1. Make up the probe mix with 8 × $10^6$ cpm/mL [$^{35}$S]-labeled RNA probe (equivalent to approx 6 ng/mL) and 100 ng/mL digoxigenated EBER probe keeping the volume as described for [$^{35}$S]-labeled probes (Chapter 7).
2. After hybridization, perform washes including the RNase A step as described in Chapter 7, **Subheading 3.3.3., steps 5–9.**
3. Transfer slides to TBS.
4. Detect digoxignated EBER probe in a single step using an AP-conjugated anti-digoxigenin-$F_{ab}$ fragments (diluted in TBS up to 1:1000) for 20 min at RT.
5. Wash with TBS 3 times for 5 min each at RT.
6. Visualize alkaline phosphatase with new fuchsin as described earlier.
7. Dehydrate through graded ethanols, taking care not to dissolve the new fuchsin precipitates.
8. The slides are ready for autoradiography as described in Chapter 7 (*see* **Note 18**).

## 4. Notes

1. In our experience, autoradiographic silver grains are best documented against the background of a red chromogen. Substrates producing a red-colored product at the site of enzymatic activity are available for both alkaline phosphatase and peroxidase, the most frequently used reporter enzymes in immunohistology. 3-amino-9-ethylcarbazole (AEC) as a substrate for peroxidase results in a bright red product which, similar to fast red for alkaline phosphatase visualization is easily dissolved in ethanol and other solvents,

whereas new fuchsin is more stable and permits dehydration through graded ethanols. We are thus providing a protocol for detection of alkaline phosphatase activity with new fuchsin.

When detecting two targets by nonradioactive methods, the two colors should give a good contrast and should be distinguishable when co-localized. A good contrast is obtained for alkaline phosphatase/new fuchsin (red signal) and peroxidase/DAB (brown signal). However, if the antigen is detected by immunostaining and the nucleic acid is visualized by nonradioactive methods, a mixed color product may arise that is difficult to distinguish if both targets localize to the same cellular compartment. From the technical point of view, this combination has a number of advantages over other substrate combinations and the problem of mixed colors is not important for transcripts with predominantly nuclear localization such as EBER and BHLF1 RNA. This combination is also best for triple-labeling procedures combining IH with radioactive as well as nonradioactive ISH (ISH-ISH) labeling procedures. Moreover, it is compatible with the use of hematoxilin for nuclear counterstaining. We are therefore restricting ourselves to peroxidase and DAB as a second substrate for two-color nonisotopic immunochemistry.

2. IH/ISH dilution buffer is made up under sterile conditions with 10X RPMI 1640 (with phenol red serving as a useful pH indicator, similar buffer solutions will suffice as well), sterile filtered BSA stock solution, heparin, and yeast tRNA. The pH is adjusted to pH 7.5 prior to reaching the final volume with $DEPCH_2O$. Aliquots may be kept frozen.
3. The most commonly applied procedure is the application of ISH subsequent to IH, which requires precautions to be taken to prevent loss of cellular RNA targets. In principle, it is possible to perform the ISH in sequence prior to immunohistology. Many epitopes, however, even when resistant to formalin-fixation and paraffin embedding, do not tolerate the denaturing conditions with high formamide concentrations present during hybridization, and the heat denaturation when detecting DNA or using DNA probes. This results in reduced or, often in case of monoclonal antibodies, loss of reactivity.
4. When immunohistology precedes the ISH labeling step, it is important to protect the cellular RNA from attack of endogenous and exogenous RNases. This is achieved by the addition of yeast-tRNA and heparin to all antibody preparations *(8)*. Moreover, it is equally important to reduce all incubation times to an absolute minimum. In most cases, incubation times of less than 20 min will suffice. If the APAAP procedure is repeated, the incubation periods may be further reduced to 5–10 min.
5. Label the baked and APES-coated glass slides as thoroughly as possible on their frosted area with a lead pencil in order to avoid unnecessary handling later on. Use gloves and take care to remove talcum powder with a sterile towel and $depcH_2O$, because the powder may disturb the immunoenzymatic reactions and may interfere with microscopy, particularly with darkfield illumination.

   Prepare a minimum of three (serial) sections for immunostaining and ISH with the anti-sense probe, at least one section for immunostaining and ISH with the sense (control) probe, and at least one slide for ISH with the anti-sense probe without immunohistology. The latter are developed with the last set of immunostained/anti-sense hybridized slides and permit estimating the background (sense probe) and the loss of cellular target RNA (anti-sense probe) during the course of the immunostaining procedure.
6. Frozen sections should be used immediately for best results. If this is not possible, fix them in ice-cold acetone for 10 min, air-dry, and store at –80°C in air-tight boxes. Boxes (and their contents) should be brought to RT, and sections fixed immediately in ice-cold 4% paraformaldehyde for 20 min prior to assaying.

Best results are obtained with paraformaldehyde-fixed frozen sections. However, this fixation restricts the spectrum of antibodies to those reacting with formalin-resistant epitopes. Some antibodies require extended paraformaldehyde-fixation such as the CD68-antibody PG-M1. When detecting antigens/epitopes sensitive to formalin or paraformaldehyde, sections may be precipitation fixed sequentially in acetone and chloroform for up to 30 min each. The sections are then ready for application of the primary antibody and should never dry out in subsequent immunostaining steps. Paraformaldehyde fixation may then be carried out after the enzymatic development. Unlike paraformaldehyde, acetone and chloroform do not reduce the endogenous RNase activity, so this procedure is not suitable for the subsequent ISH for RNA transcripts with the exception of the highly abundant and stable EBER molecules. The same considerations apply for cytospin preparations.

7. A variety of proteases have been recommended for *in situ* hybridization. In our hands, pronase has given reliable and reproducible results over many years. The concentrations given are meant as a guideline only. It is important to titrate the pronase to establish the conditions which will give the best signal without disrupting tissue morphology. It is possible to vary the pronase concentration, the duration of the digestion, and the temperature. In particular, when the ambient temperature in the laboratory may be variable, it is advisable to use an incubator, e.g., at 37°C. Factors which may effect the outcome of the pronase digestion are type of fixative, length of fixation, and other variables of the embedding procedure.

   Nevertheless, once the optimal pronase digestion conditions have been established, there is very little variation necessary for blocks from the same institution. Currently used concentrations in our laboratories are 0.5 mg/mL for paraffin sections and 0.125 mg/mL for frozen sections and cytospins. Higher concentrations may be required for DNA *in situ* hybridization. To identify an appropriate pronase concentration, digest tissue sections with different pronase concentrations keeping temperature and incubation time constant. Counterstain sections and identify the pronase concentration that visibly starts to damage the tissue; then, use half that concentration.

8. Irradiation of formalin-fixed paraffin sections in citrate buffer using a microwave oven has proved useful for the detection of a variety of antigens. A variety of microwaving conditions have been described including variations in energy, time, or buffer used. Alternatively, domestic pressure cookers may be used. Optimum conditions have to be determined individually in every laboratory. In our hands use of a large volume of citrate buffer (1 L) has proved useful. It requires longer microwave irradiation time than smaller quantities but makes substitution of volume lost through evaporation unnecessary. When placing slides into a beaker for microwave irradiation, make sure they are not stacked too tightly to ensure even distribution of heat.

9. The optimal concentration of the primary antibody in IH/ISH dilution buffer (including heparin, but without the expensive tRNA) has to be determined in preliminary experiments, because heparin nonspecifically binds to and inhibits not only RNase, but also immunoglobulins. For alkaline phosphatase reactions, TBS is used instead of PBS, because phosphate ions inhibit the enzyme.

10. It is recommended to dilute antibodies in TBS containing heat-inactivated serum obtained from the species from which the sectioned tissue was derived. This prevents nonspecific reactivity of secondary antibodies with serum proteins absorbed by the tissue prior to or during fixation. If the primary antibody is not a murine monoclonal antibody, but, e.g., a goat antibody, an additional incubation step ("mousification") is required employing, for

this example, mouse anti-goat immunoglobulin before proceeding with rabbit anti-mouse immunoglobulin and APAAP complex. If the primary antibody is from the rat, commercially available rabbit anti-rat immunoglobulin and rat APAAP complex may be used.

11. The APAAP procedure may be repeated to enhance the sensitivity of the IH procedure by increasing the amount of immobilized enzyme at the site of primary antibody binding. This is performed by incubating the slides with the anti-mouse immunoglobulin and, after washing, with APAAP for 5–10 min each. However, this extended exposure of the sections to endogenous and exogenous RNases may result in weaker autoradiographic signals.
12. The preparation of the new fuchsin substrate as outlined is more laborious than the preparation of the fast red substrate described in Chapter 7, but it results in a more intensively colored product *(11)*. Moreover, new fuchsin is less readily soluble in ethanol and xylene, permitting rapid dehydration through graded ethanols.
13. Treatment with Triton X-100 is optional and in our laboratories is used only for DNA *in situ* hybridization.
14. The mixture of triethanolamine and acetic anhydrid must be prepared fresh immediately before adding it to the sections. Acetylation is believed to reduce background by decreasing nonspecific probe binding to glass. Whether this actually works is uncertain. However, it is included in our protocol for *in situ* hybridization with $^{35}$S-labeled probes. We usually omit this step when working with nonradioactive probes.
15. Concentrated ethanol may remove the azo-dye precipitate, some other substrates are even more sensitive to alcohol. In this case, remove as much of the PBS as possible and proceed directly with the application of the appropriate probe mixture.
16. Alternatively, use a commercial blocking agent. Do not use methanol as this may dissolve the chromogen of the previous immunolabeling steps.
17. DAB is a possible carcinogen. The brown color can be enhanced by treatment with nickel sulfate *(12)*. Buffers must not contain sodium azide, because this will interfere with the enzymatic reaction.
18. When attempting to detect two transcripts localizing to the same cellular compartment, the probe detecting the transcript with the higher copy number should be labeled with digoxigenin, and the other one should be isotopically labeled. If both targets are of sufficiently high copy number to be detected by nonradioactive techniques, two-color immunostaining may be used to detect the immobilized probes if the they do not localize to the same cellular compartment. Target transcripts with predominantly nuclear localization such as EBER or BHLF1 are therefore well-suited for two-color techniques in conjunction with probes detecting cellular RNA transcripts. The cellular RNA with the least abundance should be detected by the sensitive APAAP method and new fuchsin as substrate, and the EBERs are then visualized in a single-step reaction with peroxidase-conjugated Fab fragments specific for digoxigenin. If the detection of both probes involves the application of primary or secondary antibodies of the same animal species, the peroxidase step is carried out with DAB development, the precipitates of which provide sufficient shielding of immune complexes from detection in the subsequent immunostaining procedures. The peroxide has to be washed out completely prior to the akaline phosphatase substrate reaction.

## Acknowledgment

We gratefully acknowledge the cooperation of O. Heinrichs, E. Steinbrecher, T. Spieker, R. Lisner, K. von Ostau, U. Tank, and D. Ung in developing and adapting these methods.

## References


1. Herbst, H., Steinbrecher, E., Niedobitek, G., Young, L. S., Brooks, L., Müller-Lantzsch, N., and Stein, H. (1992) Distribution and phenotype of Epstein-Barr virus-harboring cells in Hodgkin's disease. *Blood* **80,** 484–491.
2. Herbst, H., Foss, H. D., Samol, J., Araujo, I., Klotzbach, H., Krause, H., et al. (1996) Frequent expression of interleukin-10 in Epstein-Barr virus-harboring tumor cells of Hodgkin's disease. *Blood* **87,** 2918–2929.
3. Herbst, H., Samol, J., Foss, H. D., Raff, T., and Niedobitek, G. (1997) Modulation of interleukin-6 expression in Hodgkin and Reed-Sternberg cells by Epstein-Barr virus. *J. Pathol.* **182,** 299–306.
4. Herbst, H., Frey, A., Heinrichs, O., Milani, S., Bechstein, O. W., Neuhaus, P., and Schuppan, D. (1997) Heterogeneity of liver cells expressing procollagen types I and IV in vivo. *Histochem. Cell. Biol.* **107,** 399–409.
5. Spiecher, T. and Herbst, H. (2000) Distribution and phenotype of Epstein-Barr virus-infected cells in inflammatory bowel disease. *Am J. Pathol.* **157,** 51–57.
6. Foss, H. D., Herbst, H., Gottstein, S., Demel, G., and Stein, H. (1996) Interleukin-8 in Hodgkin's disease: preferential expression by reactive cells and association with neutrophil density. *Am. J. Pathol.* **148,** 1229–1236.
7. Voigt, C. F., Peljak, P., Müller-Mai, C., Herbst, H., Fuhrmann, G., and Gross, U. M. (1995) Topography of forming and resorbing cells on endosteal surfaces of the rabbit humerus by double-staining with in situ hybridization and tartrate resistent acid phosphatase-reaction: A new model to study the bone reaction to loading. *J. Mater. Sci. Mater. Med.* **6,** 279–283.
8. Höfler, H., Pütz, B., Ruhri, C., Wirnsberger, G., Klimpfinger, M., and Smolle, J. (1987) Simultaneous detection of calcitonin mRNA and peptide in a medullary thyroid carcinoma. *Virchows Arch* B **54,** 144–151.
9. Cordell, J. L., Falini, B., Erber, W. N., Ghosh, K. A., Abdaluziz, Z., MacDonald, S., et al. (1984) Immunoenzymatic labeling of monoclonal antibodies using immune completes of alkaline phosphatase and monoclonal anti-alkaline phosphatase (APAAP complex). *J. Histochem. Cytochem.* **32,** 219–229.
10. Cox, K. H., deLeon, D. V., Angerer, L. M., and Angerer, R. C. (1984) Detection of mRNAs in sea urchin embryos by in situ hybridization using asymmetric RNA probes. *Dev. Biol.* **101,** 485–502.
11. Stein, H., Gatter, K., Asbahr, H., and Mason, D. Y. (1985) Use of freeze-dried paraffin embedded sections for immunohistological staining with monoclonal antibodies. *Lab. Invest.* **52,** 676–683.
12. Gerdes, J., Van Baarlen, J., Pileri, S., Schwarting, R., Van Unnik, J. A., and Stein, H. (1987) Tumor cell growth fraction in Hodgkin's disease. *Am. J. Pathol.* **128,** 390–393.

# 9

# Detection of EBV Infection at the Single-Cell Level

## *Precise Quantitation of Virus-Infected Cells In Vivo*

**Gregory J. Babcock, Emily M. Miyashita-Lin, and David A. Thorley-Lawson**

## 1. Introduction

The polymerase chain reaction (PCR) has become a powerful tool in the world of molecular biology *(1)*. Using specific oligonucleotides complimentary to a known sequence of DNA in conjunction with Taq DNA polymerase, it is possible to synthesize billions of copies of that DNA from only one starting molecule. The benefits of this technique are numerous. This methodology is especially useful in the study of Epstein-Barr virus (EBV). EBV-infected cells in the peripheral blood of healthy donors are present at very low numbers in the order of 1–50 per $10^6$ B cells *(2)*. Direct detection of these infected cells is essentially impossible without PCR. Therefore, the required PCR reaction must detect 1 EBV-infected cell in a background of $10^6$ uninfected cells to be able precisely and reliably to quantitate the number of infected cells in a given donor.

By using PCR with this sensitivity, in conjunction with limiting dilution analysis, it is possible to quantitate absolute numbers of infected cells in a given population. Poisson statistics can be applied to the limiting dilution analysis yielding a specific number of infected cells contained in the population.

To isolate large numbers of specific cells from a population to test for the presence of EBV, the cells are labeled with subset specific monoclonal antibodies (MAbs). The labeled cells can then be separated using a variety of different procedures including magnetic beads (Dynal *[3]* and MACS *[4]*). We prefer the use of MACS as with this method larger numbers of cells can be isolated in a relatively short period of time and the purity of the positively selected population can be analyzed (not possible with Dynal). Isolated populations can be further subfractionated using fluorescence activated cell sorting (FACS) technology. Although this offers a high degree of specificity it is limited in the number of cells that can be processed. However, in principle any

From: *Methods in Molecular Biology, Vol. 174: Epstein-Barr Virus Protocols*
Edited by: J. B. Wilson and G. H. W. May © Humana Press Inc., Totowa, NJ

cell-fractionation technique that can be applied to the FACS can be used to enrich for the desired population. For example, staining cells with propidium iodide (PI) and the proliferation specific nuclear marker Ki67 has been used to separate resting and proliferating populations of cells with FACS prior to DNA PCR analysis *(5)*. Once a population is isolated and the sensitivity of the PCR optimized (*see* **Note 1**) quantitation of virally infected cells in that population can easily be determined.

## 2. Materials

### 2.1. Isolation of Mononuclear Cells From Peripheral Blood

1. Ficoll-Hypaque (Pharmacia).
2. 60-mL syringe.
3. Heplock buffer: 0.36 g NaCl, 0.0227 g Heparin, made up to 40 mL with distilled $H_2O$.
4. Alcohol swabs.
5. 19G butterfly needle.
6. Cotton pads.
7. Tourniquet.
8. Band-aids.
9. 0.5 *M* acetic acid.
10. 10X PBS: 80 g NaCl, 2 g KCl, 2 g $KH_2PO_4$, 11.5 g $Na_2HPO_4 \cdot 7H_2O$, made up to 1 L with distilled $H_2O$.
11. PBSA buffer: 1X PBS, 0.5% bovine serum albumin (kept ice cold).

### 2.2. MACS Cell Separation for B Cells

1. 10X PBS as in **Subheading 2.1.**
2. PBSA buffer as in **Subheading 2.1.**
3. VarioMACS magnet (Miltenyi).
4. Streptavidin-coated microbeads (Miltenyi).
5. MACS cell separation columns (Miltenyi).
6. 23G and 25G needles.
7. Biotinylated αCD19 antibody (or an alternative B-cell specific antibody).
8. αCD20-FITC antibody (DAKO).
9. FACScan (Beckton Dickinson).

### 2.3. Cell Digestion and DNA Isolation

1. Proteinase K (10 mg/mL).
2. Proteinase K digestion buffer: 0.45% Tween-20, 0.45% NP-40, 2 m*M* $MgCl_2$, 50 m*M* KCl, 10 m*M* Tris-HCl, pH 8.3, 0.5 mg/mL Proteinase K.
3. 96-well V-bottom microtiter plate (Falcon).
4. 55°C Incubator.
5. Rotor for centrifuging microtiter plates.

### 2.4. EBV-Specific PCR

1. 10X PCR buffer: 20 m*M* $MgCl_2$, 500 m*M* KCl, 100 m*M* Tris-HCl, pH 8.3.
2. 10 m*M* dNTP mix: 10 m*M* dATP, 10 m*M* dCTP, 10 m*M* dTTP, 10 m*M* dGTP.
3. 20 pM EM2 primer (CTT TAG AGG CGA ATG GGC GCC A).
4. 20 pM W1 primer (TCC AGG GCC TTC ACT TCG GTC T).
5. Taq DNA polymerase (Perkin Elmer).

6. 200 µL MicroAmp reaction tubes with caps (Perkin Elmer).
7. GeneAmp 9600/2400 thermocycler (Perkin Elmer).
8. BJAB (EBV negative) and Namalwa (EBV positive with 1–2 genomes) cell lines.

### 2.5. Isolation and Southern Blotting of PCR Products

1. Nusieve GTG agarose (FMG).
2. Seakem LE agarose (FMG).
3. 50X TAE: 968 g Tris, 228.4 mL glacial acetic acid, 148.8 g ethylenediamine-tetraacetic acid (EDTA), made up to 4 L with $H_2O$.
4. 6X DNA sample buffer: 0.25% bromophenol blue, 0.25% xylene cyanol, 30% glycerol.
5. Alkalization solution: 350.64 g NaCl, 80 g NaOH, made up to 4 L with $H_2O$.
6. Neutralization solution: 350.64 g NaCl, 484.56 g Tris, adjusted to pH 7.5, made up to 4 L with $H_2O$.
7. 20X SSC: 3506 g NaCl, 1764g Nacitrate, made up to 20 liters with $H_2O$.
8. Salmon sperm DNA (ssDNA) (10 mg/mL).
9. Nytran Plus (Schleicher and Schüll).
10. Polybags (National Bag Co.).
11. Polysealer (National Bag Co.).
12. Random primed DNA labeling kit (Boehringer Mannheim).
13. α-[$^{32}$P] dATP at 3000 Ci/m*M*.
14. α-[$^{32}$P] dCTP at 3000 Ci/m*M*.
15. 100X Denhardts solution: 10 g Ficoll, 10 g BSA, 10 g polyvinylpyrrolidone, made up to 500 mL with $H_2O$.
16. Prehybridization solution: 6X SSC, 1X Denhardts solution, 1% sodium dodecyl sulfate (SDS).
17. Hybridization solution: 6X SSC, 50% formamide, 1% SDS, 2% dextran sulfate.
18. 95% ethanol (ice cold).
19. 5% Trichloracetic acid (TCA, ice cold).
20. 10% TCA acid (ice cold).
21. Vacuum Erlenmyer flask with filter ready top.
22. Whatman filters (934-AH).
23. Wash A: 6X SSC, 0.25% SDS.
24. Wash B: 12X SSC, 0.8% SDS.
25. Kodak X-Omat AR film.
26. 42°C water bath.
27. TE8: 10 m*M* Tris-HCl, 1 m*M* EDTA, pH 8.0.

## 3. Methods

### 3.1. Isolation of Mononuclear Cells from Peripheral Blood

(*see* **Notes 2** and **3**)

1. Prepare a 60-mL syringe by filling it with 3 mL of Heplock buffer.
2. Obtain 60–240 mL of blood by routine venipuncture (*see* **Note 4**).
3. In a 50-mL conical tube, slowly layer 30 mL of blood onto 20 mL of Ficoll-Hypaque (*see* **Note 5**).
4. Centrifuge at 900*g* for 30 min at 25°C.
5. Using a Pasteur pipet under vacuum, aspirate off the top serum phase of the resulting gradient.

6. At the interface of the Ficoll and the serum a white buffy coat of peripheral blood mononuclear cells (PBMCs) should be seen. With a 25-mL pipet, remove the entire buffy coat and transfer to a new 50-mL conical tube.
7. Dilute buffy coats 1:1 in PBSA.
8. Centrifuge at 500*g* for 15 min at 4°C.
9. Pour off the supernatant of all tubes and combine PBMCs to 50 mL with PBSA.
10. To count the cells, dilute 10 µL of the cell suspension in 90 µL of 0.5 *M* acetic acid. This will lyse all red blood cells (*see* **Note 6**).
11. Centrifuge the remaining cells at 400*g* for 10 min at 4°C.
12. Resuspend the cells to $2 \times 10^7$ cells/mL in PBSA.

### 3.2. MACS Separation of B Cells (*see* Note 7)

1. Divide the cells into 1-mL aliquots ($2 \times 10^7$/mL) in microcentrifuge tubes.
2. Add αCD19 antibody to each tube (4 µL for our laboratory produced antibody) (*see* **Note 8**).
3. Incubate on a rotator for 30 min at 4°C (*see* **Note 9**).
4. Centrifuge the cells at 300*g* for 5 min at 4°C.
5. Pour off the supernatant and resuspend the cell pellets in 1 mL of PBSA.
6. Repeat **steps 4** and **5** a total of three times to wash off unbound antibody.
7. Resuspend the pellets in 180 µL of PBSA.
8. Add 20 µL of MACS streptavidin coated microbeads to each tube.
9. Incubate for 10 min at 4°C (*see* **Note 10**).
10. Wash the cells three times in PBSA as described in **steps 4** and **5**.
11. Resuspend the cells in 500 µL of PBSA.
12. Insert the MACS depletion column (AS, BS, or CS) into the VarioMACS magnet with the stopcock and side syringe attached (*see* **Note 11**).
13. Inject 1 column volume of PBSA with the side syringe.
14. Allow the PBSA to flow out of the column into a collection tube.
15. Apply 10 mL of PBSA to the top of the column and allow it to flow through. Now the column is ready for use.
16. Attach a 25G needle to the stopcock at the base of the column.
17. Apply cell suspension to the column and collect the flow through (negative fraction).
18. After all cells have passed over the column, wash the column by applying 3 column volumes of PBSA.
19. Turn the stopcock to the backflush position and remove the column from the magnet.
20. Push 1 column volume of PBSA into the column with the side syringe.
21. Reinsert the column into the magnet, replace the 25G needle with a 23G needle, and allow the column to run once again (*see* **Note 12**).
22. Collect this as your wash fraction.
23. Wash off nonspecifically bound cells by passing 3 column volumes of PBSA over the column.
24. Turn the stopcock to the backflush position and remove the needle from the column.
25. Remove the column from the magnet and inject 1 column volume from the side syringe.
26. Allow the column to run and collect cells by running a total of 10 mL of PBSA through the column (positive fraction).
27. All cell populations, pre column, negative fraction, wash fraction, and positive fraction can be analyzed for purity using a Becton Dickinson FACScan with DAKO αCD20 antibody as described by the manufacturer.

### 3.3. Digestion of B Cells

1. From the number of B cells isolated, you must determine a set of dilutions to use for limiting dilution analysis (*see* **Note 13**).
2. Aliquot appropriate cell numbers to the wells of a V-bottom microtiter plate (*see* **Note 14**).
3. Centrifuge plate at 400*g* for 15 min at 4°C.
4. Aspirate off the supernatant of each well.
5. Add 10 µL of PK digestion buffer to each well.
6. Incubate the plate at 55°C (100% humidity) for more than 2 h. We recommend using only the middle of the plate for samples while the outer wells are filled with water. The plate should also be sealed with tape and an adhesive plate cover (*see* **Note 15**).

### 3.4. EBV-Specific PCR

1. Count the number of samples you have plus negative and positive controls (*see* **Note 16**). This number (X) is used to make a master mix for PCR (*see* **Note 17**).
2. Prepare the master mix as follows: X µL of 10 m*M* dNTP mix, X µL of 20 pM EM2 primer, X µL of 20 pM W1 primer, 5 X µL of 10X PCR buffer, 32 X µL of high-performance liquid chromatography (HPLC) grade $H_2O$.
3. Vortex master mix.
4. Aliquot 8 µL of master mix to the appropriate number of 200 µL microamp reaction tubes.
5. Briefly centrifuge the microtiter plate to collect any condensation.
6. Add 5 µL of each sample from the microtiter plate to the appropriate PCR reaction tube.
7. Heat all at 95°C for 5 min.
8. Prepare the Taq reaction mix as follows:
   4.3 X µL of HPLC grade $H_2O$.
   0.5 X µL of 10 X PCR Buffer.
   0.2 X µL of Taq DNA polymerase.
9. While the tubes are still in the heat block at 95°C, open each one and add 5 µL of Taq reaction mix (*see* **Note 18**).
10. Carry the heating block with the tubes to a thermocycler preheated to 95°C.
11. Place all tubes in the thermocycler, stop the 95°C program and start a program consisting of the following steps: 95°C for 15 s, 66°C for 1 min. Repeat this for a total of 30 cycles followed by one 5-min extension step at 72°C.

### 3.5. Isolation and Detection of PCR Products (see Note 19)

1. In a microcentrifuge tube, add 2 µL of 6 X sample buffer and 10 µL of PCR reaction.
2. Pour a 2% Nuseive GTG agarose, 1% Seakem LE agarose gel in 1X TAE (*see* **Note 20**).
3. Load all PCR samples and run gel at 100 Volts for 1 h in 1X TAE.
4. Wash the gel 2X for 15 min each in alkalization solution to denature the DNA.
5. Wash the gel 2X for 15 min each in neutralization solution.
6. Wash the gel for 10 min in 2X SSC.
7. Wash the gel for 10 min in 5X SSC.
8. Transfer DNA to nytran using the capillary action method, as described by the manufacturer, overnight.
9. Bake nytran at 80°C for 30 min.
10. Place nytran in a plastic bag and add 10 mL of prehybridization solution per 40 $cm^2$ of Nytran.

11. Boil salmon sperm DNA (10 mg/mL) for 10 min to denature and quickly cool on ice.
12. Add denatured ssDNA to the prehybridization bag at a final concentration of 50 µg/mL and seal the bag (*see* **Note 21**).
13. Incubate at 42°C for >3 h.
14. Random prime label purified PCR product (*see* **Note 22**) with α-[$^{32}$P] dATP and α-[$^{32}$P] dCTP as described by the manufacturer (Boehringer Mannheim) (*see* **Note 22**).
15. Add 80 µL of TE8 to the 20 µL labeling reaction and vortex.
16. In order to count the incorporation of label into the probe DNA, place the Whatman filter on top of the erlenmeyer flask under vacuum.
17. Add 1 µL of the labeling reaction to the filter and let dry.
18. Rinse the filter with 10% TCA and let dry.
19. Rinse the filter with 5% TCA and let dry.
20. Rinse the filter with 95% ETOH and let dry.
21. Place the filter in a scintillation counter and obtain the CPM/µL.
22. Cut open the prehybridization bag and pour off the solution.
23. Add 10 mL of hybridization solution per 40 cm$^2$ of Nytran.
24. Boil the labeled probe and ssDNA for 10 minutes and quick cool on ice.
25. Add ssDNA to 50 µg/mL to the blot in the prehybridization solution.
26. Add the probe to $1 \times 10^6$ counts/mL of hybridization solution.
27. Incubate overnight at 42°C.
28. Carefully remove the hybridization solution from the bag.
29. Remove the blot from the bag.
30. Wash the blot 2 times in wash A for 15 min at room temperature.
31. Wash the blot in wash B for 30 min at 42°C.
32. Wrap the blot in plastic wrap and expose to X-Omat AR film at –70°C.

### 3.6. Frequency Calculation

1. Calculate the fraction negative for the presence of EBV at each dilution.
2. Plot the points on semilog graph paper using cell number on the linear scale and fraction negative on the log scale.
3. Where the line intersects 0.37 fraction negative, this cell number contains 1 EBV-infected cell. Extrapolate this number to get the frequency of infected cells per $10^6$ cells (*see* **Note 24**).

## 4. Notes

1. Optimization of this PCR must be done using control cell lines. As an EBV+ cell line, we use Namalwa, which contains only 2 copies of the EBV genome. For a negative control, we use BJAB. For best results, first start by purifying DNA from $1 \times 10^6$ Namalwa cells using SDS/Proteinase K digestion and phenol/chloroform extraction (*see* Chapter 35). Perform serial dilutions on the Namalwa DNA ranging from $1 \times 10^4$ to 1 cell equivalent of DNA. Perform the described PCR on each making sure all can be easily detected. Next, mixing experiments should be performed for 0.5, 1, and 2 Namalwa in a background of $10^6$ BJAB (8 samples at each Namalwa concentration: total of 24 samples). From these results, Poisson statistics can be used to determine if the expected number of positive samples was attained. Another mixing method is to aliquot $10^6$ BJAB into the wells of a microtiter plate and use a cell sorter to distribute 1 Namalwa cell in each well of the plate. Upon testing with PCR, all wells should be positive for the presence of EBV minus the error of the sorter.

2. Always treat blood products as biohazard. Using gloves, lab coat, eye protection, and a laminar flow hood is recommended. All blood product waste should be autoclaved and disposed of appropriately.
3. All protocols done prior to the completion of PCR should be conducted in a designated area that lacks the use of PCR products. This will minimize the chances of getting false positives in your PCR. Trafficking between post-PCR and pre-PCR areas should be avoided at all costs.
4. Blood should always be drawn by a trained phlebotomist.
5. When layering Ficoll, be sure not to mix the blood into the Ficoll. An interface should be maintained at all times.
6. Counting PBMCs can be made difficult if red blood cells are present.
7. All steps during the MACS separation protocol should be performed in the cold room at 4°C. At warmer temperatures, cells internalize antibodies bound to their surface (capping), preventing efficient separation of the desired population.
8. Biotinylated αCD19 antibody should first be titrated before use in the MACS system. This can be done by staining cells with a wide range of antibody concentrations and using streptavidin-PE as a secondary reagent for detection. You should use the least antibody necessary to see staining over background. Always remember that scaling up and down with antibody staining rarely works as you would expect so titrate the antibody in the same volume and same cell concentration as you will use during the real experimental staining.
9. Overincubation with antibody will lead to reduced purity in the positively selected population.
10. Overincubation with beads will lead to reduced purity in the positively selected population.
11. MACS procedures are essentially as described by the manufacturer. For more detail on columns, and stopcock positions see product insert.
12. The lower the gauge of the needle, the faster the column will run. The needles used for depletion and enrichment were chosen to obtain the maximum amount of cells with the greatest purity. The gauge used can be adjusted to suit the purpose of the user. Higher gauge needles result in less purity but better yield, and lower-gauge needles give excellent purity with minimal yield.
13. Dilutions are determined empirically. If the frequency of infected cells in the peripheral blood of a given individual is unknown, we recommend using a wide range of dilutions from $1 \times 10^6$ cells to $1 \times 10^4$ cells with two-fold dilutions in between. Once a frequency is known the dilutions to be used become obvious. Always use a minimum of 8 samples at each dilution to ensure statistical significance in your results.
14. Digestion using this method is more appropriate for primary cells given that it will work with up to $10^6$ cells per well. However, if cell culture cells are to be used, the maximum number distributed in each well should be $10^4$ cells.
15. If the humidity of the incubator is not 100% you will get significant evaporation of your samples.
16. For the PCR, negative controls are $1 \times 10^4$ BJAB cells digested in the microtiter plate along with the samples. For a positive control, we purify DNA from Namalwa cells and make a stock. The DNA from $1 \times 10^3$ Namalwa cells is then used in the PCR reaction for positive control.
17. X should actually be a few greater than the number of samples to be tested to ensure you will have enough reagents for each tube.
18. Once Taq DNA polymerase is added to the tube, it must not be allowed to cool to less than 80°C. If this happens, mispriming of undesired templates will occur. This is a critical step to ensure the performance of the PCR.

19. Once the PCR cycles are complete, never take these samples back to the area in which you purified cells and set up the PCR. This will undoubtably result in PCR contamination. Run gels and work with PCR products far from the area used pre-PCR. Also, never enter the area where pre-PCR work is done immediately after working in the area where PCR products are analyzed.
20. Other concentrations can be used depending on personal preference.
21. Bubbles should never be present in the bag. This will result in areas of the blot where prehybridization or hybridization solution did not contact. To remove bubbles, roll them out with a pipet and seal the bag before the bubbles reenter the blot area.
22. The probe DNA fragment is isolated by performing many PCR reactions on high concentrations of Namalwa DNA. PCR products are then resolved on agarose gels and fragments purified using any one of several methods, such as DEAE paper purification or Qiagen DNA isolation kits.
22. Probe should be labeled exactly as described by the manufacturer. Always follow standard protocols for the handling of radioactivity when using labeling materials.
24. The Poisson distribution is based on the formula $s = e^{-m}$ where s = the fraction negative events observed and m = the expected mean frequency of events. If an average of 1 event is occurring in the samples tested, the fraction negative will be about 0.37. This calculation can be used in any situation. For example, if you have 4 out of 8 samples positive for EBV at $3 \times 10^5$ cells tested, the frequency of EBV-infected cells will be 0.7 in $3 \times 10^5$ or 2.3 in $1 \times 10^6$. When multiple dilutions are tested, calculation of an accurate frequency is performed as follows. Using semi-log graph paper, plot the log of the fraction negative at the specific dilution versus the cell number tested. This should give a straight line through 1 at 0 cells tested. Such a straight line is confirmation that single events (a single genome in this case) are being detected. The error in the measurement can be estimated from the lower and upper boundary of the line. Alternatively, repeat analysis confirms a typical error of 30% *(2)*. For samples with too few signals to calculate an accurate frequency, the result can be expressed as the number of positive samples for the number of cells tested along with a 95% confidence limit based on the Poisson distribution. For example if a total of $10^7$ cells were tested and 1 positive signal was detected, the frequency would be 1 in $10^7$ (95% confidence limit 0.5). Consult a statistics textbook for more details on the application and use of Poisson statistics.

## References


1. Mullis, K., Faloona, F., Scharf, S., Saiki, R., Horn, G., and Erlich, H. (1986) Specific enzymatic amplification of DNA in vitro: the polymerase chain reaction. *Cold Spring Harbor Symp. Quant. Biol.* **51,** 263–273.
2. Khan, G., Miyashita, E. M., Yang, B., Babcock, G. J., and Thorley-Lawson, D. A. (1996) Is EBV Persistence in vivo a model for B cell homeostasis? *Immunity* **5,** 173–179.
3. Lea, T., Vartdal, F., Davies, C., and Ugelstad, J. (1985) Magnetic monosized polymer particles for fast and specific fractionation of human mononuclear cells. *Scand. J. Immunol.* **22,** 207–216.
4. Miltenyi, S., Muller, W., Weichel, W., and Radbruch, A. (1990) High gradient magnetic cell separation with MACS. *Cytometry* **11,** 231–238.
5. Miyashita, E. M., Yang, B., Babcock, G. J., and Thorley-Lawson, D. A. (1997) Identification of the site of Epstein-Barr virus persistence in vivo as a resting B cell. *J. Virol.* **71,** 4882–4891.

# 10

## Detection and Discrimination of Latent and Replicative Herpesvirus Infection at the Single Cell Level In Vivo

**Lisa L. Decker, Gregory J. Babcock, and David A. Thorley-Lawson**

### 1. Introduction

Herpesviruses have two distinct phases to their life cycle. Characteristically, they persist as a latent infection for the lifetime of the infected host. This usually involves a very small number of infected cells in a particular tissue where the virus is present at very low copy number and there is limited or no viral gene expression. The other phase of the life cycle involves replication of the virus to produce infectious virus. This typically involves expression of a large number of genes and high copy numbers of the viral genome, but again can be highly restricted to a small number of cells in a specific location. One characteristic that distinguishes latent and lytic infection is the form of the viral genome. In latently infected cells, the genome is circular, whereas during lytic replication the genome is linear. We have taken a gel technique where linear and circular herpesvirus DNA migrate with known and different mobilities, the Gardella gel *(1)*, and combined it with a highly sensitive DNA polymerase chain reaction (PCR) system (*2,3*, and Chapter 7 in this volume), that can be used to detect a single copy of the viral genome in $10^6$ uninfected cells. The result is a technique that can be used to determine if a single infected cell is present in a tissue sample and distinguish if the cell is latently or lytically infected. This technique has several advantages over other methods that typically involve some form of reverse transcriptase (RT)-PCR, for distinguishing latent from lytic infection. These advantages are:

1. DNA PCR is simpler and less error-prone than RT-PCR.
2. DNA PCR can be quantitated, whereas RT-PCR is not quantitative and usually less sensitive so lack of a signal by RT-PCR cannot be assumed to mean no infection.
3. Latent persistence may not be associated with expression of any specific genes, therefore a negative result from RT-PCR again cannot exclude the possibility of infection. By comparison, the Gardella PCR approach depends only on the presence of the viral genome

From: *Methods in Molecular Biology, Vol. 174: Epstein-Barr Virus Protocols*
Edited by: J. B. Wilson and G. H. W. May © Humana Press Inc., Totowa, NJ

and can be used to detect a single viral copy in $10^6$ cell genomes, therefore a negative signal is indicative of no infection.

4. The Gardella PCR technique requires only that a sequence long enough to perform PCR be known. A positive signal at the correct mobility means there is an intact herpesviral genome present. This method is critical for confirming that a DNA PCR product is derived from intact viral genomes and not from fragments of virions or viral DNA. As such the method is particularly applicable to new herpesviruses that may not have been fully sequenced and for which little or no gene expression is known.

   To perform the technique, intact cells are placed into the sample wells of a standard agarose gel. A mixture of sodium dodecyl sulfate (SDS) and pronase is then electrophoresed through the sample, causing a gentle lysis and release of the DNA, which is fractionated through low-melt agarose. The circular or episomal DNA is large and migrates at the exclusion volume of the gel, whereas linear DNA is able to "snake" through the gel, allowing it to migrate faster. The sample lane from the gel is sliced, DNA extracted from each slice, and DNA PCR for the viral genome performed to detect the genomes. By comparison to standard markers, latently infected cells for episomal DNA and virions for linear DNA, it is possible to identify precisely the slice number where each specific form of the viral genome migrates.

   In summary, this method has general applicability to all herpesviruses for which some DNA sequence is available and allows the unequivocal identification of sites of latent persistence and viral reactivation at the single cell level.

## 2. Materials

### 2.1. Sample Preparation

1. RPMI 1640.
2. 10 x PBS: 80 g NaCl, 2 g KCl, 2 g $KH_2PO_4$, 11.5 g $Na_2HPO_4 \times 7H_2O$, made up to 1 L with distilled $H_2O$.
3. 1X $TBE_{low}$: 8.9 m*M* Tris base, 8.9 m*M* boric acid, and 0.8 m*M* ethylenediaminetetraacetic acid (EDTA).
4. Gardella sample buffer: 20% Ficoll 400 and 0.01% bromophenol blue in 1X $TBE_{low}$.

### 2.2. Gel Preparation

1. IBI model HRH or comparable horizontal gel box and a 20 well 2 mm comb.
2. 4 L of cold 1X $TBE_{low}$ (*see* **Subheading 2.1.**).
3. 20% SDS in 1X $TBE_{low}$.
4. 20 mg/mL self-digested pronase in 1X $TBE_{low}$. Self-digested pronase is prepared by incubating the enzyme for 4 h at 37°C. The enzyme can then be stored in aliquots at –20°C
3. Seakem LE agarose and Seaplaque GTG agarose (FMC, ME).

### 2.3. Generation of Gel Slices

1. Paper template.
2. Sterile razor blades, number 10 scalpels, pipet tips, and microcentrifuge tubes.

### 2.4. Extraction of DNA from Gel Slices

1. 65–70° C and 42° C heat blocks
2. β-agarase and equilibration buffer (FMC).
3. 10 *M* ammonium acetate.

4. 100% and 70% ethanol.
5. Sterile distilled or HPLC water.

## 3. Methods

### 3.1. Sample Preparation

1. Wash up to $2.5 \times 10^6$ cells in 1X PBS or RPMI-1640.
2. Centrifuge at 4°C for 10 min at 200*g*.
3. Aspirate the supernatant and thoroughly, yet gently, resuspend the pellet in 50 µL Gardella sample buffer. Keep cells at 4°C (*see* **Note 1**).

### 3.2. Gardella Gel Preparation (*see* Fig. 1)

1. Set up the gel tray with a comb approx 4 cm from the top of the gel.
2. Pour 300 mL of molten 0.75% Seakem LE agarose into the gel tray and allow it to polymerize. Prepare all agarose with 1X $TBE_{low}$ (*see* **Note 2**).
3. Excise an area of the gel below the wells into which the sample will be electrophoresed (*see* **Note 3**).
4. Replace the excised gel with molten 0.75% Seaplaque agarose and allow polymerization.
5. Excise the agarose above the wells.
6. Prepare the 0.8% Seakem agarose containing 2% SDS and 1 mg/mL pronase. To do this, add 5 mL of 20% SDS to 42.5 mL of molten agarose. Swirl and allow to cool to 50–55°C. Add 2.5 mL of 20 mg/mL self-digested pronase and swirl (*see* **Note 4**).
7. Pipet the Seakem agarose containing SDS and pronase into the area above the wells. Take care not to introduce any bubbles.
8. Once polymerized, immediately place the gel tray into the gel box containing enough cold 1X $TBE_{low}$ to cover the gel.
9. Gently resuspend the cells again by pipetting up and down (*see* **Note 5**).
10. Load the gel and electrophorese for 2–3 h at 40 V followed by 12–18 h at 160 V at 4°C (*see* **Note 6**).

### 3.3. Generation of Gel Slices

1. Rinse the gel while still in the gel tray in 1X $TBE_{low}$ to remove residual SDS and place on ice.
2. Make a paper template of the gel by drawing an outline of the lane(s) (same width as the wells). At 0.5-cm increments, draw lines to denote the slices to be made within the lane(s) (*see* **Note 7**). The template should be positioned under the gel tray.
3. Using the template as a guide, excise the lane(s) using sterile razor blades and slices using sterile scalpels (**Fig. 1**). It is essential to prevent carry-over contamination during this step. To do this, cut the right hand side of the lane, starting with the outermost edge of the well, with four tandemly aligned razor blades. Move the blades, while maintaining their same orientation, to the left hand edge of the well and cut that side. Starting with the bottom of the gel, the area farthest from the comb or wells, make slices using sterile scalpels. At least four scalpels should be used to prevent carry-over contamination: use one for cutting up to the linear region, one through the linear region, one for the region between episomal and linear DNA, and one for the episomal region.
4. Sterile toothpicks or pipet tips can be used to maneuver each slice into a microcentrifuge tube. A different toothpick or pipet tip should be used for each slice.

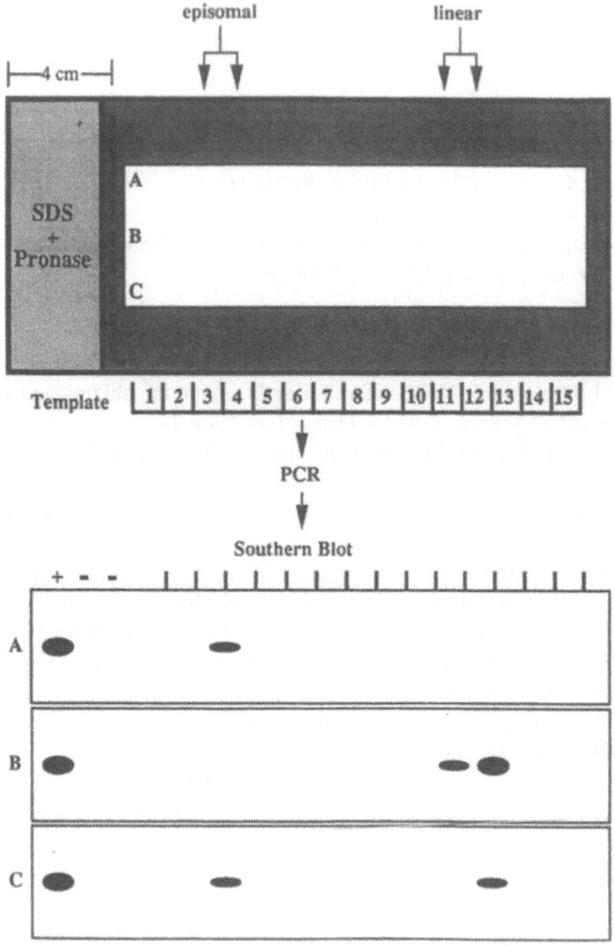


Fig. 1. Diagram of a Gardella gel analysis. An agarose gel (dark shading) is poured in an IBI model HRH horizontal gel box with the sample wells about 4 cm from the top of the gel as shown (upper panel). The region above the wells is excised and replaced with agarose containing SDS and pronase (light shading) and an area below the wells, where the samples are to be run, is excised and replaced with low melting point agarose (white area). Samples containing intact cells are loaded into alternate wells to reduce the chances of cross contamination. The approximate relative migration point following electrophoresis of episomal and linear viral genomes is indicated. Individual lanes are excised and sliced according to the template. The DNA is extracted from each slice and PCR performed for viral sequences followed by Southern blotting for the specific products (lower panel). For every experiment a positive (+) and several negative (–) PCR controls are performed. The location of the experimental samples is indicated by vertical lines. In this example, the expected results for a tightly latent cell, which should only have episomes (**A**), virion DNA, which should only have linear genomes (**B**) and a hypothetical sample with both linear and episomal DNA (**C**), are depicted. Episomal DNA migrates to slice 3–4 and linear DNA to slice 11–12.

### *3.4. Extraction of DNA from Gel Slices* (*see* **Note 9**)

1. Equilibrate the gel slice with 1 mL equilibration buffer for 1 h at room temperature.
2. Decant the supernatant and remove any residual buffer with a pipet.
3. Completely melt the gel slices at 65–70°C for 15 to 20 minutes.
4. Allow the samples to cool on the heat block to 42°C.
5. Add 1 mL of β-agarase to each tube.
6. Vortex and return the samples to the 42°C heat block to digest over night.
7. Briefly spin the samples in a microcentrifuge to collect condensation.
8. Incubate the samples on ice for at least 5 min to precipitate any undigested agarose.
9. Spin the samples in a microcentrifuge for 5 min at 13,000*g* at room temperature.
10. Transfer the supernatant to a fresh microcentrifuge tube.
11. To each sample, add 10 *M* ammonium acetate to a final concentration of 2.5 *M*.
12. Add 2.5 vol of 100% of ethanol to each tube and allow the DNA to precipitate overnight at –20°C.
13. Spin the samples at 13,000*g* for 20 min at 4°C and remove the supernatant.
14. Wash the DNA pellets in 70% ethanol.
15. Repeat **step 13** and allow the DNA to air dry for approx 1 h.
16. Solubilize the DNA in 50 µL of HPLC $H_2O$ overnight at 4°C.
17. PCR specific for the herpesvirus of interest is then performed. In the case of Epstein-Barr virus (EBV) the protocol for detection of a single genome in as many as $10^6$ uninfected cells was originally described in Miyashita et al. *(3)* and Khan et al. *(2)*. An updated version of the protocol is detailed by Babcock et al. in Chapter 7 of this volume (*see* **Note 10**).

## 4. Notes

1. It is imperative to use only fresh cells and tissues to avoid artifactually generating linear viral DNA.
2. To maintain the integrity of the wells, it is advisable not to pour the entire gel with low melting point agarose. The entire gel can be assembled in a cold room to expedite polymerization.
3. When removing the Seakem agarose, cut as close to the wells as possible without destroying them. Use a chopping motion with the razor blade, rather than sliding it along, to help prevent tearing the gel.
4. The Seakem agarose containing the SDS must be cooled to 50–55°C before the pronase is added in order to prevent destroying the enzyme. Once the SDS/pronase gel is set, the Gardella gel must be run immediately to prevent the SDS and pronase from leaching into the buffer.
5. Efficient lysis will only be obtained if the samples are thoroughly resuspended. However, this should be done gently because it is crucial to maintain the integrity of the cells in order to avoid generating artifactual linear DNA. If multiple samples are to be analyzed, load at least every other lane. This will help alleviate problems with cross-over contamination and facilitate the subsequent gel processing steps.
6. The gel must be run at 4°C to help inhibit endogenous nucleases and to prevent the gel from over-heating. Initially, the gel is run at a low voltage to allow the migrating SDS and pronase to lyse the cells. The voltage is then increased to resolve the episomal and linear DNA.
7. Slices made this size will keep the gel volume to a level where microcentrifuge tubes can be used for all subsequent manipulations.
8. Extreme care must be taken during the entire procedure to avoid contaminating the gel and slices with virus or PCR products. The gel should be assembled in an area away from

all sources of contamination. For example, do not work in an area where any of the following have been or are currently in use: constructs containing the region of the virus to be amplified by PCR, PCR products, or purified virus. A separate set of reagents and equipment should be set aside and used only for the DNA PCR-modified Gardella gel analysis (*see* Chapter 7, **Note 19**).

9. This is an adaptation of the β-agarase protocol provided by FMC. Occasionally, residual SDS within the gel slices will inactivate the enzyme and give incomplete digestion. This results in a substantial agarose contamination of the DNA that can inhibit PCR. Best results are obtained if the agarase digestion is begun as soon as the slices are generated (without gel slice storage). If agarose contamination does occur, the samples can be extracted 3 times with phenol and once with chloroform:iso-amyl alcohol (24:1). The DNA can be precipitated as described in **Subheading 3.4., steps 11–16**. Alternatively, if a relatively large number of viral copies are present within the sample (>1000), the slices can simply be melted at 70°C for 15 min and used directly for PCR. However, the reaction cannot contain more than 5–10% of the gel slice.
10. The episomal and linear regions should resolve cleanly, i.e., there should be no viral DNA in the intervening portions of the gel (*see* Fig. 1). There are several reasons why these fractions may not appear to resolve appropriately. If the cells have not lysed efficiently bound protein can alter the migration of the DNA giving rise to a smear in the Gardella gel. This generally occurs if the pronase is old, has lost activity or is from a bad batch. If too much viral DNA is present (>1000 copies), cross-over contamination can become a serious problem if the slices are not properly generated. Finally, the gel may have become contaminated with virus from an exogenous source.

## References

1. Gardella, T., Medveczky, P., Sairenji, T., and Mulder, C. (1984) Detection of circular and linear herpesvirus DNA molecules in mammalian cells by gel electrophoresis. *J. Virol.* **50,** 248–254.
2. Khan, G., Miyashita, E. M., Yang, B., Babcock, G. J., and Thorley-Lawson, D. A. (1996) Is EBV Persistence in vivo a model for B cell homeostasis? *Immunity* **5,** 173–179.
3. Miyashita, E. M., Yang, B., Lam, K. M., Crawford, D. H., and Thorley-Lawson, D. A. (1995) A novel form of Epstein-Barr virus latency in normal B cells in vivo. *Cell* **80,** 593–601.

# III

# Culture Methods

# 11

## Virus Isolation

**Lindsey M. Hutt-Fletcher and Susan M. Turk**

### 1. Introduction

There have been no reports of the direct entry of Epstein-Barr virus (EBV) into a fully permissive lytic cycle in any cell in vitro. Virus does, however spontaneously move from latency into a lytic cycle of replication in a very small percentage of the population of most B-cell lines in culture and this number can, with varying degrees of efficiency, be increased by use of inducing agents. Typically, current production methods involve induction of the lytic cycle in B cell lines and harvest of virus from spent culture medium several days after induction. There are three cell lines that are commonly used for this purpose because they respond well to induction stimuli. These lines are the B95-8 cell line, a marmoset lymphoblastoid cell line transformed by virus obtained from a patient with infectious mononucleosis *(1)*; and two lines derived from Burkitt's lymphoma tissue, the P3HR1 cell line *(2)* and the Akata cell line *(3)*. B95-8 cells and P3HR1 cells are usually induced with phorbol esters, sodium butyrate, or a mixture of the two *(4)*. In addition, replication can be induced in the Akata cell line by crosslinking cell surface immunoglobulin *(5)*.

#### *1.1. Choice of Cell Line*

The choice of cell line is determined by the amounts of virus needed and the purpose to which it is to be put. Both the B95-8 line and the Akata cell line produce transforming virus. The P3HR1 strain virus is transformation defective, but can be used to superinfect cell lines that are latently infected with EBV such as the Raji cell line *(4)*. At one end of the scale, yields of virus are greatest from the Akata cell line, probably because induction mediated by treatment with anti-human immunoglobulin induces a larger percentage of cells to enter the lytic cycle than do treatments with either phorbol esters or butyrate. Induction is also synchronous. However, the Akata strain virus has not been sequenced, as has the B95-8 strain (*6*, and *see* Chapter 1), and for some purposes this may be of consequence. At the other end of the scale, if all that is needed is sufficient virus to derive cell lines from freshly isolated human B cells

From: *Methods in Molecular Biology, Vol. 174: Epstein-Barr Virus Protocols*
Edited by: J. B. Wilson and G. H. W. May © Humana Press Inc., Totowa, NJ

(*see* Chapter 13), culture supernatant from the B95-8 cell line can frequently be used directly without induction and without concentration or purification. Phorbol esters can of course have stimulatory effects on cells and residual anti-human immunoglobulin present in preparations of Akata strain virus may be a potential confounder in some experiments. There may thus be occasions when it is preferable to use the small amounts of virus that can be recovered from the 5–10% of P3HR1 and B95-8 cells that may enter the lytic cycle spontaneously. Most cultures of Akata cells produce negligible amounts of virus without induction.

### 1.2. Concentration and Purification

Over the years several different protocols for concentration of virus from culture media have been used, including filtration and precipitation with polyethylene glycol (PEG). The most straightforward method, which requires only very basic laboratory equipment, is concentration by centrifugation, and although this may result in some loss of viability of virus, it is most appropriate for study of virus structural proteins and for isolation of virion DNA. Virus purification methods are also many and varied, but the most frequently used protocol for isolating enveloped virus, which is described here, involves repeated sedimentation in dextran gradients *(7,8)*.

## 2. Materials

### 2.1. Cell Culture and Induction

1. Complete RPMI medium: RPMI 1640 medium supplemented with 10% heat-inactivated fetal bovine serum (FBS). Penicillin (100 IU/mL) and streptomycin (100 µg/mL) may also be added if desired.
2. 12-*O*-tetradecanoylphorbol-13-acetate (TPA) stock solution: 1 mg/mL in ethanol:acetone 50:50.
3. 1 *M* sodium butyrate stock solution.
4. Affinity purified anti-human immunoglobulin G (*see* **Note 1**).
5. 150-cm$^2$ plastic tissue-culture flasks.
6. 37°C, 5% $CO_2$ humidified incubator.

### 2.2. Concentration

1. 250-mL sterile conical polypropylene centrifuge bottles (Corning).
2. 250-mL polycarbonate centrifuge bottles, which can be decontaminated by immersion in sodium hypochlorite or sterilized in an autoclave.
3. Bacitracin stock solution: 10 mg/mL in water filtered-sterilized by passage through a 0.2 µm-pore filter.
4. High speed centrifuge with rotor that will take 250-mL centrifuge bottles, e.g., Sorvall GSA rotor.
5. 0.8-µm pore filters.
6. RPMI/bacitracin: RPMI 1640 medium supplemented with 100 µg/mL bacitracin.

### 2.3. Purification

1. Dextran T-10 (Pharmacia).
2. TNB buffer: 0.01 *M* Tris-HCl, pH 7.2, 0.15 *M* NaCl, 100 µg/mL bacitracin.

3. 14 × 89-mm thin-wall polyallomer centrifuge tubes.
4. 25 × 89-mm centrifuge tubes.
5. Beckman SW 41 Ti and SW 28 rotors or equivalents.

## 3. Methods

### 3.1. Cell Culture and Induction

1. If the virus is to be concentrated, seed 20 tissue culture flasks with approx 50 mL of a suspension of cells growing in complete RPMI medium at 37°C and an atmosphere of 5% $CO_2$ (*see* **Note 2**). Feed the cells by diluting them 2–3 times/wk until the total volume of confluent cells (approx $1 \times 10^6$/mL) is 200 mL/flask. The last feed of 30–50 mL may be done with RPMI 1640 without FBS and should be done the day before induction so that the viability of the starting culture is high (>90%). Ensure that the cell density never falls below $5 \times 10^5$/mL. If the virus is not to be concentrated but used directly for transformation, much smaller volumes of culture, as needed, can be grown.
2. If P3HR1 or B95-8 cells are to be induced, on day 0 add TPA to a final concentration of 20–30 ng/mL or TPA together with sodium butyrate to a final concentration of 4 m*M* (*see* **Note 3**). Harvest the cells on d 5. Cells that are not induced should be harvested on the fifth day after reaching confluence.
3. If Akata cells are to be induced, pellet the cells in 250-mL sterile conical centrifuge bottles at 200*g* for 10 min. Resuspend the cells pelleted from each 250-mL aliquot in 25 mL complete RPMI medium at $4 \times 10^6$ viable cells per mL and 50 µg/mL anti-human immunoglobulin. Return 50 mL of concentrated cells to each of 8 of the original tissue culture flasks and reincubate them at 37°C. Four hours later, double the volume with complete RPMI medium (*see* **Note 4**) and reincubate the cells (d 0). Harvest the cultures on d 5.
4. To harvest virus from small volume cultures, centrifuge at 800*g* for 10 min at 4° C to remove the cells.
5. Filter the supernatants through a sterile 0.8 µm-pore filter to remove any remaining cells.
6. Aliquot the supernatants containing virus and store them at –80°C.

### 3.2. Concentration

1. Transfer large volume cultures to 250-mL polycarbonate centrifuge bottles (*see* **Note 5**). Centrifuge the cultures at 4000*g* for 10 min at 4°C to pellet the cells. Pour off the supernatants into clean bottles, add bacitracin to a final concentration of 100 µg/mL (*see* **Note 6**) and centrifuge the supernatants again at 16,000*g* for 90 min at 4°C to pellet the virus (*see* **Note 7**).
2. Discard the supernatants and resuspend the pellets in RPMI/bacitracin or, if the virus is to be purified, in TNB. If the virus is to be purified on dextran it is resuspended in 1/100 of the volume of the culture after induction. It can be resuspended at higher concentrations, as desired, if it is not to be layered on dextran gradients.
3. Centrifuge the concentrated virus 2–3 times at 800*g* for 10 min at 4°C to remove any remaining cell debris, discard the pellets. Filter the virus-containing supernatant through 0.8 µm-pore filters to complete removal of the cells.
4. Aliquot the virus and store at –80°C or proceed to the purification procedure.

### 3.3. Purification

1. Make up solutions of 5, 10, 15, and 30% (w/v) dextran in TNB (*see* **Note 8**).
2. Gently layer 2 mL of each dextran solution, beginning with the 30% dextran and proceeding through to the 5% dextran, in a 14 × 89-mm thin-walled polyallomer tube. Although

other tubes can obviously be used if necessary the length and breadth of this particular tube is extremely convenient and provides a good separation of interfaces.

3. Layer no more than 2 mL of concentrated virus in TNB on top of the gradient.
4. Centrifuge the gradient at 76,000*g* for 60 minutes at 4°C.
5. Remove everything down to the 15–30% interface and collect this interface.
6. Transfer the collected material to a centrifuge tube that will hold at least 30 mL and fill the tube with TNB. Pellet the virus at 60,000*g* for 60 min. As an alternative, virus can be dialyzed to remove dextran and pelleted from a smaller volume.
7. Remove and discard the supernatant and resuspend the virus pellet in 1–2 mL TNB.
8. Repeat **steps 1** through **6**.
9. Resuspend the virus pellet in the medium of choice for further use.

## 4. Notes

1. Affinity purified anti-human immunoglobulin can be obtained commercially (e.g., ICN cat. # 55049). It is, however, very expensive and investigators who anticipate a continuous need for large scale virus production might consider making their own. This can be done relatively easily by purifying immunoglobulin G from human serum on a protein A-agarose affinity column, immunizing a rabbit, purifying the rabbit immunoglobulin G on a protein A-agarose affinity column and repurifying the antibody on a column of human immunoglobulin G coupled to a substrate such as Affigel-10. A rabbit immunized with 500 µg of human immunoglobulin G might be expected, after three injections, to yield approx 30 mg affinity purified anti-human immunoglobulin from 15 mL serum.
2. The starting volume of cells to be used obviously depends on the needs of the investigator. The amount given here is merely one that the authors have found to be convenient. However, the relative amounts of anti-human immunoglobulin used and the cell concentrations should be retained for optimal results.
3. The choice to use TPA or TPA and sodium butyrate depends on the behavior of each cell line. It has been the experience of the authors that this is something that has to be determined empirically and cannot be assumed to be same for B95-8 or P3HR1 cell lines from different sources. The efficiency of virus induction is the variable that most affects virus yield and it is not a stable property of any cell line. It is therefore advisable to check the number of cells that are induced within a population before large-scale virus production is attempted. This can be done by inducing small volumes of cells and air-drying samples of induced cells on glass slides at 48 h after induction. Cells should be fixed in ice-cold acetone for 10 min and reacted in an indirect immunofluorescence assay with a monoclonal antibody (MAb) to a late virus protein to ensure as well as is conveniently possible that a complete lytic cycle has occurred. The antibody 72A1 ***(9)***, produced by hybridoma #HB168 from the American Type Culture Collection, is a good choice for this purpose as it reacts with the abundant late glycoprotein gp350/220 and provides an excellent fluorescence signal. If Akata cells have been induced with anti-human immunoglobulin care should be taken to obtain a fluorescein-conjugated second antibody that does not crossreact with the antibody used for induction. If at least 35% of cells are positive for fluorescence by this assay, a reasonable virus yield can be expected, e.g., sufficient to produce enough purified virus DNA for restriction endonuclease digestion and visualization with ethidium bromide.

   If the number of cells that are induced is low, further passage may result in an increased efficiency of induction. In general, however, it has been the experience of these authors that cells kept in continuous culture for periods of 4 or 5 mo or more become more difficult to induce over time. One approach to this problem is to single-cell clone a culture and look for individual clones that are readily induced. The second is to obtain new stock, either from other investigators or from frozen stocks. Whenever a line induces well it is advisable to freeze some cells for this purpose. When such frozen stocks are recovered they may not reach maximal levels of induction for the first 4 or 5 wk in culture, but after this time they will frequently return to the high levels of induction they showed before being frozen.

4. An induced culture of Akata cells starts out on d 0 at a concentration of approx $2 \times 10^6$ cells/mL. This cell number will increase and produces a very dense culture that may give the impression of being contaminated.
5. Concentration of virus can be carried out under sterile conditions if required. There are several brands of 250-mL centrifuge tubes on the market, however, not all are autoclavable.
6. Bacitracin is used to reduce virus aggregation.
7. All the centrifuge tube sizes and centrifugation times can of course be modified using the appropriate formulae to maintain the same separations.
8. The higher concentrations of dextran are difficult to get into solution and may take as long as 1–2 h to dissolve. The amount of dextran required to make the 30% solution has a volume almost equivalent to that of the final solution.

## References

1. Miller, G., Shope, T., Lisco, H., Stitt, D., and Lipman, M. (1972) Epstein-Barr virus: transformation, cytopathic changes, and viral antigens in squirrel monkey and marmoset leukocytes. *Proc. Natl. Acad. Sci. USA* **69,** 383–387.
2. Heston, L., Rabson, M., Brown, N., and Miller, G. (1982) New Epstein-Barr virus variants from cellular subclones of P3J-HR-1 Burkitt lymphoma. *Nature* **295,** 160–163.
3. Takada, K., Horinouchi, K., Ono, Y., Aya, T., Osato, T., Takahashi, M., and Hayasaka, S. (1991) An Epstein-Barr virus-producer line Akata: establishment of the cell line and analysis of viral DNA. *Virus Genes* **5,** 147–156.
4. Kieff, E. (1996) Epstein-Barr Virus and its Replication, in *Fields Virology,* vol. 2, (Fields, B. N., Knipe, D. M., and Howley, P. M., eds.), Lippincott-Raven, Philadelphia, pp. 2343–2396.
5. Takada, K. (1984) Cross-linking of cell surface immunoglobulin induces Epstein-Barr virus in Burkitt lymphoma lines. *Int. J. Cancer* **33,** 27–32.
6. Baer, R., Bankier , A. T., Biggin, M. D., Deininger, P. L., Farrell, P. J., Gibson, T. J., et al. (1984) DNA sequence and expression of the B95-8 Epstein-Barr virus genome. *Nature* **310,** 207–211.
7. Dolyniuk, M., Pritchett, R., and Kieff, E. (1976) Proteins of Epstein-Barr virus. I. Analysis of the polypeptides of purified enveloped Epstein-Barr virus. *J. Virol.* **17,** 935–949.
8. Nemerow, G. R., and Cooper, N. R. (1981) Isolation of Epstein-Barr virus and studies of its neutralization by human IgG and complement. *J. Immunol.* **127,** 272–278.
9. Hoffman, G. J., Lazarowitz, S. G., and Hayward, S. D. (1980) Monoclonal antibody against a 250,000-dalton glycoprotein of Epstein-Barr virus identifies a membrane antigen and a neutralizing antigen. *Proc. Natl. Acad. Sci. USA* **77,** 2979–2983.

# 12

## Generation of Lymphoblastoid Cell Lines (LCLs)

**Teresa Frisan, Victor Levitsky, and Maria Masucci**

### 1. Introduction

Epstein-Barr virus (EBV) is a lymphotropic γ herpes virus. Infection of human B cells with EBV in vitro results in their immortalization and the resulting cell lines are named lymphoblastoid cell lines (LCLs) *(1)*. In these cells, EBV establishes mainly a latent infection, characterized by the expression of a limited number of viral proteins. LCLs express 6 EBV nuclear proteins (EBNA1 to 6), 3 membrane proteins (LMP1, LMP2A, and LMP2B) and two small untranslated nuclear RNA molecules (EBER1 and EBER2) (reviewed in **refs.** *2, 3*). LCLs have the phenotype of highly activated B cells as assessed by expression of activation markers (CD23, CD39), high levels of expression of adhesion molecules (LFA1, LFA3, ICAM1) and MHC class I and II alleles (reviewed in **ref.** *4*). Owing to these characteristics, these cells are highly immunogenic (reviewed in **ref.** *5*) and provide a useful tool for reactivation of EBV-specific cytotoxic T cells (CTLs) in vitro. EBV-transformed LCLs can be obtained by explantation of blood or lymphoid tissues from EBV seropositive individuals without need for exogenous infection *(6)*. In addition, LCLs from EBV seropositive and seronegative donors can be obtained by in vitro infection of peripheral blood mononuclear cells (PBMCs) with EBV. The most commonly used strain for laboratory work is derived from the marmoset cell line B95.8 (*see* Chapter 1 and **ref.** *7*). Production of supernatant from this virus producer cell line is described in **Subheading 3.4.**

### 2. Materials

1. PBMCs obtained by Ficoll/Hipaque isolation from peripheral blood (*see* Chapter 9, **Subheading 3.1.**) or lymphnode biopsies when available (*see* **Note 1**).
2. RPMI 1640 medium (Gibco).
3. RPMI complete medium: RPMI 1640 medium supplemented with 10% fetal calf serum (FCS), 2 m*M* L-glutamine, 100 U/mL penicillin, and 100 U/mL streptomycin.
4. Spent supernatant from the virus producer cell line B95.8 (*see* **Subheading 3.4.**).
5. Cyclosporin A (Sigma).

From: *Methods in Molecular Biology, Vol. 174: Epstein-Barr Virus Protocols*
Edited by: J. B. Wilson and G. H. W. May © Humana Press Inc., Totowa, NJ

6. 48-well plates.
7. 24-well plates.
8. Tissue culture dishes (100 × 10 mm) and bottles (75 $cm^2$).
9. Sterile disposable scalpels.
10. Sterile 3-L flask for cell culture.
11. 37°C, $CO_2$, humidified incubator.

## 3. Methods

### 3.1. Spontaneous LCLs from Peripheral Blood

1. Plate 5–10 × $10^5$ PBMCs per well in a 48-well plate in 0.7–0.8 mL of RPMI complete medium with 0.1 µg/mL Cyclosporin A (*see* **Note 2**). Cultures are maintained in a 37°C, 5% $CO_2$ humidified incubator.
2. Feed the cultures weekly by replacing half of the medium with fresh medium (*see* **Note 2**). After a period of 5–8 wk, foci of EBV transformed B blasts start to grow. When the cultures are growing well (*see* **Note 3**), it is possible to expand the culture from the 48-well plate to 24-well plates and then to 75 $cm^2$ culture bottles.

### 3.2. Spontaneous LCLs from Lymphoid Tissue

1. Coat a 24-well plate with FCS by spreading a drop on the bottom of each well with a sterile Pasteur pipet. Leave the plate open for 10 min to dry (*see* **Notes 4** and **5**).
2. Place the lymphnode biopsy in a sterile tissue culture dish and finely mince it with sterile disposable scalpels into approx 1 $mm^3$ fragments.
3. Place 2–3 fragments in the FCS coated 24-well plates and add 2 mL of RPMI complete medium supplemented with 0.1 µg/mL Cyclosporin A. Culture at 37°C in a 5% $CO_2$ humidified incubator.
4. Feed the cultures weekly by replacing half of the medium with fresh medium containing Cyclosporin A during the first 15 d. After 5–8 wk, colonies of virus-transformed B cells start to grow. To expand the cultures proceed as described in **Subheading 3.1.**

### 3.3. In Vitro B95.8 Transformed LCLs

1. PBMCs infection with the B95.8 EBV strain is achieved by resuspending 3–5 × $10^6$ cells in 3–5 mL of B95.8 spent supernatant for 2 h at 37°C (*see* **Note 1**). $10^6$ cells/mL is the optimal condition for infection, although it is possible to increase this to 2 × $10^6$ cells/mL and, depending on the virus titer, up to $10^7$ cells/mL.
2. Spin down the cells at 1000*g* for 10 min and resuspend the pellet in RPMI complete medium supplemented with 0.1 µg/mL Cyclosporin A.
3. Plate 5 × $10^5$ cells/well in 0.6–0.7 mL medium/well in a 48-well plate. Culture at 37°C in a 5% $CO_2$ humidified incubator.
4. Feed the culture weekly by replacing half of the medium with fresh medium (*see* **Note 2**).
5. After 3–5 wk foci of EBV transformed B blasts start to grow. For expansion of the cultures proceed as described in **Subheading 3.1.**

### 3.4. Production of Supernatant from the B95.8 Virus Producer Cell Line

The marmoset cell line B95.8 is permissive for EBV replication and therefore is a good source of infectious viral particles *(7)*. This cell line grows in RPMI complete medium (*see* **Subheading 3.1.**). Growth in medium with low percentage of FCS favors the spontaneous activation of the lytic cycle and consequently virus production is higher.

1. Culture the B95.8 cells at a seeding concentration of $0.5 \times 10^6$ cells/mL in 1 L of RPMI incomplete medium (RPMI complete medium with 2% FCS instead of 10% FCS) at 37°C in a 5% $CO_2$ humidified incubator for 2 wk.
2. Collect the cell culture in a sterile bottle and keep the virus stock at 4°C (*see* **Note 6**).
3. The quality of the virus stock is usually evaluated by its efficiency to infect the EBV-negative cell line BJAB *(8)*. Viral infection is evaluated as percentage of EBNA-positive cells.

## 4. Notes

1. 20 mL of peripheral blood from an EBV seropositive donor are sufficient for isolating PBMCs to establish spontaneous and in vitro B95.8 transformed LCLs.
2. Cyclosporin A is essential to avoid T cell-mediated responses against EBV infected B cells. It is recommended to maintain Cyclosporin A in the medium for the first 15–21 d of culture.
3. It is important not to split the culture too early, because cell concentration is very important for cell growth, therefore just replace half of the medium twice a week and disaggregate the cell clumps by pipetting. When you see formation of big cell clumps and the culture medium turns yellow owing to the metabolic activity of the cells it is possible to expand the culture as described.
4. The FCS coating allows the biopsy fragments to adhere at the bottom of the well. In this way it is also possible to obtain autologous fibroblasts.
5. It is important to work using sterile techniques in order to avoid bacterial or fungal contamination.
6. Because the majority of the viral particles are retained inside the cells, do not discard the cell debris because this can reduce the viral titer.

## References


1. Pope, J. H., Horne, M. K., and Scott, W. (1968) Transformation of foetal human leucocytes in vitro by filtrate of a human leukemia cell line containing herpes-like virus. *Int. J. Cancer* **3,** 857–866.
2. Farrell, P. J. (1995) Epstein-Barr virus immortalizing genes. *Trends Microbiol.* **3,** 105–109.
3. Ring, C. J. A. (1994) The B cell-immortalizing functions of Epstein-Barr virus. *J. Gen. Virol.* **75,** 1–13.
4. Rickinson, A., Murray, R., Brooks, J., Griffin, H., Moss, D., and Masucci, M. (1992) T cell recognition of Epstein-Barr virus associated lymphomas, in *A New Look at Tumor Immunology,* vol. 13 (McMichael, A. and Franks, L., eds.), CSHL Press, New York, pp. 53–80.
5. Masucci, M. G. and Ernberg, I. (1994) Epstein-Barr virus adaptation to a life within the immune system. *Trends Microbiol.* **2,** 125–130.
6. Nilsson, K., Klein, G., Henle, W., and Henle, G. (1971) The establishment of lymphoblastoid lines from adult and fetal human lymphoid tissue and its dependence on EBV. *Int. J. Cancer* **8,** 443–450.
7. Miller, G. and Lipman, M. (1973) Release of infectious Epstein-Barr virus by transformed marmoset leukocytes. *Proc. Natl. Acad. Sci. USA* **70,** 190–194.
8. Menezes, J., Leibold, W., Klein, G., and Clements, G. (1975). Establishment and characterization of an Epstein-Barr virus (EBV)-negative lymphoblastoid B-cell line (BJAB) from an exceptional EBV-negative African Burkitt's lymphoma. *Biomedicine* **22,** 276–284.

# 13

# Cell Cycle Distribution of B-Lymphocytes and Cell Lines

**Alison J. Sinclair**

## 1. Introduction

Epstein-Barr virus (EBV) is able to override the mechanisms that normally regulate the proliferation of human B-lymphocytes. In the absence of other extracellular signals, EBV infects resting B-lymphocytes and drives the infected cells into the cell-division cycle. Recently, there has been much interest in defining the molecular mechanisms by which EBV reprograms the cell cycle control machinery in B-lymphocytes *(1–19)*.

This chapter will deal with three cell-cycle methods that are widely used to detect changes in cell-cycle control. Although the protocols are specifically described for primary B-lymphocytes, lymphoblastoid cell lines (LCLs), and B-lymphoma-derived cell lines, they can be readily adapted for the analysis of cell-cycle control in other cell types. The protocols allow for the identification of proliferating cells, comparisons between the rate of proliferation of different populations of cells and the identification of the proportion of cells within distinct phases of the cell cycle. None of these methods on their own are sufficient to fully describe a change in cell cycle control and two or more are frequently combined within an investigation. For example, if a decreased rate of DNA synthesis (identified by thymidine incorporation assays) is observed in combination with an increase in the proportion of cells in the G0/G1 phase of the cell cycle (identified by propidium iodide [PI] staining/fluorescence-activated cell sorting [FACS] analysis), it suggests that cells have arrested in the G1 phase, implying that a G1 cell-cycle checkpoint has been activated.

### *1.1. Distribution of Cells Within the Cell Cycle*

The DNA content within a cell changes during the cell division cycle from a 2 n content in both quiescent (G0) cells and during G1-phase, to between 2 n and 4 n during DNA synthesis (S-phase). The 4 n DNA content is maintained during G2-phase until mitosis (M-phase) is complete and the cells return to a 2 n content (**Fig. 1**).

From: *Methods in Molecular Biology, Vol. 174: Epstein-Barr Virus Protocols*
Edited by: J. B. Wilson and G. H. W. May © Humana Press Inc., Totowa, NJ

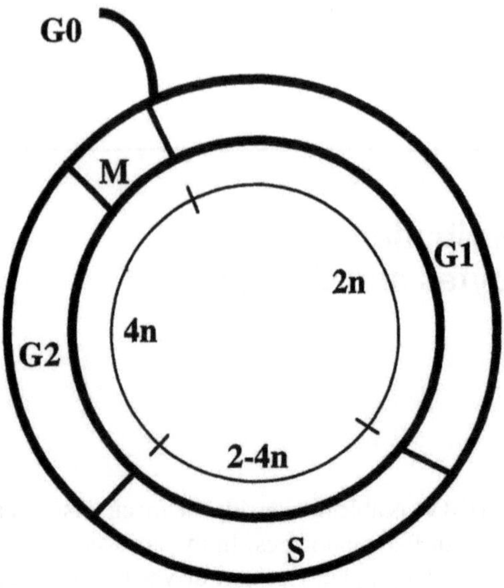


Fig. 1. The phases of the mammalian cell cycle. The phases of the mammalian cell cycle are shown, together with the DNA content present in each phase.

The distribution of cells between these phases can be readily determined using FACS analysis *(20,21)*. A fluorescent DNA binding dye, such as PI, is used to stain the DNA within a population of cells. The cells are then applied to a FACS analyzer where the fluorescent dye is excited by a laser and the deflected and emitted light are collected by a series of detectors. The resulting data is stored in the form of list mode data that typically contains between 3 and 9 pieces of information for each particle that passes through the FACS analyzer. Generally information is collected for between 2,000 and 10,000 particles for each analysis. The signals originating from cells as opposed to debris are identified by their characteristic forward and side light scattering properties and this subgroup can be gated electronically for further analysis. The emitted light is proportional to the DNA content of a cell and when the information for the subpopulation is plotted as a histogram, a profile is obtained of the number of cells with distinct DNA contents (**Fig. 2**). Calibration with a cell type of known DNA content, such as quiescent (G0) human lymphocytes, identifies the location of the 2 n signal. From this information, the location of the 4 n DNA content can be estimated with any signals between representing cells with a DNA content between 2–4 n.

### 1.2. Rate of DNA Synthesis

The rate of DNA synthesis within a population of cells can be readily measured using a radioactive analog of thymidine, Me[$^3$H] thymidine, which is incorporated into cellular DNA during replication. The theory underlying the technique is simple, Me[$^3$H] thymidine is added to the culture medium and after a defined period of time the cells are harvested onto filter mats, lysed with water, and washed extensively to

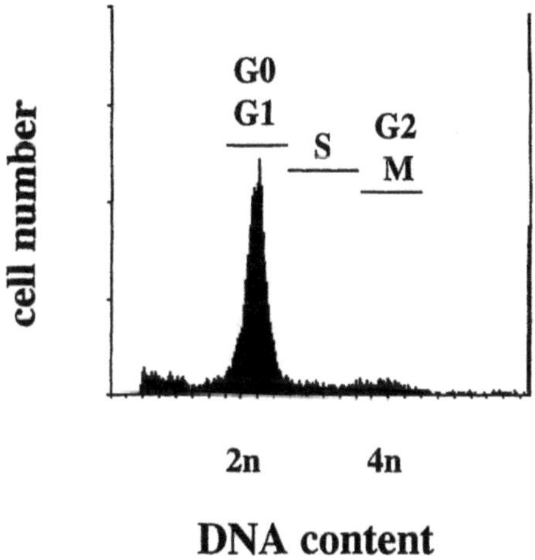


Fig. 2. DNA histogram of an EBV-immortalized LCL. The cells were stained with PI as described in **Subheading 3.1.** and analyzed on a Coulter FACS analyzer. The proportion of cells in the various phases of the cell cycle was estimated manually applying gates to the 2 n, 4 n, and 2–4 n populations as shown.

remove any "free" Me[$^3$H] thymidine. The Me[$^3$H] thymidine which has been incorporated into DNA and trapped on the filter is then quantitated by liquid scintillation counting. This technique has two major advantages over FACS analysis, (1) the sensitivity of the technique is such that it requires few cells (between 1 and $5 \times 10^4$ cells per sample) and (2) multiple samples can be analyzed simultaneously using a 96-well plate format and a semi-automatic cell harvester.

### 1.3. Estimating the Proportion of Proliferating Cells

This technique is a variation on the Me[$^3$H] thymidine incorporation assay described above. An antigenically distinct analog of thymidine, 5 Bromo-2'-deoxy-uridine (BrdU), is used to mark cells that are actively synthesizing DNA *(22)*. BrdU is added to the cell-culture medium for a defined period of time, then the cells are harvested onto glass slides and fixed. The next step is to identify the cells that have incorporated BrdU using a specific antibody. This requires cellular DNA to be accessible to the antibody and a variety of techniques have been used to achieve this.

These use either acidic conditions combined with elevated temperatures or enzymatic digestion and both approaches are thought to generate areas of single-strand DNA, which are accessible to the antibody. The use of fluorescent-labeled monoclonal antibodies to BrdU allows the percentage of positive cells to be readily determined.

## 2. Materials

### 2.1. Distribution of Cells within the Cell Cycle

1. Cell fixation solution: 80% (v/v) ethanol, store at 4°C.
2. PBS: 0.8% (w/v) NaCl, 0.02% (w/v) KCl, 0.144% (w/v) $Na_2HPO_4$, 0.024% (w/v) $KH_2PO_4$, pH 7.0.

3. PI stain: 100 µg/mL propidium iodide, 0.1% (v/v) Triton X-100 in PBS, the solution is light-sensitive, store at 4°C.
4. RNase A: 2 mg/mL in PBS, heat to 70°C for 20 min, then store at 4°C.
5. FACS, e.g., available from Beckton Dickinson or Coulter.

### 2.2. Rate of DNA Synthesis

1. Me[$^3$H] thymidine at 4 Ci/mmol, 1 µCi/µL.
2. Semi-automatic multichannel cell harvester, e.g., available from Skatron or Dynatech.
4. Filter mats for cell harvester, e.g., available from Skatron or Dynatech.
5. Multipurpose scintillation cocktail and liquid scintillation counter set for [$^3$H] e.g., Beckman LS6000 set on channels 0–400.
6. 96-well tissue culture plates.
7. Complete tissue culture medium (appropriate to cell type in use).

### 2.3. Estimating the Proportion of Proliferating Cells

1. BrdU: 10 m*M* 5-Bromo-2'-deoxy-uridine in PBS, store in aliquots at –20°C.
2. Glass slides: pre-cleaned with ethanol.
3. BrdU cell fixation solution: 70% (v/v) ethanol in 50 m*M* glycine, pH 2.0, store at –20°C.
4. Nuclease/anti-BrdU cocktail: 150 U/mL of *Eco*RI, 300 U/mL of exonuclease III, FITC-conjugated anti-BrdU antibody (dilution as recommended by the manufacturer), in 66 m*M* Tris-HCl, 0.66 m*M* $MgCl_2$, 1 m*M* 2-mercapto-ethanol, 1.0% (v/v) fetal calf serum (FCS), pH 8.0. Prepare fresh for each experiment.
5. Cell staining box: 15 × 10 cm plastic box with airtight lid, add paper tissues to base and approx 10 mL of sterile $H_2O$. Insert a small rack to lay the slides on.
6. PBS: *see* **Subheading 2.1.**
7. Mounting medium: 1.0% (w/v) DABCO in 90% (v/v) glycerol and 1X PBS, pH 8.5, store in the dark.
8. Fluorescence microscope: e.g., Zeiss axiphot with camera attachment.
9. 24-well tissue culture plates.
10. FCS: fetal calf serum.
11. Complete tissue culture medium (appropriate to cell type in use).

## 3. Methods

### 3.1. Distribution of Cells within the Cell Cycle

1. Harvest 1 × $10^6$ cells by centrifugation at 100*g* for 5 min.
2. Remove the medium and resuspend the cell pellet in the residual medium by gentle vortexing.
3. Add 1 mL of cell fixation solution and leave at 4°C for a minimum of 1 h (*see* **Note 1**).
4. Harvest cells by centrifugation at 100*g* for 5 min.
5. Remove the cell-fixation solution and resuspend the cell pellet in the residual solution by gentle vortexing.
6. Add 300 µL of PI stain and 5 µL of RNase A, then leave in the dark at room temperature for at least 30 min (*see* **Note 2**).
7. Resuspend cells by vortexing (*see* **Note 3**).
8. Analyze cells by FACS according to the manufacturer's guidelines using a laser emitting at 488 nm.
9. Forward and side scatter information can be used to exclude debris from the analysis.

10. PI bound to DNA has a peak emission maximum at 639 nm ***(20)***, which can be detected after passage through a 600 nm long-pass filter on the FL-2 and FL-3 detectors (Beckton Dickinson FACS) or the PMT-3 and PMT-4 detectors (Coulter FACS).
11. The proportion of cells with a DNA content of 2 n (the G0 and G1 populations), 4 n (the G2 and *M* populations) and 2–4 n (the S-phase population) can be determined using the manufacturer's software or by manually applying gates to the regions (*see* **Fig. 1**).

### 3.2. Rate of DNA Synthesis

1. For each sample, aliquot 200 µL of cells, in triplicate, in culture medium into three wells of a 96-well plate.
2. Prepare a dilution of Me[$^3$H] thymidine in culture medium, for example 20 µL of Me[$^3$H] thymidine added to 5 mL of culture medium is sufficient for one 96-well plate. Add 50 µL to each well. The final concentration of Me[$^3$H] thymidine in the labeling reaction is 0.8 µCi/mL.
3. Incubate at 37°C for between 1 and 4 h.
4. Harvest the cells onto filter mats 12 wells at a time, using a semi-automatic multichannel cell harvester. Wash with water for 1 min and allow the filter mats to air dry.
5. Mark the filter mats into 1 cm$^2$ grids corresponding to the location of the samples and excise the sample areas. Transfer each to a scintillation vial and add 5 mL of multipurpose scintillation cocktail.
6. Leave the vials in the dark for 12–24 h then determine the incorporation of Me[$^3$H] thymidine by the cells by counting the vials in a liquid scintillation counter set for [$^3$H].
7. Express the data as Me[$^3$H] thymidine incorporated per hour per cell.
8. Calculate the mean value and standard deviation for each sample from the triplicate values (*see* **Note 4**).

### 3.3. Estimating the Proportion of Proliferating Cells

1. For each sample, aliquot 1 mL of cells, in triplicate, in cell culture medium into three wells of a 24-well plate.
2. Prepare a dilution of bromodeoxyuridine (BrdU) in cell-culture medium, for example 25 µL of 10 m*M* BrdU added to 2.5 mL of culture medium is sufficient for one 24-well plate. Add 100 µL to each well. The final concentration of BrdU in the labeling reaction is 10 µ*M*.
3. Incubate at 37°C for between 1 and 4 h.
4. Harvest cells by centrifugation at 100*g* for 5 min.
5. Remove the cell-culture medium and resuspend the cells gently in the residual medium with a vortexer.
6. Suspend cells in 100 µL PBS supplemented with 1% (v/v) FCS. Apply 10 µL of the cell suspension as a drop to a 5 mm diameter area on each of two slides and allow to air dry (up to eight samples can be added to each slide).
7. Fix the cells by immersing the slides in BrdU cell fixation solution at –20°C for 30 minutes (*see* **Note 5**).
8. Wash the slides for 5 min in 100 mL of PBS. Repeat the wash twice more.
9. Add 100 µL of either the nuclease/anti-BrdU antibody cocktail or a nuclease only cocktail to the duplicate slides. Place the slides in the staining box in a 37°C incubator to create a warm, humid environment for between 30 and 60 min and process in parallel.
10. Wash the slides for 5 min in 100 mL of PBS. Repeat the wash twice more.
11. Add 20 µL of mounting medium to the cells and apply a coverslip.

12. View with a fluorescence microscope using phase contrast. Photograph three representative areas for each sample, first with white light to visualize the total cell population, followed by UV light to visualize the BrdU positive cells (*see* **Note 6**).
13. Count the number of BrdU positive cells and the total number of cells in a given field of view and calculate the percentage of the population that are BrdU positive.

## 4. Notes

1. Cells can be left in cell fixation solution for up to 3 mo at 4°C.
2. Cells can be left in PI stain for up to 1 wk at 4°C.
3. Clumps of cells can be disrupted by gentle mixing with a vortexer or by passing them through a 17G needle attached to a 1-mL disposable syringe.
4. The assays are usually performed in triplicate for each growth condition and/or cell type. For proliferating LCLs, 1,000–10,000 cpm of Me[$^3$H] thymidine are typically incorporated by $1 \times 10^5$ cells under these conditions.
5. Immunodetection of incorporated BrdU requires partial denaturation of cellular DNA in order to expose the incorporated BrdU. This can be achieved using further acid treatment, however, in our experience few lymphocytes survive the process, whereas the enzymatic digestion described here is more reliable. Kits containing cocktails of enzymes and antibodies are available from both Boehringer Mannheim and Amersham.
6. Incorporated BrdU appears as grainy spots within the nucleus. Cells that were not incubated with BrdU should always be included in the analysis as negative controls.

## References


1. Sinclair, A. J., Palmero, I., Peters, G., and Farrell, P. J. (1994) EBNA-2 and EBNA-LP cooperate to cause G0 to G1 transition during immortalization of resting human B lymphocytes by Epstein-Barr virus. *EMBO J.* **13,** 3321–3328.
2. Sinclair, A. J. and Farrell, P. J. (1995) Methods to study Epstein-Barr virus and p53 status in human cells, in *Methods in Molecular Genetics 7,* Academic Press, Orlando, FL, pp. 89–100.
3. Sinclair, A. J. and Farrell, P. J. (1995) Host cell requirements for efficient infection of quiescent primary B-lymphocytes by Epstein-Barr virus. *J. Virol.* **69,** 5461–5468.
4. Sinclair, A. J., Palmero, I., Holder, A., Peters, G., and Farrell, P. J. (1995) Expression of cyclin D2 in EBV positive Burkitt's lymphoma cell lines is related to methylation status of the gene. *J. Virol.* **69,** 1292–1295.
5. Allday, M. J., Sinclair, A. J., Parker, G., Crawford, D. H., and Farrell, P. J. (1995) Epstein-Barr virus efficiently immortalises human B cells without neutralising the function of p53. *EMBO J.* **14,** 1382–1391.
6. Allday, M. J., Inman, G. J., Crawford, D. H., and Farrell, P. J. (1995) DNA-damage in human B-cells can induce apoptosis, proceeding from G(1)/S when p53 is transactivation competent and G(2)/M when it is transactivation defective. *EMBO J.* **14,** 4994–5005.
7. Cannell, E. J., Farrell, P. J., and Sinclair, A. J. (1996) Epstein-Barr-virus exploits the normal-cell pathway to regulate Rb activity during the immortalization of primary B-cells. *Oncogene* **13,** 1413–1421.
8. Hollyoake, M., Stuhler, A., Farrell, P., Gordon, J., and Sinclair, A. (1995) The normal-cell cycle activation program is exploited during the infection of quiescent B-lymphocytes by Epstein-Barr-virus. *Cancer Res.* **55,** 4784–4787.
9. Palmero, I., Holder, A., Sinclair, A. J., Dickson, C., and Peters, G. (1993) Cyclins D1 and D2 are differentially expressed in human B-lymphoid cell lines. *Oncogene* **8,** 1049–1054.

10. Cayrol, C. and Flemington, E. (1996) G(0)/G(1) growth arrest mediated by a region encompassing the basic leucine-zipper (bzip) domain of the Epstein-Barr-virus transactivator zta. *J. Biol. Chem.* **271,** 31,799–31,802.
11. Cayrol, C. and Flemington, E. K. (1996) The Epstein-Barr-virus bZip transcription factor Zta causes G(0)/G(1) cell-cycle arrest through induction of cyclin-dependent kinase inhibitors. *EMBO J.* **15,** 2748–2759.
12. Chen, W. and Cooper, N. R. (1996) Epstein-Barr virus nuclear antigen 2 and latent membrane protein independently transactivate p53 through induction of NF-κB activity. *J. Virol.* **70,** 4849–4853.
13. Floettmann, J. E., Ward, K., Rickinson, A. B., and Rowe, M. (1996) Cytostatic effect of Epstein-Barr-virus latent membrane protein-1 analysed using tetracycline-regulated expression in B-cell lines. *Virology* **223,** 29–40.
14. Jiang, W. Q., Szekely, L., Wendel-Hansen, V., Ringertz, N., and Klein, G. (1991) Co-localisation of the retinoblastoma protein and the Epstein-Barr virus encoded nuclear antigen EBNA-5. *Exp. Cell Res.* **197,** 41–51.
15. Kempkes, B., Spitkovsky, D., Jansendurr, P., Ellwart, J. W., Kremmer, E., Delecluse, H. J., et al. (1995) B-cell proliferation and induction of early G(1)-regulating proteins by Epstein-Barr-virus mutants conditional for EBNA2. *EMBO J.* **14,** 88–96.
16. Kitay, M. K. and Rowe, D. T. (1996) Protein-protein interactions between Epstein-Barr virus nuclear antigen-LP and cellular gene products: binding of 70kD heat shock proteins. *Virology* **220,** 91–99.
17. Kitay, M. K. and Rowe, D. T. (1996) Cell-cycle stage-specific phosphorylation of the Epstein-Barr-virus immortalization protein EBNA-LP. *J. Virol.* **70,** 7885–7893.
18. Szekely, L., Pokrovskaja, K., Jiang, W. Q., Selivanova, G., Lowbeer, M., Ringertz, N., et al. (1995) Resting B-cells, EBV infected B-blasts and established lymphoblastoid cell lines differ in their pRb, p53 and EBNA-5 expression patterns. *Oncogene* **10,** 1869–1874.
19. Szekely, L., Selivanova, G., Magnusson, K. P., Klein, G., and Winman, K. G. (1993) EBNA-5, an Epstein-Barr virus encoded nuclear antigen binds to the retinoblastoma and p53 proteins. *Proc. Natl. Acad. Sci. USA* **90,** 5455–5459.
20. Omerod, M. G. (1994) *Flow Cytometry.* BIOS Scientific Publishers, Oxford.
21. Robinson, J. P. (1993) *Handbook of Flow Cytometric Methods.* Wiley-Liss, Inc., New York, NY.
22. Gratzner, H. G. (1982) Monoclonal-antibody to 5-bromodeoxyuridine and 5-iododeoxyuridine: a new reagent for detection of DNA-replication. *Science* **218,** 474–475.

# 14

# Introduction of Plasmid Vectors into Cells Via Electroporation

**Ann L. Kirchmaier**

## 1. Introduction

When studying the contributions of Epstein-Barr virus (EBV) to tumorogenesis, it is often advantageous to analyze the effects of the expression of one viral protein on the host cell separately from the effects of other viral proteins that are being concurrently expressed during a normal infection. Electroporation is a method of introducing a plasmid expressing the viral protein of interest into cells and, for long-term studies, generating cell lines that stably express that viral protein. This chapter will present strategies for: 1) optimizing electroporation conditions for a given cell line, 2) determining the efficiency of transfection of that cell line under those optimized conditions, and 3) selecting for cell lines that stably maintain the introduced DNA. A method for determining the susceptibility of cell lines to drug selection—a prerequisite for generating cell lines stably maintaining a desired DNA and expressing a desired protein—will also be described.

Electroporation is the process of using a high-voltage discharge to permeablize reversibly cell membranes. This method can be used to introduce foreign DNA into mammalian cells. An electroporator generally consists of an external DC power supply, one or more capacitors that can be connected in parallel by switches, a switch to allow the charged capacitor(s) to discharge, a discharge current-limiting resistor, one or more timing resistors that can also be connected in parallel by switches (or a potentiometer to vary the resistance), a monitoring system such as an oscilloscope, and a sample chamber. The capacitor(s) can be charged using the power supply and subsequently discharged through a sample chamber containing the cells plus DNA resuspended in an appropriate buffer. The operator can adjust the size of capacitance by opening or closing switches that connect multiple capacitors in parallel. Similarly, the operator can adjust the pulse length by opening or closing switches that connect the timing resistor(s) in parallel.

From: *Methods in Molecular Biology, Vol. 174: Epstein-Barr Virus Protocols*
Edited by: J. B. Wilson and G. H. W. May © Humana Press Inc., Totowa, NJ

The electric field across the chamber during electroporation can be monitored with an oscilloscope. The voltage waveform is the pattern of rise and exponential decay of voltage as the capacitors discharge. The rise time is the time required for the voltage to reach 90% of its peak value. The fall time is the time required for the voltage to fall to 37% of its peak value (the time required for the voltage to decay to 1/e [e = 2.718; the base of natural logarithms] of its peak value). The fall time is determined by the total resistance of the electroporator (the resistance from the sample chamber itself plus the resistance from the potentiometer) multiplied with the capacitance with which it is in parallel. The fall time can be controlled by varying the capacitance and by using a potentiometer to vary the resistance through the circuit. Changing the fall time affects the amount of time that the cells are exposed to an electric field. Too short a fall time could result in transient pore formation, which is insufficient to allow large DNA molecules to enter cells, whereas too long a fall time will result in the permeability of the membranes becoming irreversible and will subsequently lead to cell death. The voltage peak and fall times obtained will depend on both the electronic configuration of the electroporator used as well as the resistance provided by the sample chamber itself. For example, a 1 cm sample chamber containing 0.5 mL of 1X PBS will have a resistance of 200 ohms. The voltage selected on the electroporator will not necessarily correspond to the voltage measured across the sample upon electroporation. Therefore, when attempting to reproduce conditions of electroporation for a given cell line between electroporators from two different sources, the investigator should identify the voltage peak measured across the sample in the first machine and reproduce those conditions on the second machine. If the internal resistance and the resistance across the sample chamber for the first electroporator are known, then the voltage peak for any given voltage setting on that electroporator can be calculated using the formula $Vp = Vo \times Rc/(Rc + Ri)$ where Vp is the voltage peak, Vo is the voltage setting on the electroporator, Rc is the resistance across the chamber, and Ri is the internal resistance of the electroporator. Similarly, if one knows the internal resistance and the chamber resistance for the second machine, one can calculate the voltage setting for the second electroporator required to reproduce the voltage peak observed on the first electroporator. Thus, when reporting conditions of electroporation used, one should always state the voltage peak and the fall time of the discharge wave form, not the instrument settings. (For a detailed description of instrumentation available for electroporation and the theory of electroporation, consult **refs. *1–6***).

When optimizing electroporation conditions for a given cell line, one must take into account both the efficiency of transfection (the uptake and expression of DNA) and the efficiency of survival of cells following electroporation ***(3)***. As the voltage applied to the sample chamber increases, the percentage of cells surviving electroporation decreases ***(3)***. The optimal electroporation conditions should reflect a balance between transfection efficiency and cell survival. The percentage of cells that survive electroporation is also affected by the solution used to resuspend cells and DNA during electroporation. For example, the percentage of cells surviving electroporation is generally greater for cells electroporated in complete tissue culture medium plus buffering agent than it is for cells electroporated in complete tissue culture medium alone (B. Sugden, personal communication). Cells resuspended in complete tissue culture medium during electroporation are more likely to survive than those resuspended in phosphate-buffered saline (PBS) *(3)*. Therefore, electroporation of cells resuspended in complete tissue culture medium plus a buffering agent is recommended.

The amount of input DNA required for a given level of gene expression varies between cell lines. In addition, the linear response of increased protein expression relative to increases in input DNA varies among cell lines *(3)*. In fact, increasing the amount of DNA introduced into cells does not necessarily result in a corresponding increase in the amount of protein expressed. The introduction of large amounts of DNA into cells can sometimes specifically inhibit the expression of the reporter gene itself. For example, introduction of amounts of effector DNA encoding latent membrane protein-1 (LMP-1) that leads to its expression at physiological levels or higher can inhibit transcription from a reporter gene in a dose-dependent manner *(17)*. Additionally, some investigators have found that introduction of high concentrations of one DNA inhibits expression of a second DNA and interpreted the inhibition to result from competition for limiting cellular factors that act in *trans* *(7)*. Thus, a wide range of DNA concentrations should be tested when optimizing electroporation conditions.

When studying gene expression, investigators should be aware that the method of transfection itself can potentially affect gene expression in recipient cells. Electroporation of some cell lines derived from EBV-positive Burkitt's Lymphomas, including Raji, EB1, and EB2, results in a transient reduction of the production of endogenous LMP-1 mRNA and a corresponding transient decrease in the expression of LMP-1 protein *(8)*. Transient expression of endogenous *Bam*HI H leftward reading frame 1 (BHLF 1) is reduced following electroporation as well, whereas the level of Epstein-Barr viral nuclear antigen 2 (EBNA-2) mRNA is unaffected. In contrast, the expression of LMP-1 is not affected by electroporation in the lymphoblastoid cell lines 721, B95-8 and GM2783. This transient decrease in expression of LMP-1 in some cell lines also occurs when DNA is transfected into cells using cationic lipids *(8)*. Therefore, if electroporation of a reporter gene that is known to function under certain conditions results in the lack of expression of that reporter gene, one should consider the possibility that the transfection procedure itself has adversely affected gene expression. However, in general, electroporation serves as an efficient means of introducing foreign DNA into cells that are often otherwise resistant to transfection.

## 2. Materials

### 2.1. Culture and Preparation of Cell Lines for Electroporation

1. Appropriate complete tissue-culture medium: For example, for 143B cells *(9)*, DMEM-HG, 10% calf serum, 0.2 mg/mL streptomycin sulfate, 200 U/mL penicillin G potassium. Store at 4°C.
2. PBS: 0.137 *M* NaCl, 2.7 m*M* KCl, 5.4 m*M* $Na_2HPO_4$, 1.8 m*M* $KH_2PO_4$. Adjust pH to 7.4 and filter through a 0.2-μ filter.
3. 1X trypsin: dilute 10X trypsin (Gibco-BRL, containing 0.5% trypsin, 5.3 m*M* ethylenediaminetetraacetic acid [EDTA]-4Na) in PBS. Filter through a 0.2-μm filter and store at 4°C.
4. TCM-H: Add 1/20 vol of 1 *M* HEPES (*N*-2-hydroxyethylpiperazine-*N'*-2-ethanesulfonic acid, Gibco BRL cat. no 15630-080 or equivalent), pH 7.4–7.6, to complete tissue culture medium, giving a final concentration of 50 m*M* HEPES. Store at 4°C.

5. 1X Trypan Blue: 0.4% Trypan Blue in PBS. Filter through a 0.2-µm filter (*see* **Note 1**).
6. 1X Eosin Y: 0.1% Eosin Y, 0.2% sodium azide in PBS. Filter through a 0.2-µ filter.
7. 70% ethanol.
8. Tissue-culture flasks or dishes, e.g., 15-cm dishes (Flacon 3025 or Corning 430599), 24-well cluster dishes (1.5-cm diameter wells, Corning 3526), 60-mm gridded dishes (Corning 430196).
9. 50-mL conical tubes.
10. Hemocytometer.
11. 37°C, $CO_2$ humidified incubator.

### 2.2. Determining Transfection Efficiency of Cell Lines

1. Fixative: 1% glutaraldehyde, 100 m*M* $NaPO_4$, pH 7.0, 1 m*M* $MgCl_2$. Store at 4°C.
2. 1 *M* $K_4Fe(CN)_63H_2O$. Store at –20°C, thaw at 70°C.
3. 0.5 *M* $K_3Fe(CN)_6$. Store at –20°C, thaw at 70°C.
4. 20% X-gal. Store at –20°C.
5. X-gal cleavage buffer: 10 m*M* phosphate, pH 7.0, 150 m*M* NaCl, 1 m*M* $MgCl_2$, 3.3 m*M* $K_4Fe(CN)_6 \cdot H_2O$, 3.3 m*M* $K_3Fe(CN)_6$, 0.2% X-Gal. Make fresh for each experiment.
6. 70% glycerol in PBS or 10% glycerol in PBS (for adherent or suspension cells, respectively).

### 2.3. Drug Selection for Introduced Plamids and Cloning Selected Colonies

1. Hygromycin B: 10 mg/mL stock solution in PBS. Adjust pH to 8.0 with glacial acetic acid (drop by drop, to approximately 0.2% acetic acid). Filter through a 0.2-µm filter. Store at 4°C.
2. G418-Sulfate (Geneticin, Gibco-BRL): 100 mg/mL stock solution in PBS Filter through a 0.2-µm filter. Store at 4°C.
3. Purimycin: 1 mg/mL stock solution in PBS. Filter through a 0.2-µm filter. Store at 4°C.
4. Whatman 3 MM paper, cut into 0.5-cm squares, autoclaved.
5. 70% ethanol.
6. 3.7% formaldehyde in PBS.
7. 0.14% methylene blue in 100% ethanol.

## 3. Methods

### 3.1. Determining Cell Survival and the Transfection Efficiency of Cell Lines Following Electroporation; Optimizing the Parameters

1. Harvest the cells during exponential growth (*see* **Note 2**). For attachment-independent cells, transfer the cells in medium directly into a 50-mL conical tube. For attachment-dependent cells, remove the medium and wash the cells with PBS. Remove the PBS, then wash the cells with 1X trypsin. Remove the trypsin and incubate for approx 1 min (*see* **Note 3**). Add complete tissue-culture medium to resuspend the cells and to inactivate the trypsin. Transfer the cells in medium into a 50-mL conical tube.
2. Determine the number of viable cells by diluting a small aliquot (for example 100 µL) into 1X Trypan Blue or 1X Eosin Y in PBS and counting live (dye-excluding) vs dead (dye-absorbing) cells using a hemocytometer.
3. Pellet the cells by centrifugation at 270*g* for 10 min. Remove the medium.
4. Wash the cells with 10 mL of PBS and pellet cells as in **step 3**; remove the PBS.

5. Resuspend the cells to $1 - 2 \times 10^7$ viable cells/mL in TCM-H.
6. To a 0.5-mL aliquot of cells ($5 \times 10^6 - 1 \times 10^7$) add 10 µg of purified plasmid DNA such as CMV-βgal (CMV-βgal contains the β-galactosidase gene driven by the CMV promoter *[10]*) or an equivalent reporter plasmid (*see* **Notes 4–6**) and vortex briefly to mix.
7. Prior to electroporation, rinse the cuvets three times with $H_2O$ to clean and two times with 70% ethanol to sterilize and allow to dry in a laminar flow hood. Alternatively, after the second ethanol wash, wash cuvets three times with sterile 1X PBS, remove PBS, and use cuvets immediately (*see* **Note 7**).
8. Transfer the cells plus DNA to the sample chamber and electroporate (*see* **Note 8**).
9. Incubate the cells from one electroporated sample in 20 mL of complete tissue-culture medium in 15-cm dishes or flasks appropriate for adherent or suspension cells, respectively. Allow the cells to grow in a humidified incubator at 37°C and in 5% $CO_2$ for 24 h.
10. After electroporation, rinse the cuvets three times with $H_2O$ to remove any remaining DNA and cells. Soak the cuvets for several hours in $H_2O$, if necessary. Rinse cuvets two times with 70% ethanol and store for future re-use.
11. Following 24 h incubation, harvest and count viable cells as described in **steps 1–3**. Resuspend the cells to $1 \times 10^6$ cells/mL in fresh complete tissue culture medium.
12. Replate the cells at $1 \times 10^5$ and $5 \times 10^5$ cells per 60-mm gridded dish (or flasks for suspension cells) in 5 mL of complete tissue-culture medium. Incubate in a humidified incubator at 37°C and in 5% $CO_2$ for 24 h.
13. For attachment-dependent cell lines, remove the medium from the plate and wash the cells with 5 mL of PBS. Remove the PBS. *See* **steps 18–22** for attachment-independent cell lines.
14. Fix the cells by adding 2 mL of fixative to the plate and incubating for 15 min at room temperature. Remove the fixative.
15. Wash the cells with PBS and remove the PBS. Overlay the cells with 2 mL of X-gal cleavage buffer and incubate for 30 min to overnight at 37°C, depending on the cell line, to detect β-galactosidase expression (*see* **Note 9**) *(11)*.
16. Remove the X-gal cleavage buffer and rinse the cells with PBS. Overlay the cells with 2 mL of 70% glycerol in PBS and store at 4°C until ready to count the cells.
17. Count all of the blue and the white cells in each of 10 squares (6 $mm^2$) for each replicate of each sample and determine the percentage of blue cells present using a phase contrast or a light microscope without a filter. The percentage of blue cells detected reflects the transfection efficiency of the cell line under the electroporation conditions tested (*see* **Note 6**).
18. For attachment-independent cells, harvest, count, and pellet the cells by centrifugation at 270*g* for 10 minutes as described in **steps 1–3**. Resuspend the cells to $1 \times 10^6$ cells/mL in PBS.
19. Place a couple of drops of suspended cells on a glass slide. Allow the slide to dry.
20. Incubate the slide with the attached cells in fixative for 15 min at room temperature. Remove the fixative and rinse the slide with PBS.
21. Incubate the slide in X-gal cleavage buffer for 30 min to overnight at 37°C, depending on the cell line (*see* **Note 9**). Remove the X-gal cleavage buffer and rinse the slide with PBS.
22. Overlay the cells with a few drops of 10% glycerol in PBS. Count the cells as described in **step 17**.

### 3.2. Determining Susceptibility of Cell Lines to G418, Hygromycin B or Purimycin.

1. Harvest the cells during exponential growth and count the cells as described in **Subheading 3.1., steps 1–3**. Resuspend attachment-independent cell lines to $1 \times 10^4$ cells/mL of

complete tissue-culture medium and seed 1 × $10^4$ cells per well in a 24-well cluster dish. For attachment-dependent cell lines, plate the cells at a density of 1–5% confluency per well in a 24-well cluster dish in 1 mL of complete tissue-culture medium (approx $10^3$–$10^4$ cells/well, depending on the cell line).

2. In duplicate, add increasing concentrations of the drug of interest to each well. For G418, generate final concentrations of 0, 50, 100, 200, 300, 400, 500, 750, 1000, 1500, 2000, and 2500 µg/mL in complete tissue-culture medium. For hygromycin B, generate final concentrations of 0, 50, 100, 150, 200, 300, 400, 500, 600, 700, 800, and 1000 µg/mL in complete tissue-culture medium. For purimycin, generate final concentrations of 0, 0.1, 0.3, 1, 3, and 10 µg/mL in complete tissue-culture medium.
3. Incubate the cells in the drug at 37°C in a 6% $CO_2$ humidified incubator for 14–21 d for G418 and hygromycin B and for 4 d for purimycin and monitor the growth of the cells every second day. Cells plated in the absence of drug or in low concentrations of drug will proliferate over the course of the experiment and may eventually die owing to overcrowding and the concomitant depletion of nutrients from the medium (*see* **Note 10**).
4. Identify the lowest concentration of drug that is toxic to cells resulting in the death of all of the cells in the duplicate wells.
5. Use the next higher concentration of drug when generating stable cell lines as described in **Subheading 3.3.** (*see* **Note 11**).

### 3.3. Generating Cell Lines That Stably Maintain Introduced DNA

1. Harvest and wash the cells during exponential growth and count the cells as described in **Subheading 3.1., steps 1–4.**
2. Resuspend the cells at a concentration of 2 × $10^7$ cells/mL in TCM-H.
3. To 0.5 mL of suspended cells add 5–10 µg of cesium chloride-purified DNA of the plasmid of interest (*see* **Notes 4, 6,** and **12**), mix, transfer to cuvets (*see* **Subheading 3.1., step 4**), and put on ice. Electroporate using the conditions optimized as described in **Subheading 3.1.**
4. Incubate the cells from one electroporated sample in 20 mL of complete tissue-culture medium in 15-cm dishes or flasks appropriate for adherent or suspension cells, respectively. Allow the cells to recover and grow at 37°C in a 6% $CO_2$ humidified incubator for 24–48 h.
5. Harvest and count the cells as described in **Subheading 3.1., steps 1–3**. Resuspend the cells to 1 × $10^6$ cells/mL in complete tissue culture medium containing the appropriate concentration of the drug (as determined in **Subheading 3.2.**).
6. For attachment-dependent cells, plate the cells at 1 × $10^2$, 1 × $10^3$, 1 × $10^4$, 1 × $10^5$, and 1 × $10^6$ cells/10- or 15-cm dish in complete tissue-culture medium containing drug. After 14 to 21 d of selection, remove the medium and wash the plate with PBS. Inspect the plates to identify those containing individual colonies of at least 0.5 cm in diameter. If only smaller colonies (< 3 mm) are present, incubate the plates in medium containing drug for 2–4 more d prior to picking colonies.
7. Mark the location of the colonies to be picked, on the back of the tissue-culture plate. Sterilize a pair of forceps by dipping it in 70% ethanol and then in PBS. Use the forceps to pick up a piece of sterile Whatman paper cut into 0.5-cm squares. Dip the Whatman paper in 1X trypsin and place it on a marked colony.
8. After approx 1 min, pick up the Whatman paper (and attached cells from the colony) and transfer it to a well of a 24-well cluster dish containing 2 mL of complete tissue-culture

medium containing drug. Sterilize the forceps as described above prior to picking the next colony. Pick 10–20 drug-resistant colonies in total.

9. To determine the efficiency of colony formation, fix the remaining colonies on the plates by incubating in 10 mL of 3.7% formaldehyde for 10 min. Remove the formaldehyde. Stain with 0.14% methylene blue for 5 min, wash two times with 10 mL of water, and allow to drain and dry. Count the colonies and calculate the efficiency in terms of colonies/mg of input DNA (*see* **Note 12**).
10. For attachment-independent cells, seed 10–20 replicates of the following dilutions of cells; $1 \times 10^0$, $1 \times 10^1$, $1 \times 10^2$, $1 \times 10^3$, and $1 \times 10^4$ cells per well of a 24-well cluster dish in complete tissue-culture medium containing drug. After 14–21 d of selection, determine the well seeded at the highest dilution that contains growing cells. Transfer the cells from this well into a 10- or 15-cm tissue-culture dish and expand the cell line. As this method of generating cell lines is based on limiting dilutions, one may wish to subclone the drug resistant cell line by repeating this step to ensure that the cell line generated is clonal in origin (*see* **Note 13**).

## 4. Notes

1. Trypan Blue has to be filtered frequently to remove aggregates that accumulate and can be mistaken for cells.
2. Cells must be in their log phase of growth prior to electroporation for optimum and reproducible results. Therefore, grow cells to only 50–90% confluency prior to harvesting for electroporation.
3. Some tightly adherent cells may require longer incubation at 37°C to detach. This can be judged by gently shaking the culture dish and examining the cells under a microscope. Cells should float away from the dish surface.
4. The quality of DNA used during electroporation can dramatically affect experimental results. The use of CsCl-gradient purified DNA for electroporation is strongly recommended. One should take care to remove ethidium bromide from DNA prior to electroporation because ethidium bromide contaminated DNA is toxic to cells and will adversely affect assay results.
5. When optimizing electroporation conditions, the uptake of and expression from the reporter plasmid DNA of interest can be monitored through means other than that described in **Subheading 3.1.** For example, expression of a reporter gene driven from a constitutive promoter can be monitored using luciferase assays ***(12)***, CAT assays ***(13,14)***, green fluorescent protein (GFP) ***(15)***, indirect immunofluorescence ***(3)***, or quantitative Western blots ***(16)***.
6. In order to optimize the amount of DNA to be used in electroporation (**steps 1–22**), repeat the protocol varying the amount of reporter DNA electroporated into cells in **step 6**. For different cell lines, the range of linear response to increasing amounts of input DNA may vary. Similarly, for a given cell line, the absolute amount of different reporter plasmids or reporter and effector plasmid combinations required for a given signal may vary.
7. Do not allow the PBS to dry in the cuvets or the salt concentration of the sample will be adversely affected.
8. The heat generated owing to the resistance across the sample chamber during electroporation can reduce cell survival. Cooling the sample in the sample chamber by incubating on ice prior to and during electroporation can minimize this effect.
9. The time of incubation in X-gal cleavage buffer required for efficient staining of cells varies with each cell line. During staining, some cell lines will leach the signal from

β-galactosidase/X-gal to neighboring cells. This can be prevented by either plating fewer cells per plate, so that neighboring cells do not touch each other or by incubating in X-gal cleavage buffer for shorter periods of time.

10. This type of cell death is not owing to the toxic effects of the drug used in the experiment.
11. For example, for 143B cells grown in the presence of increasing concentrations of hygromycin B, after 21 d of incubation in hygromycin B, cell survival can be detected at 50 µg/mL hygromycin B, but no cell survival is detected in 100 µg/mL hygromycin B. Therefore, when generating 143B-based cell lines that maintain a reporter plasmid encoding hygromycin B, the cells are grown in complete tissue-culture medium containing 150 µg/mL hygromycin B.
12. When generating drug-resistant cell lines using oriP-based plasmids (under conditions where EBNA-1 is expressed from either the parental cell line itself or the oriP-based plasmid), drug-resistant colonies will be generated approx 10- to 100-fold more efficiently than with other DNAs, which require the integration of the input DNA into the chromosome for maintenance.
13. The drug-resistant cell lines generated can then be expanded and screened for the stable expression of the protein of interest encoded by the input DNA or screened for the maintenance of the input DNA as a plasmid or as DNA integrated into the host chromosome. Not all drug-resistant colonies will express the protein of interest from the input DNA (e.g., integration may have occurred within the open reading frame of the encoded protein). Also, not all cell lines generated using oriP-based plasmids will necessarily contain those DNAs as plasmids.

## Acknowledgments

I thank Tim Bloss, Donata Oertel, and Bill Sugden for their helpful comments on this manuscript. I also thank Daniel Yee for sharing his expertise regarding the electronic configuration of instrumentation used for electroporation. This endeavor was supported by Public Health Service Grants CA-22443 and CA-07175 in the laboratory of Bill Sugden at the McArdle Laboratory for Cancer Research, University of Wisconsin Medical School, Madison, WI.

## References.

1. Hofmann, G. A. (1995) Instrumentation, in *Methods in Molecular Biology, vol. 48, Animal Cell Electroporation and Electrofusion Protocols* (Nickoloff, J. A., ed.), Humana Press, Totowa, NJ, pp. 41–59.
2. Hui, S. W. (1995) Effects of Pulse length and strength on electroporation efficiency, in *Methods in Molecular Biology, vol. 48, Animal Cell Electroporation and Electrofusion Protocols* (Nickoloff, J. A., ed.), Humana Press, Totowa, NJ, pp. 29–40.
3. Knutson, J. C. and Yee, D. (1987) Electroporation: Parameters affecting transfer of DNA into mammalian cells. *Anal. Biochem.* **164,** 44–52.
4. Neumann, E., Schaefer-Ridder, M., Wang, Y., and Hofschneider, P. H. (1982) Gene transfer into mouse lyoma cells by electroporation in high electric fields. *EMBO J.* **1,** 841–845.
5. Potter, H., Weir, L., and Leder, P. (1984) Enhancer-dependent expression of human κ immunoglobulin genes introduced into mouse pre-B lymphocytes by electroporation. *Proc. Natl. Acad. Sci. USA* **81,** 7161–7165.
6. Weaver, J. C. (1995) Electroporation theory, in *Methods in Molecular Biology, vol. 48, Animal Cell Electroporation and Electrofusion Protocols* (Nickoloff, J. A., ed.), Humana Press, Totowa, NJ, pp. 3–28.

7. Brady, J. and Khoury, G. (1985) trans activation of the simian virus 40 late transcription unit by T-antigen. *Mol. Cell. Biol.* **5,** 1391–1399.
8. Gahn, T. A. and Sugden, B. (1993) Marked, transient inhibition of expression of the Epstein-Barr virus latent membrane protein gene in Burkitt's lymphoma cell lines by electroporation. *J. Virol.* **67,** 6379–6386.
9. Bacchetti, S. and Graham, F. L. (1977) Transfer of the gene for thymidine kinase to thymidine kinase-deficient human cells by purified herpes simplex viral DNA. *Proc. Natl. Acad. Sci. USA* **74,** 1590–1594.
10. Schleiss, M. R., Degnin, C. R., and Geballe, A. P. (1991) Translational control of human cytomegalovirus gp48 expression. *J. Virol.* **65,** 6782–6789.
11. Lim, K. and Chae, C.-B. (1989) A simple assay for DNA transfection by incubation of the cells in culture dishes with substrates for beta-galactosidase. *BioTechniques* **7,** 576–579.
12. de Wet, J. R., Wood, K. B., DeLuca, M., Helinski, D. R., and Subramani, S. (1987) Firefly luciferase gene: Structure and expression in mammalian cells. *Mol. Cell. Biol.* **7,** 725–737.
13. Gorman, C. M., Moffat, L. F., and Howard, B. H. (1982) Recombinant genomes which express chloramphenicol acetyl transferase in mammalian cells. *Mol. Cell. Biol.* **2,** 1044–1051.
14. Sleigh, M. J. (1986) A nonchromatographic assay for the expression of the chloramphenicol acetyltransferase gene in eukaryotic cells. *Anal. Biochem.* **156,** 251–256.
15. Zhang, G., Gurtu, V., and Kain, S. R. (1996) An enhanced green fluorescent protein allows sensitive detection of gene transfer in mammalian cells. *Biochem. Biophys. Res. Comm.* **227,** 707–711.
16. Kirchmaier, A. L. and Sugden, B. (1997) Dominant-negative inhibitors of EBNA-1 of Epstein-Barr virus. *J. Virol.* **71,** 1766–1775.
17. Sandberg, M. L. A. and Sugden, B. (2000) Latent membrane protein 1 of Epstein-Barr virus inhibits as well as stimulates gene expression. *J. Virol.* **74,** 9755–9761.

# 15

# Malignant Transformation and Immortalization Assays in Animal Cells Transfected with the BARF1 Gene

**Tadamasa Ooka**

## 1. Introduction

Epstein-Barr virus (EBV) is associated with both lymphoma (for example, Burkitt's lymphoma) and epithelial carcinoma (for example, nasopharyngeal carcinoma). Among about 90 genes encoded by the virus *(1)*, seven latent genes—(Epstein-Barr viral nuclear antigen 1 (EBNA1), EBNA2, EBNA3A, EBNA3C, latent membrane protein 1 (LMP1), and EBERs—were found to be indispensable for B cell immortalization *(2)*. LMP1 induces malignant transformation in rodent cell lines such as Rat-1 cells *(3)* and Balb/c3T3 cells *(4)*, whereas EBNA1 was recently reported to induce lymphomas in transgenic mice *(5)*. An early lytic viral gene, BARF1, was identified to have oncogenic activity in a rodent fibroblast cell line *(6)* and in the human B cell line, Louckes *(7)*.

With regard to epithelial cells, at least three genes, LMP1 *(8)*, *Bam*HI-A reading frame 0 (BARF0) *(9,10)*, and BARF1 *(11)* may be involved in immortalization and/or malignant transformation. A 40 kb subgenomic region of EBV DNA has been implicated in epithelial cell immortalization *(12)* and this region includes the BARF1 and BARF0 genes. In particular the BARF1 gene and the 40 kb subgenomic region are transcriptionally expressed in NPC tumor epithelial cells. Moreover, the BARF1 gene and the 40 kb fragment were shown to be capable of immortalizing primary monkey kidney epithelial cells *(12–14)*.

In order to demonstrate the oncogenic activity of a gene, several approaches are needed to fulfil the criteria of transformation and/or immortalization phenomena. First the gene under study must be cloned into an appropriate expression vector. This must then be transfected into primary or nontumorigenic cell lines. Subsequently, several tests may be done to determine if the cells are phenotypically changed as a consequence of the gene's expression. Parameters that can be examined include cell growth rate, adherence independent growth capacity (in soft agar), growth at low-cell concentration, serum dependence, morphological change and tumorigenicity in vivo. Moreover, pres-

From: *Methods in Molecular Biology, Vol. 174: Epstein-Barr Virus Protocols*
Edited by: J. B. Wilson and G. H. W. May © Humana Press Inc., Totowa, NJ

ence of the transfected gene must be verified and the expression levels must be assessed. For the detection of the transfected gene, polymerase chain reaction (PCR) or Southern blot analysis is usually employed. For expression, immunofluorescence, immunoblot, reverse transcriptase (RT)-PCR or Northern blot analysis may be employed.

In this chapter, assays are described that were used to test the oncogenicity of the BARF1 gene but are applicable for the analysis of many candidate oncogenes. The first protocols describe DNA transfection into cells in culture, principally a modified calcium phosphate precipitate method. **Subheading 3.2.** deals with assays that can indicate cellular immortalization or transformation.

## 2. Materials

### 2.1. Cell Culture and Transfection

1. BARF1 plasmid DNA: The BARF1 gene was cloned into the expression vector, the pZip-Neo-SV(X) 1 (*15*, and *see* **Notes 1** and **2**).
2. Dulbecco's Modified Eagle's Medium (DMEM) (Sigma) with 4000 mg/L glucose (used for both Balb/c3T3 and primary monkey kidney epithelial cells).
3. RPMI 1640 medium (Sigma; used for Louckes B cells).
4. EGF-DMEM: DMEM supplemented with 12 ng/mL epidermal growth factor (EGF; GIBCO; for primary epithelial cells).
5. Complete media: All media are supplemented with antibiotics (120 µg/mL streptomycin and 120 µg/mL penicillin) and with 10% fetal calf serum (FCS).
6. G418 (GIBCO).
7. Tissue-culture dishes or plates.
8. 2 *M* $CaCl_2$.
9. 2X HEPES buffered saline (2X HEBS): For 1 L: 10 g HEPES, 16 g NaCl, 0.74 g KCl, 7 g $Na_2HPO_4$, 2 g Dextrose. Adjust pH to 7.0.
10. 0.25% Trypsin.
11. 10X PBS (Phosphate-buffered saline): 1 L consists of 80 g NaCl, 2 g KCl, 14 g $Na_2HPO_4$ and 2 g $KH_2PO_4$. Adjust pH to 7.4 with HCl. Filter-sterilize through a 0.2-µm filter and store at 4°C.
12. DMEM-40% PEG: transfer 20 g of polyethylene glycol (PEG) (MW 6000; Merck) into a 500-mL culture bottle, incubate in boiling water to melt PEG, then add 50 mL of DMEM containing 7% sucrose to the warm PEG solution, mix well and allow the solution to cool to 37°C. Adjust pH to 7.0 with sterile 1 *N* HCl.
13. Cloning cylinders (Bellco Glass, Inc., Vineland NJ).
14. Gene Pulser II (Bio-Rad) or equivalent and cuvets.

### 2.2. Transformation and Growth Assays

1. Media and solutions as described in **Subheading 2.1.**
2. $^3H$-Thymidine (Amersham), specific activity 5 Ci/mmol.
3. 5% trichloroacetic acid (TCA).
4. Whatman GF/C glass fiber disks.
5. 95% Ethanol.
6. OPTI-Fluor 0 scintillation fluid (Packard, USA).
7. Agarose: Seaplaque FMC.
8. Giemsa dye (Sigma).
9. Newborn rats or nude mice.

## 3. Methods

### 3.1. DNA Transfection Methods

#### 3.1.1. Transfection of Recombinant Plasmid into Balb/c 3T3 Cells and Colony Cloning

This protocol is a variant of the calcium phosphate precipitate transfection method, described in detail in Chapter 5.

1. Prepare cells (Balb/c3T3) to be transfected by seeding the cells in DMEM at $0.2 \times 10^6$/100-mm Petri dish the day prior to transfection. Cuture the cells for 24 h in a 5% $CO_2$ incubator at 37°C to about 70–80% confluence.
2. Prepare the transfection mixture: solution A consists of 50 µL of 2 *M* $CaCl_2$ plus 300 µL of sterile water, solution B consists of 50 µL of plasmid (20 µg) plus 400 µL of 2X HEPES-buffered saline. All solution should be at room temperature.
3. Mix solution A and solution B by bubbling air through a Pasteur pipet into solution B while slowly adding solution A dropwise. Then vortex mixture for 10–20 s. Allow the transfection mixture to stand at room temperature for 30–40 min with agitation every 5 min.
4. Aspirate medium from the cells and save it as conditioned medium.
5. Detach log-phase growing cells from the dish using a 0.25% trypsin solution and wash with 1X PBS by gentle centrifugation at 800*g* and resuspension (*see* **Note 4**).
6. Suspend $1.5 \times 10^6$ cells in 1 mL of complete DMEM medium. Add 0.8 mL of the transfection mixture to the cells in 1 mL and mix well by pipetting.
7. Add 36 mL of plating medium (20 mL of conditioned medium from the original cell culture to be transfected (*see* **step 4**) plus 18 mL of fresh DMEM medium containing 10% FCS) plus 2.0 mL of 2X HEBS and mix by pipetting.
8. Plate 10 mL of this cell suspension per 100-mm Petri dish and incubate at 37°C for 3–4 h.
9. Aspirate the plating medium. Shock the cells for 2–3 min with 5 mL of DMEM-40% PEG per plate. Aspirate the PEG solution and wash three times with serum-free DMEM medium. Add 3 mL of 10% FCS in DMEM and incubate for 30–40 min at 37°C.
10. Aspirate DMEM and add fresh DMEM containing 10% FCS. Incubate cells in a $CO_2$ incubator at 37°C.
11. After 3 d, add 500 µg/mL of G418 (for Balb/c3T3) to each Petri dish. Maintain cells under these selective conditions for 3–4 wk with medium changes every 5 d. Generally 10–100 colonies emerge per dish.
12. Circle the chosen colonies with a marker to visualize where to place the cloning cylinders. Rinse Petri dish with 37°C PBS. Place the cylinder coated with sterile silicon (previously autoclaved in a glass Petri dish) gently around the colony (*see* **Note 5**).
13. Add 50 µL of 0.25% trypsin into the cloning cylinder. Allow this to stand for 1 min and then add 100 µL of warm medium. Pipet the contents of one cylinder in and out of a micropipet to remove the cells from the dish.
14. Seed cells into 6-well plates with 3 mL of complete DMEM medium per well and expand.

#### 3.1.2. Transfection of Recombinant Plasmid into Louckes B Cell Line

Electroporation of cell lines is described in detail in Chapter 14.

1. Seed $0.5 \times 10^6$ of Louckes cells/mL in complete RPMI-1640. Incubate for 4 d to reach approx $2 \times 10^6$ cells/mL. Add complete medium 24 h before transfection to dilute cells to $1 \times 10^6$ cells/mL.

2. For transfection, centrifuge the log-phase growing cells at 800*g* and wash with PBS. Suspend $20 \times 10^6$ cells in 0.8 mL of cold PBS without $Ca^{2+}$ and $Mg^{2+}$ and add 20 µg of recombinant BARF1 plasmid DNA (dissolved in 10 µL of sterile water), mix and allow to stand for 10 min on ice.
3. Place the mixture in a gene pulse cuvet (previously cooled to 4°C), and apply a single electric pulse delivered by a Bio-Rad gene pulser (3000 V/cm, with a capacitance of 25 µF).
4. Incubate the cell-DNA mixture for 7 min on ice. Then add to 1 mL of warm growth medium.
5. Seed the cells in two 100-mm Petri dishes with 10 mL of RPMI-1640 medium. Three days after electroporation, count cells and seed into 96-well plates at 1000 or 2000 cells in 0.25 mL of complete RPMI-1640 medium/well in the presence of 3 mg/mL G418 for selection.
6. Maintain the cells for 4 wk with medium changes once a week. Collect G418-resistant cell populations from independent wells, replate into 6-well plates with 4 mL of medium/well. The cells from each well may be considered as subclones.

#### 3.1.3. Transfection of Recombinant Plasmid into Primary Monkey Kidney Epithelial (Patas) Cells

1. Seed the primary cells in EGF-DMEM at a concentration of $0.6 \times 10^6$ cells per 100 mm Petri dish. After two passages, harvest cells by trypsinization and seed again at $0.6 \times 10^6$ cells/100-mm Petri dish.
2. Two days later, transfect cells with the BARF1 plasmid by the calcium phosphate/PEG technique as previously described (*see* **Subheading 3.1.1.**) but with the following modifications: Trypsinize cells at 30% confluence. Suspend $1.5 \times 10^6$ cells in 1 mL of complete medium and transfect with 50 µg of plasmid DNA for 20 min at room temperature and then incubate the cells at 37°C for 3–4 h in 10 mL of complete medium as described (*see* **Note 6**).
3. Count cells and plate in 100-mm dishes. Weekly, trypsinize cells and seed at $0.6 \times 10^6$ cells/100-mm dish; one passage is thus defined as a 1 wk-old culture.
4. When the cells are highly sensitive to neomycine such as Patas cells, we cannot use this selection system. Instead, for the isolation of BARF1 positive subclones, seed the transfected cells at the 12th passage at 250 or 500 cells/30-mm dish in 3 mL of complete DMEM (*see* **Subheading 3.2.3.**). Three weeks later, harvest each colony with a cloning cylinder (as described in **Subheading 3.1.1.** for Balb/c3T3). At this cell dilution of plating, no colony formation is observed with parent primary cells or with vector alone transfectants.
5. Seed cells into 6-well plates with 3 mL of DMEM medium/well. The cell culture from each colony can be considered as a subclone.

### 3.2. Phenotypic Characterization of BARF1 Expressing Cells

Before characterizing the phenotype of BARF1 transfected cells, the presence of the BARF1 gene and its expression should be verified by Southern blot and PCR (for the identification of the BARF1 sequence) and by immunofluorescence, Northern blot or immunoblot (for the expression of BARF1 gene, see **Notes 7** and **8**).

In order to examine whether the transfected cells are malignantly transformed or immortalized, the following criteria could be considered: morphological change, growth rate, growth capacity in soft agar, and tumorigenicity in newborn rat or nude mice.

#### 3.2.1. Measurement of Cell Growth Rate in the Transfected Cells

Immortalized and/or malignantly transformed cells often proliferate more rapidly than the parental cells. The transformed cells can lose contact inhibition, resulting in the formation of several cell beds (for adherent cells). For this, cell growth rate of transfected cells should be compared with that of parental or vector alone transfected cells. A protocol for $^3$H-thymidine labeling is described here as well as in Chapters 13 and 17.

1. To measure tritiated thymidine incorporation into total cell DNA, seed $0.3 \times 10^6$ cells/50-mm dish and incubate for 20 h at 37°C in 3 mL of DMEM containing 6 µCi of $^3$H-thymidine.
2. Wash cells three times with cold PBS.
3. Trypsinize cells and centrifuge at 800*g* for 5 min. Remove PBS and add 0.5 mL of ice-cold 5% TCA to the cells, mix, and incubate on ice for 30 min.
4. Filter the TCA-treated cells on Whatman GF/C glass fibre disks. Wash the filter five times with 5 mL of cold TCA and once with 5 mL of 95% ethanol. The acid insoluble fraction is retained on the filter.
5. Count the Whatman filters in a scintillation counter with 5 mL of OPTI-Fluor 0 or equivalent. The incorporated $^3$H-thymidine levels give an indication of proliferation rates.

#### 3.2.2. Growth in Soft Agar Assay

Malignantly transformed adherent cells often no longer depend on support and can grow in a semi-solid (soft agar) suspension. This assay is therefore one criterium of transformation. Anchorage-independent cell growth can be assayed in 0.3% agarose.

1. Change the culture medium 24 h before trypsinization. For the assay, trypsinize cells and count.
2. Dissolve 0.6 g of agarose in 100 mL of DMEM without serum by heating, when the agar medium is cooled to 50°C add 10% FCS. Layer 10 mL of 0.6% agarose/DMEM into a 100-mm Petri dish and allow to solidify at room temperature.
3. Mix 3 mL of complete DMEM medium containing $0.5 \times 10^6$ cells gently with 3 mL of molten, 40°C, 0.6% agarose/DMEM medium (to give a final concentration of 0.3% of agarose, *see* **Note 9**).
4. Layer 6 mL of cell/agarose suspension over the solidified 0.6% agarose. Incubate at 37°C in humid conditions (*see* **Note 10**).
5. Feed cultures regularly with two drops of complete medium twice a week. Check the colonies by microscopy every 3 d. Transformed colonies should become obvious after 2 wk.

#### 3.2.3. Growth Capacity at Low Cell Density of the Transfected Primary Epithelial Cells

For primary epithelial cells, one of the immortalization criteria is whether the cells can grow at low concentration.

1. Trypsinize the transfected primary epithelial cells after several passages (about 10 passages for monkey kidney primary epithelial cells used in our experiments).
2. Seed cells in duplicate in six well plates at the rate of 250 and 500 cells/well containing 3 mL of complete DMEM medium.
3. Two weeks later, stain the cell colonies in one of the plates with Giemsa dye and examine evidence of colony formation. Primary nonimmortalized cells are unable to grow at this cell density.

4. In order to examine the expression of the transfected gene, harvest colonies from the duplicated plate using cloning cylinders and expand into clonal cultures.

### *3.2.4. Serum Dependence Assay of the Transfected Primary Epithelial Cells*

Transformed cells are frequently less dependent upon serum for growth. As such, this assay provides another measure of a transformation parameter.

1. Seed $0.6 \times 10^6$ cells in a 100-mm dish in complete DMEM with 10% FCS. After 24 h, briefly rinse the culture three times with PBS.
2. Add DMEM medium with 10, 5, 1, and 0.1% serum. Count the cells every day for 4 d using a hemocytometer. Trypan blue exclusion should be used so as not to count dead cells.

### *3.2.5. Tumorigenicity In Vivo*

A stringent test for malignant transformation is the ability of cells to form tumors in vivo. However, it is advisable to investigate the other culture assays before embarking on this test (*see* **Note 11**).

1. Seed $0.5 \times 10^6$ of the BARF1 (or transfected gene) expressing clones in complete DMEM (for adherent cells) or RPMI 1640 (for B cells) medium. For primary epithelial cells, seed cells in EGF-DMEM medium for two passages (primary cells can divide for about 10 passages in this medium) used as control, and then in DMEM medium without EGF for 24 h before injection in nude mice (or newborn rats). Grow all cells for 24 h.
2. Harvest cells in log-phase by trypsin (for adherent cells) and count. Wash cells twice in DMEM medium without FCS, then resuspend three different aliquots of $10 \times 10^6$, $5 \times 10^6$, and $0.5 \times 10^6$ cells in 100 μL DMEM medium without FCS. Mix cells gently.
3. Inject subcutaneously 100 μL of each cell clone using a 1-mL syringe; use six animals for each of the three different cell concentrations (nude mice or newborn rats), i.e., 18 animals for each cell clone.
4. Monitor tumor development twice a week for 8 wk (*see* **Note 12**).

## 4. Notes

1. For transfections, all plasmid DNA preparations should be endotoxin-free. We purify the DNA twice using CsCl gradients.
2. The BARF1 coding sequences can be isolated from the B95-8 *BamHI* A fragment of the viral genome within a 1.1 kb *SmaI* fragment.
3. The transfection method should be chosen with regard to the cell type being used. We use a mixed method of $Ca^{2+}$ and PEG for adherent cells. PEG treatment gives an increased degree of transfection (we find threefold in comparison to without PEG) without causing any cell damage. However, at more than 40%, PEG treatment can increase the efficiency of transfection (by comparison with 40%), but some cytotoxicity is observed. As described in this chapter, the adherent cells are transfected in suspension after trypsination. We found transfection in suspension to be several times more efficient (about 10-fold) compared to transfection of cells in a monolayer.
4. We split Balb/c 3T3 cells 1:30 twice per week to avoid confluence.
5. Choose well-separated colonies for ease of cloning.
6. This transfection procedure can be immediately repeated with these cells in order to increase the transfection efficiency.

7. For the detection of BARF1 sequence by polymerase chain reaction (PCR) the following primers can be used:
   BA1: 5'-CCAGAGCAATGGCCAGGTTC-3',
   BA4: 5'-CAAGGTGAAATAGGCAAGTGCG-3',
   which prime at positions 165496 and 166192 of the *BARF1* sequence, respectively, giving a 697 bp fragment.
8. For immunofluorescence or immunoblotting, BARF1 positive human serum may be used for detection. Alternatively, use a polyclonal rabbit antiserum prepared against a synthetic peptide corresponding to a presumed epitope NGGVMKEKD (amino acids 172-180 of the p33 BARF1 protein).
9. Ensure the cells are well-separated before plating.
10. It will help to keep the plates in plastic boxes with dampened paper towels underneath the plates if the agarose shows signs of drying.
11. In vivo experiments such as this obviously require adherence to all of the necessary regulations required in your country for animal experimentation to be in place.
12. Hela cells or Melanoma B16 cells can be used as positive controls in the same way as the test clones. These will induce tumors in the first weeks of the assay.

## References


1. Baer, R., Bankier, A. T., Biggin, M. D., Deininger, P. L., Farrell, P., Gibson, T. J., et al. (1984) DNA sequence and expression of the B95-8 Epstein-Barr virus genome. *Nature* **310,** 207–211.
2. Kieff, E. (1996) Epstein-Barr virus and its replication, in *Fields Virology, 3rd ed.* (Fields, B. N., Knipe, D. M., Howley, P. M., et al., eds.), Lippincott-Raven, Philadelphia, pp. 2343-2394.
3. Wang, D., Liebowitz, D., and Kieff, E. (1985) An EBV membrane protein expressed in immortalized lymphocytes transforms established rodent cells. *Cell* **43,** 831–840.
4. Baichwal, V. R. and Sugden, B. (1988) Transformation of Balb 3T3 cells by the BNLF-1 gene of Epstein-Barr virus. *Oncogene* **2,** 461–467.
5. Wilson, J. B., Bell, J. L., and Levine, A. J. (1996) Expression of Epstein-Barr virus nuclear antigen-1 induces B cell neoplasia in transgenic mice. *EMBO J.* **15,** 3117–3126.
6. Wei, M. X. and Ooka, T. (1989) A transforming function of the BARF 1 gene encoded by Epstein-Barr Virus. *EMBO J.* **8,** 2897–2903.
7. Wei, M. X., Moulin, J. C., Decaussin, G., Berger, F., and Ooka, T. (1994) Expression and tumorigenicity of the Epstein-Barr virus BARF1 gene in human Louckes B-lymphocyte cell line. *Cancer Res.* **54,** 1843–1848.
8. Pathmanathan, R., Prasad, U., Sadler, R., Flynn, K., and Raab-Traub, N. (1995) Clonal proliferations of cells infected with Epstein-Barr Virus in preinvasive lesions related to nasopharyngeal carcinoma. *N. Engl. J. Med.* **333,** 693–698.
9. Gilligan, K. J., Rajadurai, P., Lin, J. C., Busson, P., Abdelhamid, M., Prasad, U., et al. (1991) Expression of the Epstein-Barr virus B*am*HI A fragment in nasopharyngeal carcinoma: evidence for a viral protein expressed *in vivo*. *J. Virol.* **65,** 6252–6259.
10. Hitt, M. M., Allday, M. J., Hara, T., Karran, L., Jones, M. D., Busson, P., et al. (1989). EBV gene expression in an NPC-related tumor. *EMBO J.* **8,** 2639–2651.
11. Sbih-Lammali, F., Djennaoui, D., Belaoui, H., Bouguermouh, M., Decaussin, G., and Ooka, T. (1996) Transcriptional expression of Epstein-Barr virus genes and proto-oncogenes in North african nasopharyngeal carcinoma. *J. Med. Virol.* **49,** 7–14.

12. Griffin, B. E. and Karran, L. (1984) Immortalization of monkey epithelial cells by specific fragment of Epstein-Barr virus DNA. *Nature* **309,** 78–82.
13. Wei, M., de Turenne-Tessier, M., Deacussin, G., Benet, G., and Ooka, T. (1997) Establishment of a monkey kidney epithelial cell line with the BARF1 open reading frame from Epstein-Barr virus. *Oncogene* **14,** 3073–3081.
14. Karran L., Teo, C. G., King, D., Hitt, M. M., Gao, Y., Wedderburn, N., and Griffin, B. E. (1990) Establishment of immortalized primate epithelial cells with sub-genomic EBV DNA. *Int. J. Cancer* **45,** 763–772.
15. Cepko, C. L., Bryan, E. R., and Mulligan, R. C. (1984) Construction and applications of a highly transmissible murine retrovirus shuttle vector. *Cell* **37,** 1053–1062.

# 16

# Transient Gene Expression and MACS Enrichment

**Dieter Kube and Martina Vockerodt**

## 1. Introduction

The analysis of the effects of expression of one viral protein on the host cell separately from the effect of other viral proteins is often limited by the efficiency of the transfection method. Lymphoid cells are effectively transfected by electroporation *(1–4)*. However, the transfection efficiency varies usually between 5 and 20% of the living cells, depending on the cell line used. In the case of primary lymphoid cells, the transfection efficiency is below 5% *(5–7)*. Thus the analysis of the influence of viral genes on the expression of cellular proteins is often impossible because of the predominance of untransfected cells. In addition, some viral genes could result in cytostasis, such as latent membrance protein 1 (LMP1; *8*). The establishment of cell lines, where the viral gene is expressed constitutively or in an inducible fashion, is one way to try to address the problem, but is associated with a selection process *(8,9)*. This selection process prevents the analysis of early effects of expressed viral genes and could also lead to secondary cell culture effects not associated with the viral gene. Often, inducible gene expression systems are difficult to modulate and can be leaky. To overcome these problems, it is useful to analyze transiently transfected cells and enrich them to obtain pure cell populations without a selection process. A number of methods exist, with magnetic- or fluorescence-activated cell sorting (MACS/FACS) being the most common approaches used *(10)*. FACS and MACS are powerful and sophisticated methods for efficient purification of cells expressing a specific immunological marker molecule. Since the introduction of the green fluorescence protein (GFP) the purification of cells by FACS is no longer limited to immunological-stained proteins, which thus opens new applications for this approach.

In this chapter the transfection and enrichment of transfected cells by high gradient magnetic separation will be described *(11,12)*. This method is based on the cotransfection of two plasmids, one coding for the viral gene of interest and the other for a gene suitable for selection (which is not expressed in the untransfected cells) followed by high gradient magnetic cell enrichment. The genes used for selection frequently

From: *Methods in Molecular Biology, Vol. 174: Epstein-Barr Virus Protocols*
Edited by: J. B. Wilson and G. H. W. May © Humana Press Inc., Totowa, NJ

encode truncated surface antigens without intracellular domains or hybrid genes coding for a protein tagged with a synthetic peptide (termed here the selection molecule; ***6,13,14***). The cells are transfected with both plasmids, e.g., by electroporation, maintained in media, and separated through a magnetic enrichment process at an appropriate time point.

By introducing a magnetic label specific for the selection molecule, complex mixtures of cells can be fractionated. This magnetic label usually consists of an antibody coupled to small colloidal magnetic particles. The small size of the colloidal particles minimizes their interference in assays and allows the cells to grow in culture. In addition, it is possible to evaluate and control the quality of separation by flow cytometry and light microscopy simultaneously. However, the use of small colloidal magnetic particles requires high gradient magnetic separation techniques. For this purpose columns filled with thin plastic-coated ferromagnetic fibers/particles are used, which are magnetized in the field of a strong permanent magnet ***(10)***.

The magnetic enrichment process usually involves the binding of a specific antibody directed against the selection molecule expressed on the surface of the transfected cell. If the separated cells are analyzed only by molecular biological methods and there is no need to culture them after the separation process, intracellular molecules could also be used for cell enrichment. This approach with magnetic beads is limited because it is necessary to fix cells with formaldehyde for labeling ***(15)***. The selection process depends on the molecule used, the promotor defining the expression kinetics, and thus the optimal separation time point. The specific antibody used for selection is usually directly coupled to the magnetic beads. In addition, modification of the small colloidal magnetic particles with, for example, streptavidin allows the use of biotinylated antibodies for this cell separation method. It is also possible to label and separate cells indirectly using α-Ig-specific microbeads or α-Digoxigenin beads. The bead-labeled cells are then separated in a column fixed within a high magnetic field. After release of the separation columns from the magnetic field the labeled cells are eluted and can be either analyzed directly, cultured further, selected with antibiotics, or enriched again. This process of magnetic enrichment can be repeated several times on the same day (to enhance purity), at different time points after the first separation (to maintain the purity) or with different labels, thus allowing enrichment of subfractions of transfected cells induced by the viral gene. When establishing cell lines stably expressing foreign genes, such an enrichment is also useful in reducing the time and cost of selection.

## 2. Materials

### 2.1. Transfection by Electroporation

1. Supplemented RPMI: RPMI-1640 supplemented with 20 m*M* glutamine, 200 U/mL penicillin, 0.2 mg/mL streptomycin, and 10% fetal calf serum (FCS) (Sigma Aldrich). Store at 4°C in the dark.
2. Cell lines: We use L428, a cell line established from patients with Hodgkin's disease; BL2 and BL41, Burkitt's lymphoma cell lines; IARC171, a lymphoblastoid cell line (LCL) derived from normal blood of the same patient as BL41; and Jurkat, a T-cell line

*(16–18)*. Maintain the cell lines at cell densities between $3 \times 10^5$ and $1 \times 10^6$ cells /mL (*see* **Note 1**).

3. Trypan Blue: 0.4% Trypan Blue in PBS (Sigma Aldrich).
4. RPMI1640 containing 10% FCS and 25 m*M* HEPES, pH 7.5.
5. RPMI1640 containing 10% FCS and 10 m*M* HEPES, pH 7.5.
6. Plasmids, in 10 m*M* Tris-HCl, pH 8.0, 1 m*M* ethylenediaminetetraacetic acid (EDTA), at 1 mg/mL: pMACS4.1 or $_p$MACS $K^k$ (Miltenyi Biotec GmbH, Bergisch Gladbach, Germany,), which encode truncated CD4 or H-$2K^k$ molecule (the murine major histocompatibility complex), respectively, for selection of transfected cells. Expression plasmids for eukaryotic cells: pSG5 and pBK-RSV (Stratagene, La Jolla, CA), pCDNA (Invitrogen, USA) or equivalent, and recombinant variants thereof containing your gene of interest (*see* **Note 2**).
7. Easy-jet electroporator (Equibio, UK) or equivalent.
8. Electroporation cuvets: 50 × 4 mm (Eurogentec, Belgium) or equivalent.
9. Tissue-culture flasks.
10. 15-mL and 50-mL conical tubes.
11. 37°C, $CO_2$ humidified incubator.
12. Hemocytometer or other means of counting cell number.

## 2.2. Magnetic Enrichment of Transfected Cells

1. Phosphate-buffered saline (PBS): 58 m*M* $Na_2HPO_4$, 17 m*M* $NaH_2PO_4$, 68 m*M* NaCl, pH 7.4, prepared by using one tablet (Sigma Aldrich) in 200 mL of $H_2O$; usually no pH adjustment needed.
2. PBS-EDTA (2 m*M*), ice cold: Take 4 mL of a 0.5 *M* EDTA solution, pH 8.0, and five PBS tablets to prepare 1 L.
3. PBS-BSA-EDTA: dissolve 0.5 g BSA (*see* **Note 3**) in 100 mL of PBS containing 2 m*M* EDTA and de-gas with a vacuum pump immediately before use, keep this buffer at 4°C.
4. α-CD4 beads, α-H-$2K^k$ beads (Miltenyi Biotec GmbH, 551-01), 1:5 dilution.
5. α-CD4-PE (Immunotech, France, PN IM449), 1:10 dilution or α-H-$2K^k$-PE antibody (Becton-Dickinson BD-Pharmingen, San Diego, CA, 06055A) 1:10 dilution.
6. Mini-MACS columns (Miltenyi Biotec GmbH, Germany).
7. Mini-MACS magnets (single magnets or octo-MACS) and multi-stand (Miltenyi Biotec GmbH, Germany).
8. Column-prefilters (Dako, Clostrup, Denmark).

## 2.3. Immunofluorescence Analysis Using Flow Cytometry

1. PBS-BSA: PBS supplemented with 0.5% bovine serum albumin (BSA).
2. Fluorescein (FITC)- or phycoerythrin (PE)- conjugated monoclonal antibodies (MAbs): IgG1 FITC/PE (Becton-Dickinson BD, San Jose, CA, 349526) 1:10 dilution (as isotype control), CD54-PE (ICAM-1) (Becton-Dickinson BD, San Jose, CA, 347977) 1:10 dilution, CD54-FITC (ICAM-1) (Diaclone, Besancon, France, 852.691.010) 1:10 dilution, CD40-FITC, H-$2K^k$ - PE (Becton-Dickinson BD-Pharmingen, San Diego, CA, 33074x, 06055A) 1:10 dilution, CD4-PE (Immunotech France, PN IM449), 1:10 dilution.
3. Propidium-Iodide (PI): 2 mg/mL in PBS, store at –20°C. The working solution (100 μg/mL) is made by 20-fold dilution in PBS and stored at 4°C in the dark (*see* **Note 4**).
5. FACS-Calibur (Becton Dickinson BD, San Jose, CA) with Cellquest Software or equivalent instrument.

## 3. Methods

### 3.1. Transfection by Electroporation

1. On the day before transfection, resuspend the cells in supplemented RPMI at a cell density of $5 \times 10^5$ cells/mL.
2. Harvest approx $2 \times 10^7 - 2 \times 10^8$ cells and wash them with cold RPMI by centrifugation at 600*g* for 10 min. Transfer the cells into 50-mL conical tubes on ice. Count the viable cells with a hemacytometer using trypan blue to exclude dead cells. More than 90% of cells should be viable. Keep the cells on ice from now on (*see* **Note 5**).
3. Resuspend the cells in RPMI/10% FCS/25 m*M* HEPES at 4°C at the appropriate cell density (*see* **Note 6**): BL2 and BL41 at $1 \times 10^7$ cells/250 µL, L428 and Jurkat at $1 \times 10^7$ cells/500 µL. Incubate on ice for 20 min.
4. Cool sterile electroporation cuvets on ice for 20 min and add DNA to the cuvets (*see* **Notes 7** and **8**).
5. Prepare cell-culture flasks containing RPMI/10% FCS/10 m*M* HEPES to take $1 \times 10^7$ cells/10 mL after electroporation (**step 9**).
6. Add the appropriate amount of cell suspension to the cuvets: 250 µL of BL2 or BL41, 500 µL of L428 or Jurkat.
7. Mix the cell suspension and DNA within the cuvet by shaking and transfer the cuvet to the electroporator.
8. Pulse the cells: BL2 and BL41 at 250 V/1350 µF, L428 at 250 V/1650 µF, Jurkat at 250 V/2100 µF.
9. Transfer the electroporated cells immediately into media at room temperature (prepared in **step 5**, *see* **Note 9**).
10. Transfer the cell culture flask with the transfected cells into an incubator at 37°C with 5% $CO_2$. Grow the cells for 24–48 h.

For additional details on electroporation *see* also Chapter 14.

### 3.2. Magnetic-Enrichment of Transfected Cells

1. Dilute cells 24 h after transfection with 3 vol of ice-cold PBS-EDTA and pellet by centrifugation at 600*g*, 4°C, for 10 min. Start de-gassing of PBS-BSA-EDTA (*see* **Notes 3, 10–13**).
2. Wash cells twice with PBS-BSA-EDTA at 4°C .
3. Resuspend cells in de-gassed PBS-BSA-EDTA at 4°C at $1 \times 10^7$ cells/80 µL (*see* **Note 15**). Add 20 µL of α-CD4 or α-H-2K$^k$ beads (*see* **Notes 16** and **17**).
4. Incubate cells with magnetic beads in a fridge at 10°C for 15 min (*see* **Note 18**).
5. Dilute cells 10-fold with PBS-BSA-EDTA and pellet by centrifugation at 600*g*, 4°C, for 10 min (*see* **Note 19**).
6. Resuspend cells in 500 µL of de-gassed PBS-BSA-EDTA per Mini-MACS column (at $1 \times 10^7$ cells positive for the selection marker, see **Notes 20** and **21**).
7. During the centrifugation steps, equip Mini-MACS columns with pre-filters and wash once with 500 µL of ice-cold and de-gassed PBS-BSA-EDTA (*see* **Note 22**). Fit columns into the magnet.
8. Pass 500 µL of cell suspension over the MiniMACS column.
9. Wash three times with 500 µL of PBS-BSA-EDTA.
10. Take the column out of the magnet and add 500 µL of PBS-BSA-EDTA to elute the cells.
11. Count the cells and wash the cells with RPMI/10 m*M* HEPES/10% FCS.

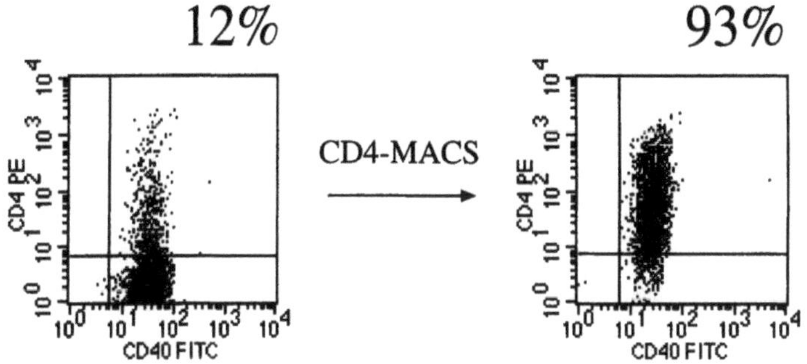


Fig. 1. Representative flow cytometric dot blot analysis of BL2 cells transfected with pSG5-LMP1 and ΔCD4 (pMACS 4.1) expression vectors before and after positive selection of ΔCD4-expressing cells. The vertical axis indicates ΔCD4 expression visualized by α-CD4 PE staining, the horizontal axis shows CD40 expression (α-CD40 FITC). Quadrant statistics revealed 12% of the cells stained with α-CD4 PE before magnetic separation and 93% after the enrichment.

12. Resuspend cells in medium at 3–5 × $10^5$ cells/mL. Culture the cells for a further 3–5 d (*see* **Note 23**).
13. Determine the purity of the enriched cells by FACS using α-CD4-PE or α-II-$2K^k$-PE antibodies (*see* later) (**Fig. 1**).
14. You can obtain supernatants for enzyme-linked immunosorbent assay (ELISA), cells for Western blot, RNA, or flow cytometry analysis every 24 h after MACS (**Figs. 2** and **3**; for additional detail on Western blotting, *see also* Chapters 25 and 26).

### 3.3. Immunofluorescence Analysis

1. For detection of cell-surface antigen expression, wash 1 × $10^5$ cells/measurement twice in PBS-BSA (*see* **Note 19**) (**Fig. 3**).
2. Resuspend cells in 45 µL of PBS-BSA and add 5 µL of antibody. For direct immunofluorescence staining use fluorescein (FITC)- or phycoerythrin (PE)- conjugated MAbs (*see* **Notes 24** and **25**).
3. Incubate cells for 10 min on ice in the dark.
4. Wash cells twice with PBS-BSA and resuspend in 500 µL of PBS-BSA.
5. Add PI to the stained sample immediately before measurement (diluted 1:100, *see* **Note 4**).
6. Analyze cells by flow cytometry using a FACS-Calibur or an equivalent instrument. Data can be presented as specific mean linear fluorescence intensity after subtraction of background staining with isotype-matched control. Exclude dead cells by propidium-iodide staining (*see* **Notes 25–29** and **Figs. 1** and **3**).

## 4. Notes

1. L428 cells are growing well at high cell densities. Maintain them at a minimum of 3 × $10^5$ cells/mL. A density of up to 2 × $10^6$ cells /mL is possible. Grow the BL2 and BL41 cell lines at between 2 × $10^5$ and 1 × $10^6$ cells/mL.
2. In our cell lines, the pSG5 vector is for high levels and the pBK-RSV vector for low levels of expression (see Figs. 2 and 3). The pCDNA vector allows intermediate expression levels of EBV genes. Miltenyi Biotec GmbH optimized the pMACS vectors. The name of the new vectors are pMACS 4-IRES and pMACS Kk.II. The new vectors are

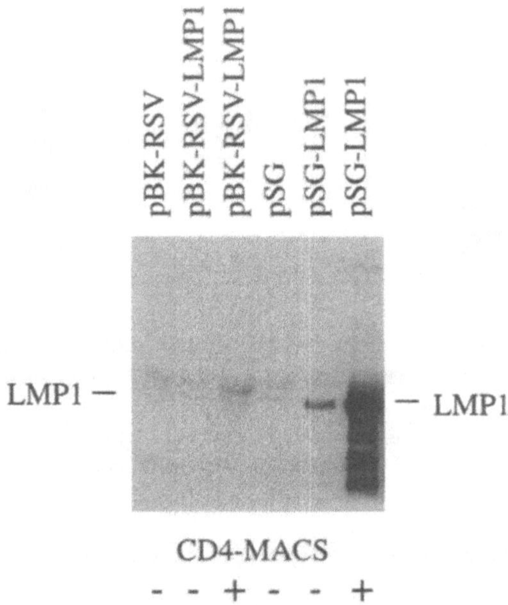


Fig. 2. Representative Western blot analysis using a mouse monoclonal α-LMP1 antibody of BL41 cells transfected with pBK-RSV, pBK-RSV-LMP1 or pSG5, pSG5-LMP1, and ΔCD4 (pMACS 4.1) before (–) and after (+) MACS.

recommended in preference to the older one. The pMACS Kk.II, especially, is much better compared to the first vector released. For details contact Miltenyi Biotec GmbH (*see* **Subheading 2.1.**).

3. For magnetic enrichment of cells that are to be cultured afterwards, use cell-culture-grade BSA. In all other experiments, standard molecular biology-grade BSA (fraction V) is sufficient.
4. Use PI to gate out dead cells by scatter (FSC/SSC) and the FL3 channel fluorescence gate for quality control. PI is highly carcinogenic; always wear gloves.
5. The electroporation buffer RPMI/10% FCS/25 m*M* HEPES, pH 7.5 is optimal in our hands to minimize the heat and pH-shift generated in the electroporation chamber. Cooling the sample in the chamber on ice before electroporation is also essential.
6. The number of cells transfected with expression vector depends on the question asked. For standard experiments we transfect $3 \times 10^7$ cells. The amount of cells could be increased up to $2 \times 10^8$ cells, if it is necessary to prepare nuclear extracts. We do not recommend transfecting higher numbers of cells because of the time scale of the cell-enrichment procedure. When high numbers of cells are to be transfected in more than 5 cuvets we use DNA concentrations at 5 µg/µL.
7. In our experiments we use a ratio of expression to selection plasmids of 1:1. In other cases a ratio of expression plasmid/selection marker plasmid between 10:1 and 3:1 may be required. We used CsCl- as well as Qiagen-prepared DNA with the same efficiency.
8. For transient expression assays we transfect cells with 10 µg of pMACS4.1 or pMACS$2^{kk}$ and 10 µg of one of the expression vectors pBK-RSV/pBK-RSV-LMP1 or pSG5/pSG5-LMP1/pSG5-EBNA2/pSG-LMP2. pMACS $K^k$ can be used for selection of Jurkat cells

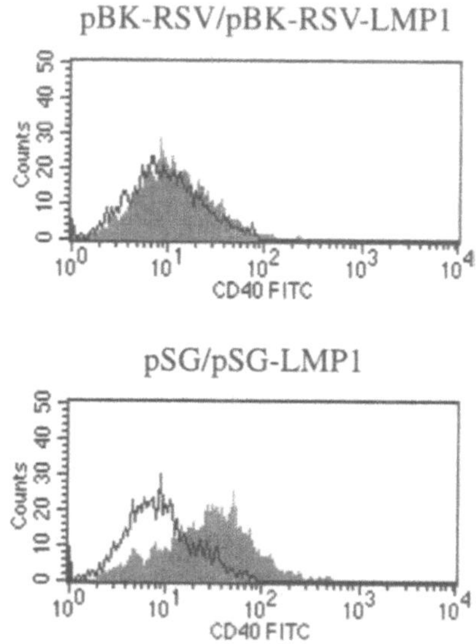


Fig. 3. LMP1 dose-dependent activation of CD40 in BL41 cells. Representative flow cytometric analysis of BL41 cells transfected with pBK-RSV-LMP1 or pSG5-LMP1 and ΔCD4 (pMACS 4.1) after positive selection of ΔCD4 expressing cells. The vertical axis indicates the relative cell number, the horizontal axis indicates CD40 expression. Vector controls are (–), LMP1 expression plasmids (gray).

that express CD4 ***(19)***. pMACS4.1 can be used for B-cell lines that are CD4 negative. Cells should be analyzed by flow cytometry for the expression of the selection marker.

9. After electroporation cuvets can be washed, incubated in an ultrasound water bath, air dried and gas-sterilized. Keep sterile cuvets in a hood for 10 min before adding DNA and cells to ensure that no remaining sterilization gas is in the chamber.
10. The earliest time-point for magnetic enrichment is about 12 h after transfection. We obtained the best results in enrichment and cell number 24 h after transfection. It is important to establish an individual time-curve for the expression of the selection marker for every cell line. It is possible that in some cell lines the SV40 promoter used for CD4 or $2H^{kk}$ expression is not effective enough.
11. For magnetic enrichment of cells that are to be cultured afterward, use only sterile reagents.
12. Sometimes it is required to separate dead cells before performing the magnetic separation (for example by Ficoll-separation using Ficoll hypaque, Amersham-Pharmacia, UK). Dead cells significantly reduce the efficiency and purity of the magnetic separation.
13. Dilution of the cultured cells with 3 vol of PBS-EDTA helps to reduce the formation of large cell aggregates.
14. If you want to measure the influence of your gene of interest on ion channels, do not use EDTA-containing buffers.
15. Use only de-gassed ice-cold PBS-BSA-EDTA. It is important to avoid air bubbles when resuspending cells. We recommend a 200-1000 µL micropipet for resuspension of cells.

16. To enrich cells using other selection markers, corresponding direct beads should be used. If direct beads are not available indirect selection via Streptavidin/Digoxigenin and α-Ig is possible. If you are using a selection molecule, where the corresponding antibody for selection is not in common use, titrate the antibody conjugated with FITC or PE to determine the best concentration for cell separation. The antibody concentration required for cell separation is frequently the same as that used for fluorochrome labeling in flow cytometry analysis.
17. Microbeads can be sterilized by filtration through 0.2-μm filters, however, this is usually not necessary.
18. Increased temperature and prolonged incubation time for staining may result in nonspecific cell labeling. We recommend the use of "Multisort-beads" if available because they give better enrichments of cells transfected with LMP1. In addition, the colloidal particle can be removed and the cells can be selected with beads for another surface antigen.
19. Cells should be diluted with a 10-fold volume of PBS-BSA-EDTA and pelleted by centrifugation to wash out unbound magnetic microbeads.
20. We usually transfect $3 \times 10^7$ cells and then use one Mini-MACS column. In case of high transfection efficiency and low numbers of dead cells we recommend to use only $2 \times 10^7$ cells per Mini-MACS column. We only use single-use Mini-MACS columns, even for large-scale separations. For good enrichments of cells, use as small columns as possible. Overloading is advantageous for better enrichment of positive cells.
21. It is important to use de-gassed buffer for the columns. Air bubbles can reduce the efficiency of magnetic separation by blocking the column.
22. It is important to use prefilters on the Mini-MACS columns to ensure that the cells are in a single cell suspension when passing through the column. Cell aggregates could lead to an obstruction of the column. The prefilters have to be wet to avoid loss of cells by attaching to dry filter mesh. We usually pipet the column washing buffer onto these filters. For L428 cells, we use mesh sizes of 75 μm; for BL and Jurkat cells we use 30 μm filters.
23. If you obtain only bad purity, try faster flow rates, lower concentrations of reagents, or add a second step of enrichment. In case of poor recovery of positive cells in the elution fraction, try slower flow rates, use columns with larger capacity, remove dead cells by ficoll separation, or improve magnetic labeling and count how many stained cells are in your flow-through fraction.
24. To evaluate the separation process, we stain the cells after elution from the magnetic column using antibody fluorochrome staining with an antibody directed against a different epitope from the selection antibody. This can reduce the amount of fluorochrome antibody required. Presence of the microbead antibody may impair antibody fluorochrome staining when the antibodies are of the same specificity.
25. Check your transfection efficiency by measuring the amount of CD4 or $2H^{kk}$ before starting the cell separation. In case of very low transfection efficiency, measure 10,000 events. After enrichment it is enough to count 2000–3000 events on the flow cytometer. We prefer PE-modified antibodies because of their brighter staining.
26. Before starting FACS analysis and cell enrichment, it is important to adjust the configuration of the flow cytometer for both channels (FL1 (FITC/GFP) and FL2 (TRITC, Phycoerytrin), FL3 for propidium-iodide) using antibodies directed against well-expressed surface antigens. Use antibodies that give a clear but not too intense signal.
27. If you have a flow cytometer with multiple lasers, you can analyze the cells by multicolor analysis. Always include PI in the sample.
28. Do not forget to use isotype controls.

29. For the analysis of LMP1 dependent CD54 expression we used the α-CD54-FITC instead of α-CD54-PE. This is to measure the changes more accurately, because the fluorescence of the bound α-CD54-PE is often too intensive to measure changes in the expression of CD54. We used the antibodies at 1:10 dilution, but sometimes it is necessary to titrate them to define the right dilution to avoid nonspecific staining.

## References


1. Zhdanov, R. I., Kutsenko, N. G., and Fedchenko, V. I. (1997) Non-viral gene transfer in gene therapy. *Vopr. Med. Khim.* **43,** 3–12.
2. Andreason, G. L. (1993) Electroporation as a technique for the transfer of macromolecules into mammalian cell lines. *J. Tissue Culture Methods* **15,** 56–62.
3. Fouillard, L. (1996) Physical method for gene transfer: An alternative to viruses. *Hematol. Cell. Ther.* **38,** 214–216.
4. Lurquin, P. F. (1997) Gene transfer by electroporation. *Mol. Biotechnol.* **7,** 5–35.
5. Peng, M. and Lundgren, E. (1995) Transient expression of the Epstein-Barr virus LMP1 gene in human primary B cells induces cellular activation and DNA synthesis. *Oncogene* **7,** 1775–1782.
6. Pilon, M., Gullberg, M., and Lundgren, E. (1991) Transient expression of the CD2 cell surface antigen as a sortable marker to monitor high frequency transfection of human primary B cells. *J. Immunol.* **146,** 1047–1051.
7. Liljeholm, S., Hughes, K., Grundström, T., and Brodin, P. (1998) NF-κB only partially mediates Epstein-Barr virus latent membrane protein 1 activation of B cells. *J. Gen. Virol.* **79,** 2117–2125.
8. Floettmann, J. E., Ward, K., Rickinson, A. B., and Rowe, M. (1996) Cytostatic effect of Epstein-Barr virus latent membrane protein-1 analyzed using tetracycline-regulated expression in B cell lines. *Virology* **223,** 29–40.
9. Wang, F., Gregory, C., Sample, C., Rowe, M., Liebowitz, D., Murray, R., et al. (1990) Epstein-Barr virus latent membrane protein (LMP1) and nuclear proteins 2 and 3C are effectors of phenotypic changes in B lymphocytes: EBNA-2 and LMP1 cooperatively induce CD23. *J. Virol.* **64,** 2309–2318.
10. Miltenyi, S., Mueller, M., Weichel, W., and Radbruch, A. (1990) High gradient magnetic cell separation with MACS. *Cytometry* **11,** 231–238.
11. Kube, D., Vockerodt, M., Weber, O., Hell, K., Wolf, J., Haier, B., et al. (1999) Expression of Epstein-Barr Virus Nuclear Antigen 1 is associated with enhanced expression of CD25 in the Hodgkin cell line L428. *J. Virol.* **73,** 1630–1636.
12. Vockerodt, M., Haier, B., Buttgereit, P., Tesch, H., Kube, D. (2001) The Epstein-Barr virus latent membrane protein 1 induces Interleukin-10 in Burkitt's lymphoma cells but not in Hodgkin's cells involving the p38/SAPK2 pathway. *Virology*, in press.
13. Ichijo, H., Nishida, E., Irie, K., Ten, D. P., Saitoh, M., Moriguchi, T., et al. (1997) Induction of apoptosis by ASK1, a mammalian MAPKKK that activates SAPK/JNK and p38 signaling pathways. *Science* **275,** 90–94.
14. Chesnut, J. D., Baytan, A. R., Russell, M., Chang, M. P., Bernard, A., Maxwell, I. H., and Hoeffler, J. P. (1996) Selective isolation of transiently transfected cells from a mammalian cell population with vectors expressing a membrane anchored single-chain antibody. *J. Immunol. Methods* **193,** 17–27.
15. Martin, V. M., Siewert, C., Scharl, A., Harms, T., Heinze, R., Oehl, S., et al. (1998) Immunomagnetic enrichment of disseminated epithelial tumor cells from peripheral blood by MACS. *Exp. Hematol.* **26,** 252–264.

16. Falk, M. H., Tesch, H., Stein, H., Diehl, V., Jones, D. B., Fonatsch, C., and Bornkamm, G. W. (1987) Phenotype versus immunoglobulin and T-cell receptor genotype of Hodgkin-derived cell lines: activation of immature lymphoid cells in Hodgkin's disease. *Int. J. Cancer* **40,** 262–269.
17. Kube, D., Platzer, C., von Knethen, A., Straub, H., Bohlen, H., Hafner, M., and Tesch, H. (1995) Isolation of the human interleukin 10 promoter. Characterization of the promoter activity in Burkitt's lymphoma cell lines. *Cytokine* **7,** 1–7.
18. Murray, R., Young, L., Calendar, A., Gregory, C., Rowe, M., Lenoir, G., and Rickinson, A. (1988) Different patterns of EBV gene expression and of cytotoxic T-cell recognition in B cell lines infected with transforming (B95.8) or nontransforming (P3HRI) virus strain. *J. Virol.* **62,** 894–901.
19. Izumi, K. M. and Kieff, E. D. (1997) The Epstein-Barr virus oncogene product latent membrane protein 1 engages the tumor necrosis factor receptor-associated death domain protein to mediate B lymphocyte growth transformation and activate NF-κB. *Proc. Natl. Acad. Sci. USA* **94,** 12,592–12,597.

# 17

## In Vitro Assays to Study Epithelial Cell Growth

**Christopher W. Dawson and Lawrence S. Young**

### 1. Introduction

The inability to directly infect epithelial cells in vitro with Epstein-Barr virus (EBV) *(1)* has led to the development of epithelial cell-culture models to examine virus-induced growth transformation and productive infection.

A number of cell-culture model systems have been developed to study virus:epithelial-cell interactions, all of which make use of established cell lines rather than primary epithelial cells. Unlike primary cells, which are relatively difficult to grow and have a finite lifespan in tissue culture, established cell lines are easier to propagate, more amenable to transfection, and can be maintained in vitro indefinitely.

For studies examining EBV growth transformation, the introduction of EBV genes into epithelial cells provides a powerful approach for studying the functions of these genes and their effects on epithelial cell behavior *(2–12)*. Similarly, targeting expression of CR2 (the receptor used by EBV) to epithelial cells has allowed investigators to examine the outcome of EBV infection in cells that are normally refractory to EBV infection in vitro *(13,14)*.

The model system that we have used to examine the effects of EBV proteins on growth transformation involves the use of an established epithelial cell line, SCC12F, a nontumorigenic subclone of the carcinoma-derived SCC12 cell line *(2,11,15)*. This cell line, although not of nasopharyngeal origin, retains several characteristics of normal cultured epidermal keratinocytes, which render it useful for this type of study. Such properties include a requirement for fibroblast feeder support and responsiveness to terminal differentiation stimuli. Other squamous epithelial-cell lines that have been used in this type of study include RHEK-1, an SV40 immortalized epidermal keratinocyte cell line *(16)*; HaCat, a spontaneously immortalized epidermal keratinocyte line *(17)*; and C33A, a cell line derived from a cervical carcinoma *(18–21)*. Other, nonsquamous-derived cell lines that have been used in transfection studies include the Hela and EJ cell lines *(22,23)*

From: *Methods in Molecular Biology, Vol. 174: Epstein-Barr Virus Protocols*
Edited by: J. B. Wilson and G. H. W. May © Humana Press Inc., Totowa, NJ

A number of assays are available for assessing the effects of EBV gene expression on epithelial cell growth. The suitability of each assay will depend on the characteristics of the cell line used. For epithelial cell lines which comprise fairly homogeneous populations of carcinoma-derived cells such as Hela, EJ, and C33A, a greater number of assays can be applied. For epithelial cell lines derived from stratified squamous epithelia such as SCC12F, HaCat, and RHEK-1, the choice may be restricted owing to technical limitations of a given methodology when applied to more complex epithelial cell types. Cell-proliferation assays can either directly measure cell growth (e.g., by counting total cell number), or measure it indirectly by analyzing: (1) the incorporation of radioactive precursors into cells (e.g., [$^3$H]thymidine), or (2) measure the metabolic activity of cellular enzymes in viable cells (e.g., MTT assay).

### 1.1. Determination of Cell Number by Direct Cell Count

Perhaps the easiest and most straightforward way of analyzing cell growth is to measure the increase in cell number as a function of time. In this protocol, cell growth is determined over a defined period and viable cell number estimated by trypan blue exclusion and hemocytometer counting. Although labor-intensive, this approach is both simple and inexpensive. However, this method can only provide a measure of the growth of a population of cells, which may result (in some cell populations and under certain conditions) from a balance between cell proliferation and cell death.

### 1.2. [$^3$H]Thymidine Incorporation

The incorporation of [$^3$H]thymidine is a well-established assay for measuring cell proliferation and is particularly useful for measuring cellular responses to exogenous growth factors (*see* also Chapter 13 for suspension cells). The assay involves the pulsing of cells with radiolabeled thymidine [$^3$H-TdR] and measuring the extent of incorporation into cellular DNA. This assay gives an indication of the number of cells within the total cell population that are actively replicating DNA (i.e., the number of cells going through S phase). Although this technique is useful for certain epithelial cell lines, it may not be the best way of measuring the proliferation of keratinocytes or cell lines derived from squamous epithelia owing to their ability to catabolize thymidine ***(24)***. Under normal circumstances, cells are analyzed after reaching mid-log phase in their growth, and pulsed for between 1–4 h. There may be instances, however, when it is desirable to pulse for longer periods, e.g., when cells are at a higher cell density or when the rate of DNA synthesis is low.

### 1.3. MTT Tetrazolium and Other Colorimetric-Based Assays

Colorimetric-based assays are viable alternatives to $^3$H-thymidine incorporation, and do not have its associated difficulties. The MTT assay is a rapid colorimetric assay for determining viable cell numbers in proliferation, cytotoxicity, and apoptosis assays ***(25)***. This assay utilizes the ability of dehydrogenases in active mitochondria in living cells to cleave the tetrazolium ring off the MTT substrate (3-(4,5-dimethylthiazol-2-yl)-2,5-diphenyl tetrazolium bromide) releasing purple formazan crystals, which are dissolved in dimethyl sulfoxide (DMSO) or acid isopropanol ***(26)***. The intensity of color obtained, which is relative to the number of viable cells, is subsequently measured by a microtiter plate reader OD at 550–570 nm. A number of alternative tetrazolium dyes, XTT and XTS, are now available that have the additional benefit of being water-soluble *(27,28)*.

### *1.4. Alamar Blue Assay for Cell Growth and Viability*

Alamar Blue is a reagent that is becoming increasingly popular as an alternative to MTT, having the benefits of being water-soluble and nontoxic *(29,30)*. Alamar Blue is a fluorogenic redox indicator, turning red upon reduction in living cells. Unlike the oxidized blue form, which has little intrinsic fluorescence, the reduced red form is highly fluorescent. Cell viability can therefore be assessed either by OD or fluorescence intensity.

Like the MTT assay, the Alamar Blue assay is simple to perform and requires the addition of the indicator towards the end of the incubation test period; however, unlike MTT, further manipulations such as solubilization of the product are not required.

## 2. Materials

### *2.1. Tissue-Culture Reagents and Equipment*

1. Incubator: 37°C with 5% $CO_2$.
2. Tissue-culture media: Dulbecco's Modified Eagle's Medium (DMEM, Gibco) with L-glutamine added to a final concentration of 2 m*M*. Ham's F12 with L-glutamine (final concentration 2 m*M*).
3. Complete growth medium: appropriate tissue-culture medium, 5–10% (depending on cell type) fetal calf serum (Gibco), 0.2 mg/mL streptomycin sulfate, 200 U/mL penicillin G potassium.
4. Hydrocortisone (Sigma).
5. Tissue-culture plates: 96-well flat-bottomed plates (Nunc).
6. PBS (Phosphate buffered saline): 58 m*M* $Na_2HPO_4$, 17 m*M* $NaH_2PO_4$, 68 m*M* NaCl.

### *2.2. Solutions*

#### *2.2.1. Trypan Blue Exclusion Assay Reagents*

1. 0.4% trypan blue solution.

#### *2.2.2. Thymidine Incorporation Assay Reagents*

1. [5'-$^3$H] thymidine aqueous solution 1 mCi/mL (37 MBq/mL) (Amersham).
2. [5'-$^3$H] thymidine stock: dilute [5'-$^3$H] thymidine in complete growth medium to 17.2 Ci/mMol.
3. Lysis buffer: 0.1% Triton-X-100 in $H_2O$. Store at 4°C.

#### *2.2.3. MTT Assay Reagents*

1. MTT substrate: 5 mg/mL MTT (3-(4,5-dimethylthiazol-2-yl)-2,5-diphenyl tetrazolium bromide) (Sigma) in PBS.
2. Phosphate-buffered saline (PBS): 58 m*M* $Na_2HPO_4$, 17 m*M* $NaH_2PO_4$, 68 m*M* NaCl.
3. DMSO.
4. Sorenson's buffer: 0.1 *M* glycine, 0.1 *M* NaCl, pH 10.5.

#### *2.2.4. Alamar Blue Assay Reagent*

1. Alamar Blue solution (Serotec).

### 2.3. Equipment

1. Enzyme-linked immunosorbent assay (ELISA) plate reader (with filter set for 570 nm and 600 nm).
2. Beta-plate reader.
3. Cytofluoroscan, with filter set for FITC (excitation 560 nm and emission 590 nm).
4. Hemocytometer.

## 3. Methods

### 3.1. Determination of Cell Number by Cell Counting (Using Trypan Blue Exclusion)

1. Harvest cells in the log phase of growth by trypsination and suspend (to an estimated $1 \times 10^6$ cells/mL) in complete growth medium (*see* **Note 1**).
2. Take 40 µL of cell suspension and mix with 160 µL of 0.4% trypan blue in the well of a microtiter plate. Transfer an aliquot to a hemocytometer and count the number of viable cells. Viable cells can be differentiated from nonviable or dead cells as viable cells exclude the blue dye. Calculate the total viable cell number taking the dilution factor (1:5) into account.
3. Seed single-cell suspensions into 6-well plates at an appropriate cell number in complete growth medium. The input density will depend on the cell line being used and its doubling time. (We routinely use between $10^4$ and $5 \times 10^4$ cells/well for SCC12F cells; *see* **Note 2**.) Incubate at 37°C 5% $CO_2$ for 24 h.
4. Aspirate the medium to remove unattached cells and add fresh complete growth medium. If serum responses are to be measured, then add medium containing various amounts of serum at this stage. If very low concentrations of serum are to be used, it may be necessary to wash the wells with serum-free medium prior to addition of fresh medium to remove all traces of serum.
5. Assess cell growth at 24- or 48-h intervals by trypsinization of one well at a time and counting the cells as described in **step 2** (*see* **Note 3**).

### 3.2. $^3$H-Thymidine Incorporation

1. Harvest cells in the log phase of growth and count viable cells as described in **Subheading 3.1., steps 1–2.**
2. Seed between $10^3$ and $10^4$ cells (depending upon the cell type being used) into the wells of a 96-well plate in 200 µL of complete growth medium (Each sample condition or time-point should be conducted in triplicate, using a different plate for different time points) and incubate for 24 h at 37°C, 5% $CO_2$.
3. Aspirate the medium to remove unattached cells and add fresh complete growth medium. If serum or growth factor responses are to be measured, then add medium containing various amounts of serum (or growth factor) at this stage. If very low concentrations of serum are to be used it may be necessary to wash the cell wells with serum-free medium prior to addition of fresh medium to remove all traces of serum.
4. At the end of the period of study (time-points between 1–4 d), add 20 µL of a 17.2 Ci/m*M*ol [$^3$H]thymidine stock solution to each well (final concentration 0.33 µCi/well) and incubate the plates for 4 h at 37°C, 5% $CO_2$ (*see* **Note 5**).
5. Aspirate the medium into an appropriate container and dispose according to the practices for radioactive disposal at the institution. Rinse cells twice with PBS.
6. Add 200 µL of lysis buffer to each well and allow the plates to stand for 5 min.

7. The amount of radioactivity is determined by scintillation counting.
8. Calculate the mean and standard deviation of each set of triplicates for comparison of proliferation between cell sets or medium conditions (*see* **Notes 6** and **7**). Plot comparative proliferation curves for the study period.

### 3.3. Determination of Viable Cell Number by MTT Assay

1. Follow **steps 1–3** of **Subheading 3.2.**, to plate $10^3$–$10^4$ cells per well of a 96-well plate, incubating for 24 h prior to the study period.
2. At the end of the period of study (time points between 2–5 d), aspirate the medium and add 200 µL of fresh complete growth medium.
3. Add 20 µL of MTT substrate (5 mg/mL) to each well and incubate the plate for 4 h at 37°C, 5% $CO_2$, to allow formazan crystals to form.
4. Aspirate the medium with a 21G needle and syringe, leaving the formazan crystals. Add 200 µL DMSO to dissolve the crystals (*see* **Note 8**).
5. Add 25 µL of Sorenson's buffer to each well.
6. Measure absorbance at 550–570 nm immediately on an ELISA plate reader using DMSO as a blank.
7. Calculate the mean and standard deviation for each set of triplicates for comparison of growth between cell sets or medium conditions and plot a growth curve for the study period (*see* **Notes 7** and **9**).

### 3.4. Determination of Viable Cell Number Using Alamar Blue

1. Follow **steps 1–3** of **Subheading 3.2.**, to plate $10^3$–$10^4$ cells per well of a 96-well plate, incubating for 24 h prior to the study period.
2. At the end of the study period (time points between 2–5 d), add 20 µL of Alamar Blue reagent to each well (1/10th of the total volume), and incubate for 3 h at 37°C, 5% $CO_2$.
3. Measure the spectrophotometric absorbance at 570 nm and 600 nm on an ELISA plate reader using cell free wells containing medium as a blank. Determine the reaction values by subtracting the background reading (absorbance at 600 nm) from the reading obtained at 560 nm. Alternatively, the plates can be read spectrofluorimetrically on a cytofluorimeter (560 nm excitation and 590 nm emission wavelength).
4. Calculate the mean and standard deviation for each set of triplicates for comparison of growth between cell sets or medium conditions and plot a growth curve for the study period (*see* **Notes 7** and **9**).

## 4. Notes

1. To ensure this, do not harvest cells over 90% confluency. More details on trypsination of cells are provided in Chapter 14.
2. It may be important to check that the cell lines being analyzed have similar plating efficiencies to ensure that any observed differences in growth kinetics are real and not the result of differences in the number of adherent cells in the starting population.
3. If the investigation requires the counting of both viable and total cell number, care should be taken to ensure that any desquamated or unattached cells are also collected at the time of sample analysis and included in the total cell count.
4. [$^3$H]thymidine uptake may not be the best method for analyzing the growth of primary keratinocytes or epithelial cell lines derived from stratified squamous epithelium owing to the unusual manner in which keratinocytes metabolize thymidine.
5. It may be necessary to adjust the amount of radioactive label if cells are grown in media that contain high levels of thymidine (e.g., Ham's F10 or F12).

6. Problems may be encountered if comparisons are being made between cell lines that have marked differences in the duration of their S-phase, i.e., cells with a longer S-phase will incorporate more label during the pulse.
7. If standard deviation values are large, each cell type/condition must be analyzed in more than triplicate to produce meaningful values.
8. When solubilized, the formazan crystals are not stable for lengthy periods of time. It is advisable to read the plates within 10 min of solubilizing the formazan crystals.
9. The MTT and Alamar Blue assays are dependent on enzymatic activity. As the cellular activities will vary from one cell line to another, it is important to optimize the parameters of the assay for each cell type being tested (i.e., dilution of the substrate and the incubation time). Calibration curves should be constructed to identify the range of cell numbers that give a linear relationship between od/fluorescence intensity and cell density.

## References

1. Niedobitek, G. and Young, L. S. (1994) Epstein-Barr-Virus persistence and virus-associated tumors. *Lancet* **343,** 333–335.
2. Dawson, C.W, Rickinson, A. B., and Young, L. S. (1990) Epstein-Barr-Virus Latent Membrane-Protein inhibits Human epithelial-cell differentiation. *Nature* **344,** 777–780.
3. Fahraeus, R., Rymo, L., Rhim, J. S., and Klein, G. (1990) Morphological transformation of Human keratinocytes expressing the LMP gene of Epstein-Barr-virus. *Nature* **345,** 447–449.
4. Hu, L. F., Chen, F., Zheng, X., Ernberg, I., Cao, S. L., Christensson, B., et al. (1993) Clonability and Tumorigenicity of Human epithelial-cells expressing the EBV-encoded membrane-protein LM P1. *Oncogene* **8,** 1575–1583.
5. Zheng, X., Yuan, F., Hu, L. F., Chen, F., Klein, G., and Christensson, B. (1994) Effect of B-Lymphocyte-derived and NPC-derived EBV-LMP1 gene expression on in-vitro growth and differentiation of Human epithelial-cells. *Intl. J. Cancer* **57,** 747–753.
6. Dawson, C. W., Eliopoulos, A. G., Dawson, J., and Young, L. S. (1995) BHRF1, a viral homolog of the Bcl-2 oncogene, disturbs epithelial-cell differentiation. *Oncogene*, **10,** 69–77.
7. Lu, J. J. Y., Chen, J. Y., Hsu, T. Y., Yu, Y. C. Y., Su, I. J., and Yang, C. S. (1996) Induction of apoptosis in epithelial-cells by Epstein-Barr-Virus Latent Membrane-Protein-1. *J. General Virol.* **77,** 1883–1892.
8. Fries, K. L., Miller, W. E., and Raab-Traub, N. (1996) Epstein-Barr-Virus Latent Membrane-Protein-1 blocks p53–mediated apoptosis through the induction of the A20 gene. *J. Virol.* **70,** 8653–8659.
9. Sheu, L. F., Chen, A., Meng, C.L, Ho, K.C, Lee, W. H., Leu, F. J., and Chao, C. F. (1996) Enhanced malignant progression of nasopharyngeal carcinoma-cells mediated by the expression of Epstein-Barr nuclear antigen-1 in-vivo. *J. Pathol.* **180,** 243–248.
10. Kawanishi, M. (1997) Epstein-Barr Virus BHRF1 protein protects Intestine 407 epithelial cells from apoptosis induced by Tumor Necrosis Factor a and anti-Fas antibody. *J. Virol.* **71,** 3319–3322.
11. Nicholson, L. J., Hopwood, P., Johannessen, I., Salisbury, J. R., Codd, J., Thorley-Lawson, D., and Crawford, D. H. (1997) Epstein-Barr Virus latent membrane protein does not inhibit differentiation and induces tumorigenicity of Human epithelial cells. *Oncogene* **15,** 275–283.
12. Lu, J. J. Y., Chen, J. Y., Hsu, T. Y., Yu, W. C. Y., Su, I. J., and Yang, C. S. (1997) Cooperative interaction between bcl-2 and Epstein-Barr virus latent membrane protein 1 in the growth transformation of Human epithelial cells. *J. General Virol.* **78,** 2975–2985.

13. Li, Q. X., Young, L. S., Niedobitek, G., Dawson, C. W., Birkenbach, M., Wang, F., and Rickinson, A. B. (1992) Epstein-Barr-Virus infection and replication in a Human epithelial-cell system. *Nature* **356,** 347–350.
14. Knox, P. G., Li, Q. X., Rickinson, A. B., and Young, L. S. (1996) In-vitro production of stable Epstein-Barr Virus-positive epithelial-cell clones which resemble the virus-cell-interaction observed in Nasopharyngeal carcinoma. *Virol.* **215,** 40–50.
15. Parkinson, E. K., Grabham, P., and Emmerson, A. (1983) A subpopulation of cultured human keratinocytes which is resistant to the induction of terminal differentiation-related changes by phorbol, 12-myristate, 13-acetate—evidence for an increase in the resistant population following transformation. *Carcinogenesis* **4,** 857–861.
16. Rhim, J. S., Arnstein, P., Price, F. M., Sanford, K. K., and Aaronson, S. A. (1984) Neoplastic transformation of human epidermal keratinocytes by the combined action of Adeno 12-SV40 virus and kirsten murine sarcoma-virus. *Proc. Am. Assoc. Cancer Res.* **25,** 390.
17. Boukamp, P., Petrussevka, R. T., Breitkreutz, D., Hornung, J., Markham, A., and Fusenig, N. E. (1988) Normal keratinisation in a spontaneously immortalised aneuploid Human keratinocyte cell line. *J. Cell Biol.* **106,** 761–771.
18. Scheffner, M., Munger, K., Byrne, J. C., and Howley, P. M. (1991) The state of the p53 and retinoblastoma genes in human cervical-carcinoma cell-lines. *Proc. Natl. Acad. Sci USA* **88,** 5523–5527.
19. Miller, W. E., Earp, H. S., and Raab-Traub, N. (1995) The Epstein-Barr-Virus latent membranc-protein 1 induces expression of the epidermal growth-factor receptor. *J. Virol.* **69,** 4390–4398.
20. Paine, E., Scheinman, R. I., Baldwin, A. S., and Raab-Traub, N. (1995) Expression of LMP1 in epithelial-cells leads to the activation of a select subset of NF-kappa-B/rel family proteins. *J. Virol.* **69,** 4572–4576.
21. Miller, W. E., Mosialos, G., Kieff, E., and Raab Traub, N. (1997) Epstein-Barr-Virus LMP1 induction of the epidermal growth-factor receptor is mediated through a TRAF signaling pathway distinct from NF-kappa-B activation. *J. Virol.* **71,** 586–594.
22. Eliopoulos, A. G., Dawson, C. W., Mosialos, G., Floettmann, J. E., Rowe, M., Armitage, R. J., et al. (1996) CD40-induced growth-inhibition in epithelial-cells is mimicked by Epstein-Barr Virus-encoded LMP1: Involvement of TRAF3 as a common mediator. *Oncogene* **13,** 2243–2254.
23. Eliopoulos, A. G., Stack, M., Dawson, C. W., Kaye, K. M., Hodgkin, L., Sihota, S., et al. (1997) Epstein-Barr Virus-encoded LMP1 and CD40 mediate IL-6 production in epithelial cells via an NF-Kappa-B pathway involving TNF receptor-associated factors. *Oncogene* **14,** 2899–2916.
24. Dover, R. and Potten, C. S. (1983) Cell-cycle kinetics of cultured human epidermal-keratinocytes. *J. Invest. Dermatol.* **80,** 423–429.
25. Sieuwerts, A. M., Klijn, J. G. M., Peters, H. A., and Foekens, J. A. (1995) The MTT tetrazolium salt assay scrutinized: how to use this assay reliably to measure metabolic-activity of cell-cultures in-vitro for the assessment of growth-characteristics, $IC_{50}$-values and cell-survival. *Euro. J. Clin. Chem. Clin. Biochem.* **33,** 813–823.
26. Mosmann, T. (1983) Rapid colorimetric assay for cellular growth and survival: application to proliferation and cyto-toxicity assays. *J. Immunologic. Methods* **65,** 55–63.
27. Scudiero, D. A., Shoemaker, R. H., Paull, K. D., Monks, A., Tierney, S., Nofziger, T. H., et al. (1988) Evaluation of a soluble tetrazolium formazan assay for cell-growth and drug sensitivity in culture using human and other tumor-cell lines. *Cancer Res.* **48,** 4827–4833.

28. Goodwin, C. J., Holt, S. J., Downes, S., and Marshall., N. J. (1995) Microculture tetrazolium assays: a comparison between two new tetrazolium salts, XTT and MTS. *J. Immunologic. Methods* **179,** 95–103.
29. Fields, R. M., and Lancaster, M. V. (1993) Dual attribute continuous monitoring of cell proliferation/cytotoxicity. *Am. Biotechnol. Lab.* **11,** 48.
30. Nakayama, G. R., Caton, M. C., Nova, M. P., and Parondoosh, Z. (1997) Assessment of the Alamar Blue assay for cellular growth and viability in vitro. *J. Immunologic. Methods* **204,** 205–208.

# 18

# In Vitro Assays to Study Epithelial Cell Differentiation

**Christopher W. Dawson and Lawrence S. Young**

## 1. Introduction

The development of in vitro systems for the culture of human epithelial cells has aided the study of epithelial cell transformation by the epitheliotrophic papillomaviruses *(1)*. Although long-term proliferation of keratinocytes in vitro can now be achieved, the tissue-culture environment is not optimal for differentiation, hampering the study of virus:cell interactions in differentiating epithelial cells.

Although differentiation can be achieved by depriving keratinocytes of substrate attachment (so-called suspension culture), the expression of differentiation-specific proteins is usually limited to proteins that are expressed at only the very earliest stages of the differentiation process such as involucrin *(2)*.

Considerable progress in enhancing the differentiation of keratinocytes in vitro has been achieved through the development of more complex culture systems. The growth of keratinocytes at an air-liquid interface on a physiological substrate such as collagen or a dermal equivalent ("organotypic raft culture") is a reliable system where both the histo-morphological and biochemical properties of keratinocyte terminal differentiation can be reproduced in vitro *(3,4)*. In much the same way as investigators have used these systems to investigate papillomavirus:epithelial cell interactions, the same systems can be used to study the effects of Epstein-Barr virus (EBV) on epithelial cell differentiation.

Cell lines established from stratified squamous epithelia tend to retain an ability to differentiate in vitro, albeit to a lesser degree than normal keratinocytes *(5)*. Although cell lines such as SCC12F and HaCat are not as responsive as normal keratinocytes to terminal differentiation stimuli, their ability to attain a substantial degree of differentiation renders them useful in studies aimed at investigating the ability of EBV genes to interfere with the differentiation process *(6,7)*. A number of assays are available for testing the competence of keratinocytes to differentiate in vitro. The expression of differentiation-specific proteins such as high molecular weight keratins or involucrin, a component of the crosslinked envelope, are useful markers for identifying terminally

From: *Methods in Molecular Biology, Vol. 174: Epstein-Barr Virus Protocols*
Edited by: J. B. Wilson and G. H. W. May © Humana Press Inc., Totowa, NJ

differentiating cells *(8)*. The availability of antibodies allows the detection of these proteins by conventional immunohistochemistry or by Western blotting.

### 1.1. Suspension-Induced Terminal Differentiation

A standard assay for inducing terminal differentiation is to deprive keratinocytes of matrix attachment; so-called suspension culture *(2,9)*. Under such conditions, keratinocytes undergo cell-cycle withdrawal and initiate the differentiation process. The ability of terminally differentiating keratinocytes to assemble all of the components necessary for crosslinked envelope formation can be assayed either by immunostaining for envelope proteins *(2)*, or by inducing the assembly of the crosslinked envelope using calcium ionophore *(9,10)*.

### 1.2. Organotypic Raft Culture

Although suspension-induced differentiation is a useful protocol for assessing the ability or competence of keratinocytes to terminally differentiate, the growth of keratinocytes on collagen rafts provides a reliable system where both the histo-morphological and biochemical properties of keratinocyte terminal differentiation can be reproduced in vitro *(3,4)*.

## 2. Materials

### 2.1. Suspension-Induced Differentiation

1. 9-cm bacteriological Petri dishes (Sterilin).
2. poly-HEMA solution: 0.1% (w/v) Poly-(methacrylsaeure-2-hydroxy-ethylester) (Aldrich) in ethanol.
3. Methyl cellulose (Aldrich).
4. Calcium ionophore A23187 (Sigma): use at 50 µg/mL in Dulbecco's Modified Eagle's Medium (DMEM)-H.
5. Polyclonal rabbit antisera to involucrin (Biogenesis).
6. Phosphate-buffered saline (PBS): 58 m*M* $Na_2HPO_4$, 17 m*M* $NaH_2PO_4$, 68 m*M* NaCl.
7. Tissue-culture medium appropriate to cell type (e.g., DMEM) including any required additives, apart from serum.
8. Foetal calf serum (Gibco-BRL).
9. Hemocytometer.
10. 37°C, 5% $CO_2$ incubator.
11. 4% paraformaldehyde: add 4 g paraformaldehyde (BDH, cat. no. 294474L) to PBS to a final volume of 100 mL. Stir overnight to dissolve. Foil-wrap and store for up to 1 mo.
12. Methanol, cooled to –20°C.
13. DMEM-H: DMEM + HEPES at a concentration of 25 m*M*, pH 7.4 (Gibco, cat. no. 13016-035).
14. Differentiation medium: DMEM-H with 2% bovine serum, 2 m*M* glutamine, penicillin (1000 U/mL), streptomycin (1 mg/mL).
15. Complete growth medium: DMEM with 5% fetal calf serum (FCS), 2 m*M* glutamine, 0.4 µg/mL hydrocortisone, penicillin (1000 U/mL), streptomycin (1 mg/mL).
16. 5-mL polypropylene tubes.
17. Sodium dodecyl sulfate-dithiothreitol (SDS-DTT): 2% SDS, 40 m*M* DTT.
18. Antibody to involucrin: Biogenesis, cat. no. 5391–0006.
19. FITC-labeled goat anti-rabbit antibodies (Sigma, cat. no. F-0382).

20. DABCO solution: 90% glycerol, 10% PBS, 2.5% (w/v) 1,4-dizabicyclo(2,2,2)octane, pH 8.6.
21. UV-fluorescence microscope: Olympus or equivalent.
22. Tissue-culture dishes.

### 2.2. "Organotypic" Raft Culture

1. Rat tail collagen type IA: use at 5 mg/mL (Collaborative Research).
2. Raft salt solution: 2.2 g $NaHCO_3$, 4.77 g HEPES in 100 mL of 0.05 *M* NaOH.
3. 10X DMEM (Gibco).
4. Stainless steel grids/mesh: Orme (cat. No. G34–150) 150 × 150-mm squares. Cut to 60–70-mm diameter circles.
5. Cryo-M-Bed: (Bright Instrument Co. Ltd, Merck BDH, cat. no. 404/0144/25).
6. Hemocytometer.
7. 3.5 and 9-cm bacteriological Petri dishes.
8. Complete growth medium: tissue-culture medium appropriate for the cell type with required additives.
9. Differentiation medium: DMEM-H with 2% bovine serum, 2 m*M* glutamine, 1000 U/mL penicillin, 1 mg/mL streptomycin.
10. Aluminum foil.
11. Isopentane.
12. Nickel crucible (Orme, cat. no. B15-520).
13. Cryostat.
14. Acetone, cooled to –20°C.

## 3. Methods

### 3.1. Suspension-Induced Terminal Differentiation

#### 3.1.1. Preparation of Poly-HEMA Coated Plates

1. Aliquot 2 mL of poly-HEMA solution into 9-cm bacteriological Petri dishes and allow to dry overnight in a laminar flow cabinet.
2. Prior to use, rinse the plates with several changes of PBS.

#### 3.1.2. Preparation of 1.6% Methyl Cellulose Medium

1. Measure 8 g of methyl cellulose powder into a 500-mL flat bottomed bottle containing a magnetic stirrer and autoclaved at 120°C for 30 min.
2. Add 475 mL of serum-free tissue-culture medium, preheated to 60°C, and allow the methyl cellulose to dissolve overnight on a stirring platform at 4°C.
3. Transfer the contents to a sterile centrifuge bottle and centrifuge at 4500*g* at 4°C for 30 min to pellet undissolved material.
4. Decant the semi-solid medium into sterile bottles (~100-mL aliquots).
5. Add serum to a final concentration of 5% (5 mL) and store the complete medium at –20°C.

#### 3.1.3. Preparation of Cells

1. Harvest cells in the log phase of growth (less than 90% confluent) by trypsinization (*see* **Note 1**), resuspend in tissue-culture medium, and count cell numbers using a hemocytometer. If keratinocyte cultures have been grown on irradiated 3T3 cells, rinse the cells free of the 3T3 fibroblasts. After aspiration of the growth medium, rinse plates twice with PBS. A dilute solution of ethylediamine tetraacetic acid (EDTA) (0.02%) is then added and incubated for 30–60 s. The surface of the plates are then washed with the EDTA

solution, which selectively removes the fibroblasts. After another wash in PBS, the remaining keratinocytes can be recovered by trypsinization.

2. In triplicate for each test, pellet $10^6$ cells by centrifugation at 500*g* for 5 min, and resuspend in 10 mL of 1.6% methyl cellulose medium. Dispense each 10-mL sample into a poly-HEMA coated 9 cm bacteriological Petri dish. Incubate at 37°C, 5% $CO_2$ for 24–72 h to allow differentiation (*see* **Note 2**).
3. Collect and dilute the cell suspension at least 10-fold in PBS (to reduce the viscosity). Recover the cells by centrifugation at 500*g* for 5 min.
4. Wash cell 2–3 times in PBS (centrifuge to remove PBS wash).
5. For immunostaining, smear an aliquot of cells onto glass slides and allow to air-dry. For Western blotting analysis, cell pellets can be processed.
6. Fix air-dried slides in 4% para-formaldehyde for 20 min followed by cold methanol (–20°C) for 5 min. The samples are now ready for immunostaining.
7. Rehydrate samples in PBS for 5 min. Stain with undiluted rabbit antibody against involucrin and incubate at 37°C for 60 min. Wash slides twice for 15 min in PBS. Stain with secondary FITC conjugated goat anti-rabbit antibody, diluted 1:75 in PBS. Wash slides in PBS and mount samples in DABCO solution. Examine under a UV fluorescent microscope.
8. Count the number of involucrin positive cells and express as a percentage of the total population. Count between 100–200 cells per field.

### *3.1.4. Cross-Linked Envelope Formation*

1. Induce cells to differentiate by suspension culture and collect by centrifugation as described in **Subheading 3.1.3., steps 1–3.**
2. Wash cells twice in serum free DMEM by centrifugation, removing the wash, and count using a hemocytometer.
3. Pellet $10^6$ cells and resuspend in 0.5 mL DMEM-H containing 50 µg/mL of A23187 ionophore. Transfer to a sterile 5-mL polypropylene tube. Incubate at 37°C, 5% $CO_2$ for 3–4 h.
4. Add 0.5 mL of SDS-DTT and mix the cell suspension thoroughly.
5. Heat the samples to 100°C for 5 min and allow to cool.
6. Remove an aliquot of the sample and examine by phase-contrast microscopy. Score cross-linked envelopes by appearance (cell ghosts). Data is expressed as the mean (± SEM) percentages of ionophore-treated cells that formed cornified envelopes from assays performed on triplicate cultures of each of the cell lines examined (*see* **Notes 3** and **4**).

## *3.2. Organotypic Raft Culture Systems*

The procedure for preparing collagen rafts is outlined schematically in **Fig. 1**. The typical appearance of a collagen raft culture is shown in **Fig. 2**.

### *3.2.1. Preparation of NIH 3T3 Cells (see **Note 5**) and the Collagen Matrix*

1. Harvest subconfluent cultures of NIH 3T3 cells by trypsinization and count cell numbers.
2. Pellet $10^6$ cells by centrifugation at 500*g* for 5 min, and allow the pellet to cool on ice for 10 min prior to incorporation into the collagen matrix.
3. All of the reagents required for the preparation of the collagen rafts must be kept on ice prior to raft formation. Mix 8 mL of collagen type IA (rat tail) with 1 mL of 10X serum-free DMEM and 1 mL of raft salt solution (*see* **Note 6**).
4. Carefully resuspend the pelleted 3T3 cells in this mixture (to $10^5$ cells/mL) and mix thoroughly. Aliquot 2 mL/dish into 3.5-cm Petri dishes.

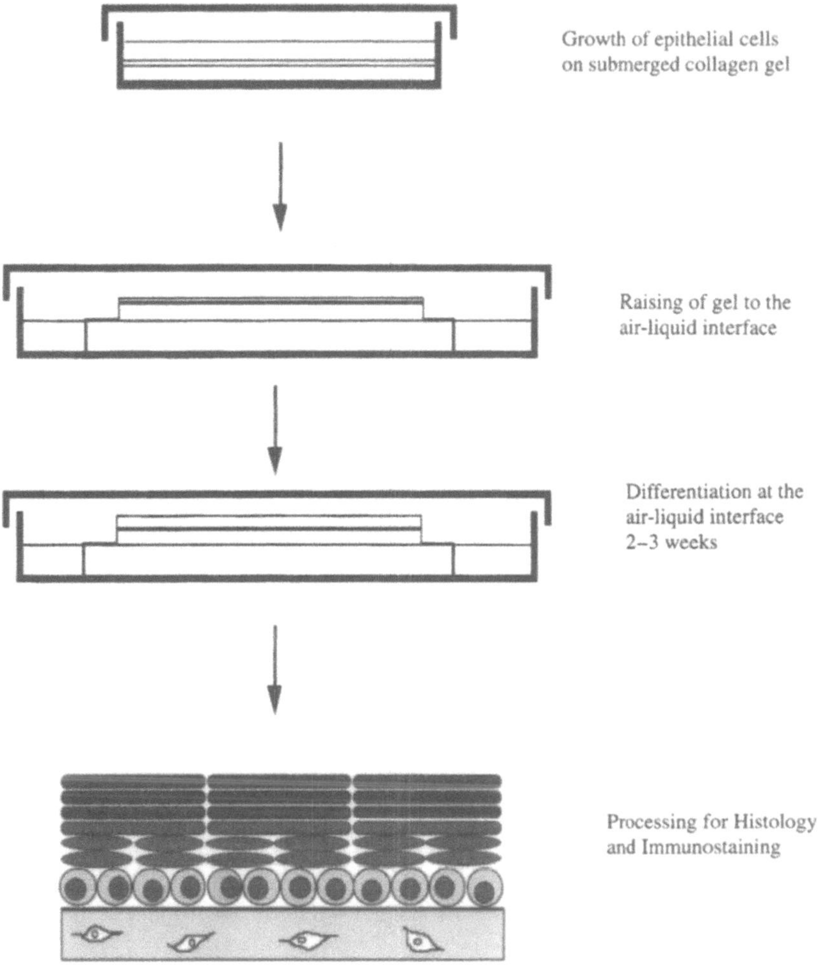


Fig. 1. Schematic representation of the steps involved in generating collage raft cultures.

5. Allow the collagen rafts to gel at 37°C for at least 30 min. Add 1 mL of complete growth medium to each dish to cover the gel.

### 3.2.2. Seeding of the Collagen Rafts

1. Harvest primary keratinocytes or squamous cell carcinoma-derived cell lines by trypsinization and count cells. Seed between 2 and $5 \times 10^5$ cells onto the surface of the collagen raft. Incubate for 24 h at 37°C, 5% $CO_2$ (*see* **Note 7**).
2. Aspirate the medium to remove unattached cells and replace with fresh complete growth medium.
3. Replace medium every 2 d until the keratinocytes form a confluent monolayer. This usually takes between 7–10 d.

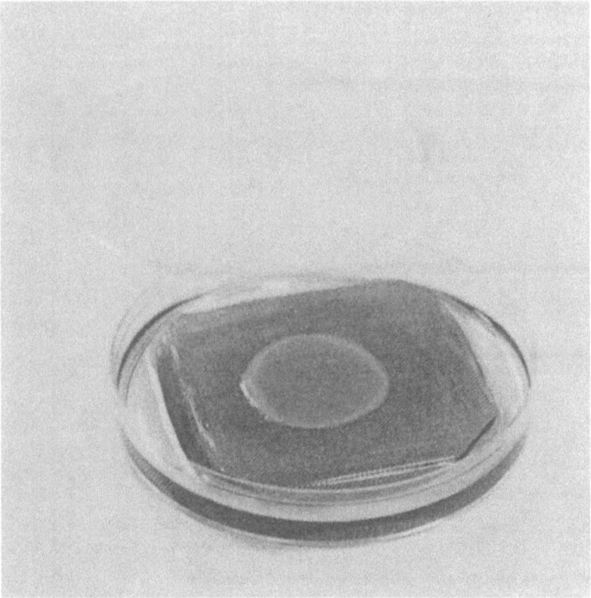

Fig. 2. The typical appearance of a collagen raft culture.

### 3.2.3. Induction of Differentiation

To induce a program of terminal differentiation, keratinocytes are cultured at the air:medium interface.

1. Using a spatula, carefully pull away the edge of the collagen raft from the edge of the Petri dish and lift the whole raft onto a stainless-steel grid placed in the center of a 9-cm Petri dish.
2. Add 10–15 mL of differentiation medium such that the surface of the collagen raft is kept dry. Replace medium at two daily intervals and maintain collagen rafts for 2–3 wk at 37°C, 5% $CO_2$ (*see* **Note 8**).

### 3.2.4. Processing of Collagen Rafts

1. After 2–3 wk of incubation, remove the collagen rafts from the surface of the stainless-steel grids with the aid of fine forceps.
2. Immerse the rafts in 2–3 mL of Cryo-M-Bed that has been coated on the surface of a 5-$cm^2$ strip of aluminum foil. Place the raft with the top (exposed) surface of the epithelium facing downward and smooth out.
3. Freeze the rafts by lowering the foil onto the surface of isopentane contained in a small nickel crucible floating on the surface of liquid nitrogen (*see* **Note 9**). After freezing, store the rafts at –70°C.
4. Cut 5-µm sections on a cryostat and fix in cold acetone (–20°C) for 10 min prior to immunostaining with antibodies specific for differentiation-associated proteins such as involucrin, and high-molecular weight keratins (**Fig. 3**, *see* **Notes 10** and **11**).

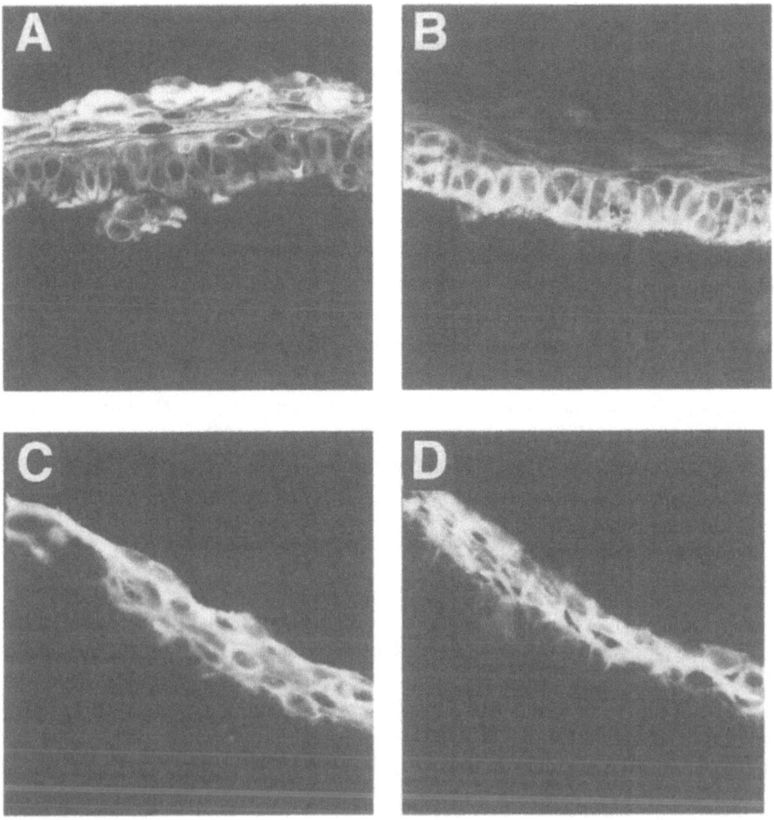


Fig. 3. Representative sections from a culture of SCC12F cells grown at the air:liquid interface for 3 wk and stained for expression of differentiation specific proteins: **(A)** staining with a pan-keratin antibody, AE1. **(B)** Staining with the P1E6 antibody, specific for $\alpha_2\beta_1$ integrin, which stains only basal cells. **(C)** Staining with the 8.60 antibody, specific for the differentiation specific keratins K1/10, which are expressed in suprabasal cells. **(D)** Staining with a rabbit polyclonal antibody against involucrin, which is only expressed in suprabasal cells.

## 4. Notes

1. Details on trypsinizing adherent cells are given in Chapter 14.
2. The time required for differentiation in suspension culture may vary considerably between cell lines. Cells can be incubated for up to 10 d.
3. Calcium ionophores activate the calcium-dependent enzyme transglutaminase that catalyzes the formation of the crosslinked envelope. In theory, only keratinocytes that have assembled all of the proteins necessary for envelope formation will form cross-linked envelopes, whereas those that have not will be lysed in SDS.
4. Solubilization of ionophore-treated cells results in the release of DNA. This may lead to excessive clumping of the envelopes and make quantitation difficult. The addition of 0.1 mg/mL DNAse may reduce envelope aggregation.

5. If 3T3 fibroblasts are not available then human skin fibroblasts can be used as an alternative.
6. Certain suppliers recommend the use of lower concentrations of collagen (1–3 mg/mL). In this case the collagen solution should be diluted with sterile 0.02 *N* HCl to give the desired concentration.
7. As certain epithelial cell lines migrate very poorly on collagen rich gels, it may be necessary to plate out greater than $5 \times 10^5$ cells onto the collagen raft at the initial seeding.
8. Care should be taken not to cover the surface of the exposed epithelium at any time during this period as this will interfere with terminal differentiation. However, there may be instances when the aim of the experiment is to recapitulate the in vivo differentiation of wet-stratified squamous epithelium. In this case, the surface of the differentiating epithelium must be bathed in serum-free medium at every re-feeding.
9. Care should be taken when snap-freezing the collagen rafts, as too rapid freezing results in poor morphology and "break-up" of the raft.
10. As the growth of keratinocytes on the surface of the collagen raft may be uneven, it is advisable to take sections from at least 3 different areas of the raft.
11. As an alternative to snap-freezing, collagen rafts can be fixed in 4% para-formaldehyde and processed as for conventional histology. This has the benefit of preserving the architecture of the raft.

## References

1. Chow, L. T. and Broker, T. R. (1997) In vitro experimental systems for HPV: epithelial raft cultures for investigations of viral reproduction and pathogenesis and for genetic analyses of viral proteins and regulatory sequences. *Clin. Dermatol.* **15,** 217–227.
2. Watt, F. M. (1983) Involucrin and other markers of keratinocyte terminal differentiation. *J. Investig. Dermatolo.* **81,** S100–S103.
3. Asselineau, D., Bernhard, B., Bailly, C., and Darmon, M. (1985) Epidermal morphogenesis and induction of the 67-kd keratin polypeptide by culture of human keratinocytes at the liquid-air interface. *Exp. Cell Res.* **159,** 536–539.
4. Kopan, R., Traska, G., and Fuchs, E. (1987) Retinoids as important regulators of terminal differentiation-examining keratin expression in individual epidermal-cells at various stages of keratinization. *J. Cell Biol.* **105,** 427–440.
5. Rheinwald, J. G. and Beckett, M. A. (1981) Tumorigenic keratinocyte lines requiring anchorage and fibroblast support cultured from Human squamous-cell carcinomas. *Cancer Res.* **41,** 1657–1663.
6. Parkinson, E. K., Grabham, P., and Emmerson, A. (1983) A subpopulation of cultured human keratinocytes which is resistant to the induction of terminal differentiation-related changes by phorbol, 12-myristate, 13-acetate—evidence for an increase in the resistant population following transformation. *Carcinogenesis* **4,** 857–861.
7. Ryle, C. M., Breitkreutz, D., Stark, H. J., Leigh, I. M., Steinert, P. M., Roop, D., and Fusenig, N. E. (1989) Density-dependent modulation of synthesis of keratin-1 and keratin-10 in the Human keratinocyte line HaCat and in ras-transfected tumorigenic clones. *Differentiation* **40,** 42–54.
8. Fuchs, E. (1990) Epidermal differentiation: the bare essentials. *J. Cell Biol.* **111,** 2807–2814.
9. Green, H. (1977) Terminal differentiation of cultured Human epidermal cells. *Cell* **11,** 405–416.
10. Rubin, A. L. and Rice, R. H. (1986) Differential regulation by retinoic acid and calcium of transglutaminases in cultured neoplastic and normal human keratinocytes. *Cancer Res.* **46,** 2356–2361.

# 19

# Cell Sensitivity Assays

## *Quantitative Detection of Apoptotic Cells In Vitro Using the TUNEL Assay*

**Neil A. Jones and Caroline Dive**

## 1. Introduction

### *1.1. Principles of Flow Cytometry*

Flow cytometry allows rapid multi-parameter analyses of individual cells. Cells are illuminated with incident laser light of a specific wavelength. Resultant light-scatter signals and fluorescence-emission signals from fluorochromes contained at the surface of the cell or within it are detected by an array of photomuliplier tubes. For example, fluorochrome-conjugated antibodies and DNA interchelating dyes can be used to acquire information on protein expression and DNA ploidy (via fluorescence signals) together with information on cell size and structure (via light-scatter signals).

### *1.2. Chromatin Changes During Apoptosis*

Apoptosis is a process whereby cells die via an ordered cellular program and is therefore often referred to as programmed cell death. Apoptosis is important in the maintenance of tissue homeostasis and during animal development *(1,2)*. Many currently used cytotoxic drugs kill tumor cells because of their ability to induce apoptosis *(3)* and apoptosis is increasingly being studied in the context of drug resistance. Despite the wide variety of stimuli that can induce apoptosis, most cells undergoing the process exhibit a similar series of changes, suggesting that these signals converge to engage a common pathway, which is required for the execution of cell death. One of the most widely studied biochemical process that occurs during apoptosis is the non-random cleavage of genomic DNA. This cleavage is owing to the activation of specific endogenous endonucleases and results in the formation of a large numbers of DNA strand breaks *(4)*. The separation of DNA from these apoptotic cells by agarose gel electrophoresis and subsequent visualization using ethidium bromide reveals a characteristic "ladder" pattern *(4)*. Such "ladders" consist of multiples of ~200 base

From: *Methods in Molecular Biology, Vol. 174: Epstein-Barr Virus Protocols*
Edited by: J. B. Wilson and G. H. W. May © Humana Press Inc., Totowa, NJ

pairs, and occur as a result of cleavage of DNA between nucleosome histone complexes (or bundles). In some cells, such nucleosomal DNA laddering is not seen, and in these cases high molecular weight (50 or 300 kbp) DNA fragments may be produced *(5–7)*.

These high molecular weight DNA fragments are thought to arise as a result of the release of chromatin from the nuclear matrix. The identification of such DNA fragmentation by agarose gel electrophoresis, although indicative of apoptosis, cannot be used as a quantitative assay. In addition, apoptosis of mammalian cells in culture, although regulated, is often asynchronous and therefore accurate determination of levels and rates of apoptosis is difficult using the aforementioned assay.

An alternative methodology that can be used to rapidly detect and quantitate DNA strand breaks in individual cells undergoing apoptosis utilizes flow cytometry *(8)*. This has the advantage of simultaneous detection of the DNA strand breaks and cell-cycle distribution in individual cells. In addition, this methodology has been used to detect DNA strand breaks in clinical samples before and after treatment with cytotoxic drugs *(8,9)*.

During cell death there is an alteration in the ability of cells to scatter light at a forward angle reflecting cell size and at 90° reflecting cell granularity. These changes can be detected using flow cytometry. Such changes can be used to discriminate between live cells, dead cells, and cells that are undergoing apoptosis *(10)*. As mentioned earlier, apoptotic cells characteristically exhibit DNA strand breaks and these can be detected using terminal deoxynucleotidyl transferase *T*dT mediated d*U*TP *N*ick *E*nd *L*abelling (TUNEL) and flow cytometry *(8)*. Exogenous terminal deoxynucleotidyl transferase is used to incorporate either BrdUTP or biotinylated dUTP to the 3' end of single-stranded DNA. Fragmented DNA can then be detected by using FITC-conjugated antibody or FITC-labeled avidin to reveal the incorporation of labeled nucleotide. By counterstaining with propidium iodide (PI), information on cell-cycle distribution can also be obtained within the same cell. We shall outline the methodology, which can be used to label strand breaks in suspension or adherent tissue-culture cells induced to undergo apoptosis, using both of these deoxynucleotides.

## 2. Materials (*see* Note 1)

1. Phosphate-buffered saline (PBS): 10X PBS tablets can be obtained from Oxoid. 1X PBS is made by dissolving 1 tablet in every 100 mL of $dH_2O$. PBS should be made weekly and kept at 4°C.
2. Fixatives: (i) 1% (v/v) formaldehyde in PBS. Formaldehyde is normally supplied as a 20% or 40% solution and should therefore be diluted fresh for each experiment and kept on ice. The formaldehyde should be methanol free and can be purchased from Polysciences Inc. (ii) 100% ethanol and PBS should be prechilled on ice.
3. Terminal deoxynucleotidyl transferase (TdT): Can be purchased from Boehringer Mannheim and is supplied as 25 U/μL and stored at –20°C.
4. TdT reaction buffer: Supplied with the TdT enzyme as a 5X concentrated solution (5X concentrated = 1 *M* potassium cacodylate, 125 m*M* Tris-HCl, pH 6.6, 1.25 mg/mL BSA) and stored at –20°C.

5. Cobalt Chloride ($CoCl_2$): Supplied as a 25 m*M* solution with the enzyme and is stored at –20°C.
6. 20X SSC: Dissolve 17.5 g NaCl and 8.8 g tri sodium citrate in 80 mL $dH_2O$. Adjust pH to 7.0 and make up to 100 mL with $dH_2O$. This should be autoclaved and can then stored at room temperature.
7. BrdUTP solution: BrdUTP powder (Sigma) is prepared as a 2 m*M* solution in 50 m*M* Tris-HCl, pH 7.5, and stored at –20°C.
8. Biotin-16-dUTP (bt-dUTP) solution: Obtained from Boehringer Mannheim as a 50 n*M* solution and stored at –20°C.
9. FITC (fluorescein isothiocyanate) conjugated anti BrdU antibody: Purchased from Becton Dickinson.
10. FITC-conjugated anti-BrdU antibody-staining solution: Make a solution of PBS + 0.1% Triton X-100 + 1% BSA + 0.1 µg/mL FITC conjugated anti BrdU antibody. This is made up fresh for each experiment and kept on ice.
11. Avidin-FITC stock (1000X): Obtained from Sigma. Made as a 5 mg/mL solution in PBS. This stock solution should be aliquoted and stored at –20°C. Working stock solutions can be stored at 4°C but should be used within a month and should only be diluted to a working dilution when required.
12. Avidin-FITC solution: 4X SSC (diluted from 20X SSC using $dH_2O$) + 0.1% (v/v) Triton X-100 and 5% (w/v) fat-free dried skimmed milk (Marvel) + 5 µg/mL avidin-FITC (purchased from Sigma). Make up fresh for each experiment.
13. Washing solution: PBS + 0.1% (v/v) Triton X-100 + 5 mg/mL BSA, make fresh for each experiment.
14. PI staining solution: PBS + 5 µg/mL PI (Molecular Probes) + 200 µg/mL DNase free RNase (Sigma), make up fresh immediately before use. The RNase can be made as a stock of 20 mg/mL in $H_2O$ and stored in aliquots at –20°C.
15. Flow cytometer: We use a Becton Dickinson FACS Vantage instrument. Whatever flow cytometer you have access to, the machine must be set up appropriately; because dual color detection will be used the machine may require color-compensation adjustment (*see* **Subheading 3.3.**). It is important therefore that control reactions are included in each experiment (*see* **Note 2**). It is wise to use an experienced flow cytometry user to undertake such adjustments unless you know what you are doing. The data analysis shown in **Fig. 1** was obtained using Lysis II software supplied with the instrument.

## 3. Methods

We will describe the two basic methodologies of the TdT assay, which can be used to detect DNA strand breaks in cells undergoing apoptosis (*see* **Note 3**). Both methods are essentially identical except that Method A utilizes brdUTP to label DNA ends, whereas Method B uses biotin-16-dUTP; bt-dUTP. Incorporation of both the nucleotides is obtained using exogenous terminal deoxynucleotidyl transferase. Detection of incorporation of these nucleotides is achieved using a FITC-conjugated BrdU antibody or FITC-labeled avidin (avidin binds to the biotin conjugated onto the nucleotide). Control reactions must also be carried out in addition to experimental samples. These are used to determine nonspecific binding of detection reagents and allow the flow cytometer to be adjusted to compensate for such binding. These control reactions are highlighted in the notes section (*see* **Note 2**)

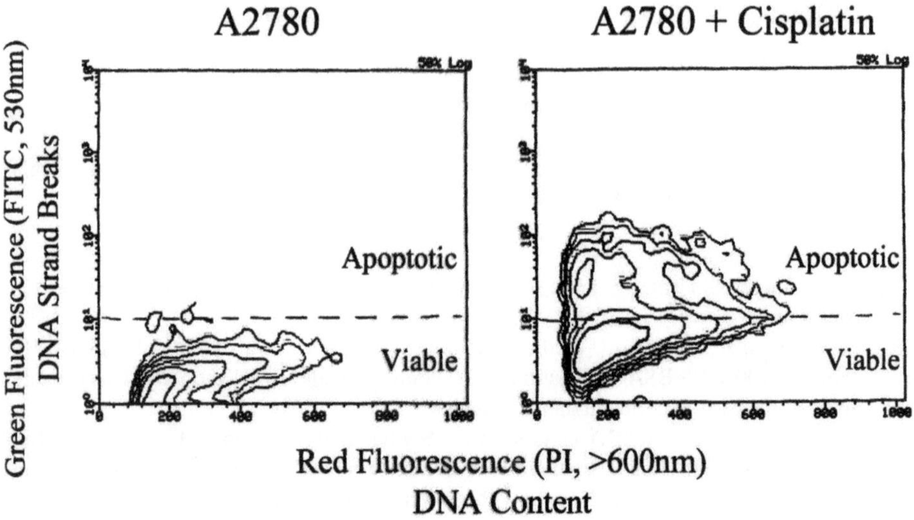


Fig. 1. Incorporation of bt-dUTP by exogenous TdT into the DNA of human ovarian carcinoma cells exposed to the DNA damaging agent cisplatin. Two-dimensional frequency contour plots of red fluorescence (*x*-axis; PI stained DNA) vs green fluorescence (*y*-axis; bt-dUTP labeled with avidin-FITC). Untreated human A2780 ovarian carcinoma cells and these cells exposed to 20 μ*M* cisplatin for 1 h and then incubated for 96 h at 37°C were then processed using method B. Cells with green fluorescence above the dotted line are considered to be positive for incorporation of labeled nucleotide by exogenous TdT and therefore undergoing apoptosis.

### 3.1. Method A: Using BrdUTP to Label the DNA Strand Breaks

1. Harvest cells and count using a hemocytometer (*see* **Note 4**). Place aliquots of $1 \times 10^6$ cells into flow cytometer tubes. Wash once in ice-cold PBS, pour off the PBS, leaving the pellet with a small amount of fluid. Cells are pelleted at 200*g* for 5 min.
2. Vortex the cell pellet at the same time as adding 1 mL of the formaldehyde fixative solution (*see* **Note 5**). Vortexing at the same time as adding the fixative will reduce cell clumping which may block the flow cytometer. Leave the cells to fix on ice for 15 min.
3. Pellet cells and wash once with 2 mL PBS. Resuspend the pellet in 300 μL of ice cold PBS. Add 700 μL of ice-cold ethanol, again while the cells are being vortexed. The cells can now be stored in the fridge for up to 2 wk; if the cells are to be used immediately, they must be in this ethanol fixative for at least 30 min on ice. The ability to keep the fixed cells for a period of time means that time-course experiments can be undertaken and the samples then processed for end labeling at the same time.
4. On the day of the end-labeling experiment, spin the cells down and remove the ethanol solution. The cells should then be rehydrated in 1 mL of PBS for 15 min. It is a good idea to look at the cells by microscopy now to make sure there are no large clumps of cells.
5. Spin cells down (*see* **Note 6**), resuspend the pellets in 50 μL of 1X TdT reaction buffer (the 5X concentrated stock is diluted to 1X with $dH_2O$). Add 1 μL TdT (5 U; the enzyme is supplied at 25 U/μL and should be diluted to 5 U/μL with 1X reaction buffer) and 2 μL brdUTP. Incubate at 37°C for 40 min.

6. Add 2 mL of washing buffer to each tube and spin down (*see* **Note 6**).
7. Resuspend the pellet in 50 µL of the FITC-conjugated BrdU antibody solution and incubate at room temperature for 30 min in the dark.
8. Add 2 mL of washing buffer to each tube and spin down.
9. Resuspend the cell pellet in 1 mL of PI staining solution and incubate for 30 min at room temperature again in the dark.
10. Analyze the cells by flow cytometry (*see* **Note 2**).

### 3.2. Method B: Using Biotin-16-dUTP to Label the Strand Breaks

1. Harvest cells and count using a hemocytometer (*see* **Note 4**). Place aliquots of $1 \times 10^6$ cells into flow cytometer tubes. Wash once in ice-cold PBS, pour off the PBS leaving the pellet with a small amount of fluid. Cells are pelleted at 200*g* for 5 min.
2. Vortex the cell pellet and add 1 mL of the formaldehyde fixative (*see* **Note 5**). Vortexing at the same time as adding the fixative will reduce cell clumping, which may block the flow cytometer. Leave the cells to fix on ice for 15 min.
3. Pellet cells and wash once with 2 mL PBS. Resuspend the pellet in 300 µL of ice-cold PBS. Add 700 µL of ice-cold ethanol, again while the cells are being vortexed. The cells can now be stored in the fridge for up to 2 wk, if the cells are to be used immediately they must be in this ethanol fixative for a minimum of 30 min on ice.
4. On the day of the labeling experiment, spin the cells down and remove the ethanol solution. The cells should then be rehydrated in 1 mL PBS for 15 min. Look at the cells now by microscopy to make sure there are no large clumps of cells.
5. Spin cells down (*see* **Note 6**), resuspend the pellets in 50 µL of TdT reaction buffer (the 5X concentrated stock is diluted to 1X with $H_2O$). Add 1 µL TdT (5 U; the enzyme is supplied at 25 U/µL and should be diluted to 5 U/µL with 1X reaction buffer) and 0.5 µL of bt-dUTP (0.5 n*M* final concentration). Incubate at 37°C for 40 min.
6. Add 2 mL of washing buffer to each tube and spin down (*see* **Note 6**).
7. Resuspend the pellet in 50 µL of the avidin-FITC solution containing 5 µg/mL avidin-FITC (1 in 1000 dilution of the stock solution). Incubate in the dark at room temperature for 30 min.
8. Add 2 mL of washing buffer to each tube and spin down.
9. Resuspend the cell pellet in 1 mL of PI staining solution and incubate for 30 min at room temperature again in the dark.
10. Analyze the cells by flow cytometry (*see* **Note 2**)

### 3.3. Data Analysis

Light-scatter properties are used to discriminate large cell clumps and cellular debris by pacement of an electronic gate around intact fixed cells on a scatter plot prior to analysis of DNA fragmentation. Such gating should be done when running the control samples (*see* above and **Note 2**). To measure the binding of FITC-labeled antibody to incorporated nucleotide at the same time as cell-cycle distribution via propidium binding to DNA, the following laser wavelengths should be used.

The samples should be illuminated with a 488 nm laser line. 10,000 cells are analyzed per sample with a flow rate of 300–500 cells per second. Green fluorescence of the FITC is detected using a 530 nm ± 20 nm band pass filter. Red fluorescence of the propidium bound to DNA is measured at 630 ± 22 nm band pass filter. The green and red fluorescence should be separated using a 560 nm short-pass dichroic filter. Check to see whether color compensation is required by analysis of green only, and then red only, fluorescing cells. Two cells in $G_1$ phase of the cell cycle passing the laser together can be discriminated from a single cell in $G_2$ using pulse-width analysis *(11)*.

A typical two-dimensional profile of green and red fluorescence is shown in **Fig. 1.** For each cell that passes in single file through the laser both red fluorescence and green fluorescence are measured. The amount of PI binding to DNA, which indicates phase of cell cycle, is plotted on the x axis. The y axis shows the amount of green fluorescence displayed by the cells and therefore indicates the extent of incorporation of the labeled nucleotide. Elevated green fluorescence exhibited by the cells is taken as a measure of the number of strand breaks and therefore the extent of apoptosis in the cells. The percentage of cells exhibiting high green fluorescence is determined using a gate positioned above the green fluorescence levels observed in control samples.

## 4. Notes

1. There are now a number of commercially available kits with which to undertake this assay; they can be obtained from, e.g., Appligene Oncor, Boehringer Mannheim, Pharmingen, or Promega.
2. It is essential that control reactions are included in every experiment; this allows the flow cytometer to be set up and adjusted as necessary. The following samples are needed in addition to the experimental samples you want to run: Using control healthy cells with no strand breaks:
   1. Blank (just cells);
   2. TdT only (no BrdU antibody or avidin-FITC or PI);
   3. BrdU antibody or avidin-FITC only (no TdT enzyme or PI);
   4. TdT and BrdU antibody or avidin-FITC (no PI);
   5. PI only (no TdT or BrdU antibody or avidin-FITC);

   Dying cells with strand breaks:

   6. TdT and BrdU antibody or avidin-FITC; and
   7. PI only.
3. In our experience, quantification of apoptosis using this assay in apoptotic cells that fail to produce a 200 bp ladder but that do produce 30 and 500 kb DNA fragments is much more difficult, although not impossible *(12)* because there are fewer DNA strand breaks and therefore fewer free DNA ends with which to label. It is therefore worthwhile to determine if your chosen cell type does undergo nucleosomal DNA laddering when they apoptose; this can be determined using conventional agarose gel electrophoresis.
4. All samples should contain equal cell numbers ($1 \times 10^6$ or more is ideal because of the inevitable loss of cells during the washing steps) to ensure that the reagents are not limiting for efficient labelling of the DNA.
5. Cell fixation using cross-linking agents is essential; this prevents loss of small DNA fragments during the labeling and detection reactions and after the washes. Vortexing of the cells when adding the fixatives is vital, particularly when using cells that normally grow as adherent monolayers in vitro; this reduces cell clumping that, if high, will block the flow of sample in the flow cytometer. It is therefore worthwhile to check by microscopy that the cell suspension contains single cells and not as clumps before running the samples through the flow cytometer. Very fragile cells may not survive these procedures and so this may not be an ideal method with which to measure apoptosis; empirical determination of the suitability of this method to detect strand breaks for different cell types must

therefore be carried out. Alternatively, try the Annexin V binding assay on fixed cells ***(13)***, or the Hoeschst assay on unfixed cells ***(14)***.

6. During washes make sure the wash buffer is completely removed and that the pelleted cells are as dry as possible. The small reaction volumes used means that any wash buffer that does remain with the pellets after washing will dilute the enzyme or antibody reaction mixes, which may therefore reduce the efficiency of incorporation of nucleotides into the strand breaks and their subsequent detection.

## References


1. Raff, M. C. (1992) Social controls on cell survival and cell death. *Nature* **356,** 397–399.
2. Williams, G. T. and Smith, C. A. (1993) Molecular recognition of apoptosis: genetic controls on cell death. *Cell* **74,** 777–779.
3. Hickman, J. A. (1992) Apoptosis induced by anticancer drugs. *Cancer Metastasis Rev.* **11,** 121–139.
4. Wyllie, A. H. (1994) Apoptosis: death gets a break. *Nature* **369,** 272, 273.
5. Anthoney, D. A., McIlwrath, A. J., Gallagher, W. M., Edlin, A. R. M., and Brown, R. (1996) Microsatellite instability, apoptosis and loss of p53 function in drug-resistant tumour cells. *Cancer Res.* **56,** 1374–1381.
6. Ormerod, M. G., O'Neill, C. F., Robertson, D., and Harrap, K. (1994) Cisplatin induced apoptosis in a human ovarian carcinoma cell line without concomitant internucleosomal degradation of DNA. *Exp. Cell Res.* **211,** 231–237.
7. Oberhammer, F., Wilson, J. W., Dive, C., Morris, I. D., Hickman, J. A., Wakeling, A. E., et al. (1993) Apoptotic death in epithelial cells: cleavage of DNA to 300 and/or 50 kb fragments prior to or in the absence of internucleosomal fragmentation. *EMBO J.* **12,** 3679–3684.
8. Gorczyca, W., Gong, J., and Darzynkiewicz, Z. (1993) Detection of DNA strand breaks in individual apoptotic cells by the in situ terminal deoxynucleotidyl transferase and nick translation assays. *Cancer Res.* **53,** 1945–1951.
9. Gorczyca, W., Bigman, K., Mitterman, A., Ahmed, T., Gong, J., Melamed, A. R., and Darzynkiewicz, Z. (1993) Induction of DNA strand breaks associated with apoptosis during the treatment of leukaemias. *Leukaemia* **7,** 659–670.
10. Gregory, C. D., Dive, C., Henderson, S., Smith, C. A., Williams, G. T., Gordon, J., and Rickinson, A. B. (1991) Activation of Epstein Barr Virus latent genes protects human B cells from death by apoptosis. *Nature* **249,** 612–614.
11. Ormerod, M. G. ed. (1990) *Flow Cytometry: A Practical Approach.* IRL Press, Oxford.
12. Chapman, R. S., Chresta, C. M., Herberg, A. A., Beere, H. M., Heer, S., Whetton, A. D., et al. (1995) Further characterisation of the in situ terminal deoxynucleotidyl transferase (TdT) assay for the flow cytometric analysis of apoptosis in drug resistant and drug sensitive leukaemic cells. *Cytometry* **20,** 245–256.
13. Vermes, I., Haanen, C., and Reutelingsperger, C. (1995) A novel assay for apoptosis based upon flow cytometric detection of phosphatidylserine on the cell surface with use of FITC-labelled annexin V. *Clin. Chem.* **41,** 91.
14. Dive, C., Gregory, C. D., Phipps, D. J., Evans, D. L., Milner, A. E., and Wyllie, A. H. (1992) Analysis and discrimination of necrosis and apoptosis (programmed cell death) by multi parameter flow cytometry. *Biochim. Biophys. Acta* **1133,** 275–285.

# 20

# Qualitative Detection of Apoptotic Cells Assessed by DNA Fragmentation

**Amanda J. McIlwrath**

## 1. Introduction

The techniques presented in this chapter describe the experimental procedure for the identification of the nonrandom DNA fragmentation associated with apoptosis. The major benefits of this method are its ability to detect a low level of DNA fragmentation and its ability to detect large DNA fragments (50 kb and 300–1000 kb) as opposed to the internucleosomal DNA ladder. It is a qualitative technique although it can be of limited quantitative value. It can be used to detect apoptosis in cell lines following exposure to a wide variety of agents.

In most cells that are undergoing apoptosis, the DNA is broken down into 180–200 bp internucleosomal fragments known as the DNA ladder *(1)*. The DNA ladder can be visualized by ethidium bromide staining of DNA which has been subjected to agarose gel electrophoresis. The DNA ladder is not always observed and in some apoptosing cells only the large DNA fragments of 50 kb and/or 300–1000 kb are produced *(2)*. The appearance of these large fragments is thought to be a precursor to DNA laddering. Apoptotic morphology may also be observed in the absence of DNA fragmentation *(3,4)*. The absence of DNA fragmentation therefore is not necessarily diagnostic of lack of apoptosis although this appears to be an infrequent observation.

Because fragments of 50 kb and 300–1000 kb cannot be discriminated using normal agarose gel electrophoresis, field inversion gel electrophoresis must be employed. In order to sensitize the detection of DNA from potentially low numbers of apoptotic cells Southern blotting and detection of the DNA with a radiolabeled probe is the preferred method. The Southern blot is hybridized with randomly sheared human DNA that is $^{32}$P-labeled by random priming. This allows visualization of the total human DNA that is present on the membrane owing to hybridization of the probe to repetitive DNA sequences. Before attempting to detect the large DNA fragments, it is worth trying to detect the DNA ladder as this is a more rapid means for demonstrating the presence of apoptotic cells.

From: *Methods in Molecular Biology, Vol. 174: Epstein-Barr Virus Protocols*
Edited by: J. B. Wilson and G. H. W. May © Humana Press Inc., Totowa, NJ

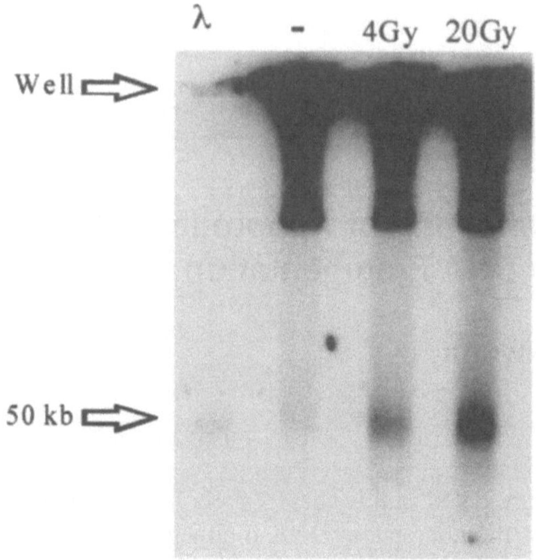


Fig. 1. FIGE of unirradiated (–), 4 GY, and 20 GY irradiated A2780 cells (total cell population, 72 h after treatment). Lane 1 contains full-length, linearized Lambda DNA.

The protocol, as described, refers to irradiated, adherent, monolayer tissue culture cells but may be equally applied to many cell types under a range of treatments with little modification. **Figure 1** shows an irradiation dose-dependent induction of DNA fragmentation in the A2780 ovarian adenocarcinoma cell line as measured by the appearance of 50 kb fragments. No evidence of internucleosomal, nonrandom DNA fragmentation was observed in the DNA from irradiated A2780 cells. Field inversion gel electrophoresis enabled discrimination between genomic DNA and 50 kb DNA fragments in irradiated A2780 cells. This method was also used to demonstrate reduced levels of cisplatin-induced apoptosis in cisplatin-resistant derivatives of A2780 cells *(5)*. Instead of the lambda DNA marker a lambda ladder marker (available from Promega Corp.) can be used. This covers the range of 50–1000 kb, which allows for the confirmation of size for both the 50 kb band and the larger, 300–1000 kb band.

## 2. Materials

All solutions are made using double distilled water (dd $H_2O$).

1. L Buffer: 100 m*M* EDTA, pH 8.0, 10 m*M* Tris-HCl, pH 7.6, 20 m*M* NaCl.
2. TAE: 40 m*M* Tris-acetate, 1 m*M* ethylenidiaminetetraacetic acid (EDTA); for 1 L of 50X concentrated stock: 242 g Tris base, 57.1 mL Glacial acetic acid, 100 mL 500 m*M* EDTA, pH 8.0.
3. Denaturation buffer: 500 m*M* NaOH (20 g/L), 1.5 *M* NaCl (87.7 g/L).
4. Neutralization buffer: 1 *M* Tris-HCl, pH 7.4 (121.2 g/L), 1.5 *M* NaCl (87.7 g/L).
5. Genescreen buffer: 500 m*M* $Na_2HPO_4$ (345.9 g/5 L), 500 m*M* $NaH_2PO_4$ (390.02 g/5 L).

6. Hybridization buffer: 50 m*M* PIPES, pH 6.8 (7.6 g/500 mL), 50 m*M* $NaH_2PO_4 \times 2H_2O$ (3.9 g/500 mL), 50 m*M* $Na_2HPO_4$ (3.8 g/500 mL), 100 m*M* NaCl (2.9 g/500 mL), 1 m*M* EDTA (1 mL of 500 m*M* EDTA/500 mL), 5% SDS (25g/500 mL).
7. 20X SSC: 3 *M* NaCl (175.3 g/L), 300 m*M* tri-Sodium citrate (88.2 g/L), pH 7.0.

## 3. Methods

### 3.1. Preparation of DNA

The following protocol was used in the experiment described earlier. It therefore refers to monolayer tissue-culture cells, which were irradiated and trypsinized 72 h after treatment. **Steps 1–3** may vary according to the treatment required and the type of cells under investigation.

1. Seed cells into 10-cm sterile tissue-culture plates at a density that will allow for exponential growth of control cells for the duration of the experiment.
2. Irradiate cells and harvest by trypsinization. The suspension cells are retained along with the monolayer cells (*see* **Note 1**).
3. Centrifuge at 200*g*, remove medium and resuspend cells in ice-cold PBS at $4 \times 10^6$ cells/100 µL. Transfer cell suspension to Eppendorf tubes and keep on ice.
4. Melt 2% low-gelling temperature (lgt) agarose in L buffer and keep at 42°C (*see* **Note 2**). Warm the cell suspensions to 42°C and add agarose to each tube to halve the cell concentration, i.e., to give a final concentration of $2 \times 10^6$ cells/100 µL 1% agarose.
5. Pipet cell suspension into a disposable plug mold (available from Bio-Rad) and allow to set at 4°C for 5–10 min (*see* **Note 3**). Transfer plugs into 500 m*M* EDTA, pH 8.0 in bijou bottles and store at 4°C until all plugs are ready for the lysis step (e.g., until the time-course is complete).
6. Lyse agarose-embedded cells in L buffer containing 1 mg/mL proteinase K and 1% SDS in bijou bottles at 50°C (*see* **Note 4**). Lyse a maximum of $10^7$ cells in 5 mL of buffer. Lyse for 48 h replacing with fresh buffer after 24 h.

### 3.2. Field Inversion Gel Electrophoresis

1. Either lambda ladder (Promega Ltd) or denatured λ DNA (Life Technologies Ltd) can be run as a size marker (*see* **Note 5**). Firstly linearize the λ DNA. Heat 5 µg of λ DNA at 56°C for 5 min and add 1% lgt agarose in L buffer to make up to 200 µL. Pipet into a plug mold, cool at 4°C, and store in 500 m*M* EDTA, pH 8.0, as for cell plugs. Run approx 1 µg λ DNA per lane. The lambda ladder is supplied as an agarose plug (follow the manufacturers instructions).
2. Make a large (approx 450 mL volume, 24 cm wide × 20 cm long) horizontal 1% agarose gel in 1X TAE buffer. While the gel is setting, rinse agarose/cell plugs in 500 m*M* EDTA and make up 5–10 mL of 1% lgt agarose (keep at 42°C until needed).
3. Load equal volumes of the plugs (i.e., approx equal cell numbers) into the wells (*see* **Note 6**). Load appropriate molecular weight markers and fill up all wells with 1% lgt agarose to prevent the plugs from floating out.
4. Place the gel in a large, horizontal gel electrophoresis tank and fill with 1X TAE. Run the gel at 4–15°C using a mini-pump to recirculate the buffer. Run the gel in a refrigerated room or, if this is unavailable, by using an electrophoresis tank with a cooling maze below the gel platform (*see* **Note 7**). Run the gel at 7–10 V/cm in 1X TAE for 48 h using a 500 V power supply and a Minipulse Polarity Switching System (IBI).

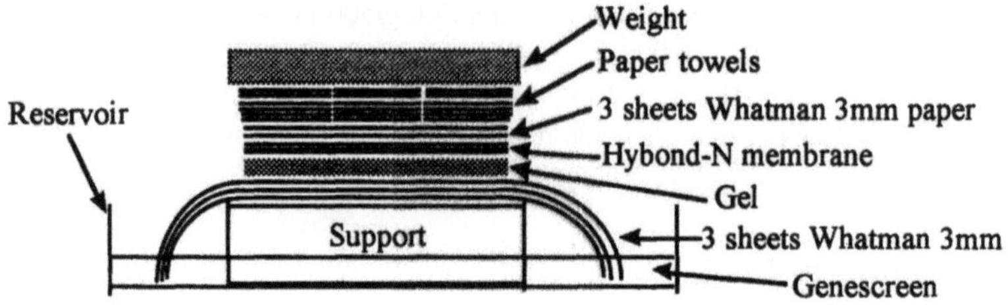


Fig. 2. Scheme for a Southern blot (*see* **Note 9**).

Use the following parameters: A, initial reverse time: 0.1 s; B, reverse increment: 0; C, initial forward time: 0.3 s; D, forward increment: 0; E, number of steps: 51; F, reverse increment increment: 0.02 s; G, forward increment increment: 0.06 s. These parameters allow for resolution to 1600 kb emphasizing the lower range (*see* **Note 8**).

### 3.3. Southern Blotting of DNA

1. Place the gel in a Tupperware box and denature gel for 15 min in denaturation buffer. Change denaturation buffer and denature for a further 15 min.
2. Discard the denaturation buffer and rinse the gel with a small volume of neutralization buffer. Neutralize for 30 min in neutralization buffer. Change buffer and neutralize for a further 30 min.
3. Southern blot onto Hybond-N membrane. Using Genescreen buffer rinse the gel and wet the nylon membrane. Set up the blot according to the cartoon shown in **Fig. 2** (*see* **Note 9**). Transfer for at least 18 h (overnight).
4. Wrap the damp membrane in Saran wrap or clingfilm, crosslink the DNA using a UV crosslinker or UV box and store at 4°C until ready to hybridize (*see* **Note 10**).

### 3.4. Random Priming

Human double-stranded DNA and λ DNA are randomly sheared using a hypodermic needle and end-labeled with [$\alpha^{32}$P]dCTP using the Prime-It kit (Stratagene, Cambridge, UK; contains Klenow, primers, primer buffer without dCTP [also primer buffer without dATP], and Stop mix).

1. Shear some suitable DNA (e.g., human, mouse, λ) at a concentration of 10 ng/µL into random fragments with a disposable, 25-gauge hypodermic needle (*see* **Note 11**).
2. Take 5 µL of sheared DNA (i.e., 50 ng) and add 19 µL dd $H_2O$ and 10 µL primers (from Prime-It kit). Boil for 5 min to denature the DNA.
3. Add 10 µL of primer buffer without dCTP, 8 µL [$\alpha^{32}$P]dCTP (Amersham International plc, Little Chalfont, Bucks, UK) and 1 µL Klenow. Mix thoroughly with a pipet tip and incubate for a minimum of 1 h at 37°C (*see* **Note 12**).
4. Add 2 µL of Stop mix.
5. Separate unincorporated [$\alpha^{32}$P]dCTP from labeled DNA using a disposable Sephadex G50 NICK column (Pharmacia Biotech). Wash column with 0.8 mL dd $H_2O$ and dispose of eluent. Apply probe to center of column and wash with 0.4 mL dd $H_2O$ collecting eluent as waste. With a fresh Eppendorf tube under the column, add a further 0.4 mL dd $H_2O$ and collect this fraction containing labeled DNA. Check the counts from 4 µL of the probe in a liquid scintillation analyzer (should be about 1–2 × $10^5$ cpm/mL).

6. Probes are denatured before hybridization by adding 0.1 vol of 3 *M* NaOH for 5 min at room temperature followed by 0.05 vol of 1 *M* Tris-HCl, pH 7.5 for 5 min on ice. Lastly add 0.1 vol of 3 *M* HCl for a further 5 min on ice.

### 3.5. Hybridization of Probes

All hybridization steps at 65°C are carried out in a hybridization oven containing a rotisserie.

1. Roll up the membrane and put in a hybridization bottle (*see* **Note 13**). Pour in 30 mL of hybridization buffer and pre-hybridize the membrane for 1 h at 65°C.
2. Add all of both probes to 10 mL of hybridization buffer and add to the bottle, having discarded the pre-hybridization buffer. Hybridize overnight at 65°C.
3. Wash with 1X SSC, 5% SDS 3 times: once for 15 min, once for 30 min and once for 60 min (*see* **Note 14**).
4. Expose the side of the membrane that was next to the gel to X-ray film (usually for about 6 h minimum) and develop (*see* **Note 15**).

## 4. Notes

1. The number of apoptotic cells in a culture at any one time may be very low since the execution of apoptosis is rapid. The time over which one can detect any one particular apoptotic cell may be as little as 30 min *(6)*. To produce as quantitative a result as possible, total cell cultures (suspension cells and trypsinized, monolayer cells) are resuspended and analyzed, thereby allowing the detection of apoptotic DNA fragments relative to the total amount of DNA obtained from the culture.
2. DNA extracted from cell cultures by phenol/chloroform is susceptible to random degradation and shearing during handling, resulting in a smear of DNA on the autoradiograph. To minimize random shearing, embed cells in agarose plugs before lysing to liberate the DNA. Embed in molten agarose at a concentration of $2 \times 10^6$ cells/100 µL. An approximately equal volume of agarose is then loaded in each well (try to get about $10^6$ cells/well). Lgt agarose melts at approx 65°C and gels at approx 30°C. The lgt agarose must be kept at 42°C to prevent gelling while the cell suspensions are being prepared. The most convenient way of achieving this is by using a dry block set to 42°C.
3. The 1% agarose blocks are quite delicate and it is therefore easiest to do all manipulations involving them in a 4°C room.
4. Proteinase K and SDS must be added fresh to the L buffer. Make sure that the proteinase K is DNase-free (store at –20°C). The very high concentration of proteinase K is required because the cells are embedded in agarose. This is ten times the concentration that is used for cells in suspension. Agarose plugs should not be kept un-lyzed for more than 72 h.
5. Although λ DNA is used as a size marker for the 50 kb fragments it is actually 48.5 kb in length. The lambda ladder is a 20-step ladder ranging in size from approx 50–1000 kb. It is constructed from λ DNA concatamerized into oligomers. Again, each step actually differs by 48.5 kb. Store the markers at 4°C.
6. Cut equal volumes off each agarose plug using a scalpel on a glass plate in a 4°C room. Load into the wells of the gel with the aid of a small spatula.
7. Rubber tubing can be attached to adapters on the gel tank and to a cold water supply thereby allowing cold water to be pumped through the maze, cooling the gel above. One such electrophoresis unit incorporating a cooling maze is available from IBI. A mini-pump is required to recirculate the TAE in order to maintain the buffering capacity of the

buffer. Place one end of the pump's tubing in one reservoir of the electrophoresis tank and the other end of the tubing in the second reservoir. Make sure that the valve between the two reservoirs is open.

8. Run on program 7 of IBI Minipulse Polarity Switching System. If you have a different switching system the instruction manual may have a list of pre-programmed parameters allowing resolution of 50–1000 kb. Alternatively use the parameters listed in **Subheading 3.2., step 4** to program your system.
9. Mark the side of the nylon membrane that is next to the gel and make sure that the gel, the membrane, the Whatman 3MM paper on top of the membrane and paper towels are all exactly the same size to ensure efficient capillary transfer. If, for example, the paper towels are overhanging and in contact with the Whatman 3MM paper below the gel, the Genescreen buffer will bypass the gel and the DNA will not be transferred onto the nylon membrane. To ensure that this is avoided cut strips off an unwanted autoradiograph and place around the gel on the lower layer of Whatman 3MM paper. This will prevent accidental "shorting" of the system. The setup and volume of Genescreen buffer depends on the size of your gel. You may find that you need to balance a support on top of two reservoirs with one end of the Whatman paper hanging in each reservoir. Use about 2 L of Genescreen buffer for a 20 cm × 20 cm gel.
10. If a UV crosslinker is not available, expose the side of the membrane carrying the DNA to a total of 1.5 J/cm$^2$ on a UV light box. Alternatively, membranes may be baked in an oven between two sheets of 3MM paper for 30 min to 2 h.
11. You will need a probe to hybridize to the DNA from your treated cells and also a probe to recognize the $\lambda$ marker.
12. Appropriate safety guidelines for handling radioactivity should be followed. Use laboratory space that is designated for work involving the use of radioactive substances. Use protective screening and wear 2 pairs of gloves. Monitor the work bench before and after use and decontaminate any spills. Dispose of radioactive waste (e.g., contaminated Sephadex column) according to safety guidelines.
13. Place the hybridization bottle on the rotisserie so that the membrane sticks to the sides of the bottle when it rotates. If it is on the wrong way round the membrane will form a tight roll and hybridization will be uneven. If you are only hybridizing one blot remember to put another bottle on the rotisserie for balance.
14. Wash the membrane until there is a low background activity. Take the membrane out of the bottle after the third wash and lay it on a piece of Whatman 3MM paper. Check the radioactive signal using a Geiger counter. If there is a high count coming from the bottom of the membrane (where there should be no DNA and therefore no hybridization of the probe) put the membrane back in the bottle and perform further washes until this is reduced.
15. We use Fuji photographic film and a Kodak, automated X-ray developer. Other X-ray films of similar quality are suitable.

## References


1. Wyllie, A. H. (1980) Glucocorticoid-induced thymocyte apoptosis is associated with endogenous endonuclease activation. *Nature* **284,** 555, 556.
2. Oberhammer, F., Wilson, J. W., Dive, C., Morris, I. D., Hickman, J. A., Wakeling, A. E., et al. (1993) Apoptotic death in epithelial cells: cleavage of DNA to 300 and/or 50 kb fragments prior to or in the absence of internucleosomal fragmentation. *EMBO J.* **12,** 3679–3684.

3. Sun, D. Y., Jiang, S., Zheng, L. M., Ojcius, D. M. and Young, J. D. (1994) Separate metabolic pathways leading to DNA fragmentation and apoptotic chromatin condensation. *J. Exp. Med.* **179,** 559–568.
4. Cohen, G. M., Sun, X. M., Snowden, R. T., Dinsdale, D. and Skilleter, D. N. (1992) Key morphological features of apoptosis may occur in the absence of internucleosomal DNA fragmentation. *Biochem. J.* **286,** 331–334.
5. Anthoney, D. A., McIlwrath, A. J., Gallagher, W. M., Edlin, A. R. M. and Brown, R. (1996) Microsatellite instability, apoptosis and loss of p53 function in drug resistant tumour cells. *Cancer Res.* **56,** 1374–1381.
6. Evan, G. I., Wyllie, A. H., Gilbert, C. S., Littlewood, T. D., Land, H., Brooks, M., et al. (1992) Induction of apoptosis in fibroblasts by c-myc protein. *Cell* **69,** 119–128.

# IV

## Immune Assays

# 21

## Regression Assay

**Teresa Frisan, Victor Levitsky, and Maria Masucci**

### 1. Introduction

In Epstein-Barr virus (EBV)-seropositive individuals, cell-mediated immunity against EBV can be monitored in vitro as the capacity of T-cell lymphocytes to inhibit virus-induced proliferation of autologous B cells. In vitro infection of peripheral blood mononuclear cells (PBMCs) from EBV-seronegative and EBV-seropositive donors is accompanied by the appearance of foci of proliferating cells expressing the EBV nuclear antigens (EBNAs) within 7–14 d postinfection. These cells continue to expand giving rise to EBV-transformed lymphoblastoid cell lines (LCLs) in cultures from EBV-seronegative individuals. In corresponding cultures from EBV-seropositive donors, the initial proliferation is followed by a regression of growth, seen preferentially at high cell concentration, that culminates within 1 mo in the complete degeneration of the culture *(1)*. This phenomenon has been termed regression or outgrowth inhibition and can be monitored by the regression assay. The strength of the regression can be quantitatively expressed as the minimal number of cells required for 50% growth inhibition.

### 2. Materials

1. PBMCs obtained by Ficoll/Hipaque isolation from peripheral blood (*see* **Note 1** and Chapter 9, **Subheading 3.1.** for protocol details).
2. Supernatant from the virus producer cell line B95.8 (*see* Chapter 12, **Subheading 3.4.**).
3. RPMI complete medium: RPMI 1640 (Gibco) with 10% fetal calf serum (FCS), 2 m*M* L-glutamine, 100 U/mL penicillin, 100 U/mL streptomycin.
4. Fetal calf serum (FCS).
5. Flat-bottom microtiter plates and tissue culture flasks.

### 3. Methods

#### *3.1. Regression Assay Set-Up*

1. To remove the macrophages from isolated PBMCs, incubate 2.5–3 × $10^7$ PBMCs for 2 h in 10 mL of RPMI complete medium in a 125 $cm^2$ culture bottle at 37°C, 5% $CO_2$. After

From: *Methods in Molecular Biology, Vol. 174: Epstein-Barr Virus Protocols*
Edited by: J. B. Wilson and G. H. W. May © Humana Press Inc., Totowa, NJ

**Table 1**
**Regression Assay for Donor JT**

| Donor | Incidence of B-cell Transformation[a] | | | | | | | |
|---|---|---|---|---|---|---|---|---|
| | 8[b] | 4 | 2 | 1 | 0.5 | 0.25 | 0.12 | 0.006 |
| JT | 0/10 | 0/10 | 0/10 | 0/10 | 0/10 | 0/10 | 4/1 | 10/10 |
| EBV+[c] | 0/10 | 0/10 | 0/0 | 0/10 | 7/10 | 10/10 | 10/10 | 10/10 |
| EBV−[c] | 10/10 | 10/10 | 10/10 | 10/10 | 10/10 | 10/10 | 10/10 | 10/10 |

[a]Cultures were scored at 4 wk postinfection.
[b]Number of cells per well (× $10^5$).
[c]EBV seropositive and EBV seronegative controls, respectively.

2 h incubation, decant the nonadherent cells (the macrophages should adhere to the plastic).

2. To infect PBMCs with the B95.8 EBV strain, resuspend $1.6 \times 10^7$ nonadherent cells in 16 mL of spent supernatant from the B95.8 cell line for 2 h at 37°C, 5% $CO_2$ as described in Chapter 12, **Subheading 3.4.** $10^6$ cells/mL is the optimal condition for infection, although it is possible to increase this to $2 \times 10^6$/mL (*see* **Notes 2** and **3**).
3. Seed the cells doubling dilutions from $8 \times 10^5$ to $0.6 \times 10^4$ PBMCs. Set up 10 replicates for each dilution. For this purpose, resuspend $1.6 \times 10^7$ cells in 5 mL of RPMI complete medium and distribute 250 µL/well in 10 microwells, corresponding to a cell concentration of $8 \times 10^5$ cells/well. For the next dilution, add 2.5 µL of RPMI complete medium to the remaining cell suspension, distribute 250 µL/well in 10 replicates and proceed in the same way for the remaining dilutions. Maintain cultures in a 37°C, 5% $CO_2$ humidified incubator.
4. Feed the culture weekly by replacing 100 µL of the growth medium with fresh RPMI complete medium.

### 3.2. Evaluation of the Assay

1. After 4–5 wk, evaluate the cell transformation visually using the following scoring system (all positive scores are considered transformed, the number of pluses indicates the dimension of the cell clumps): +, single blasts; ++, small clumps (5–10 cells/clump); +++, big clumps (more than 10 cells/clump); ++++, overgrowth; –, no growth.
2. Calculate the percentage of wells where B-cell transformation occurred, for each cell dilution as indicated in **Table 1**. By plotting the % inhibition on the Y axis and the number of cells/well on the X axis, it is possible to evaluate the number of cells required to induce 50% inhibition, as described in **Fig. 1**.

## 4. Notes

1. 40–50 mL of peripheral blood in heparin-coated tubes from each donor is sufficient to set up a regression assay.
2. For each experiment, PBMCs from an EBV seropositive and an EBV-seronegative donor are tested in parallel in order to assess the T-cell activity and the efficiency of B-cell infection, respectively.

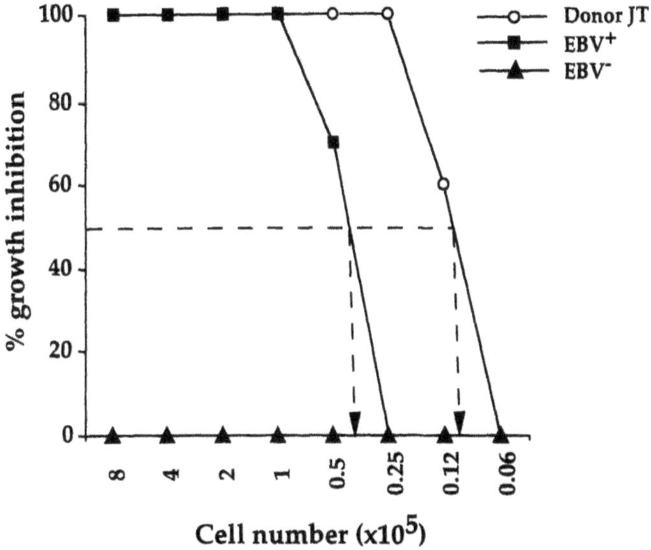


Fig. 1. Growth inhibition graph for donor JT.

3. Failure to induce growth of EBV-transformed B cells from the EBV seronegative donor is likely to be owing to low virus titers in the spent B95.8 supernatant used. If such a situation occurs, use a different batch of B95.8 supernatant.

## References


1. Moss, D. J., Rickinson, A. B., and Pope, J. H. (1978) Long-term T-cell-mediated immunity to Epstein-Barr virus in man. I. Complete regression of virus-induced transformation in culture of seropositive donor leukocytes. *Int. J. Cancer* **22,** 662–668.

22

# Generation of Polyclonal EBV-Specific CTL Cultures and Clones

Victor Levitsky, Teresa Frisan, and Maria Masucci

## 1. Introduction

Although Epstein-Barr virus (EBV) infection elicits both CD4- and CD8-positive T-cell responses, a considerable body of experimental evidence indicates that the latter responses play a major role in controlling the number of EBV-infected cells and proliferation of EBV-transformed B-blasts in vivo *(1,2)*. Recently, cytotoxic T-cells (CTLs) were introduced into clinical practice as an efficient tool for treatment of EBV-associated malignancies *(3,4)*. This chapter is focused on describing the generation and characterization of EBV-specific CD8-positive cytotoxic T-cells. Primarily, techniques that are used to generate CTLs specific for EBV proteins expressed in EBV-transformed lymphoblastoid cell lines (LCLs) will be discussed.

The process of generation and characterization of EBV-specific CTLs includes four major steps:

1. Stimulation and expansion of EBV-specific memory T-cells in vitro;
2. Characterization of HLA restriction;
3. Characterization of antigen specificity; and
4. Mapping of cognate peptide epitope(s).

Each of these steps involve several basic techniques (e.g., standard cytotoxicity assay, immunoblotting, etc.), detailed descriptions of which can be found in *Current Protocols in Immunology* *(5)* or similar technical manuals.

The majority of methods used for the generation and characterization of EBV-specific CTLs utilize EBV transformed LCLs as antigen-presenting and stimulator cells. LCLs express high levels of MHC class I and different co-stimulatory molecules (such as B7.1, B7.2, LFA, ICAM-1, etc.) along with the 10 viral proteins: EBNA 1 to 6, LMP1, LMP2A, LMP2B *(1,2)* and protein(s) encoded by the *Bam*HI A fragment of the EBV genome *(6)*. Exposure of peripheral blood mononuclear cells (PBMCs) from

From: *Methods in Molecular Biology, Vol. 174: Epstein-Barr Virus Protocols*
Edited by: J. B. Wilson and G. H. W. May © Humana Press Inc., Totowa, NJ

EBV-seropositive individuals to autologous LCLs leads to the reactivation and expansion of EBV-specific memory T-cells in vitro. It should be stressed, however, that naive CD8 positive T-cells from EBV-seronegative individuals cannot be activated in the same way and no reliable protocols have been developed so far to achieve this. CTLs specific to all EBV proteins expressed in LCLs, with the exception of the *Bam*HI A encoded protein(s), have been described.

Although the generation of CTL clones is a laborious and time-consuming procedure, usually it greatly facilitates the characterization of MHC restriction, protein and peptide specificity of EBV-specific CTLs. CTL clones are also much more useful than polyclonal CTL cultures as a tool for the investigation of immunogenicity and presentation of EBV-specific peptide epitopes.

In the EBV system, CTL clones can not be obtained by direct cloning of PBMCs and can only be generated from polyclonal CTL cultures established by several rounds of in vitro restimulation.

## 2. Materials

1. Ficoll.
2. Phosphate-buffered saline (PBS): 0.137 *M* NaCl, 2.7 m*M* KCl, 5.4 m*M* $Na_2HPO_4$, 1.8 m*M* $KH_2PO_4$. Adjust pH to 7.4 and filter through a 0.2-µm filter.
3. AIM-V medium.
4. Fetal calf serum (FCS).
5. Complete medium: RPMI 1640 with 10% FCS, penicillin 100 U/mL, streptomycin 10 µg/mL.
5. Autoclaved carbonyl iron powder (Fluka Chemie AG, Switzerland).
6. Purified phytohemagglutinin (PHA) (e.g., PHA-L, Boehringer Mannheim, cat. no. 1 249 738).
7. 3% solution of glutamine in PBS. Use as 100 times concentrated stock solution.
8. Supernatant of gibbon lymphoma cell line MLA 144 ***(6)***; grow MLA 144 cells in 225 $cm^2$ flasks in complete medium to the density of $1.5 \times 10^6$ cells/mL. Collect the cell suspension and centrifuge for 10 min. at 1000*g*. Collect the supernatant and distribute it into 50-mL Falcon tubes (45 mL/tube). Store the material at –20°C. Thaw and filter the supernatant through 0.2-µm filter before use.
9. IL2 medium: 45 mL supernatant of MLA 144 cells, 90 mL RPMI-1640, 15 mL FCS, 10 U/mL recombinant IL2.
10. PHA activated blasts: isolate PBMCs of the donor by Ficoll separation of the peripheral blood. Resuspend the PBMCs in complete medium at $1 \times 10^6$ cells/mL. Add 1 µg/mL of PHA and seed the cell suspension in a 24-well plate (1.5 mL/well). Incubate the cells for 3 d at 37°C in a humidified $CO_2$ incubator. Exchange the culture medium for IL2 medium and let the blasts expand.
11. Plastic laboratory ware: culture flasks, 15-mL disposable sterile plastic tubes, 24-well flat-bottom microtiter plates with lids.
12. A set of instruments for bleeding, including vacuum tubes containing heparin, vacuum needles and needle holders, arm belt, sterile wads, 70% ethanol.
13. $CO_2$ incubator (37°C, 5% $CO_2$, maximal humidity).
14. 1 mg/mL PHA: in PBS, filter-sterilize.
15. Ionizing radiation source (60Co or 137Cs γ-irradiator).

## 3. Methods

### 3.1. Generation and Characterization of EBV-Specific Polyclonal CTL Cultures

1. Take about 50 mL of blood from a selected donor into heparin containing tubes.
2. Dilute the blood with PBS 1:1 and perform ficoll separation of PBMC in 15-mL tubes by centrifugation for 30 min at 2000*g*.
3. Collect the ring(s) of white blood cells retained on the interface between ficoll and plasma and wash the cells three times in 10 mL of PBS by centrifugation for 5–10 min at 1000*g*.
4. Resuspend the cell pellet in complete medium to achieve a final cell density of $2 \times 10^6$ cells/mL.
5. Transfer 10 mL of the suspension to a 50 mL flask, add a bit of iron powder at the tip of a scalpel, shake gently, and incubate the flask in a horizontal position for 1 h at 37°C.
6. Bring a strong magnet into the contact with the flask (iron particles will be trapped on the wall by the magnetic field together with phagocytes that have engulfed some of these particles) and transfer the suspension into 15-mL tubes.
7. Pellet the cells by centrifugation for 5–10 min at 1000*g*, wash them once, and resuspend in 10 mL AIM-V medium (add glutamine to the medium if required).
8. Count the cells and dilute the suspension with AIM-V to $1 \times 10^6$ cells/mL.
9. Irradiate $2–3 \times 10^6$ autologous LCL with 4000 Rad using a source of ionizing irradiation. Wash the cells twice in PBS and resuspend in 5 mL of AIM-V medium.
10. Add the suspension of LCL to PBMCs at a 1:40 ratio.
11. Distribute the suspension into a 24-well plate at $1.5 \times 10^6$ cells/well and incubate in $CO_2$ incubator at 37°C.
12. After 1 wk, count the number of viable cells by the trypan blue exclusion method (*see* Chapter 42, Subheading 3.4.) and restimulate the culture with LCL as described in **steps 9–10**.
13. On d 10–12 add FCS to the wells to 10% final concentration (v/v).
14. Repeat the restimulation on d 14 as described in **step 12**.
15. Five to seven days after the second stimulation, replace 50% of cell-culture medium with IL2 medium and repeat the restimulation procedure (*see* **Note 2**).
16. Continue to expand the culture by feeding it as frequently as required with IL2 medium.
17. Five to seven days after the third stimulation, test the culture for EBV specificity and predominant HLA restriction(s) using a standard cytotoxicity assay (*see* **Note 3**).
18. Repeat the stimulation procedure every 1–2 wk, if required (*see* **Note 4**).

### 3.2. Generation and Characterization of EBV-Specific CTL Clones

1. Separate PBMCs from an allogeneic blood donor and wash cells 3 times in PBS. Either peripheral blood or a concentrated preparation of leukocytes can be used as a source. The required amount depends on the number of microtiter plates that are to be used for cloning.
2. After the last wash, resuspend the PBMCs in 5 mL of complete medium. The cell density should be in the range of $10–20 \times 10^6$ PBMCs/mL. Add 50 µL of 1 mg/mL PHA (final concentration 10 µg/mL). Incubate the suspension for 1 h at 37°C.
3. Pellet the cells by centrifugation for 5–10 min at 1000*g* and resuspend them in 5 mL of complete medium.
4. Prepare a suspension of autologous (for the donor of CTLs) LCL in complete medium.
5. Irradiate the PBMCs with 3000 Rad and the LCL with 4000 rad, using a source of γ-irradiation. Wash the cells twice in PBS.

6. Resuspend the cells in complete IL2 medium and mix them to prepare a cell suspension containing $1 \times 10^6$ PBMC and $1 \times 10^5$ LCL cells/mL. Distribute 100 µL of the suspension to each well of U-bottom 96-well plates as feeder cells.
7. Prepare a single cell suspension of CTLs. Dilute CTLs to densities of 100, 30, and 10 cells/mL. Distribute 100 µL of these suspensions to the plates containing feeder cells. Incubate the plates in a $CO_2$-incubator changing 30% of the medium once a week until the growth of CTL clones becomes apparent (usually 2–6 wk) (*see* **Note 5**).
8. Transfer each CTL clone culture to two flat-bottom wells of a 96-well plate. CTLs do not firmly attach but spread over the surface more or less homogeneously. As soon as you see a rather "confluent" culture in both wells, transfer CTLs into one well of 48- or 24-well plate. Continue to expand the culture by stimulating it with irradiated autologous LCL at an effector/stimulator ratio of 10:1. Split the culture into new wells. Do not transfer CTLs to culture flasks.
9. As soon as you have sufficient numbers of cells, test the cultures for EBV specificity and HLA restriction in a standard cytotoxicity assay (*see* **Notes 2** and **6**).

## 4. Notes

1. The bleeding must be performed by a qualified person (MD or nurse) in accordance with technical and ethical regulations accepted in your country and institution.
2. After the third stimulation and addition of IL2, EBV-specific T-cells begin to expand and can be used for functional assays. The aforementioned protocol cannot be followed precisely as described in each case; sometimes the addition of FCS or IL-2 has to be performed earlier than suggested to avoid massive cell death.
3. EBV specificity and HLA restriction of polyclonal CTLs can be determined in the same experiment by testing the ability of the culture to lyse a panel of target cells in a standard cytotoxicity assay. An ideal panel should include the following targets:
   a. An autologous LCL;
   b. Allogeneic LCLs matched with the autologous cell line by a single HLA class I allele;
   c. Mismatched LCLs;
   d. Autologous EBV-negative cells; and
   e. Natural Killer (NK)-sensitive targets such as the K562 cell line.

   Usually, fibroblasts and PHA activated T-blasts of the donor serve as EBV-negative targets because they are relatively easy to obtain and propagate in vitro.

   In practice, many CTL cultures generated by stimulation with autologous LCL exhibit clear EBV specificity reflected in the killing of autologous and some single matched LCLs without recognition of EBV-negative autologous cells. However, the predominant HLA restriction of the cultures may be more difficult to determine owing to a number of reasons. First, the culture can possess a high level of NK activity and kill mismatched, single allele-matched, and NK-sensitive targets. Second, certain MHC peptide combinations may be presented efficiently only by some but not all LCLs expressing the relevant MHC allele *(8)*. This may considerably complicate the evaluation of the data. Third, a similar problem may be observed owing to a subtype polymorphism of several HLA alleles that may affect T-cell recognition *(9)*.

   If the data generated in the assay is difficult to interpret in terms of MHC restriction, the specificity of the culture may be increased by additional rounds of restimulation as described. In some cases, HLA restriction may be clearly determined only for CTL clones (*see* Chapter 23).

4. The specificity of the resulting culture is determined by a number of factors that cannot be easily controlled (such as the frequency of EBV-specific precursors in the peripheral blood of the donor, the range of peptides presented by the LCL, the immunogenicity of these epitopes, etc.). Lowering the LCL/PBMC ratio during the restimulations and withdrawal of IL2 from the culture for as long as the viability of T-cells can be maintained, may increase the specificity. This promotes the proliferation of EBV-specific cells and restrains the proliferation of other cells stimulated through different nonspecific or bystander effects.
5. One of the critical steps of the cloning procedure is the selection of an appropriate seeding density of CTLs. Theoretically, seeding of 0.3 cell/well should ensure the true clonality of CTLs obtained from such a plate. In practice, seeding at this density very seldom results in the growth of CTLs. For some CTL cultures, more than 10 cells per well should be seeded to observe the growth of CTL clones. Our experience indicates that CTL cultures obtained from a plate with 30% yield are usually monoclonal. We recommend to prepare microtiter plates with three different seeding densities: 1, 3, and 10 cells per well and analyze clones that are derived from a plate with 30% or lower yield of clones.
6. It was reported that CTL clones may be unable to recognize the LCL that was used for restimulation of these CTLs in culture ***(10)***.

   The reasons underlying this phenomenon remain unclear. Though in our laboratory we observe this phenomenon rather as an exception than a rule, it should be taken in consideration during the screening of CTL clones for peptide specificity. CTL clones with this type of activity can be screened with an autologous LCL prepulsed with a relevant synthetic peptide or infected with recombinant vaccinia virus encoding for a relevant EBV protein.

## References


1. Masucci, M. G. and Ernberg, I. (1994) Epstein-Barr virus: adaptation to a life within the immune system. *Trends Microbiol.* **2,** 125–130.
2. Rickinson, A. B. and Kieff, E. (1996) Epstein-Barr virus, in *Fields Virology,* vol. 2 (Fields, B. N., Knipe, D. M., and Howley, P. M., eds.), Lippincott-Raven, Philadelphia, pp. 2397–2446.
3. Heslop, H. E., Ng, C. Y. C., Li, C., Smith, C. A., Loftin, S. K., Krance, R. A., et al. (1996) Long-term restoration of immunity against Epstein-Barr virus infection by adoptive transfer of gene-modified virus-specific T lymphocytes. *Nature Med.* **2,** 551–555.
4. Rooney, C. M., Smith, C. A., Ng, C. Y. C., Loftin, S., Li, C., Krance, R. A., Brenner, M. K., and Heslop, H. E. (1995) Use of gene-modified virus-specific T lymphocytes to control Epstein-Barr-virus-related lymphoproliferation. *Lancet* **345,** 9–13.
5. Coligan, T. E., KruisBeck, A. M., Margulies, D. H., and Strobek, W. (1996) *Current Protocols in Immunology,* in 3 volumes, National Institutes of Health, John Wiley and Sons Inc., New York, NY.
6. Fries, K. L., Sculley, T. B., Webster-Cyriaque, J., Rajadurai, P., Sadler, R. H., and Raab-Traub, N. (1997) Identification of a novel protein encoded by the BamHI A region of the Epstein-Barr virus. *J. Virol.* **71,** 2765–2771.
7. Rabin, H., Hopkins, R. F., Ruscetti, F. W., Neubawer, R. H., Brown, R. L., and Kawakami, T. G. (1981) Spontaneous release of a factor with properties of T-cell growth factor from a continuous line of primate tumor T cells. *J. Immunol.* **127,** 1852–1856.
8. Levitsky, V., Zhang, Q.-J., Levitskaja, J., and Masucci, M. G. (1996) The life span of major histocompatibility complex-peptide complexes influences the efficiency of presen-

tation and immunogenicity of two class I-restricted cytotoxic T lymphocyte epitopes in the Epstein-Barr virus nuclear antigen 4. *J. Exp. Med.* **183,** 915–926.

8. Khanna, R., Burrows, S. R., Neisig, A., Neefjes, J., Moss, D. J., and Silins, S. L. (1997) Hierarchy of Epstein-Barr virus-specific cytotoxic T-cell responses in individuals carrying different subtypes of an HLA allele: implications for epitope-based antiviral vaccines. *J. Virol.* **71,** 7429–7435.
9. Hill, A. B., Lee, S. P., Haurum, J. S., Murray, N., Yao, Q.-Y., Rowe, M., et al. (1995) Class I major histocompatibility complex-restricted cytotoxic T lymphocytes specific for Epstein-Barr virus (EBV) nuclear antigens fail to lyse the EBV-transformed B lymphoblastoid cell lines against which they were raised. *J. Exp. Med.* **181,** 2221–2228.

# 23

# Determination of Antigen and Fine Peptide Specificity of EBV-Specific CTLs

**Victor Levitsky, Teresa Frisan, and Maria Masucci**

## 1. Introduction

Currently, the antigen specificity of Epstein-Barr virus (EBV)-specific cytotoxic T cells (CTLs) can be determined using a set of recombinant vaccinia viruses expressing individual EBV proteins. These recombinant viruses are used to infect EBV-negative target cells, which are then tested for recognition by CTLs in standard cytotoxicity assay. Autologous fibroblasts are the most frequently used target cells for this type of experiment.

After the protein specificity of a CTL culture is determined, epitope mapping can be performed. There are two alternative approaches to achieve this. First, if the human leukocyte antigen (HLA) restriction of CTLs is unambiguously defined, peptides comprising the binding motif of the relevant HLA class I molecule can be synthesized and tested for recognition by CTLs. This approach has two drawbacks: (1) binding motifs are not known for a number of MHC alleles; (2) even the best algorithms used to define potential CTL epitopes can predict only about 70% of the immunogeneic peptides that are actually recognized by the immune system.

The second approach involves the generation of a set of 15 amino acid long peptides (15-mers) that overlap with each other by 5 amino acid residues and represent the entire sequence of the protein in question. Such peptides can be loaded on autologous EBV-negative cells (e.g., phytohemagglutinin [PHA] activated blasts) and tested for their ability to induce CTL lysis.

For the final mapping of cognate epitopes, 15-mers which exhibit activity in the assay are selected and short peptides overlapping their sequence are synthesized. At this stage, information concerning the binding motif of the relevant MHC molecule may be very useful in selecting sequences that can potentially represent the cognate peptide contained within the 15-mer. If no information on the binding motif is available, sets of 8-, 9-, 10-, and 11-mer peptides representing the entire sequence of the 15-mer should be synthesized and tested in a cytotoxicity assay.

From: *Methods in Molecular Biology, Vol. 174: Epstein-Barr Virus Protocols*
Edited by: J. B. Wilson and G. H. W. May © Humana Press Inc., Totowa, NJ

## 2. Materials

1. Phosphate buffered saline (PBS): 0.137 *M* NaCl, 2.7 m*M* KCl, 5.4 m*M* $Na_2HPO_4$, 1.8 m*M* $KH_2PO_4$. Adjust pH to 7.4 and filter through a 0.2-µm filter.
2. Fetal calf serum (FCS).
3. Dimethyl sulfoxide (DMSO).
4. Complete medium: RPMI-1640 with 10% fetal calf serum (FCS), penicillin 100 U/mL, streptomycin 10 µg/mL.
5. AIM-V medium (Gibco).
6. IL2 medium: 45 mL supernatant of MLA 144 cells, 90 mL RPMI 1640, 15 mL FCS, 10 U/mL recombinant IL2.
7. PHA-activated blasts (*see* Chapter 22, Subheading 2.10.).
8. Plastic laboratory ware.
9. $CO_2$ incubator (37°C, 5% $CO_2$, maximal humidity).
10. 1X trypsin: Dilute 10X trypsin (Gibco-BRL, containing 0.5% Trypsin, 5.3 m*M* ethylenediamine tetraacetic acid [EDTA]-4Na) in PBS. Filter through a 0.2-µm filter and store at 4°C.
11. Preparations of recombinant vaccinia viruses (*see* **Note 1; ref.** ***1***).
12. Hemocytometer.
13. Sonication waterbath.

## 3. Methods

### 3.1. Characterization of Antigen Specificity of EBV-Specific CTLs

1. Rinse a flask containing a confluent culture of fibroblasts twice in PBS. Add 5 mL of 1X trypsin and incubate the flask at 37°C until the cells are completely detached (10–15 min).
2. Collect the suspension of fibroblasts into a 15-mL plastic tube and add 5 mL of complete medium (serum contained in the medium will neutralize the activity of trypsin). Pellet cells by centrifugation at 1000*g* for 5 min, remove the supernatant, wash cells once in PBS, and pellet cells again.
3. Resuspend cells in PBS and count cells using a hemocytometer. Distribute the cells to 5-mL plastic tubes adding $1 \times 10^6$ cells/tube. Centrifuge the tubes for 5 min at 1000*g* and remove the supernatant.
4. Thaw an aliquot of vaccinia virus stock in a 37°C water bath and snap freeze it again in liquid nitrogen (it is convenient to use Eppendorf tubes to prepare aliquots of the virus). Repeat this freeze/thaw procedure three times. Thaw the stock after the final freezing and sonicate it in a sonication water bath for 3 min (*see* **Note 2**).
5. Add the required amount of vaccinia viral stock (usually 5–10 µL) to the cell pellets. Add 50 µL of AIM-V medium and incubate tubes at 37°C for 1 h.
6. Add 1 mL of complete medium and incubate the tubes overnight at 37°C (*see* **Note 3**).
7. Pellet cells by centrifugation at 1000*g* for 5 min, remove the supernatant and after labeling with radioactive chromium, use the cells as targets in a standard chromium release assay (*see* **Note 4**).

### 3.2. Mapping of CTL Cognate Epitopes Using Synthetic Peptides

1. Dissolve preparations of synthetic peptides in DMSO and measure the concentration of peptide in the solution (*see* **Note 5**).
2. Adjust the concentration of the solution to 10 mg/mL. Prepare 50 µL aliquots of this solution in 0.5-mL Eppendorf tubes and keep both the stock and aliquots at –20°C.

3. Dilute the peptide stock to $1 \times 10^{-4}$ *M* in PBS. This solution can be kept at +4°C for 4 wk without any significant loss of activity.
4. Dilute the $1 \times 10^{-4}$ *M* stock solution to $1 \times 10^{-6}$ *M* in complete medium.
5. Mix 20 µL of $1 \times 10^{-6}$ *M* peptide solution with 20 µL of target cell suspension, corresponding to 4000 cells, in complete medium.
6. Preincubate the mixture of target cells and peptide for 1 h at 37°C in a $CO_2$ incubator.
7. Add effector cells (*see* **Note 6**) and run a standard cytotoxicity assay.

## 4. Notes.

1. The generation of recombinant vaccinia viruses and preparation of viral stocks are described elsewhere *(1)*.
2. Vaccinia virus tends to form large aggregates that can lead to irregular attachment of the virus to the target cells. This may leave many cells uninfected while infected ones may have very different levels of expression of virus-encoded EBV protein. The described procedure prevents the formation of aggregates and ensures a relatively uniform expression of target protein in the infected cells.
3. The time of infection can be reduced to 6 h.
4. PHA-activated blasts can be infected in essentially the same way by following **steps 4–6** of the protocol. If new stocks of recombinant vaccinia viruses are used, we recommend to test the expression of relevant proteins in infected cells by immunoblotting. Store aliquoted viral stocks at –70°C and do not allow more than five rounds of freezing/thawing of the same sample.
5. Any colorimetric test such as the Biuret assay can be used *(2)*.
6. In peptide pulsing experiments, we usually use 10:1 effector/target ratio for polyclonal CTL cultures and 3:1 or 1:1 effector/target ratios for CTL clones.

## References

1. Murray, R. J., Kurilla, M. G., Griffin, H. M., Brooks, J. M., Mackett, M., Arrand, J. R., et al. (1990) Human cytotoxic T cell responses against Epstein-Barr virus nuclear antigens demonstrated using recombinant Vaccinia viruses. *Proc. Natl. Acad. Sci. USA* **87,** 2906–2910.
2. Hirs, C. and Timasheff, S. (1977) Methods of peptide synthesis, in *Enzyme Structure,* vol. XLVII (Hirs, C. H. W. and Timesheff, S. N., eds.), Academic, New York, pp. 501–617.

24

# Limiting Dilution Assay

**Teresa Frisan, Victor Levitsky, and Maria Masucci**

## 1. Introduction

Limiting dilution assays (LDA) are designed to define an unknown frequency of effector cells in a population. LDA are dose-response assays that allow detection of an all-or-none (positive or negative) immunoresponse in each individual culture within replicates that vary in the number of responder cells tested (reviewed in **ref. *1***). The frequency of positive cultures is not informative because it is never clear whether one or more precursors in the culture well are giving the positive response. The negative response instead demonstrates that there are no precursors of a given specificity. Therefore, the evaluation of the cell frequency in the original population is possible by determining the number of cultures that are negative in the experiment. Multiple cultures are set up at different cell concentrations and the larger the number of replicates used for each cell concentration, the more precise the estimate will be. If the percentage of negative cultures is converted to its negative logarithm, the results can be plotted graphically. The fraction of negative cultures is plotted on the ordinate while the cell concentration is plotted on the abscissa to give a straight line. Suitable statistic tests are used to fit this line, including regression analysis and the least square method *(2,3)*.

To determine the precursor frequency of Epstein-Barr virus (EBV)-specific cytotoxic T cells ($CTL_p$), peripheral blood mononuclear cells (PBMCs) are distributed in graded numbers from 500–64,000 cells per well and stimulated with $10^4$ irradiated cells of an autologous lymphoblastoid cell line (LCL) (4000 rad). Cytotoxicity is measured by $^{51}Cr$ release assays ***(4)***. The protocol presented here describes the evaluation of precursor frequency of EBV-specific CTLs restricted through HLA-A, -B, or C alleles and CTLs specific for characterized CTL epitopes.

## 2. Materials

1. PBMCs obtained by Ficoll/Hipaque isolation from peripheral blood (*see* **Note 1** and Chapter 9 for protocol).

From: *Methods in Molecular Biology, Vol. 174: Epstein-Barr Virus Protocols*
Edited by: J. B. Wilson and G. H. W. May © Humana Press Inc., Totowa, NJ

2. Autologous, HLA single matched and mismatched
3. Autologous PHA blasts (*see* Chapter 22).
4. AIM-V medium (Gibco).
5. Fetal calf serum (FCS).
6. RPMI complete medium: RPMI-1640, 10% FCS, 2 m*M* L-glutamine, 100 U/mL penicillin, and 100 U/mL streptomycin.
7. Human recombinant interleukin-2 (rIL-2).
8. 96-well round-bottom microtiter plates.
9. $CO_2$ incubator.
10. Ionizing radiation source ($^{60}Co$ or $^{137}Cs$ γ-irradiator).

## 3. Methods

### 3.1. Stimulation

1. One round-bottom microtiter plate is set up for each cell dilution. Resuspend $12.4 \times 10^6$ PBMCs after plastic adherence (*see* Chapter 21, Subeading 3.1.) in 19.2 mL of AIM-V medium and distribute 100 μL/well of the cell suspension in a 96 round-bottom microtiter plate. This will correspond to the highest concentration of 64,000 cells/well. For the next dilution, which corresponds to 32,000 cells/well, add 9.6 mL of AIM-V medium to the remaining cell suspension and distribute 100 μL/well in a microtiter plate. Follow the same procedure for all the subsequent dilutions.
2. Irradiate $9 \times 10^6$ autologous LCL cells with 4000 rad, using a source of ionizing irradiation. Wash the cells once in AIM-V by centrifugation at 1000*g* for 10 min. Resuspend the cell pellet in 44 μL of AIM-V medium and aliquot 50 μL/well in each of the 8 plates containing the PBMC dilutions plus one plate containing only irradiated LCL that will serve as negative control for the cytotoxicity test. Maintain cultures in a humidified 37°C, 5% $CO_2$ incubator.
4. On d 3, add 50 μL/well of AIM-V medium containing 40 U/mL rIL-2 and 40% FCS. The total volume per well will be 200 μL with a final concentration of 10 U/mL rIL-2 and 10% FCS.

### 3.2. CTLp for EBV-Specific CTLs Restricted Through HLA-A, -B, and -C Alleles

On d 10, perform the first cytotoxicity test, using 24 replicates for each dilution. To evaluate the CTLp of EBV-specific CTLs restricted through HLA class I alleles, it is sufficient to test cell dilutions from 500 cells/well to 8000 cells/well (*see* **Note 2**).

1. Use 4,000 target cells per well in 100 μL RPMI complete medium. The target cells are $^{51}Cr$-labeled autologous, MHC class I single matched and mismatched LCLs. Twenty-four replicates can be tested simultaneously against a maximum of three different targets, using 50 μL of the effector cells (split-well analysis). Always include the mismatched LCL in order to discriminate between specific and nonspecific responses. **Figure 1** illustrates the split-well analysis for a single cell dilution when five cell lines are used as targets.
2. Calculate the background level of $^{51}Cr$ release as the mean of the spontaneous $^{51}Cr$ release in 24 control replicates containing only the irradiated autologous LCL and the target cell.
3. Score the cultures as positive when the specific $^{51}Cr$ release is higher than the background plus 3 standard deviations (SD).

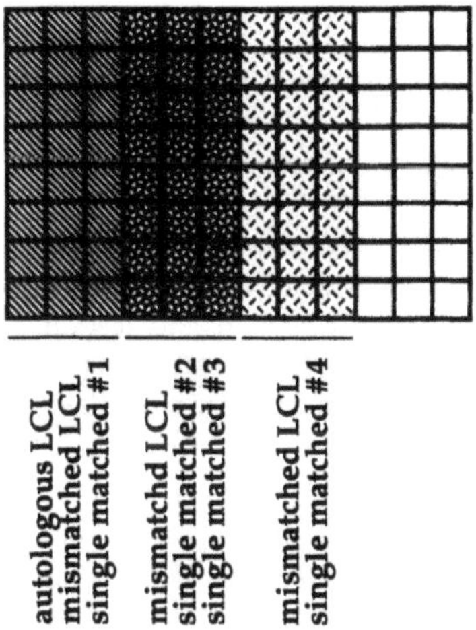


Fig. 1. Split-well analysis. The microtiter plate containing 1000 cells/well was tested against 5 different targets. A maximum of 3 targets were tested for each 24 replicates.

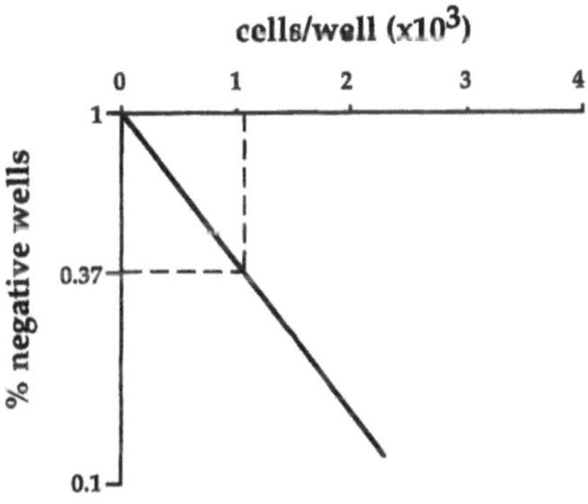


Fig. 2. Evaluation of CTLp specific for the autologous LCL in donor EA.

4. Evaluation of CTLp for each target is performed by plotting the logarithm of the percentage of negative wells on the Y axis and the cell dilution on the X axis. The zero term of the Poisson equation predicts that when 37% of the test cultures are negative there is an average of one precursor cell per well, therefore the frequency of a given precursor can be extrapolated directly from the graph as shown in **Fig. 2**.

### 3.3. CTLp for Individual Peptide Epitopes

A broader range of cell dilutions is required to evaluate the CTLp for individual peptide epitopes (from 1000 cells/well up to 64,000 cells/well).

1. The target cells are $^{51}$Cr-labeled autologous PHA blasts untreated or pulsed with the peptide epitope of interest at $10^{-6}$ *M* concentration. Split-well analysis and evaluation of the CTLp frequency is performed as described in **Subheading 3.2.** (*see* **Note 3**).

## 4. Notes

1. 30–40 mL of peripheral blood in heparin-coated tubes from each donor is sufficient to set up a limiting dilution assay.
2. At the highest cell concentrations the number of wells with nonspecific responses is very high.
3. It is possible that one stimulation is not enough to detect CTLs specific for single peptide epitopes. In this case, the cultures can be restimulated once or twice with 5,000 irradiated autologous LCL at d 7 and d 21. The cytotoxicity test can be performed 7 d after the last stimulation. The cultures should be fed weekly by replacing 100 µL of RPMI complete medium (*see* **Subheading 3.2.**) supplemented with 10 U/mL rIL-2.

## References


1. Sharrock, C. E. M., Kaminski, E., and Man, S. (1990) Limiting dilution analysis of human T cells: a useful clinical tool. Immunol. *Today* **11,** 281–286.
2. de St Groth, S. F. (1982) The evaluation of limiting dilution assays. *J. Immunol. Methods* **49,** R11–R23.
3. Taswell, C. (1981) Limiting dilution assays for the determination of immunocompetent cell frequencies. *J. Immunol.* **126,** 1614–1619.
4. Svedmyr, E. A. and Jondal, M. (1975) Cytotoxic effector cells specific for B cell lines transformed by Epstein-Barr virus are present in patients with infectious mononucleosis. *Proc. Natl. Acad. Sci. USA* **72,** 1622–1626.

# V

# Viral Protein Detection

# 25

## Antibodies for Detecting EBV Latent Proteins

**Martin Rowe and Anja Mehl**

### 1. Introduction

Antibodies to many Epstein-Barr virus (EBV) gene products are present in sera from infected human carriers. Historically, the ready demonstration of antibodies to lytic cycle proteins in particular allowed the seroepidemiological studies, which implicated EBV as a factor in various diseases *(1–4)*. However, human sera also contain antibodies to EBV latent gene products, as first demonstrated in an immunofluorescence test that detected predominantly EBNA1 *(5)*. Subsequently, human sera proved to be remarkably useful reagents for detecting and characterizing various latent EBV proteins in Western blot assays (e.g., **refs.** ***6–8***). Indeed, even now that monoclonal antibodies (MAbs) are available to many of the EBV latent proteins, human sera continue to be useful for "EBNotyping" assays in which EBV isolates can be distinguished by virtue of the characteristic fingerprint of variable-sized EBNA proteins (e.g., **refs.** ***9–12***). An example of EBNotyping is shown in **Fig. 1**.

Human sera, although useful in certain applications, do have considerable limitations. Thus, although nearly all immune sera can be demonstrated by Western blotting to contain antibodies to EBNA1, and a significant proportion also contain antibodies to EBNA2, only rare sera contain antibodies of suitable titer reactive with the other EBNAs, whereas human antibodies to LMP1 and LMP2 are not detected using ordinary Western blotting procedures *(13)*. There is also the problem that many sera show crossreactivities with normal cell proteins at the serum dilutions necessary to detect EBV latent proteins; this is particularly true of sera from rheumatoid arthritis and Burkitt's lymphoma patients, which are otherwise useful because they more frequently contain antibodies to the weakly immunogenic EBNA3A, 3B, and 3C proteins. This latter problem can be overcome by affinity purifying specific antibodies from human sera (*see* **Subheading 2.1.**). However, it is usually more practical to use experimental animal sera or, better still, MAbs. This chapter summarizes the monospecific reagents that have been generated to EBV latent proteins, with a particular emphasis placed on MAbs.

From: *Methods in Molecular Biology, Vol. 174: Epstein-Barr Virus Protocols*
Edited by: J. B. Wilson and G. H. W. May © Humana Press Inc., Totowa, NJ

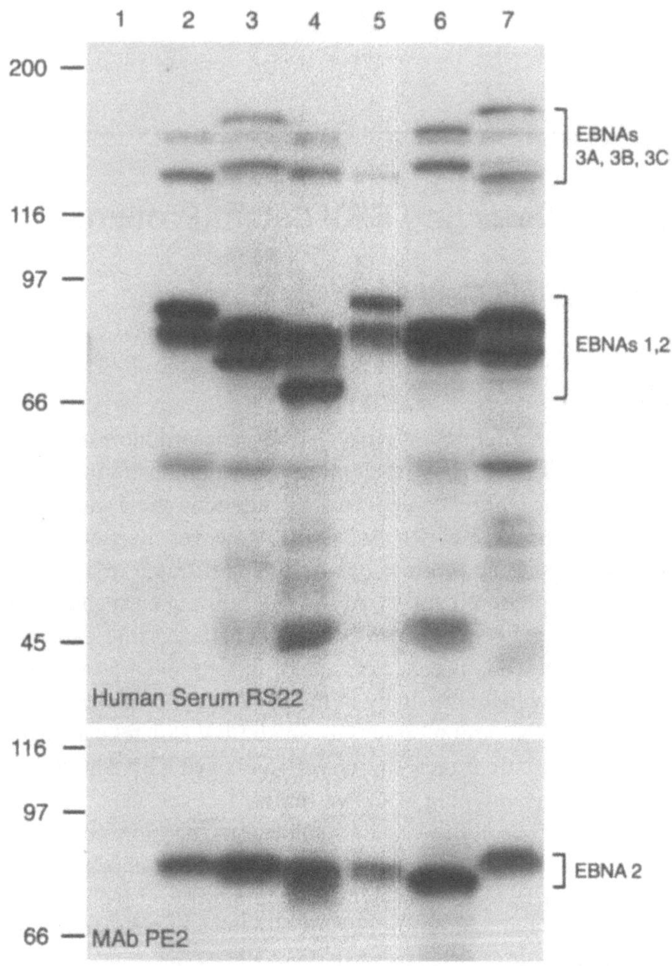


Fig. 1. EBNotyping of EBV-transformed B cell lines. Proteins from $10^6$ cells were separated by Laemmli SDS-PAGE on a 7.5% acrylamide resolving gel in a large-format slab gel apparatus giving 16 × 16 cm gels. Lane 1 contains protein from an EBV-negative B cell line, and lanes 2 through 7 contain proteins from 6 lymphoblastoid cell lines, each transformed with a different EBV isolate. The upper blot was probed with a serum from a juvenile rheumatoid arthritis patient which showed reactivity with EBNAs 1, 2, 3A, 3B, and 3C, and that was unusual in showing little crossreactivity with cellular proteins. Variations in the size of the EBNA proteins between different EBV isolates produces a characteristic fingerprint, or EBNotype, that allows different EBV isolates to be distinguished. The lower blot of a second gel run in parallel with the first, was probed with a MAb, PE2, reactive with EBNA2. Comparison of the two blots enables the EBNA1 and EBNA2 bands to be identified in the upper blot, and in this panel of cell lines it is apparent that the EBNA1 proteins show considerable size variation. EBNA1 usually has a lower MWt than EBNA2, but these samples include two EBV isolates (lanes 2 and lane 5) where the EBNA1 protein clearly migrates more slowly than the EBNA2 band.

## 2. Materials

### 2.1. Affinity-Purified Antibodies From Human Sera

Although rarely used nowadays, affinity purified human antibodies have in the past played an important role in characterizing the EBNA proteins. The methods employed for affinity-purification have included: adsorption to a synthetic peptide antigen cross-linked to agarose beads *(14)*, adsorption to recombinant fusion protein antigen cross-linked to agarose beads *(11,15,16)*, or adsorption to antigen from EBV-transformed cells that had been separated by sodium dodecyl sulfate-polyacrylamide gel electroporation (SDS-PAGE) and electroblotted onto nitrocellulose membranes *(13,17)*. These methods are tedious when considering the limited amount of antibody that is recovered. However, it should be noted that Western blot protocols have since improved in sensitivity with the introduction of chemiluminescent detection methods, so that the antibody probes can be used at least 10-fold more dilute and, therefore, the limited amount of valuable reagents produced by affinity purification would now serve for many more experiments.

### 2.2. Animal Immune Sera

There have been several reports of rabbit polyclonal antibodies being raised to synthetic peptides *(14,18–21)*, to bacterial recombinant fusion proteins *(22–25)*, or to recombinant baculovirus proteins expressed in insect cells *(26)*. While these sera have proved to be useful experimental reagents, they do suffer some of the drawbacks of human sera that render them unsuitable for more general use. Thus, they are available in finite amounts only, and they often show additional nonspecific reactivities that may require that the antibodies be affinity-purified before use. Furthermore, these reagents show batch-to-batch variations in specificity and titer.

### 2.3. Monoclonal Antibodies

Since 1984, the availability of MAbs to EBV latent proteins has steadily increased. **Table 1** summarizes the characteristics of many of these MAbs.

## 3. Notes

1. All of the MAbs listed in **Table 1** are reported to work in immunoprecipitation experiments, and most will work in Western blots. Although many of the antibodies are reported to work in immunofluoresence or immunohistochemistry, many are not sensitive enough to render them suitable for routine immunohistochemical staining of biopsy tissues. Those MAbs that have been used for routine immunohistochemistry include: OT1X and 1H4 (EBNA1), PE2, 1E6, R3 and 3E9 (EBNA2), CS.1-4, S12 and LMP024 (LMP1), and 8C3 (LMP2A). Often, special manipulations, such as microwave or enzymatic pretreatment, are necessary to increase the sensitivity of detection of antigen.
2. The usefulness of some MAbs is limited by the restricted specificity for the viral antigen from different isolates of EBV. This can be severe, as with some of the EBNA1 MAbs that recognize only a minority of natural EBNA1 variants (e.g., 3E4, 4D3, 1-150, 3-78, and 3-207). In other cases, the restricted specificity correlates with one of the two major subtypes of EBV (e.g., R3 and 3E9 MAbs to EBNA2, and E3C.A10 MAb to EBNA3C), and this can be advantageous.

**Table 1**
**Summary of Monoclonal Antibodies Reactive with EBV Latent Proteins**

| Antibody | Epitope | Ig type[a] | Applications[b] | Comments | Source[c] | Refs. |
|---|---|---|---|---|---|---|
| **EBNA1 MAbs** | | | | | | |
| OT1X | aa 430-440 | m, IgG1 | WB, IP, IH | | A | *(27–29)* |
| 1H4 | aa 461-464 | r, IgG2a | WB, IP, IH | | B | *(30,31)* |
| 2B4-1 | aa 7-37,420-607 | r, IgG1 | WB, IP, IH | | – | *(30,31)* |
| A2E8 | aa 1-59,429-641 | m, IgG | IP | | – | *(32,33)* |
| A3C7 | aa 1-59,429-641 | m, IgG | IP | | – | *(32,33)* |
| A5A12 | aa 1-59,429-641 | m, IgG | IP | | – | *(32,33)* |
| H6A12 | aa 1-59,429-641 | m, IgG | IP | | – | *(32,33)* |
| P135 | Gly/Ala repeats | m, IgM | WB, IP, IH | Crossreactive with a cell protein (*see* **Note 3**) | – | **(34,35)** |
| E95.4 | aa 610-640 | m, IgG2 | WB, IP, IH | | V | *(36)* |
| E98.1 | | m, IgG2 | WB, IP, IH | | V | *(36)* |
| E1-297 | aa 460-488 | m, IgG | WB, IP | – | *(37)* | |
| 3E4 | aa 8-39,439-641 | m, IgG1 | IP, IH | Restricted strain recognition (*see* **Note 2**) | – | *(38)* |
| 4D3 | aa 8-39,439-641 | m, IgG1 | IP, IH | Restricted strain recognition (*see* **Note 2**) | – | *(38)* |
| 1-150 | aa 442-530 | m, IgG1 | IP | Restricted strain recognition (*see* **Note 2**) | – | *(39)* |
| 2-79 | aa 442-530 | m, IgG1 | IP | – | *(39)* | |
| 3-78 | aa 442-530 | m, IgG1 | IP | Restricted strain recognition (*see* **Note 2**) | – | *(39)* |
| 3-207 | aa 442-530 | m, IgG1 | IP | Restricted strain recognition (*see* **Note 2**) | – | *(39)* |
| **EBNA2 MAbs** | | | | | | |
| PE2 | aa 405-480 | m, IgG1 | WB, IP, IH | Reacts with type-1 and -2 EBNA2 | D, N | *(40–42)* |
| 1E6 | aa 438-453 | r, IgG2a | WB, IP, IH | Reacts with type-1 and -2 EBNA2 | B | *(43)* |
| R3 | aa 450-464 | r, IgG2a | WB, IP, IH | Reacts with type-1 EBNA2 only (*see* **Note 2**) | – | *(43)* |
| 3E9 | C-terminal 79aa[d] | r, IgG2a | WB, IP, IH | Reacts with type-2 EBNA2 only (*see* **Note 2**) | – | *(43)* |
| 115E | aa 471-487 | m, IgG1 | WB, IP | EBV-type specificity not determined | – | *(44,45)* |

| | | | | | | |
|---|---|---|---|---|---|---|
| **EBNA3A MAbs** | | | | | | |
| T2.78 | aa 643-792 | m, IgG1 | WB, IP | Reacts with type-1 and -2 EBNA3A | – | *(11)* |
| **EBNA3C MAbs** | | | | | | |
| E3C.A10 | aa 682-686 | m, IgG1 | WB, IP | Reacts with type-1 EBNA3C only. In IP, it also co-precipitates type-1 EBNA2 (*see* **Notes 2** and **5**) | – | *(41,46)* |
| E3C.D8 | aa 736-781 | m, IgG1 | IP | Reacts with type-1 EBNA3C only (*see* **Note 2**) | – | *(41)* |
| **EBNA-LP MAbs** | | | | | | |
| JF186 | aa 4-12 of W1 repeat | m, IgG2a | WB, IP, IH | Reacts with only 35% EBV isolates (*see* **Note 6**) | – | *(17)* |
| **LMP1 MAbs** | | | | | | |
| CS.1 | aa 372-382 | m, IgG1 | WB, IP, IH | | D, N | *(47–49)* |
| CS.2 | aa 197-386 | m, IgG1 | WB, IP, IH | | D, N | *(47–49)* |
| CS.3 | aa 252-298 | m, IgG1 | WB, IP, IH | Crossreacts with cell protein (*see* **Note 4**) | D, N | *(47–49)* |
| CS.4 | aa 252-298 | m, IgG1 | WB, IP, IH | Crossreacts with cell protein (*see* **Note 4**) | D, N | *(47–49)* |
| S12 | aa 289-317 | m, IgG2a | WB, IP, IH | Crossreacts with cell protein? (*see* **Note 4**) | P | *(50)* |
| LMP024 | aa 351-386 | m, IgG1 | IP, IH | | – | *(42)* |
| 1G4 | | r, IgG2a | WB, IP, IH | | B | – |
| **LMP2A MAbs** | | | | | | |
| 4E11 | aa 21-36 | r, IgG1 | WB, IP,IH | | B | *(51,52)* |
| 14B7 | aa 36-64 | r, IgG2a | WB, IP | | – | *(51,52)* |

[a]Species of Ig is indicated by m, (mouse) or r, (rat).

[b]Applications for which the antibodies have been tested and found suitable are: WB, Western blot; IP, immunoprecipitation and/or DNA supershift assays; IH, immunohistochemistry and/or immunofluorescence staining of fixed cells.

[c]Antibodies that are available from commercial sources are indicated by: A, Advanced Biotechnologies Incorporated, Columbia MD; B, Biotest AG, Dreieich, Germany; D, DAKO Ltd, High Wycombe, UK; N, NovoCastra Laboratories, Newcastle, UK; P, Pharmingen, San Diego, CA; V, Virostat, Portland, Maine. Where no source is given, the antibodies are often available from the authors of the cited references.

[d]The epitope for the 3E9 antibody is contained within the Jijoye strain EBNA2 sequence. Epitopes for all other MAbs refer to the B95.8 strain EBNA2 sequence.

3. Some antibodies show crossreactivities with cellular proteins. The first reported example of this was the P135 MAb to the Gly/Ala repeats of EBNA1 that crossreacts with a 62 kDa cellular protein.
4. The CS3 and CS4 MAbs to LMP1 recognize a 42/44kD doublet of cellular proteins in Western blots; this crossreactivity dilutes out before the reactivity with LMP1, and the relative intensity of the cellular bands will, therefore, depend on the dilution of CS.3/CS.4 used to probe the blots. The cellular crossreactivity is not observed by immunofluorescence staining of acetone/methanol-fixed cells. However, in immunohistochemical staining of routine paraffin sections, crossreactivities with EBV-negative cells are sometimes observed even when antibody dilutions are optimized for LMP1 staining. The S12 anti-LMP1 antibody, which also detects an epitope flanking the repeat region of LMP1, does not show cellular crossreactivity in Western blots, but may show crossreactivity in immunohistochemistry of some tissue sections. The CS.1, CS.2, CS.3, and CS.4 pool of MAbs are usually employed as a pooled CS.1-4 reagent in order to ensure that all natural sequence variants of LMP1 are detected. However, MAbs directed to epitopes at the extreme C-terminus of LMP1 (e.g., CS.1 or LMP024) appear to be less problematic with regard to crossreactivities with cellular proteins. Because this domain of LMP1 is highly conserved among different EBV isolates, there is a case for using these antibodies individually in immunohistochemistry. It should be noted that the CS.1 and LMP024 antibodies are not as sensitive as other LMP1 antibodies in Western blots.
5. The E3C.A10 MAb to EBNA3C shows an unusual crossreactivity. Although it is highly specific in Western blots, and recognizes EBNA3C from about 80% of type-1 EBV isolates, in immunopreciptation experiments it also reacts strongly with type-1 EBNA2.
6. The published IgG1 isotype of the JF186 MAb to EBNA-LP is an error. As indicated in **Table 1**, the JF186 is a mouse IgG2a antibody.

## References

1. Henle, W., Henle, G., Burtin, P., Cachin, Y., Clifford, P., et al. (1970) Antibodies to EBV virus in nasopharyngeal carcinoma, other head and neck neoplasms and control groups. *J. Natl. Cancer Inst.* **44,** 225–231.
2. Henle, G. and Henle, W. (1966) Immunofluorescence in cells derived from Burkitt's lymphoma. *J. Bacteriol.* **91,** 1248–1256.
3. de The, G., Geser, A., Day, N. E., Tukei, P. M., Williams, E. H., Beri, D. P., et al. (1978) Epidemiological evidence for causal relationship between Epstein-Barr virus and Burkitt's lymphoma from Ugandan prospective study. *Nature* **274,** 756–761.
4. Mueller, N., Evans, A., Harris, N. L., Comstock, G. W., Jellum, E., Magnus, K., et al. (1989) Hodgkin's disease and Epstein-Barr virus. Altered antibody pattern before diagnosis. *N. Engl. J. Med.* **320,** 689–695.
5. Reedman, B. M. and Klein, G. (1973) Cellular localization of an Epstein-Barr virus (EBV)-associated complement-fixing antigen in producer and non-producer lymphoblastoid cell lines. *Int. J. Cancer* **11,** 499–520.
6. Kallin, B., Dillner, J., Ernberg, I., Ehlin-Henriksson, B., Rosen, A., Henle, W., et al. (1986) Four virally determined nuclear antigens are expressed in Epstein-Barr virus-transformed cells. *Proc. Natl. Acad. Sci. USA* **83,** 1499–1503.
7. Rowe, D. T., Rowe, M., Evan, G. I., Wallace, L. E., Farrell, P. J., and Rickinson, A. B. (1986) Restricted expression of EBV latent genes and T-lymphocyte-detected membrane antigen in Burkitt's lymphoma cells. *EMBO J.* **5,** 2599–2607.

8. Strnad, B. C., Schuster, T. C., Hopkins, R. F. d., Neubauer, R. H., and Rabin, H. (1981) Identification of an Epstein-Barr virus nuclear antigen by fluoroimmunoelectrophoresis and radioimmunoelectrophoresis. *J. Virol.* **38,** 996–1004.
9. Falk, K., Gratama, J. W., Rowe, M., Zou, J.-Z., Khanim, F., Young, L. S., et al. (1994) The role of repetative DNA sequences in the size variation of Epstein-Barr virus (EBV) nuclear antigens, and the identification of different EBV isolates using RFLP and PCR analysis. *J. Gen. Virol.* **76,** 779–790.
10. Gratama, J. W., Oosterveer, M. A., Klein, G., and Ernberg, I. (1990) EBNA size polymorphism can be used to trace Epstein-Barr virus spread within families. *J. Virol.* **64,** 4703–4708.
11. Rowe, M., Young, L. S., Cadwallader, K., Petti, L., Kieff, E., and Rickinson, A. B. (1989) Distinction between Epstein-Barr virus type A (EBNA 2A) and type B (EBNA 2B) isolates extends to the EBNA 3 family of nuclear proteins. *J. Virol.* **63,** 1031–1039.
12. Yao, Q. Y., Tierney, R. J., Croom-Carter, D., Dukers, D., Cooper, G. M., Ellis, C. J., et al. (1996) Frequency of multiple Epstein-Barr virus infections in T-cell-immunocompromised individuals. *J. Virol.* **70,** 4884–4894.
13. Rowe, M., Finke, J., Szigeti, R., and Klein, G. (1988) Characterisation of the serological response in man to the latent membrane protein (LMP) and the six nuclear antigens (EBNA 1-6) encoded by the Epstein-Barr virus. *J. Gen. Virol.* **69,** 1217–1228.
14. Dillner, J., Sternås, L., Kallin, B., Alexander, H., Ehlin-Henriksson, B., Jörnvall, H., et al. (1984) Antibodies against a synthetic peptide identify the Epstein-Barr virus-determined nuclear antigen. *Proc. Natl. Acad. Sci. USA* **81,** 4652–4656.
15. Hennessy, K., Wang, F., Bushman, E. W., and Kieff, E. (1986) Definitive identification of a member of the Epstein-Barr virus nuclear protein 3 family. *Proc. Natl. Acad. Sci. USA* **83,** 5693–5697.
16. Petti, L., Sample, J., Wang, F., and Kieff, E. (1988) A fifth Epstein-Barr virus nuclear protein (EBNA3C) is expressed in latently infected growth-transformed lymphocytes. *J. Virol.* **62,** 1330–1338.
17. Finke, J., Rowe, M., Kallin, B., Ernberg, I., Rosén, A., Dillner, J., and Klein, G. (1987) Monoclonal and polyclonal antibodies against Epstein-Barr virus nuclear antigen 5 (EBNA-5) detect multiple protein species in Burkitt's lymphoma and lymphoblastoid cell lines. *J. Virol.* **61,** 3870–3878.
18. Dillner, J., Kallin, B., Alexander, H., Ernberg, I., Uno, M., Ono, Y., et al. (1986) An Epstein-Barr virus (EBV)-determined nuclear antigen (EBNA5) partly encoded by the transformation-associated Bam WYH region of EBV DNA: preferential expression in lymphoblastoid cell lines. *Proc. Natl. Acad. Sci. USA* **83,** 6641–6645.
19. Ricksten, A., Kallin, B., Alexander, H., Dillner, J., Fahraeus, R., Klein, G., et al. (1988) BamHI E region of the Epstein-Barr virus genome encodes three transformation-associated nuclear proteins. *Proc. Natl. Acad. Sci. USA* **85,** 995–999.
20. Modrow, S. and Wolf, H. (1986) Characterization of two related Epstein-Barr virus-encoded membrane proteins that are differentially expressed in Burkitt lymphoma and in vitro-transformed cell lines. *Proc. Natl. Acad. Sci. USA* **83,** 5703–5707.
21. Moorthy, R. and Thorley-Lawson, D. A. (1990) Processing of the Epstein-Barr virus-encoded latent membrane protein p63/LMP. *J. Virol.* **64,** 829–837.
22. Billaud, M., Busson, P., Huang, D., Mueller-Lantzch, N., Rousselet, G., Pavlish, O., et al. (1989) Epstein-Barr virus (EBV)-containing nasopharyngeal carcinoma cells express the B-cell activation antigen blast2/CD23 and low levels of the EBV receptor CR2. *J. Virol.* **63,** 4121–4128.

23. Sauter, M. and Mueller-Lantzsch, N. (1987) Characterization of an Epstein-Barr virus nuclear antigen 2 variant (EBNA 2B) by specific sera. *Virus Res.* **8,** 141–152.
24. Baichwal, V. R. and Sugden, B. (1987) Posttranslational processing of an Epstein-Barr virus-encoded membrane protein expressed in cells transformed by Epstein-Barr virus. *J. Virol.* **61,** 866–875.
25. Hennessy, K. and Kieff, E. (1983) One of two Epstein-Barr virus nuclear antigens contains a glycine-alanine copolymer domain. *Proc. Natl. Acad. Sci. USA* **80,** 5665–5669.
26. Sample, C. and Parker, B. (1994) Biochemical characterization of Epstein-Barr virus nuclear antigen 3A and 3C proteins. *Virology* **205,** 534–539.
27. Wang, Y., Finan, J. E., Middeldorp, J. M., and Hayward, S. D. (1997) P32/TAP, a cellular protein that interacts with EBNA-1 of Epstein-Barr virus. *Virology* **236,** 18–29.
28. Chen, M. R., Middeldorp, J. M., and Hayward, S. D. (1993) Separation of the complex DNA binding domain of EBNA-1 into DNA recognition and dimerization subdomains of novel structure. *J. Virol.* **67,** 4875–4885.
29. Wagner, H. J., Hornef, M., Middeldorp, J., and Kirchner, H. (1995) Characteristics of viral protein expression by Epstein-Barr virus- infected B cells in peripheral blood of patients with infectious mononucleosis. *Clin. Diagn. Lab. Immunol.* **2,** 696–699.
30. Murray, P. G., Niedobitek, G., Kremmer, E., Grasser, F., Reynolds, G. M., Cruchley, A., et al. (1996) In situ detection of the Epstein-Barr virus-encoded nuclear antigen 1 in oral hairy leukoplakia and virus-associated carcinomas. *J. Pathol.* **178,** 44–47.
31. Grasser, F. A., Murray, P. G., Kremmer, E., Klein, K., Remberger, K., Feiden, W., et al. (1994) Monoclonal antibodies directed against the Epstein-Barr virus-encoded nuclear antigen 1 (EBNA1): immunohistologic detection of EBNA1 in the malignant cells of Hodgkin's disease. *Blood* **84,** 3792–3798.
32. Orlowski, R., Polvino-Bodnar, M., Hearing, J., and Miller, G. (1990) Inhibition of specific binding of EBNA 1 to DNA by murine monoclonal and certain human polyclonal antibodies. *Virology* **176,** 638–642.
33. Hearing, J. C., Lewis, A., and Levine, A. J. (1985) Structure of the Epstein-Barr virus nuclear antigen as probed with monoclonal antibodies. *Virology* **142,** 215–220.
34. Luka, J., Kreofsky, T., Pearson, G. R., Hennessy, K., and Kieff, E. (1984) Identification and characterization of a cellular protein that cross-reacts with the Epstein-Barr virus nuclear antigen. *J. Virol.* **52,** 833–838.
35. Fox, R., Sportsman, R., Rhodes, G., Luka, J., Pearson, G., and Vaughan, J. (1986) Rheumatoid arthritis synovial membrane contains a 62,000–molecular-weight protein that shares an antigenic epitope with the Epstein-Barr virus-encoded associated nuclear antigen. *J. Clin. Invest.* **77,** 1539–1547.
36. http://members.tripod.com/~herpesvirus/research/moabs.htm
37. Inoue, N., Harada, S., Honma, T., Kitamura, T., and Yanagi, K. (1991) The domain of Epstein-Barr virus nuclear antigen 1 essential for binding to oriP region has a sequence fitted for the hypothetical basic- helix-loop-helix structure. *Virology* **182,** 84–93.
38. Wrightham, M. N., Stewart, J. P., Janjua, N. J., Pepper, S. D., Sample, C., Rooney, C. M., and Arrand, J. R. (1995) Antigenic and sequence variation in the C-terminal unique domain of the Epstein-Barr virus nuclear antigen EBNA-1. *Virology* **208,** 521–530.
39. Iwakiri, D., Nakamura, H., Ono, Y., and Fujiwara, S. (1997) Antigenic variation of the Epstein-Barr virus nuclear antigen EBNA1 as revealed by monoclonal antibodies. *Virus Res.* **50,** 139–149.
40. Young, L., Alfieri, C., Hennessey, K., Evans, H., O'Hara, C., Anderson, K. C., et al. (1989) Expression of Epstein-Barr virus transformation-associated genes in tissues of patients with EBV lymphoproliferative disease. *N. Engl. J. Med.* **321,** 1080–1085.

41. Maunders, M. J., Petti, L., and Rowe, M. (1994) Precipitation of the Epstein-Barr virus protein EBNA 2 by an EBNA 3c-specific monoclonal antibody. *J. Gen. Virol.* **75,** 769–778.
42. Niedobitek, G., Agathanggelou, A., Rowe, M., Jones, E. L., Jones, D. B., Turyaguma, P., et al. (1995) Heterogeneous expression of Epstein-Barr virus latent proteins in endemic Burkitt's lymphoma. *Blood* **86,** 659–665.
43. Kremmer, E., Kranz, B. R., Hille, A., Klein, K., Eulitz, M., Hoffmannfezer, G., et al. (1995) Rat monoclonal antibodies differentiating between the Epstein-Barr virus nuclear antigens 2A (EBNA2A) and 2B (EBNA2B). *Virology* **208,** 336–342.
44. Dillner, J., Wendel-Hansen, V., Kjellstrom, G., Kallin, B., and Rosen, A. (1988) Purification and characterization of the Epstein-Barr virus nuclear antigen 2 using monoclonal antipeptide antibodies. *Int. J. Cancer* **42,** 721–727.
45. Randahl, H., Fahraeus, R., and Klein, G. (1992) Biochemical characterization of Epstein-Barr virus nuclear antigen 2A and an associated ATPase activity. *Eur. J. Biochem.* **207,** 55–59.
46. Yao, Q. Y., Tierney, R. J., Croom-Carter, D., Cooper, G. M., Ellis, C. J., Rowe, M., and Rickinson, A. B. (1996) Isolation of intertypic recombinants of Epstein-Barr virus from T-cell-immunocompromised individuals. *J. Virol.* **70,** 4895–4903.
47. Rowe, M., Evans, H. S., Young, L. S., Hennessy, K., Kieff, E., and Rickinson, A. B. (1987) Monoclonal antibodies to the latent membrane protein of Epstein-Barr virus reveal heterogeneity of the protein and inducible expression in virus-transformed cells. *J. Gen. Virol.* **68,** 1575–1586.
48. Gregory, C. D., Rowe, M., and Rickinson, A. B. (1990) Different Epstein-Barr virus (EBV)-B cell interactions in phenotypically distinct clones of a Burkitt lymphoma cell line. *J. Gen. Virol.* **71,** 1481–1495.
49. Pallesen, G., Hamilton-Dutoit, S. J., Rowe, M., and Young, L. S. (1991) Expression of Epstein-Barr virus latent gene products in tumour cells of Hodgkin's disease. *Lancet* **337,** 320–322.
50. Mann, K. P., Staunton, D., and Thorley-Lawson, D. A. (1985) Epstein-Barr virus-encoded protein found in plasma membranes of transformed cells. *J. Virol.* **55,** 710–720.
51. Fruehling, S., Lee, S. K., Herrold, R., Frech, B., Laux, G., Kremmer, E., et al. (1996) Identification of latent membrane protein 2A (LMP2A) domains essential for the LMP2A dominant-negative effect on B-lymphocyte surface immunoglobulin signal transduction. *J. Virol.* **70,** 6216–6226.
52. Niedobitek, G., Kremmer, E., Herbst, H., Whitehead, L., Dawson, C. W., Niedobitek, E., et al. (1997) Immunohistochemical detection of the Epstein-Barr virus-encoded latent membrane protein 2A in Hodgkin's disease and infectious mononucleosis. *Blood* **90,** 1664–1672.

# 26

# Detection of EBV Latent Proteins by Western Blotting

**Martin Rowe and Matthew Jones**

## 1. Introduction

Western blotting is a well established technique for identifying Epstein-Barr virus (EBV)-encoded proteins in lysates from cell lines or biopsy material. The basic technique involves separation of proteins by sodium dodecyl sulphate-polyacrylamide gel electrophoresis (SDS-PAGE) and transfer onto a support membrane such as nitrocellulose or polyvinylidine difluoride (PVDF), followed by immunostaining with specific antibody reagents. The initial SDS-PAGE separation procedure is essentially similar to the method originally described by Laemmli *(1)*, except that vertical slab gels are used instead of the original tube gels. Until recently, the slab gels commonly used were relatively large (approx 16 × 16 cm), but now it has become popular to use "mini" slab gels (approx 7 × 8 cm) because the electrophoresis and blotting times are considerably reduced and there is a significant saving in the amounts of the reagents required.

The principle of transfer of proteins from SDS-PAGE gels onto membrane supports for subsequent immunostaining was developed by several groups *(2–5)*, but the electroblotting method commonly employed now is essentially that described by Towbin *(3)*. For many years, the choice of membranes for Western blotting was almost exclusively limited to nitrocellulose-based supports that, over the years, have been improved with respect to their quality and characteristics. More recently, PVDF membranes have gained in popularity because of their higher protein-binding capacities, their greater physical strength, and the improved sensitivity in certain chemiluminescence-based immunodetection protocols. Furthermore, the characteristics of PVDF membranes make them a preferred choice when it is intended to strip the membranes of bound antibodies and to re-probe with a second set of antibodies *(6,7)*.

There are a variety of immunodetection methods available for Western blotting. The original method employed rabbit antisera followed by $^{125}$I-labeled Protein A and autoradiography. The detection of murine monoclonal antibodies (MAbs) by this method is inefficient unless an intermediate rabbit anti-mouse Ig is used to improve

From: *Methods in Molecular Biology, Vol. 174: Epstein-Barr Virus Protocols*
Edited by: J. B. Wilson and G. H. W. May © Humana Press Inc., Totowa, NJ

the binding of Protein A. This detection method is reliable, and we have used it over a period of several years to detect specific binding of rabbit sera, human sera, or murine MAbs to blotted membranes (e.g., ***8–11***). However, $^{125}$I-labeled probes are not suitable for laboratories that only perform occasional Western blots, because the half-life of $^{125}$iodine necessitates that the probe be used within 4 wk of purchase; this is an expensive and wasteful option if only a small amount of probe is used each month. Alkaline phosphatase-conjugated secondary antibodies followed by colorimetric development with tetrazolium salts ***(12)*** show a comparable sensitivity to radiolabeled probes, and they have the advantage that the enzyme-conjugated antibodies are stable and cost-effective. Horseradish peroxidase conjugated secondary antibodies can also be used with colorimetric substrates. We and others have previously used the enzyme conjugated secondary antibodies with colorimetric substrates for the detection of EBV proteins (e.g., ***13–16***).

Although the aforementioned immunodetection methods are quite adequate for most purposes, they are now losing ground to methods based on chemiluminiscent substrates for phosphatase or peroxidase-conjugated secondary antibodies ***(17–22)***. Chemiluminescent substrates have several advantages over equivalent colorimetric substrates, including: (1) vastly superior sensitivity, typically being able to detect at least 10× less protein; (2) the antibodies are used much more dilute, thus conserving valuable reagents; (3) several exposure times can be recorded on photographic film so that both weak and strong bands can be examined on the same blot; and (4) the photographic film exposures provide a permanent hard copy of the results, which is not subject to the fading that can occur with blots developed with some colorimetric substrates.

Of the chemiluminescence methods, the luminol-based assays for peroxidase-conjugated antibodies (e.g., ECL, Amersham Pharmacia) are widely used throughout the research community. However, similar results can be obtained with chemiluminescence-based substrates for alkaline phosphatase-conjugated enzymes, and the protocol that we describe here is one such method using the CDP-Star™ substrate. In practical terms, there is little to choose between the peroxidase- and phosphatase-detection protocols. However, alkaline phosphatase has the advantage of being more stable than horseradish peroxidase, and is not inhibited by sodium azide. The CDP-Star reaction produces a light signal within minutes, and this gradually increases in intensity for up to 2 h; light then continues to be produced until the substrate is exhausted. In contrast, the ECL light reaction peaks more sharply within minutes, then decays more rapidly than does the alkaline phosphatase substrate. Therefore, the CDP-Star detection method for alkaline phosphatase allows a more predictable degree of exposure over a longer period of time, which may be critical if there is a scramble for the use of the darkroom. The CDP-Star™ detection method described here is 10–40 times more sensitive than methods employing higher concentrations of antibody followed by development with colorimetric substrates. This sensitivity is illustrated in **Fig. 1**; the CDP-Star method with the CS.1-4 anti-LMP1 murine MAbs is able to detect LMP1 from as few as $5 \times 10^3$ EBV-transformed B lymphoblastoid cells at typical development times (up to 5 min), and as few as $1.5 \times 10^3$ cells if development is extended

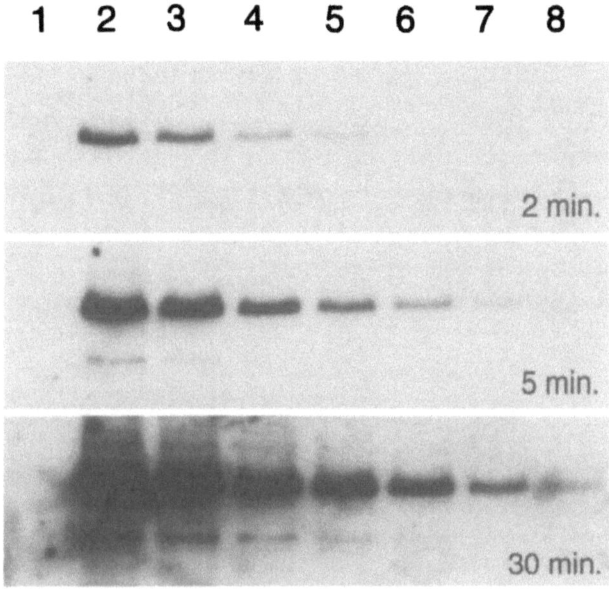


Fig. 1. Sensitivity of CDP-Star™ Western blot for detecting LMP1. Doubling dilutions of a cell lysate from a lymphoblastoid cell line transformed with the B95.8 isolate of EBV were loaded onto an 8% polyacrylamide resolving gel: lane 2, $10^5$ cells; lane 3, $5 \times 10^4$ cells; lane 4, $2.5 \times 10^4$ cells; lane 5, $1.3 \times 10^4$ cells; lane 6, $6.3 \times 10^3$ cells; lane 7, $3.1 \times 10^3$ cells; lane 8, $1.5 \times 10^3$ cells. Lane 1 was loaded with $10^5$ cells from an EBV-negative B cell line. The separated proteins were blotted onto a PVDF membrane and immunostained with 0.5 µg/mL CS.1-4 for 1 h, then detected with alkaline phosphatase conjugated goat anti-mouse IgG and developed with CDP-Star substrate. Three sequential exposures of 2, 5, and 30 min were made to Kodak X-Omat LS photographic film.

to 30 min. In our hands, equivalent immunodetection using BCIP/NBT colorimetric substrate for alkaline phosphatase will not detect LMP1 from less than $5 \times 10^4$ cells.

One refinement of the Western blotting procedure is the option of stripping and re-probing the blots with a different antibody. This may be particularly desirable when protein samples are obtained from limited amounts of precious biopsy material. The results in **Fig. 2A,B** illustrate the sequential staining of a blot with antibodies to different EBV antigens.

## 2. Materials

### 2.1. Sample Preparation for SDS-PAGE

1. Phosphate buffered saline (PBS): 58 m*M* $Na_2HPO_4$, 17 m*M* $NaH_2PO_4$, 68 m*M* NaCl.
2. Rippa buffer: 150 m*M* NaCl, 0.5% Nonidet P40 detergent, 0.5% sodium deoxycholate, 0.1% sodium dodecyl sulfate (SDS), 5 m*M* EDTA, 20 m*M* Tris-HCl, pH 7.5.
3. Protease inhibitors: 100X stock solution prepared from Sigma protease inhibitor cocktail (cat. # P2714) by dissolving the lyophilized powder in 1 mL $H_2O$ at 0°C. Single-use aliquots of 50 µL are stored frozen at –70°C.

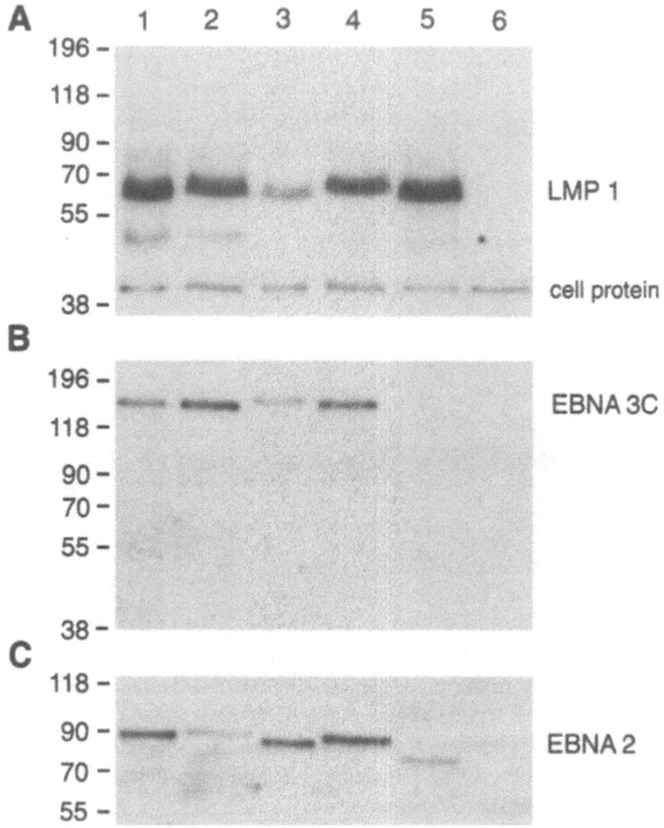


Fig. 2. Detection of LMP1, EBNA3C and EBNA2 from different EBV isolates. Each lane of an 8% polyacrylamide resolving gel was loaded with lysates from $2 \times 10^5$ cells: lanes 1 through 4, four EBV-transformed lymphoblastoid cell lines each carrying a different type-1 EBV isolate; lane 5, an EBV-transformed lymphoblastoid cell line carrying a type-2 EBV isolate; lane 6, an EBV-negative B cell line. **(A)** Blot probed with the anti-LMP1 MAbs, CS.1-4 (Dako), diluted to 0.5 µg/mL and incubated for 1 hour at room temperature. **(B)** After development, blot A was stripped and re-probed with the anti-EBNA3C MAb, E3C.A10, diluted to 1 µg/mL and incubated overnight at 4°C. **(C)** A parallel blot was probed with the anti-EBNA2 MAb, PE2, diluted to 0.2 µg/mL and incubated overnight at 4°C. Note that the stripped blot B shows no sign of the LMP1 bands from the first round of detection. The E3C.A10 reacts only with EBNA3C from type-1 EBV isolates, hence the lack of a band in lane 5 of blot B. In contrast, the CS.1-4 and PE2 antibodies react respectively with LMP1 (blot A) and EBNA2 (blot C) from all EBV isolates.

4. 2X gel sample buffer (GSB): 125 m*M* Tris-HCl, pH 6.8, 20% glycerol, 10% β-mercaptoethanol, 4% SDS, 0.004% bromophenol blue (*see* **Note 1**). Store short-term at 4°C, or longer term as frozen aliquots below –20°C. If the SDS precipitates during storage, re-dissolve by incubating for 5–10 min in a 37°C water bath.

5. Hemocytometer. For safety reasons, disposable plastic hemocytometers are recommended, e.g., Kova Glasstic® Slide 10 with Grids, obtained from Hycor Biomedical Inc (cat.# 87144).
6. Motorized tissue homogenizer.
7. Sonicator, with 3-mm tip probe.
8. Electric heating block with Eppendorf tube adapter.

### 2.2. SDS-PAGE

1. Ethanol.
2. Acrylamide solution: purchased as a ready-mixed 40% stock solution containing acrylamide and bis-acrylamide at a ratio of 37.5:1 (*see* **Note 2**).
3. Ammonium persulphate: 15% solution prepared fresh.
4. Resolving gel buffer, 4X stock solution: 1.5 *M* Tris-HCl, pH 8.8, 0.24% *NNN'N*-tetramethyl-ethylenediamine (TEMED), 0.4% SDS. Store at 4°C for up to 1 mo.
5. Stacking gel buffer, 2X stock solution: 0.25 *M* Tris-HCl, pH 6.8, 0.24% TEMED, 0.2% SDS. Store at 4°C for up to 1 mo.
6. 10X Electrophoresis Running buffer: 0.25 *M* Tris-base, 1.92 *M* glycine, 1% SDS. Prepare 1 L by dissolving 30.3 g Tris base, 14.42 g glycine, and 10 g SDS in $H_2O$. Do not adjust pH (*see* **Note 3**). Store at room temperature.
7. Prestained molecular weight markers (e.g., Sigma; cat # SDS-7B).
8. Vertical gel electrophoresis apparatus and power pack (*see* **Note 4**).
9. Gel-application disposable tips (e.g., P200 Gel-Load tip from Greiner; cat # 770290).

### 2.3. Electroblotting

1. PVDF (polyvinylidene difluoride) membranes cut according to the size of gels (*see* **Notes 5** and **6**). For minigels, 7.5 × 9 cm is appropriate.
2. Whatman 3MM filter paper, cut to size of blotting apparatus (*see* **Note 6**). For the BioRad Transblot apparatus, a 15 × 20 cm size is appropriate; two sheets are required for each cassette (*see* **Note 7**).
3. Analytical-grade methanol (*see* **Notes 8** and **9**).
4. Transfer buffer: 25 m*M* Tris-base, 192 m*M* glycine, 20% methanol. Prepare 1 L by dissolving 3.03 g Tris base, 14.42 g glycine, and 200 mL methanol in $H_2O$. Do not adjust the pH (*see* **Note 3**). Store at room temperature in sealed container.
5. Blotting apparatus and power pack (*see* **Note 7**).

### 2.4. Immunodetection

1. 10X PBS: 0.58 *M* $Na_2HPO_4$, 0.17 *M* $NaH_2PO_4$, 0.68 *M* NaCl. Autoclave, and store at room temperature. Make sufficient 1X working solution fresh for each experiment.
2. 10X PBS-T (PBS with Tween-20): 2% Tween-20 in 10X PBS. Store at room temperature, and make sufficient 1X working solution fresh for each experiment.
3. Blocking buffer (*see* **Note 10**): 0.4% casein, 0.1% Tween-20, 0.02% $NaN_3$ in PBS. Prepare 200 mL of blocking buffer by microwaving 180 mL $H_2O$ for 45 s, adding 20 mL of 10X PBS, then stirring in 0.8 g casein powder until the mixture has cooled and the casein is dissolved (*see* **Note 11**). Finally, when the solution has cooled completely, add 0.2 mL Tween-20 and 0.4 mL of a 10% $NaN_3$ stock solution (*see* **Note 12**). Store at 4°C for up to 2 wk.
4. Primary antibody: MAbs are typically diluted to 0.2–1 μg/mL in Blocking buffer; human sera are typically diluted 1/1000–1/5000 in Blocking buffer; immune rabbit sera are typically diluted 1/2000–1/10,000 in Blocking buffer (*see* **Note 13**).

5. Alkaline phosphatase conjugated secondary antibody: typically diluted 1/10,000–1/40,000 in Blocking buffer (*see* **Note 14**).
6. 10X APA (alkaline phosphatase assay) buffer: 1 *M* diethanolamine, pH 9.5, 10 m*M* $MgCl_2$. To make 100 mL of 10X APA buffer, 11 mL of diethanolamine is mixed with 80 mL of $H_2O$ and the pH adjusted with concentrated HCl before adding 0.2 g $MgCl_2$ and additional $H_2O$ to give a final volume of 100 mL (*see* **Note 15**). Store 10X APA buffer at 4°C for up to 6 mo, and make sufficient 1X working solution fresh for each experiment.
7. CDP-Star™ development reagent: purchased as a ready-to-use substrate mix, e.g., from TROPIX Inc. (cat # MS100R). Store at 4°C.
8. Polyethylene lay-flat film: e.g., 204-mm width roll available from Jencons (cat # 295-003).
9. Heavy duty heat-sealing apparatus for making bags and envelopes from polyethylene sheets.
10. Rocking apparatus.

### 2.5. Stripping and Re-Probing Western Blots

1. MESNA stripping buffer: 62.5 m*M* Tris-HCl, pH 6.8, 2% SDS, 50 m*M* sodium 2-mercapto-ethansulfonate (*see* **Note 1**).
2. SDS wash buffer: 62.5 m*M* Tris-HCl, pH 6.8, 2% SDS.

## 3. Methods

### 3.1. Sample Preparation of Cell Lines for SDS-PAGE

1. Harvest approx $2 \times 10^6$ to $2 \times 10^7$ cells, and wash in ice-cold PBS by centrifugation.
2. Resuspend in 2 to 20 mL ice-cold PBS, and take an aliquot for counting in a hemocytometer.
3. Centrifuge, and resuspend pellet in 1 mL of ice-cold PBS containing protease inhibitors.
4. Transfer to 1.8 mL Eppendorf tube and pellet cells by centrifugation.
5. Resuspend in a predetermined volume of ice-cold PBS containing protease inhibitors, to give a suspension of $2 \times 10^7$ cells/mL.
6. Add an equal vol of 2X GSB, giving a lysate equivalent to $10^7$ cells/mL.
7. Sonicate for up to 5 s to shear DNA and thus reduce the viscosity.
8. Transfer to heating block at 100°C for 3 min.
9. Store samples frozen below –20°C until required.

### 3.2. Sample Preparation of Cell Lines for Immunoprecipitation and SDS-PAGE

1. Harvest at least $2 \times 10^7$ cells, and wash in ice-cold PBS by centrifugation.
2. Resuspend in ice-cold PBS, and take an aliquot for counting in a hemocytometer.
3. Cool Rippa buffer on ice, and add 1% protease inhibitors immediately before use.
4. Centrifuge cells, and resuspend pellet at $4 \times 10^7$ cells/mL in ice-cold Rippa buffer containing protease inhibitors.
5. Sonicate for up to 5 s to shear DNA and thus reduce the viscosity.
6. Incubate on ice for 15–20 min, then re-sonicate.
7. Clarify by centrifugation at 10,000*g* for 2 min (*see* **Note 16**).
8. To an aliquot of the clarified lysate, add one volume of 2X GSB plus two vol of 1X GSB, giving a lysate equivalent to $10^7$ cells/mL.
9. Transfer to heating block at 100°C for 3 min.
10. Store samples frozen below –20°C until required.

**Table 1**
**Recipes for Resolving Gel Solutions with Different Percentages of Acrylamide**

| | Volume (mL) of component stock solutions | | | |
|---|---|---|---|---|
| Stock solution | 8% gel | 10% gel | 12% gel | 15% gel |
| $H_2O$ | 6.15 | 5.60 | 5.10 | 4.20 |
| 4X Resolving buffer | 2.80 | 2.80 | 2.80 | 2.80 |
| 40% Acrylamide/bis mix | 2.25 | 2.80 | 3.40 | 4.20 |
| 15% Ammonium persulphate | 0.044 | 0.044 | 0.038 | 0.038 |

### 3.3. Sample Preparation of Tissue Biopsies for SDS-PAGE

1. Cool Rippa buffer on ice and add 1% protease inhibitors immediately before use.
2. Weigh snap-frozen tissue biopsies (*see* **Note 17**).
3. Add Rippa buffer, with protease inhibitors, to the pieces of frozen biopsy to give a 5% w/v ratio of biopsy/Rippa, then homogenize for 10–15 s on ice to produce a fine homogenate.
4. Incubate on ice for 15 min, with periodic mixing of the homogenate.
5. Clarify lysate by centrifugation at 10,000*g* for 2 min at 4°C.
6. Add 1 vol of 2X GSB, then 3 vol of 1X GSB, to give a final lysate equivalent to 10 mg biopsy/mL.
7. Sonicate for up to 5 s.
8. Transfer to heating block at 100°C for 3 min.
9. Store samples frozen below –20°C until required.

### 3.4. SDS-PAGE Using 8 × 10-cm Mini-Gels

1. Clean the glass plates with ethanol, dry with tissue, and assemble according to the manufacturer's instructions (*see* **Note 18**).
2. Prepare resolving gel solution of the desired percentage acrylamide by following a recipe in **Table 1** (*see* **Note 19**). These quantities are sufficient for two mini-gels.
3. For 1.0 mm thick gels, pipet 4.5 mL of resolving gel mix into each plate sandwich.
4. Overlay the acrylamide mix with 200 μL water-saturated butan-2-ol, and allow to set on a level bench for 30–60 min.
5. Rinse the butanol off the resolving gels with $H_2O$, and use a 3MM filter paper to dry the inside of the glass plates above the gel.
6. Prepare a 4% acrylamide stacking gel mix with the following components: 3.1 mL $H_2O$, 3.9 mL Stacking gel buffer, 0.8 mL 40% acrylamide/bisacrylamide solution, 78 μL 15% ammonium persulfate. Gently mix, then pipet onto the resolving gel.
7. Insert a well-forming comb into each stacking gel (*see* **Note 20**), and allow the gel to set for at least 30 min.
8. Carefully remove combs from the stacking gels, and rinse the wells with electrophoresis running buffer.
9. Fill the wells with electrophoresis running buffer.
10. If cell samples in GSB have been stored frozen, thaw by heating to 100°C in a heating block.
11. Using special gel-application disposable tips, carefully pipet 20 μL cell sample (i.e., equivalent to $2 \times 10^5$ cells) or 5 μL pre-stained molecular weight markers into each well.
12. Assemble the gels into the electrophoresis tank according to the manufacturer's instructions, and add electrophoresis buffer to the cathode and anode reservoirs.

13. Connect to power-pack, and run at a constant 180 V for 40–45 min until the bromophenol blue dye front reaches the bottom of the resolving gel (*see* **Note 21**).

### 3.5. Electroblotting onto PVDF Membranes

1. Pre-wet PVDF membrane by soaking in methanol for 1 min, then equilibrate in Blotting buffer for 5 min (*see* **Notes 6, 8, 9,** and **22**).
2. Place a Transblot cassette, with clear side (anode) down in a tray of blotting buffer.
3. Soak the fiber pads of the Transblot apparatus in blotting buffer, and place one in the open cassette submerged in blotting buffer.
4. Soak a sheet of 3MM filter paper and lay onto the fiber pad.
5. Lay a sheet of wetted PVDF membrane onto the filter paper, and add sufficient blotting buffer to the tray so that the PVDF membrane is just covered but not floating.
6. Disassemble the SDS-PAGE apparatus according to the manufacturer's instructions (*see* **Note 23**).
7. Wet your gloved fingers with blotting buffer, and pick up the gel by two corners, peeling the gel away from the glass plate.
8. Dip the gel into transfer buffer, then layer the gel onto the PVDF membrane, ensuring that no air bubbles form (*see* **Note 24**).
9. Set up a second PVDF membrane and gel adjacent to the first if required.
10. Layer a sheet of pre-soaked 3MM filter paper onto the gel(s), followed by a pre-soaked fiber pad.
11. Close the cassette, and engage the locking mechanism.
12. Place the cassette into a Transblot tank containing blotting buffer, ensuring that the clear side (PVDF membrane side) faces the anode.
13. If required, set up a second cassette in the same manner and place in the same Transblot apparatus.
14. Connect to the power pack, and blot for 1 h at a constant 65 V (*see* **Note 25**).
15. Switch off power, and disassemble the Transblot apparatus.
16. Open up the cassette, and remove the top fiber pad and filter paper.
17. Lift the gel away from the PVDF membrane and check that transfer of the pre-stained MWt markers has taken place (*see* **Notes 25** and **26**).

### 3.6. Immunodetection of Protein on PVDF Blots

1. Rinse the blotted membrane twice in PBS-T, then incubate with 15 mL Blocking buffer in a sealed plastic bag on a rocking platform overnight at 4°C (*see* **Note 27**).
2. Cut open the bag along the top edge, and decant the blocking buffer. Replace with 10 mL of primary antibody diluted in Blocking buffer (*see* **Note 13**). Reseal, and incubate the bag on a rocking platform for 1–2 h at room temperature.
3. Decant antibody solution and wash the membrane twice with 20 mL of PBS-T for 5–10 min each wash.
4. Incubate with 20 mL Blocking buffer for 20 min.
5. Decant Blocking buffer, and replace with 10 mL of alkaline-phosphatase secondary antibody diluted in Blocking buffer (*see* **Note 14**). Reseal bag, and incubate on a rocking platform for 1 h at room temperature.
6. Decant antibody solution and wash membrane three times with 20 mL of PBS-T for 5–10 min each.
7. Decant PBS-T solution and wash membrane twice with 20 mL of APA buffer for 5 min each.

8. Prepare development envelopes from the polyethylene sheeting by cutting a square from one folded edge to create an envelope open on three sides. The size of envelope for developing two membranes simultaneously should be about 20 × 15 cm.
9. Drain the membrane of excess APA buffer by touching an edge to a paper towel, and place in the open polyethylene envelope.
10. Pipet 0.5 mL CDP-Star™ substrate onto the surface of each membrane, then gently lower top sheet of polyethylene onto the membrane, ensuring that the membrane is uniformly wetted with a film of substrate and that no air bubbles are formed.
11. Allow to incubate at room temperature for 10–20 min, then open the envelope and lift out the membranes with forceps. Drain away excess substrate by touching an edge to a paper towel, and place in a new development envelope (*see* **Note 28**).
12. In a darkroom, place the development envelope against a sheet of standard X-ray photographic film (e.g., Kodak X-Omat LS) in an autoradiography cassette, and expose for 2 min.
13. Develop the film and determine the optimum exposure time, which is typically in the range 10 s to 15 min. Re-expose the membrane to a fresh sheet of photographic film for the desired length of time (*see* **Note 29**).

### *3.7. Stripping Western blots for Re-Probing*

1. Remove the PVDF membrane from the development envelope and rinse with PBS-T (*see* **Note 30**).
2. Pre-heat some MESNA Stripping buffer in a 55°C water bath.
3. Place the membrane in a sealed polyethylene bag with 20 mL MESNA stripping buffer and incubate in a water bath at 55°C for 30 min (*see* **Note 31**).
4. Remove the membrane from the bag, and rinse with SDS wash buffer to remove the excess stripping buffer.
5. Wash twice at room temperature for 20 min each in PBS-T.
6. Block and re-probe according to the method described in **Subheading 3.6.** (*see* **Note 32**).

## 4. Notes

1. Sodium 2-mercaptoethanesulfonate has been described as an odorless alternative to β-mercaptoethanol *(23)*.
2. Unpolymerized acrylamide/bis-acrylamide is a recognized neurotoxin in humans, and the effects are cumulative. An early sign of over-exposure is peeling of skin of fingers. More severe exposure causes peripheral neuropathy, and sometimes central nervous system (CNS) damage. It may also cause adverse reproductive effects. The risks from exposure are substantially reduced by purchasing ready-mixed solutions, because exposure to dust during weighing is eliminated. The remaining risks can be controlled by wearing latex gloves when preparing acrylamide gels in order to prevent skin contact. Polymerized acrylamide is relatively nonhazardous.
3. The Tris-glycine buffer is formulated to give pH 8.3 without the need for further adjustment by addition of acid or alkali. It is essential that HCl is not used in the electrophoresis running buffer because the presence of chloride ions will interfere with the separation of proteins on Laemmli gels.
4. There are many commercially available apparatus for SDS-PAGE of proteins. The essential features are similar, but they predominantly fall into two size categories. The larger apparatus produce gels of approx 16 × 16 cm, while the smaller apparatus produce gels of approx 7 × 8 cm. The thickness of the gels is determined by the set of spacers used, and

are usually available in the range 0.5–1.5 mm. Although the resolution between similar sized bands tends to be better on the larger gels, for most applications the mini-gels are adequate; because the smaller gels also lead to a significant reduction in the required amounts of expensive reagents, the mini-gel apparatus has become the popular choice for most researchers. The method described in this chapter is tailored to 1-mm thick gels run in the BioRad mini-gel apparatus.

5. PVDF membranes are used in preference to nitrocellulose because of their superior signal-to-noise performance with the CDP-Star chemiluminescent substrate for alkaline phosphatase. Nitrocellulose can be used with this detection system provided that an additional enhancer reagent is used, but the results do not match those obtained with PVDF. The PVDF membranes also have a greater protein-binding capacity, and have better physical strength than nitrocellulose, which renders them particularly suitable for stripping and re-probing with a different set of antibodies.
6. Special care should be taken to keep the PVDF membranes and filter papers clean and free of finger prints. Gloves should be worn, and clean, sharp scissors or a scalpel should be used to cut the membranes and paper in a clean area. Clean forceps should be used for subsequent handling of the PVDF membranes at their edges only.
7. The method described here is for a large tank blotting apparatus, such as the BioRad Transblot with wire electrodes. Smaller tanks can be purchased specifically for transfer of mini gels, but the larger tanks have the benefit of versatility in being able to transfer a larger number of mini-gels simultaneously and/or being able to transfer larger 16 × 16 cm gels if necessary. Semi-dry blotting apparatus are also available, and these can give perfectly acceptable results: they have the advantage of using smaller volumes of buffer, but this also makes them unsuitable for extended transfer times that may sometimes be required.
8. It is essential that the methanol be of highest purity, otherwise problems can arise in transfer and immunodetection.
9. Methanol is highly flammable and is toxic. It may be absorbed through skin. Inhalation of high concentrations of methanol vapor may cause dizziness, stupor, cramps, and digestive disturbance, whereas lower levels may cause headache and nausea. Chronic effects include damage to the nervous system (especially the optic nerve) and internal organs. Exposure limits are specified: OES 260 mg/m$^3$ (8 h TWA), 310 mg/m$^3$ (15 min TWA).
10. We use highly purified casein that is screened for minimal alkaline phosphatase contamination, e.g., "I-Block™" from TROPIX Inc. (cat # AI300). The commonly used "Blotto" based on 5% nonfat skimmed milk does not give as good results in the alkaline phosphatase/CDP-Star detection method described here.
11. Care should be taken not to add the casein to boiling buffer. When prepared correctly, the casein solution will be opaque, but the solids should be dissolved.
12. Sodium azide ($NaN_3$) is very toxic. It forms detonable salts with many metals, especially heavy metals, and contact with acids liberates a very toxic gas. There is evidence that sodium azide has mutagenic effects. An exposure limit is specified: OES 0.3 mg/m$^3$ (8 h TWA). Especial care should be taken when preparing and handling 10% stock solutions of sodium azide. Toxic gas may be formed when sodium azide initially dissolves in $H_2O$, so the preparation of the stock solution should be carried out in a fume cupboard. The more dilute 0.02% working solutions are less hazardous, but contact with skin should be avoided and proper care should be taken with disposal.
13. The optimum dilution of antibody will depend on the affinity of the antibody being used. In our experience, the dilutions of primary antibody for the alkaline phosphatase/CDP-

Star detection method are comparable to dilutions that are used in peroxidase/ECL detection methods, and at least 10X more dilute than the concentrations required for methods involving colorimetric substrates, or for methods employing radiolabeled protein A. We routinely use purified MAbs to EBV antigens at 0.5 µg/mL, and incubate for 2 hr at room temperature; in many cases, the antibodies can be used more dilute without loss of sensitivity. Lower affinity antibodies may benefit from extended incubation times with the blotted membranes, e.g., overnight at 4°C. MAb presented as culture supernatants have less consistent amounts of antibody, and it will necessary to determine the optimum dilution of each batch by experimentation; as a rough guide, a 1/20–1/40 dilution may be appropriate. For low avidity MAbs, it may be better to increase the incubation time (e.g., overnight at 4°C) than to use more concentrated. The diluted antibody solutions in Blocking buffer may be re-used several times without noticeable loss of reactivity. They may be stored in the short-term at 4°C, or frozen at below –20°C for longer-term storage.

14. The optimum dilution of alkaline phosphatase-conjugated secondary antibody will depend on the commercial source, and will typically be in the range 1/10,000–1/40,000. As a general rule, they should be used 5–10× more dilute than if being used for colorimetric detection methods. The anti-mouse Ig (cat # 170-6461), anti-human Ig (cat # 170-6462) and anti-rabbit Ig (cat # 170-6460) conjugates from BioRad should be used at 1/10,000 in the CDP-Star detection protocol. The anti-rabbit Ig (cat # AC11R) from TROPIX, and the anti-human Ig (cat #A9544) from Sigma can likewise be used at 1/10,000. We have also used alkaline phosphatase conjugated Protein A (Sigma; cat # P-9650) at 1 ng/mL to detect primary antibodies from human sera. It is not recommended that these secondary reagents be re-used.
15. It is important to add the $MgCl_2$ to the buffer after adjustment of the pH with concentrated HCl, otherwise precipitation may occur.
16. At this stage, the lysates may be used for immunoprecipitation studies if desired. It is also possible to determine protein concentrations of these lysates, using commercially available assay kits. For this reason, the Rippa method of sample preparation described here may be preferred to the direct lysis in GSB that is described in **Subheading 3.1.**
17. Snap-freezing is achieved by cutting the biopsy into small pieces, ideally less than 3-mm cubes, and placing in a polypropylene tube, which is then submerged in liquid nitrogen. The frozen tissues should be stored below –70°C.
18. It is essential that the glass plates be clean. Deposits of dried acrylamide gel from a previous experiment are a common cause of problems with removing the new gel from the plates after electrophoresis. Therefore, immediately after use, the plates should be submerged in a detergent solution. When cleaning, scratching of the plates should be avoided, and this is best achieved by wearing latex gloves and wiping the plates with your fingers in a detergent bath; in this way it is possible to feel whether any gel deposits remain on the glass. The detergent must be thoroughly rinsed from the glass using filtered, deionized water. Care must be taken to prevent the edges of the glass being chipped, because this will impair the seal formed with the rubber gaskets when assembling and pouring the gels.
19. A gel with 8% acrylamide will be suitable for most of the EBV latent genes, which migrate with apparent molecular weights between 50 and 180 kDa. However, for proteins with apparent molecular weights below 40 kDa (e.g., some EBNA-LP species, and the BZLF1 immediate-early protein) a 10 or 12% acrylamide resolving gel is required. Add the ingredients in the order listed in **Table 1**. Mix thoroughly, but gently to avoid creating bubbles, and pipet into the casting apparatus without delay. The gel should polymerize within 10–20

min; this can be monitored, without disturbing the gel apparatus, by examining the surplus resolving gel mix kept in a capped bottle. The amount of TEMED and/or ammonium persulphate may be varied to adjust the setting time if it is unacceptably rapid or slow. Degassing the buffers under vacuum may give more reliable polymerization, but this is not essential. Remember that unpolymerized acrylamide is hazardous and that gloves should be worn during handling of these solutions (*see* **Note 2**).

20. Combs producing 10 sample wells are ideal for mini-gels; combs producing a greater number of wells may lead to unsatisfactory separations of total cell lysates. Likewise, with larger 16 × 16 cm gels, 15 wells is the maximum advisable. Remember that unpolymerized acrylamide is hazardous and that gloves should be worn during handling of these solutions (*see* **Note 2**).
21. The exact running time will vary according to the physical design of the gel apparatus, the thickness of the gels, and the percentage of acrylamide; typically, mini-gels will require 40–60 min. The larger 16 × 16 cm gels should be run at voltage/amp settings recommended by the manufacturers, and will typically run for 4.5–6 h with cooling, or they may be set to run overnight at lower power without cooling.
22. This pre-wetting step is important. After the PVDF membrane has been wetted in aqueous solutions, care should be taken to ensure that it remains wet throughout the immunodetection protocol; if the membrane inadvertently dries out, it must be pre-wetted again in 100% methanol and re-equilabrated with aqueous buffers before continuing. Manipulations of the PVDF membrane should be carried out using clean forceps to grip the edges of the membrane only.
23. Lay the gel plate sandwich flat, and insert a scalpel blade at one corner in between the gel and the upper plate before attempting to lever away the upper plate at that point using one of the spacers removed from the sides of the gel sandwich. This will ensure that the gel always remains on the lower plate, ready to be picked up with gloved fingers and transferred onto the PVDF membrane in the Transblot cassette.
24. Bubbles will prevent the transfer of proteins onto that area of the membrane. Before laying the gel onto the PVDF membrane, ensure that there is a film of blotting buffer on the membrane, and that any bubbles have been smoothed away with a wet gloved finger. If bubbles do form, lift the gel away, re-soak in blotting buffer, and re-lay onto the PVDF membrane.
25. In the standard BioRad Transblot apparatus, 65 V for 1 h is sufficient for efficient transfer of all proteins of less than 100 kDa from a 1-mm thick mini-gel of 8% acrylamide. However, under these conditions, only about 80% of the 180–200 kDa pre-stained markers may transfer. With higher percentage gels, and for more complete transfer of high MWt proteins, the blotting times may need to be extended to up to 2.5 h. Alternatively, the voltage may be increased to 80 V, but cooling is then advisable.
26. It is also advisable to mark the membranes at this stage in order that the orientation of the gel and the antibody combination may be identified subsequently. This can be done by cutting specified corners and/or edges of the membrane, or by writing around the edge with a ball-point pen.
27. If preferred, the blocking may be performed at room temperature for as little as 1 h. This option allows the gel separation, blotting, and immunodetection to be performed in a single day.
28. Self-adhesive fluorescent labels (e.g., Sigma, cat# L5149) may be stuck on the outside of the development envelope. This will assist the precise superimposition of the developed

photographic film with the PVDF membrane that is necessary to locate the positions of the molecular weight markers. These strips may be re-used repeatedly.

29. Excessive, even background on the developed gel is indicative of the antibody concentrations being too high, and/or the washing steps being too short. Smeared, uneven excessive background may be owing to incomplete blocking; the re-blocking step just prior to addition of the secondary antibody (**Subheading 3.6., step 4**) appears to be particularly crucial with membranes that have been stripped and re-probed. Dark spots randomly distributed across the blot may be owing to aggregates of primary or secondary antibody; this can be eliminated by centrifugation of the antibody solutions.
30. The membrane should not be allowed to dry. If the membrane should inadvertently dry out, it must be pre-wetted again in 100% methanol and re-equilibrated with PBS-T before continuing.
31. This protocol usually results in complete removal of both the secondary and the primary antibody probes, as illustrated in **Fig. 2B**. However, it is possible that traces of primary antibody may remain that will only be detected after the membrane has been re-probed with the alkaline phosphatase secondary antibody. If this is the case, the incubation temperature of the stripping process may be increased to 60°C. Many published protocols for equivalent β-mercaptoethanol/SDS stripping buffers suggest stripping at 70°C, but in our experience this is unnecessarily harsh and will lead to significant loss of electroblotted proteins from the PVDF membrane.
32. Blots may be stripped and re-probed several times without serious loss of electroblotted protein. However, some antigens may be adversely affected by repeated stripping, leading to loss of sensitivity.

## References


1. Laemmli, U. K. (1970) Cleavage of structural proteins during the assembly of the head of bacteriophage T4. *Nature* **227,** 680–685.
2. Renart, J., Reiser, J., and Stark, G. R. (1979) Transfer of proteins from gels to diazobenzyloxymethyl-paper and detection with antisera: a method for studying antibody specificity and antigen structure. *Proc. Natl. Acad. Sci. USA* **76,** 3116–3120.
3. Towbin, H., Staehelin, T., and Gordon, J. (1979) Electrophoretic transfer of proteins from polyacrylamide gels to nitrocellulose sheets: procedure and some applications. *Proc. Natl. Acad. Sci. USA* **76,** 4350–4354.
4. Erlich, H. A., Levinson, J. R., Cohen, S. N., and McDevitt, H. O. (1979) Filter affinity transfer. A new technique for the in situ identification of proteins in gels. *J. Biol. Chem.* **254,** 12,240–12,247.
5. Burnette, W. N. (1981) "Western blotting": electrophoretic transfer of proteins from sodium dodecyl sulfate: polyacrylamide gels to unmodified nitrocellulose and radiographic detection with antibody and radioiodinated protein A. *Anal. Biochem.* **112,** 195–203.
6. Kaufmann, S. H., Ewing, C. M., and Shaper, J. H. (1987) The erasable Western blot. *Anal. Biochem.* **161,** 89–95.
7. Tesfaigzi, J., Smith-Harrison, W., and Carlson, D. M. (1994) A simple method for reusing western blots on PVDF membranes. *BioTechniques* **17,** 268–269.
8. Rowe, M., Rowe, D. T., Gregory, C. D., Young, L. S., Farrell, P. J., Rupani, H., and Rickinson, A. B. (1987) Differences in B cell growth phenotype reflect novel patterns of Epstein-Barr virus latent gene expression in Burkitt's lymphoma. *EMBO J.* **6,** 2743–2751.

9. Rowe, M., Young, L. S., Cadwallader, K., Petti, L., Kieff, E., and Rickinson., A. B. (1989) Distinction between Epstein-Barr virus type A (EBNA 2A) and type B (EBNA 2B) isolates extends to the EBNA 3 family of nuclear proteins. *J. Virol.* **63,** 1031–1039.
10. Rowe, M., Young, L. S., Crocker, J., Stokes, H., Henderson, S., and Rickinson, A. B. (1991) Epstein-Barr virus (EBV)-associated lymphoproliferative disease in the SCID mouse model: implications for the pathogenesis of EBV-positive lymphomas in man. *J. Exp. Med.* **173,** 147–158.
11. Yao, Q. Y., Tierney, R. J., Croom-Carter, D., Dukers, D., Cooper, G. M., Ellis, C. J., et al. (1996) Frequency of multiple Epstein-Barr virus infections in T-cell-immunocompromised individuals. *J. Virol.* **70,** 4884–4894.
12. Blake, M. S., Johnston, K. H., Russell-Jones, G. J., and Gotschlich, E. C. (1984) A rapid, sensitive method for detection of alkaline phosphatase-conjugated anti-antibody on Western blots. *Anal. Biochem.* **136,** 175–179.
13. Sauter, M. and Mueller-Lantzsch, N. (1987) Characterization of an Epstein-Barr virus nuclear antigen 2 variant (EBNA 2B) by specific sera. *Virus Res.* **8,** 141–152.
14. Finke, J., Rowe, M., Kallin, B., Ernberg, I., Rosén, A., Dillner, J., and Klein, G. (1987) Monoclonal and polyclonal antibodies against Epstein-Barr virus nuclear antigen 5 (EBNA-5) detect multiple protein species in Burkitt's lymphoma and lymphoblastoid cell lines. *J. Virol.* **61,** 3870–3878.
15. Kallin, B., Dillner, J., Ernberg, I., Ehlin-Henriksson, B., Rosen, A., Henle, W., Henle, G., and Klein, G. (1986) Four virally determined nuclear antigens are expressed in Epstein-Barr virus-transformed cells. *Proc. Natl. Acad. Sci. USA* **83,** 1499–1503.
16. Martin, J. and Sugden, B. (1991) Transformation by the oncogenic latent membrane protein correlates with its rapid turnover, membrane localization, and cytoskeletal association. *J. Virol.* **65,** 3246–3258.
17. Whitehead, T. P., Kricka, L. J., Carter, T. J., and Thorpe, G. H. (1979) Analytical luminescence: its potential in the clinical laboratory. *Clin. Chem.* **25,** 1531–1546.
18. Kricka, L. J. (1991) Chemiluminescent and bioluminescent techniques. *Clin. Chem.*, **37,** 1472–1481.
19. Mattson, D. L. and Bellehumeur, T. G. (1996) Comparison of three chemiluminescent horseradish peroxidase substrates for immunoblotting. *Anal. Biochem.* **240,** 306–308.
20. Bronstein, I., Edwards, B., and Voyta, J. C. (1989) 1,2–dioxetanes: novel chemiluminescent enzyme substrates. Applications to immunoassays. *J. Biolumin. Chemilumin.* **4,** 99–111.
21. Bronstein, I., Voyta, J. C., Murphy, O. J., Bresnick, L., and Kricka, L. J. (1992) Improved chemiluminescent western blotting procedure. *BioTechniques* **12,** 748–753.
22. Akhavan-Tafti, H., Schaap, A. P., Arghavani, Z., DeSilva, R., Eickholt, R. A., Handley, R. S., et al. (1994) CCD camera imaging for the chemiluminescent detection of enzymes using new ultrasensitive reagents. *J. Biolumin. Chemilumin.* **9,** 155–164.
23. Singh, R. (1994) Odorless SDS-PAGE of proteins using sodium 2-mercaptoethanesulfonate. *BioTechniques* **17,** 263–265.

# 27

# Biosynthetic Radiolabeling of Virus Glycoproteins for Immunoprecipitation and Electrophoretic Analysis

**Lindsey M. Hutt-Fletcher and Susan M. Turk**

## 1. Introduction

There are many different approaches to a biochemical analysis of virus glycoproteins. However, because Epstein-Barr virus (EBV) does not replicate to high titer in any cell line, several of these are compromised by the relatively small amounts of glycoprotein that are made. For example, unless expressed to high levels under the control of a heterologous promotor, most EBV glycoproteins are not made in sufficient quantity to be detected by Western blotting. Virus expression is not induced at high enough levels in the maximal amount of cell protein that can be reasonably loaded on a standard one dimensional gel (equivalent to approx two million cells). Likewise, the inability to induce virus replication in the majority of latently infected cell lines in a highly synchronous manner makes it difficult to incorporate sufficient amounts of radiolabel into glycoproteins in a short period of time in order to perform pulse chase analyses. Long-term biosynthetic radiolabeling of glycoproteins does, however, allow for analysis by immunoprecipitation and electrophoresis and in combination with inhibitors of glycosylation such as tunicamycin or glycosidases such as endoglycosidase N and endoglycosidase F can provide a considerable amount of useful information about the processing and biochemical characteristics of a glycoprotein species. Glycoproteins have been analyzed in each of the cell lines that can be induced to produce virus. However, the Akata cell line *(1)*, which can be induced in a relatively synchronous manner *(2)* by treatment with anti-human immunoglobulin to support virus replication in more than 30% of cells *(3)*, provides the best results.

### *1.1. Choice of Label*

The choice of radioactive compound to be incorporated into a virus glycoprotein depends obviously on the amino acid composition of the protein, the use to which the labeled glycoprotein is to be put and the speed with which a result is needed. The cost of purchase and disposal of the label may also be of concern. One of the major problems

From: *Methods in Molecular Biology, Vol. 174: Epstein-Barr Virus Protocols*
Edited by: J. B. Wilson and G. H. W. May © Humana Press Inc., Totowa, NJ

with biosynthetic radiolabeling of EBV proteins is that even in cultures in which relatively high percentages of cells have been successfully induced into the lytic cycle a significant percentage of cells remain uninduced. These uninduced cells continue to synthesize cell proteins and incorporate labeled precursors. A considerable amount of labeled precursor will thus never make its way into virus-encoded products. The large number of labeled cell proteins also increases the amount of nonspecifically immunoprecipitated material that is visualized in an electrophoretic analysis.

Labeling with [$^3$H]glucosamine typically produces the best results. It reduces nonspecific background because many cell proteins are not glycosylated. It also has the advantage of facilitating detection of virus glycoproteins that may not be abundant and are made in multiple differentially glycosylated forms. Such proteins may be almost impossible to visualize with labeled amino acids. The disadvantages of [$^3$H]glucosamine as a label are its high cost and the very long exposures of gels to X-ray film that may be necessary (for example, *see [4]*). It is also obviously not much use for experiments seeking to look at the protein backbone of a molecule in the absence of sugar modification.

Labeling with [$^{35}$S]methionine is probably the next best choice if the protein in question includes a significant number of methionine residues (several EBV glycoproteins have none *[5]*). Methionine is an essential amino-acid that allows for reasonably effective depletion of intracellular pools by eliminating or reducing methionine in growth media. Other labels that are commonly used include [$^{35}$S]cysteine and [$^3$H]leucine. Both are likely to be incorporated less efficiently than methionine or glucosamine, but are relatively cheap and for some glycoproteins may be the only choice.

## 2. Materials

1. Akata cells.
2. Complete RPMI medium: RPMI 1640 medium supplemented with 10% heat-inactivated fetal bovine serum (FBS). Penicillin (100 IU/mL) and streptomycin (100 μg/mL) may also be added if desired.
3. Deficient RPMI medium: RPMI 1640 medium deficient in the appropriate amino acid or glucose and supplemented with 2% heat-inactivated, dialyzed FBS. Penicillin (100 IU/mL) and streptomycin (100 μg/mL) may also be added if desired.
4. Trypan blue solution: 0.4% Trypan Blue in PBS. Filter through a 0.2-μm filter.
5. Affinity purified anti-human immunoglobulin G.
6. 25 cm$^2$ tissue-culture flasks.
7. Radioactive precursors. For example, the following Amersham products can be used: D-[6-$^3$H]glucosamine hydrochloride in sterile aqueous solution, 15–35 Ci/mmol; L-[$^{35}$S]methionine in sterile aqueous solution stabilized with 0.1% 2-mercaptoethanol and 15 m*M* pyridine 3,4-dicarboxylic acid, >1000 Ci/mmol; L-[$^{35}$S]cysteine, in aqueous solution containing potassium acetate and dithiothreitol (DTT) (5 m*M*), stabilized with 15 m*M* pyridine 3,4-dicarboxylic acid, >600 Ci/mmol; L-[4,5-$^3$H]leucine in sterile aqueous solution, 120-190 Ci/mmol.
8. Radioimmunoprecipitation buffer (RIPA): 50 m*M* Tris-HCl, pH 7.2, 0.15 *M* NaCl, 1% sodium deoxycholate, 0.1% sodium dodecylsulfate (SDS), 1 m*M* phenylmethylsulfonyl fluoride (PMSF), 100 U of aprotinin/mL (*see* **Note 1**).

9. 50% Protein A-Sepharose beads: Protein A-Sepharose CL4B beads (e.g., Sigma). Swell 1 g overnight in 10 mL RIPA, wash the beads five times in RIPA and resuspend them 1:1 (v/v) in RIPA.
10. Antibody (*see* **Note 2**).
11. Bench paper.
12. 37°C, 5% $CO_2$ humidified incubator.
13. Sonicating waterbath.
14. Microfuge tubes and microfuge (e.g., Eppendorf).

## 3. Methods

1. Feed the cells lightly the day before they are to be used. Check the viability of the cells by trypan blue exclusion (*see* Chapter 12) and do not use them unless their viability is at least 90% and at least 30% of the population can be induced to enter the lytic cycle (*see* **Note 3**).
2. Centrifuge the cells at 400*g* for 5 min and resuspend them in complete RPMI medium at a concentration of $10^6$ cells/mL. Ten mL is a convenient starting volume, which will provide enough labeled cells for at least 10 samples to be analyzed on a standard 16 cm SDS-polyacrylamide gel. To this volume of cells, add 1 mg affinity purified anti-human immunoglobulin and incubate the cells at 37°C in 5% $CO_2$.
3. Six h later centrifuge the cells again at 400*g* for 5 min and resuspend them in 10-mL deficient RPMI medium. Incubate the cells at 37°C in 5% $CO_2$.
4. After the 2-h incubation add the radioactive precursor using 100 µCi for $10^6$ cells. Incubate the cells wrapping the bottles loosely in bench paper (*see* **Note 4**) for 20 h at 37°C in 5% $CO_2$ (*see* **Note 5**).
5. Harvest the cells later (20 h) by centrifugation at 400*g* for 5 min. The supernatant media can be stored at –80°C. Pooling the supernatants from at least 4 experiments and centrifuging them at 60,000*g* for 60 min will provide enough virus to lyse in 1 mL RIPA and use for one or two immunoprecipitations. Before immunoprecipitation it is advisable to purify the virus at least once over a dextran gradient (*see* Chapter 11 for a purification protocol).
6. Lyse the cell pellet in up to 5 mL of an immunoprecipitation buffer such as RIPA by vortexing periodically on ice for 30–60 min. Lysed material should then be bath sonicated for 1 min and clarified by centrifugation at 20,000*g* for 30 min at 4°C.
7. Place 500 µL lysate in a microfuge tube, add up to 100 µg antibody and incubate overnight on a rocking platform at 4°C. Add 100–200 µL 50% protein A-sepharose beads and incubate for another 1–2 h.
8. Centrifuge the material for 1–2 min in a microfuge at full speed (e.g., 16,000g) to pellet the beads. Remove and discard the supernatant. To wash the immunoprecipitation add 1 mL RIPA to the beads, vortex the beads and pellet them again. Repeat this washing step 3 times.
9. Add 100–200 µL of electrophoresis sample buffer to the beads and either boil them for 1–2 min or put them at 37°C for 30–60 min to release the immunoprecipitated proteins (*see* **Note 6**).
10. Briefly centrifuge each sample to pellet the beads and load the supernatant into the wells of a stacking gel for SDS-PAGE and fluorography (*see* Chapter 26 for details on SDS-PAGE). Retain 5–10 µL of each sample to count the amount of radioactivity that has been loaded and provide an estimate of the length of time for which the dried gel, impregnated with a fluorographic reagent, will need to be exposed to X-ray film.

## 4. Notes

1. The choice of lysing buffer depends primarily on the affinity of the antibody to be used and can only be determined empirically. Many of the MAbs to EBV glycoproteins will immunoprecipitate well in RIPA and use of RIPA will minimize contamination with nonspecifically precipitated proteins. However, some glycoprotein complexes may not be stable in SDS and a lysing buffer from which the SDS has been omitted can also be used.
2. Whole serum or hybridoma supernatant can be used. However, cleaner and more reproducible results can be obtained if the antibody is first purified by affinity chromatography on protein A-Sepharose.
3. If lytic virus replication can only be induced in fewer than 30% of cells it will be very difficult to incorporate sufficient label into viral glycoproteins to get a distinguishable signal from an electrophoretic analysis. The extent to which a particular batch of cells can be induced can be tested by inducing a small number with an appropriately reduced amount of anti-human immunoglobulin and examining glycoprotein expression by indirect immunofluorescence as outlined in Chapter 11.
4. All appropriate precautions necessary for safe handling of radioisotopes should of course be taken. Bottles are routinely wrapped in bench paper, but the major concern here is for use of [$^{35}$S]-labeled compounds, which are volatile and will contaminate the incubator. Wrapping bottles will reduce, but not eliminate this problem.
5. The times given for starvation, addition of label and harvest have been optimized for analysis of late glycoproteins whose synthesis becomes readily detectable at approx 8 h postinduction *(2)*. The optimal time for labeling of other proteins would have to be determined empirically.
6. Glycoproteins with multiple domains that span the membrane frequently aggregate on boiling and will not enter a polyacrylamide gel.

## References

1. Takada, K., Horinouchi, K., Ono, Y., Aya, T., Osato, T., Takahashi, M., and Hayasaka, S. (1991) An Epstein-Barr virus-producer line Akata: establishment of the cell line and analysis of viral DNA. *Virus Genes* **5,** 147–156.
2. Takada, K. and Ono, Y. (1989) Synchronous and sequential activation of latently infected Epstein-Barr virus genomes. *J. Virol.* **63,** 445–449.
3. Takada, K. (1984) Cross-linking of cell surface immunoglobulin induces Epstein-Barr virus in Burkitt lymphoma lines. *Int. J. Cancer* **33,** 27–32.
4. Wang, X., Kenyon, W. J., Li, Q. X., Mullberg, J., and Hutt-Fletcher, L. M. (1998) Epstein-Barr virus uses different complexes of glycoproteins gH and gL to infect B lymphocytes and epithelial cells. *J. Virol.* **72,** 5552–5558.
5. Li, Q. X., Turk, S. M., and Hutt-Fletcher, L. M. (1995) The Epstein-Barr virus (EBV) BZLF2 gene product associates with the gH and gL homologs of EBV and carries an epitope critical to infection of B cells but not of epithelial cells. *J. Virol.* **69,** 3987–3994.

# VI

# Protein-Protein, Protein-DNA, and Protein-RNA Interactions

# 28

# The Yeast Two-Hybrid Assay to Identify Interacting Proteins

**Kenneth M. Izumi**

## 1. Introduction

The yeast two-hybrid assay invented by Stanley Fields and Stephen Elledge *(1–4)* is a powerful tool to investigate protein-protein interactions, the essence of many biological processes. Owing to the adaptability of the assay procedure, the ease of manipulating and cultivating *Saccharomyces cerevesiae*, and the speed with which interacting proteins and their genes can be identified and characterized, this assay has been widely utilized and directly responsible for major discoveries in signal transduction and gene regulation *(5–7)*.

The basic principle of the assay is that the yeast transcriptional activating protein GAL4 can be divided into two functional domains: a DNA binding domain (DBD) and activation domain (ACT). The bait, the gene product of interest, is cloned in frame in a yeast expression vector of GAL4 DBD and the prey, a degenerate cDNA library, is cloned into a yeast expression vector of GAL4 ACT. Both DNA vectors are introduced into millions of yeast cells, but those cDNAs that encode a protein that interacts with the gene product of interest are selected because a hybrid GAL4 protein forms. The hybrid GAL4 protein transactivates a nutritional marker gene which spares the yeast cell from nutrient auxotrophy. Further, the hybrid GAL4 protein transactivates a β-galactosidase reporter gene that simplifies the identification of yeast clones with the sought after cDNAs.

To screen a cDNA library, first the bait or yeast expression vector of GAL4 DBD fused to the gene of interest is constructed. This vector is cloned and amplified in *Escherichia coli* by standard molecular biology methods. Once cloned, the bait vector is characterized for expression, endogenous transactivation potential and sensitivity to

From: *Methods in Molecular Biology, Vol. 174: Epstein-Barr Virus Protocols*
Edited by: J. B. Wilson and G. H. W. May © Humana Press Inc., Totowa, NJ

selection. Once a suitable bait vector expressed in yeast is defined, then a cDNA library can be screened. The resulting clones of the library screen are then characterized for prey cDNA that have been trapped by the assay.

This procedure applied towards the Epstein-Barr virus (EBV) oncogene product latent membrane protein 1 (LMP1) was pivotal to recent results demonstrating that LMP1 mediates transforming signals by engaging the tumor necrosis factor (TNF) receptor associated factors (TRAFs) through a core sequence Pro-X-Gln-X-Thr *(8)*. This core was genetically defined as a transformation effector site (TES1) and NF-κB C-terminal activation region (CTAR1). The yeast two-hybrid procedure also played a critical role in characterizing a second transformation effector site (TES2), which coincides with a second NF-κB C-terminal activation region (CTAR2). LMP1 carboxyl terminal residues engage the TNF receptor associated death domain protein (TRADD) to mediate growth transformation and activate NF-κB *(9)*.

The choice of bait was essential to the success in analyzing LMP1 and was guided by published results. LMP1 interactions with TRAFs and TRADD were revealed respectively with GAL4 DBD fused to 45 and 32 residues from the 200 residue carboxyl terminal tail. Both domains were defined by recombinant virus genetic analysis as transformation effector sites and by transient transfection expression assays as NF-κB C-terminal activation regions. Investigations of other EBV latency proteins with the yeast two-hybrid assays have not been as productive. More genetic analysis to define transforming domains is required and physiological assays need to be developed. Yeast two-hybrid assays with full-length proteins have been attempted, but using the entire LMP1 protein in a yeast two-hybrid assay would be unlikely to be revealing because about 130 residues form six consecutive hydrophobic, membrane spanning domains that constitutively aggregate LMP1 in the plasma membrane. Further, TRADD binds LMP1 much more weakly than TRAF3 does. Thus, the 200 residue carboxy tail as bait in a library screen efficiently retrieves TRAF3 but not TRADD. The full cytoplasmic tail, the 45-residue TRAF binding site, and the 32-residue TRADD binding site do not activate β-galactosidase expression in yeast. In contrast, the TRADD binding site with 21 or 46 upstream residues does activate β-galactosidase expression thus obviating any further use.

Owing to the power of the assay to identify interacting proteins and aid in characterizing protein interactions for specificity and strength, there is the temptation to associate positive results in this assay with biological relevance or significance. Investigators who plan to use the yeast two-hybrid assay are cautioned to have other assays well in hand before embarking because the sensitivity of the yeast two-hybrid assay often leads to enormous numbers of potentially interacting proteins from which the true positive candidates must be selected by other criteria. In the case of LMP1, the knowledge concerning the ability of mutated vs wild-type LMP1 to transform and induce NF-κB were used to screen positive interacting proteins. TRADD was selected because it was the only protein that interacted with wild-type transforming, NF-κB activating LMP1 but not with a mutated, nontransforming, nonactivating LMP1. TRAF3 was selected because TNF receptors activate NF-κB upon binding of TNF-α ligand.

## 2. Materials

### 2.1. Preparing Frozen, Transformation Competent Y190

1. *S. cerevesiae* strain Y190 (Clontech).
2. YPD: Yeast extract, peptone, and dextrose. Prepared medium is available from BIO-101 and Clontech.
3. Sterile distilled water.
4. LiTE: 0.1 *M* Lithium acetate, 10 m*M* Tris-HCl, pH 8.0, 1 m*M* ethylenediamine tetraacetic acid (EDTA). Filter-sterilize through a 0.22-μm filter.
5. Dimethyl sulfoxide (DMSO).

### 2.2. Transformation of Y190 with Bait Vector

1. GAL4 DBD vector pAS1 or equivalent (Clontech).
2. HT DNA: dissolve and denature 20 mg/mL herring testis DNA (Sigma) in distilled water by boiling for 10 min. While hot, dispense 0.2-mL aliquots into sterile microcentrifuge tubes.
3. LiSORB: 0.1 *M* lithium acetate, 1.0 *M* sorbitol, 10 m*M* Tris-HCl, pH 8.0, 1 m*M* EDTA. Filter-sterilize through a 0.22-μm filter.
4. PEG/LiTE: dissolve 4 g polyethylene glycol (PEG) (MW avg 3350) (Sigma) in LiTE to a final total volume of 10 mL. Filter-sterilize through a 0.22-μm filter.
5. DOB-Trp drop-out: Drop-out based medium with complete supplement mixture lacking tryptophan (BIO-101, Clontech).
6. DOBA-Trp drop-out: 100-mm Petri dishes with drop-out base medium and agar with complete supplement mixture lacking tryptophan (BIO-101, Clontech).

### 2.3. Protein Expression Analysis

1. Glass beads: 425–600 micrometer diameter, acid washed (Sigma).
2. SDS/PAGE sample buffer: 125 m*M* Tris-HCl, pH 6.8, 0.04 g/mL sodium dodecyl sulfate (SDS), 20% (v/v) glycerol, 10% (v/v) 2-mercapto-ethanol.

### 2.4. β-Galactosidase and Nutritional Selection Assay

1. DOBA-Trp, His drop-out: 100-mmPetri dishes with drop-out base medium and agar with complete supplement mixture lacking tryptophan and histidine (BIO-101, Clontech) and supplemented with 0, 15, 25, 35, or 50 m*M* 3-amino-triazol. Cool autoclaved agar media to 50°C before adding 3-amino-triazole.
2. 3-amino-triazole: dissolve in water and filter-sterilize through a 0.22-μm filter.
3. Nitrocellulose: 100-mm diameter circles, 0.45-μm pore size.
4. Whatman 3MM paper: 100-mm diameter circles.
5. Z buffer: 10 mL phosphate buffer (60 m*M* $Na_2HPO_4$, 40 m*M* $NaH_2PO_4$, 10 m*M* KCl, 0.12 m*M* $MgSO_4$ adjusted to pH 7.0 and stored at 22°C), 1 mg/mL X-gal (Stock solution of 100 mg/mL 5-chloro-4-bromo-3-indolyl-β-galactopyanoside dissolved in dimethylformamide and stored –20°C shielded from light. Prepare in small quantities), 27 μL 2-mercapto-ethanol.

### 2.5. Library Screen

1. cDNA library: cDNA library cloned into GAL4 ACT vector pACT or equivalent (Clontech).
2. DOB-Trp, His, Leu drop-out: drop-out based medium and agar with complete supplement mixture lacking tryptophan, histidine, and leucine (BIO-101, Clontech).

3. DOBA-Trp, Leu drop-out: 100-mm Petri dishes with drop-out based medium and agar with complete supplement mixture lacking tryptophan and leucine (BIO-101).
4. DOBA-Trp, His, Leu drop-out: 150-mm Petri dishes with drop-out based medium and agar with complete supplement mixture lacking tryptophan, histidine, and leucine (BIO-101, Clontech) and supplemented with the selective level of 3-amino-triazole (Sigma).

### 2.6. Recovery of cDNAs

1. DOB-Leu drop-out: Drop-out base medium with complete supplement mixture lacking leucine (BIO-101, Clontech).
2. STE : 0.25% (w/v) SDS, 10 m*M* Tris-HCl, pH 8.0, 1 m*M* EDTA.
3. Phenol: Adjust the acidity of water saturated phenol by vigorously shaking with 1/5 volume of 1.0 *M* Tris-HCL, pH 8.0, centrifuging 5 min at 500*g*, removing the aqueous supernatant, adding sterile water and shaking, centrifugation, and repeating the water extraction step. Store unused phenol with a layer of water at 4°C protected from light for no more than 3 wk. Discolored phenol is unusable.
4. Chloroform/Isoamyl alcohol: 96% chloroform (v/v) and 4% isoamyl alcohol.
5. 5.0 *M* NaCl.
6. Ethanol.

### 2.7. Introduction of cDNAs into E. coli

1. *E. coli* strain XL-1 Blue or equivalent.
2. LB medium: For 1 L, dissolve 10 g tryptone, 5 g yeast extract, and 10 g NaCl. Adjust to pH 7.5. For agar plates add 15 g agarose. Sterilize by autoclaving. Cool media to 48°C before adding antibiotics.
3. Sterile distilled water: Chill to 4°C.
4. 10% glycerol: 10% (v/v) glycerol in distilled water. Filter-sterilize through a 0.22-μm filter.
5. Electroporation cuvets: 1-mm gap.
6. Electroporator, e.g., BTX Transporator, Invitrogen Electroporator II.
7. TB medium: For 1 L, dissolve 12 g tryptone, 24 g yeast extract, and 4 mL glycerol. Sterilize by autoclaving. Once cooled to 22°C, add 20 mL of 3.6 *M* $K_2HPO_4$, 0.85 *M* $KH_2PO_4$ prepared separately and sterilized by autoclaving. Supplement with antibiotics when required

## 3. Methods

### 3.1. Preparing Frozen, Transformation Competent Y190

(*see* **Notes 1** and **2**)

1. Inoculate Y190 into 30 mL of YPD medium in a 125-mL culture flask that has aeration baffles. Incubate at 30°C on an orbital shaker at 200–250 rpm. After 2 d, a stationary culture will have an optical density at 600 nm wavelength between 1–2.
2. Subculture Y190 into 500 mL of fresh YPD medium in a 1 L culture flask that has aeration baffles so that the initial optical density (OD) is between 0.1–0.2.
3. Incubate at 30°C on an orbital shaker at 200–250 rpm until the OD is between 0.6–0.8.
4. Transfer yeast to a sterile centrifuge bottle and centrifuge for 5 min at 2000*g* at 22°C. Aspirate off spent medium.
5. Resuspend cells in 100 mL of distilled sterile water at 22°C by pipetting up and down.
6. Centrifuge yeast for 5 min at 2000*g* at 22°C. Aspirate off water.

7. Resuspend in 5 mL of LiTE at 22°C by pipetting up and down. Note the total volume of resuspended yeast plus LiTE.
8. Add sufficient sterile DMSO to a final concentration of 10% (v/v).
9. Pipet 0.5 mL of Y190 suspension into screw-capped microtubes and freeze rapidly in a dry ice/acetone bath.
10. Store at –80°C.

### 3.2. Introduction of the Bait Vector into Transformation Competent Y190

1. Prepare bait vector by cloning full length or part of gene of interest into GAL4 DBD vector pAS1 or equivalent and amplify by standard molecular biology methods (*see* **Note 3**).
2. Prepare carrier by incubating 0.2 mL HT DNA at 95–100°C for 5 min, adding 0.8 mL LiSORB, and immediately and vigorously vortexing for 30 s. The resulting mixture must be homogeneous.
3. After carrier has cooled to 22°C, pipet 50 µL of carrier into a microcentrifuge tube and then add 5 µg of bait vector DNA. Mix well.
4. Thaw frozen competent yeast at 22°C. Add 50 µL to the bait vector/carrier DNA and mix by gentle pipetting (*see* **Note 4**).
5. Incubate at 30°C for 30 min.
6. Add 450 µL of PEG/LiTE solution and mix by gentle pipetting.
7. Incubate at 30°C for 30 min.
8. Heat-shock cells by incubating at 42°C for 10 min.
9. Spin down cells in a microcentrifuge for 5 s at 13000*g*.
10. Use a pipet to remove the viscous PEG/LiTE supernatant.
11. Resuspend cells in 1 mL of DOB-Trp drop-out. Incubate cells at 30°C for 1 h to recover.
12. Spin down cells in a microcentrifuge for 5 s at 13000*g*. Remove supernatant.
13. Resuspend in 0.5 mL of DOB-Trp drop-out. Pipet 50, 100, and 200 µL onto dishes of DOBA-Trp drop-out and spread with a sterile glass rod. Invert plates and incubate at 30°C.
14. Colonies are visible after 2–3 d. Individual clones are then characterized for suitability in a library screen.

### 3.3. Characterization of Yeast: Protein Extracts for Western Immunoblot Analysis

1. With a sterile loop, inoculate individual colonies into 20 mL of DOB-Trp drop-out in 125-mL culture flasks and incubate at 30°C on an orbital shaker at 200–250 rpm for 2–3 d until stationary.
2. For short-term storage (weeks), refrigerate yeast at 4°C. For indefinitely long storage, transfer 1.4 mL of yeast suspension to a microcentrifuge tube and add 150 µL of sterile DMSO. Freeze at –80°C. Yeast can be retrieved by scraping off a sample and inoculating into liquid medium or onto agar medium plates.
3. For protein analysis, transfer 10 mL of the culture to a centrifuge tube and centrifuge for 5 min at 2000*g*.
4. Aspirate off medium. Resuspend yeast in 1 mL of sterile water and transfer cells to a screw-capped microcentrifuge tube containing 0.15–0.25 mL of glass beads.
5. Spin down cells in a microcentrifuge for 5 s at 13,000*g*. Remove supernatant.
6. Add 0.3 mL of SDS/PAGE sample buffer. Cap tube securely and vortex vigorously for 1 min.
7. Boil samples for 5 min.

8. Assess protein expression by Western immunoblot of size-separated proteins (*see* **Note 5** and Chapter 26).

### 3.4. Characterization of Yeast: Endogenous Transactivation Potential

1. Dilute a fresh culture of yeast (*see* **Subheading 3.3., step 1**) 1/100 in fresh medium and pipet and spread 0.1–0.3 mL on DOBA-Trp drop-out (growth control) or DOBA-Trp, His drop-out supplemented with 0, 15, 25, 35, or 50 m*M* 3-amino-triazole. Invert plates and incubate at 30°C.
2. At least 50 colonies/plate should grow on the DOBA-Trp drop-out plates and be still well separated by 3 d. The goal is to have actively growing yeast. A crowded plate will deplete nutrients and give spurious β-galactosidase results.
3. Determine the minimal concentration of 3-amino-triazole needed to inhibit colony growth on DOBA-Trp, His drop-out dishes. There is usually small colony growth on the 50 m*M* 3-amino-triazole plates, but colonies less than 0.3-mm diameter after 5 d at 30°C are adequately inhibited.
4. To test endogenous β-galactosidase activity, overlay yeast colonies growing on DOBA-Trp drop-out with a dry nitrocellulose filter circle. When wetted, remove filter with attached yeast colonies and freeze at –80°C for at least 10 min colony side up in a Petri dish. Thaw at 37°C for 5 min, then freeze again.
5. Cut Whatman 3MM chromatography paper into 100-mm diameter circles, place in Petri dish, wet with 3 mL Z buffer, and pour off excess buffer. Overlay with the thawed nitrocellulose filter of yeast with the colonies on top. Seal the dish with Parafilm and incubate at 37°C. Check at hourly intervals for the appearance of blue colored yeast. A usable clone remains white to pink in all of the colonies for at least 5 h.

### 3.5. cDNA Library Transformation of Y190 Expressing the Bait

1. Inoculate 0.5 mL of Y190 containing the bait vector into a 250-mL culture flask with 50 mL of DOB-Trp drop-out. Incubate at 30°C on an orbital shaker at 200–250 rpm. After overnight growth the OD at 600 nm will be 1–2.
2. Add enough cells to 500 mL YPD in a 2 L culture flask for an OD of 0.1–0.2. Incubate at 30°C on an orbital shaker at 200–250 rpm until the OD is between 0.6–0.8.
3. Transfer yeast to a sterile-centrifuge bottle and centrifuge yeast for 5 min at 2000*g* at 22°C. Aspirate off YPD.
4. Resuspend yeast in 40 mL sterile distilled water and transfer to a capped centrifuge tube. Centrifuge yeast for 5 min at 2000*g* at 22°C. Aspirate off water.
5. Resuspend yeast in 40 mL of LiSORB. Incubate yeast for 30 min at 30°C.
6. Prepare carrier DNA by incubating 0.2 mL HT DNA between 95 to 100°C for 5 min, adding 0.8 mL LiSORB, and immediately and vigorously vortexing for 30 s. The resulting mixture must be homogeneous.
7. Let carrier DNA cool to less than 30°C before mixing 100 μg of pACT-cDNA library DNA with 900 μL of carrier DNA.
8. Centrifuge yeast 5 min at 2000*g*. Aspirate off LiSORB.
9. Resuspend yeast in 1.4 mL LiSORB.
10. Add pACT-cDNA library/carrier mixture to cells and gently mix. Incubate the mixture for 30 min at 30°C. Note the volume of resuspended yeast.
11. Add 9 volumes of PEG/LiTE solution (about 20 mL) and mix. Incubate the mixture for 30 min at 30°C.

12. Heat shock the yeast by incubating the cells at 42°C for 15 min.
13. Centrifuge yeast for 10 min at 2000*g*.
14. Use a pipet to remove the viscous supernatant containing PEG.
15. Resuspend cells in 100 mL of DOB-Trp, His, Leu drop-out and transfer to a 500 mL culture flask. Incubate at least 1 h at 30°C on an orbital shaker at 200–250 rpm.
16. Transfer yeast to a centrifuge bottle and centrifuge yeast for 5 min at 2000*g*. Remove all but 10 mL of medium.
17. Resuspend yeast in the remaining medium.
18. Remove a 25 µL aliquot of yeast and dilute with 25 mL of sterile water. Mix well by vortexing. With a sterile glass rod, spread 25, 50, and 100 µL of diluted yeast on DOBA-Trp, Leu drop-out agar plates. Invert and incubate at 30°C. After 3 d, count the number of colonies to determine transformation efficiency, which should be greater than one million yeast double-transformed with bait and cDNA vectors.
19. Spread the remaining 10 mL of transformed yeast in 0.5 mL aliquots onto 150-mm agar plates of DOBA-Trp, His, Leu drop-out supplemented with the predetermined selective level of 3-amino-triazole. Invert plates and incubate at 30°C for 3–5 d.

### 3.6. Isolation of Interacting cDNAs

1. Pick individual colonies with a sterile loop and transfer to a fresh 100-mm agar plates of DOBA-Trp, His, Leu drop-out supplemented with the selective level of 3-amino-triazole. Eight colonies per 100-mm plate can be grown if plates are marked into sectors with a felt-tip pen. Generally, start with the colonies larger than 3 mm diameter before testing smaller ones. Invert plates and incubate at 30°C for 2–3 d.
2. The resulting yeast growth is not intended to be individual colonies but a line of growing cells. With a sterile loop, pick up a sample of yeast and transfer to a wet nitrocellulose filter on top of a 100-mm Petri dish of DOBA-Trp, His, Leu drop-out. Spread out the yeast into 3–5-mm diameter circles.
3. Once a sample of all the yeast colonies is transferred, remove the nitrocellulose filter and place in an empty Petri dish with the colonies facing up.
4. Freeze at –80°C and thaw at 37°C twice and then score for β-galactosidase (*see* **Subheading 3.4., step 5**).
5. Colonies that turn blue within 0.5 h may indicate a strong protein interaction. Colonies that take longer are still worth pursuing because the copy number of the two plasmids may be low, the two-hybrid proteins may be present in nonoptimal stoichiometry, or their interaction may be weak (*see* **Note 6**).

### 3.7. Recovery of cDNA

1. Inoculate a colony that is both positive for β-galactosidase and growth on DOBA-Trp, His, Leu drop-out supplemented with the selective level of 3-amino-triazole into 15 mL of DOB-Leu drop-out and incubate at 30°C for 2 d on an orbital shaker at 200–250 rpm.
2. When yeast growth is dense, centrifuge 10 mL of culture for 5 min at 2000*g*.
3. Aspirate off medium and resuspend yeast in 10 mL of sterile distilled water. Centrifuge cells again.
4. Aspirate off water. Resuspend yeast in 1 mL of sterile-distilled water and transfer to a screw capped 2.0 mL microcentrifuge tube containing about 0.2 mL of glass beads. Centrifuge yeast in a microcentrifuge at 13,000*g* for 5 s.
5. Aspirate off water, add 0.5 mL of STE and vortex vigorously for 3 min.
6. Add 0.5 mL of phenol and vortex vigorously for 1 min. Separate phases by centrifuging for 1 min at 13,000*g*.

7. Remove the lower phenol phase and repeatedly extract by adding 0.5 mL of phenol, vortexing, and centrifuging.
8. Once the interface material is mostly extracted, add 0.5 mL of chloroform/isoamyl alcohol, vortex for 15 s, and centrifuge at 13,000*g* for 30 s. Repeat once.
9. Transfer the aqueous supernatant to a new tube. Adjust the supernatant to 0.1 *M* NaCl by adding 1/50 vol of 5.0 *M* NaCl. Add two volumes of 100% ethanol to precipitate.
10. Precipitate DNA by centrifugation for 20 min at 13,000*g* at 4°C. Pellets are sometimes dark red colored.
11. Carefully aspirate off ethanol then remove residual salts by adding 1.5 mL of 70% ethanol, mixing to wash the DNA pellet, and centrifuging the tubes at 13,000*g* for 10 min.
12. Aspirate off ethanol, air dry and dissolve the pellet in 20 μL of TE.

### 3.8. Introduction of cDNA into E. Coli by Electroporation

1. Inoculate an appropriate *E. coli* strain (e.g., XL-1 Blue) into 400 mL of LB medium in a 1-L culture flask and grow at 37°C on an orbital shaker at 200–250 rpm until the OD at 600 nm is 0.6–0.8.
2. Centrifuge bacteria 10 min at 10,000*g* at 4°C.
3. Aspirate off medium. Resuspend bacteria in 300 mL of sterile-distilled water chilled to 4°C and centrifuge. Repeat chilled water wash three more times.
4. Aspirate off water. Resuspend bacteria in 2 mL of chilled 10% glycerol. Pipet about 0.3 mL of bacteria into capped microtubes. Bacteria are now electroporation competent.
5. Electroporation competent bacteria can be used immediately, otherwise freeze bacteria rapidly in a dry ice/acetone bath and store at –80°C for later use.
6. Thaw bacteria on ice.
7. Chill 1-mm gap electroporation cuvets and microcentrifuge tubes on ice.
8. Transfer 1 μL of cDNA (*see* **Subheading 3.7., step 12**) to a chilled microcentrifuge tube, add 50 μL of bacteria, mix by gentle pipetting, and transfer to a cuvet. Dry off the exterior of the cuvet before placing in the electroporation chamber.
9. Follow the manufacturer's directions for operating electroporation equipment. Electroporate the bacteria at an electrical potential of 1500V (If using the Invitrogen unit additional settings of 50 μF capacitance and 150 ohm load resistance are required). There must not be any electrical arcing.
10. Working quickly, resuspend the bacteria in 1 mL of LB medium and transfer to a 15-mL capped culture tube. Incubate bacteria at 37°C for 1 h to allow for antibiotic resistance genes to be expressed.
11. With a glass rod, spread 0.5, 0.3, and 0.1 mL of bacteria onto LB agar plates supplemented with the appropriate selective antibiotic (usually ampicillin at 50 μg/mL). Invert plates and incubate at 37°C.
12. After 18 h, individual bacterial clones can be picked, inoculated and amplified in TB medium supplemented with antibiotic, and mini-preparations of plasmid DNA can be isolated by standard molecular biology methods. However, for the first round of bacterial isolates, it is recommended that all of the clones be pooled by pipetting 5 mL of TB onto the plates and resuspending bacteria with a glass rod. Amplify bacteria for a few hours at 37°C on an orbital shaker if the culture is not dense before preparing DNA.

### 3.9. Verification of the Protein-Protein Interaction

1. Mini-preparations of the cDNA plasmid are suitable for re-transformation. Estimate the quantity of DNA by agarose gel electrophoresis and ethidium bromide staining of nucleic acids.

2. Transform competent Y190 with both the GAL4 DBD bait vector DNA and GAL4 ACT cDNA (*see* **Subheading 3.2.**). Grow yeast on dishes of DOBA-Trp, His, Leu drop-out supplemented with the selective level of 3-amino-triazole and on DOBA-Trp, Leu drop-out to score for transformation efficiency. Invert plates and incubate at 30°C for 3–5 d.
3. Score for β-galactosidase activity by nitrocellulose lifts of yeast colonies (*see* **Subheading 3.4., steps 4** and **5**). Orient the filter with needle marks through the filter.
4. Pick positive colonies and inoculate into DOB-Leu drop-out. Recover cDNA plasmid as described in **Subheading 3.7.** and introduce and amplify in bacteria as described in **Subheading 3.8.**

### 3.10. Identification of the cDNA

1. Once the protein encoded by the cDNA has been verified to interact with the bait protein and the gene has been amplified in bacteria, the insert is characterized by DNA sequencing. Choose primers appropriate for the GAL4 ACT plasmid in use. For the pACT plasmid, the oligonucleotide 5'-atggatgatgtatataactatctattcg-3' is suitable for sequencing the coding strand. Pay particular attention to the open reading frame amino acid sequence and the fusion between the GAL4 ACT and the c-DNA. The oligonucleotide 5'-tgagatggtgcacgatgcacagttg-3' is suitable for the template strand.

## 4. Notes

1. For this method, *S. cerevesiae* stain Y190, yeast GAL4 DBD vector pAS1, and yeast GAL4 ACT vector pACT are discussed. Other vectors can be used so long as the nutritional markers allow for selection in Y190. Packaged kits from Clontech have compatible elements. Care should be exercised with regards to nutritional markers.
2. Batches of frozen, transformation competent Y190 can be prepared ahead of time and are convenient for generating bait expressing yeast and assaying protein interactions with mutated genes. They are less transformation competent once frozen and thawed and hence not best suited for screening cDNA libraries.
3. The construction of the bait vector is critical to the success of the experiment. Many investigators assume that full-length clones of the gene of interest when fused to GAL4 DBD cast the widest net to capture interacting proteins. For several possible reasons, full-length clones are not necessarily superior in library screens. Larger proteins may not fold properly in yeast, yeast may not tolerate the foreign protein, improperly folded or poorly tolerated proteins may be degraded, very large proteins may interfere with the dimerization or nuclear localization of GAL4 DBD and large proteins may have cryptic transcriptional activation domains. Screening with functional domains is more likely to be productive because of the focused nature of the investigation.
4. Unused thawed yeast can be frozen again, although transformation efficiency declines.
5. Western immunoblots are best analyzed with an antibody against the protein of interest. Alternatives include antibodies against the GAL4 DBD (Santa Cruz Biotechnology) or an antibody against a tag included in some yeast bait vectors such as the hemagglutinin epitope (BAbCo). Protein extraction is rather inefficient because the rigid yeast cell wall has to be pulverized.
6. Positive and negative controls for β-galactosidase detection included in commercial kits can be included in the screen. Try to obtain yeast strains containing known interacting proteins from other investigators.

## References


1. Fields, S. and Song, O. (1989) A novel genetic system to detect protein-protein interactions. *Nature* **340,** 245–246.
2. Chien, C. T., Bartel, P. L., Sternglanz, R., and Fields, S. (1991) The two-hybrid system: a method to identify and clone genes for proteins that interact with a protein of interest. *Proc. Natl. Acad. Sci. USA* **88,** 9578–9582.
3. Bai, C. and Elledge, S. J. (1997) Gene identification using the yeast two-hybrid system. *Methods Enzymol.* **283,** 141–156.
4. Bartel, P. L. and Fields, S.(1995) Analyzing protein-protein interactions using two-hybrid system. *Methods Enzymol.* **254,** 241–263.
5. Rothe, M., Wong, S. C., Henzel, W. J., and Goeddel, D. V. (1994) A novel family of putative signal transducers associated with the cytoplasmic domain of the 75 kDa tumor necrosis factor receptor. *Cell* **78,** 681–692.
6. Hsu, H., Xiong, J., and Goeddel, D. V. (1995) The TNF receptor 1–associated protein TRADD signals cell death and NF-kappa B activation. *Cell* **81,** 495–504.
7. Regnier, C. H., Song, H. Y., Gao, X., Goeddel, D. V., Cao, Z., and Rothe M. (1997) Identification and characterization of an IkappaB kinase. *Cell* **90,** 373–383.
8. Mosialos, G., Birkenbach, M., Yalamanchili, R., VanArsdale, T., Ware, C., and Kieff, E. (1995) The Epstein-Barr virus transforming protein LMP1 engages signaling proteins for the tumor necrosis factor receptor family. *Cell* **80,** 389–399.
9. Izumi, K. M. and Kieff. E. D. (1997) The Epstein-Barr virus oncogene product latent membrane protein 1 engages the tumor necrosis factor receptor-associated death domain protein to mediate B lymphocyte growth transformation and activate NF-kappaB. *Proc. Natl. Acad. Sci. USA* **94,** 12,592–12,597.

29

# Identification of Transactivation, Repression, and Protein-Protein Interaction Domains Using GAL4-Fusion Proteins

**James J.-D. Hsieh and S. Diane Hayward**

## 1. Introduction

The Epstein-Barr viral nuclear antigen 2 (EBNA2) latency protein is a transcriptional activator that plays a critical role in regulation of Epstein-Barr virus (EBV) latency gene expression and in EBV-induced B-cell immortalization. GAL4-fusion constructions have been instrumental in elucidating the mechanism of action of EBNA2 *(1–4)*. Regulatory proteins are modular in structure with separate domains for functions such as promoter targeting, transcriptional activation, transcriptional repression, and protein-protein interactions. Functional chimeras can be generated by fusing domains from different proteins. In the case of transcriptional activation, the transactivator protein must be targeted to the responsive promoter and contain an activation domain that either directly or indirectly interacts with the core cellular transcriptional machinery to increase transcriptional efficiency. Early work on transcriptional transactivators demonstrated the modular nature of these proteins by showing that the DNA binding domain of the yeast transcriptional activator GAL4, GAL4 (aa1-147) could be fused to a variety of yeast, cellular, bacterial, and viral sequences to reconstitute functional transcriptional activator proteins *(5,6)*. Subsequently, GAL4-fusions became the standard experimental approach for identifying activation domains.

Transient expression assays are used to assess the function of the GAL4-fusion protein. DNA plasmids expressing the GAL4-fusion protein are co-transfected into tissue culture cells with target plasmids expressing a readily assayable protein such as bacterial chloramphenicol acetyltransferase (CAT; *7*) or firefly luciferase (Luc; *8*) under the control of a promoter containing binding sites for GAL4 located in the upstream regulatory sequences. The fusion protein is targeted to the reporter by GAL4 binding to its recognition sequences in the promoter. Activation of expression of the reporter gene above the levels observed in the presence of the parental GAL4 vector

From: *Methods in Molecular Biology, Vol. 174: Epstein-Barr Virus Protocols*
Edited by: J. B. Wilson and G. H. W. May © Humana Press Inc., Totowa, NJ

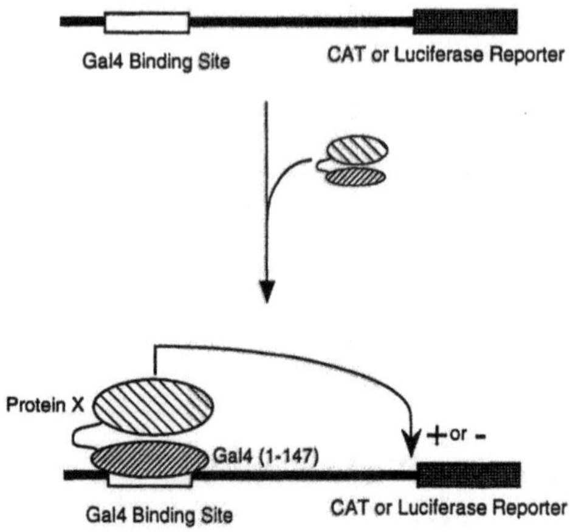


Fig. 1. Schematic representation of activation or repression mediated by Gal4 fusion proteins.

provides evidence that a transcriptional activation domain has also been brought to the promoter within the fused sequences (**Fig. 1**). Additional constructions containing overlapping segments of these sequences can then be generated to map the active domain.

In addition to their initial use in identifying and mapping the location of transcriptional activation domains within proteins, GAL4-fusions are also valuable tools for identifying transcriptional repression domains and protein-protein interaction domains. Demonstrating the presence of a transcriptional repression domain within a test protein using GAL4-fusions is directly comparable in rationale and practice to an assessment of transcriptional activation except that the read-out is loss of expression of the reporter, rather than increased expression (**Fig. 1**). GAL4-fusions can also be employed in a mammalian cell variation of the yeast two-hybrid assay to identify protein-protein interactions (**Fig. 2**). The yeast-two hybrid assay *(9)* has as its basis the recognition that the modular nature of transactivators can be extended and transactivation can be obtained when the promoter targeting domain and transcriptional activation domain are not only of heterologous origin but are also encoded within completely separate proteins, providing these two proteins interact to bring both functional domains to the promoter. In this version of the assay, protein X is fused to the GAL4 DNA binding domain (DBD), while protein Y is fused to a known transcriptional activation domain such as that from the EBV EBNA2 protein (E2TANLS; [*E*BNA*2* *T*rans*A*ctivation and *N*uclear *L*ocalization *S*ignal domains]). Tissue-culture cells are cotransfected with the expression vectors for GAL4 DBD-protein X and for protein Y-E2TANLS along with a reporter containing upstream GAL4 DNA binding sites. The GAL4 DNA binding domain targets protein X to the GAL4 sites in the reporter plasmid. If proteins X and Y interact, then the activation domain fused to protein Y will also be tethered to the promoter, leading to increased expression of the reporter. Again, the generation of derivative plasmids containing segments of proteins X and Y allows mapping of the individual interaction domains.

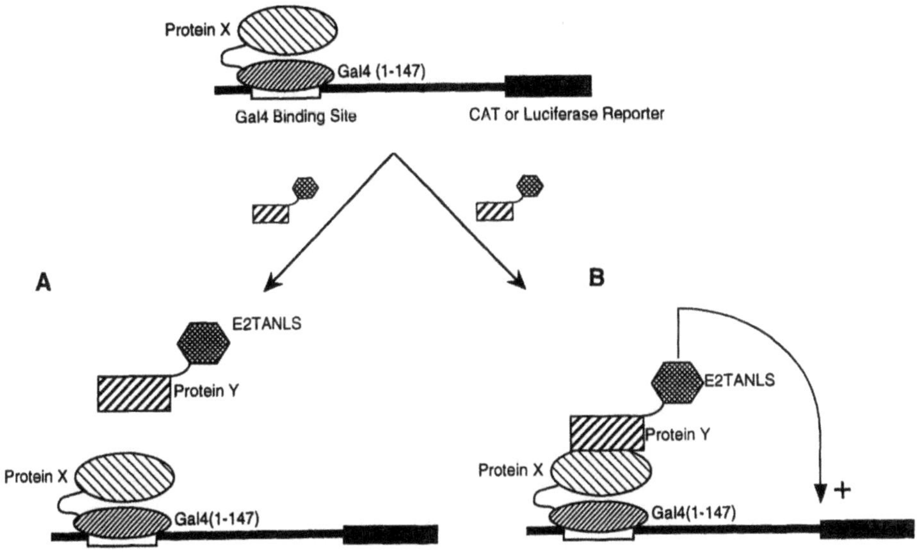


Fig. 2. Mammalian two-hybrid assay using Gal4 fusions to measure protein–protein interactions.

### 1.1. GAL4-Fusion Proteins

An example of a vector series used to express proteins fused to the GAL4 DNA binding domain (aa1-147) is shown in **Fig. 3**. These vectors express the fusion protein from the SV40 early promoter and contain cloning sites that allow in frame fusion of the open reading frame for the test protein to codon 147 of GAL4. The plasmids pGH250, pGH251, and pGH252 are identical except for the reading frame of the *Bgl*II and *Sac*I sites in the multiple cloning sequence. The choice of vector is solely dependent on the requirement to maintain a continuous open reading frame from the GAL4 DNA binding domain through the inserted heterologous protein coding sequence. Cloning into the *Bgl*II site of these vectors with fragments bounded at one end by a *Bam*HI restriction enzyme site and at the other by a *Bgl*II restriction site has the advantage of simplifying the determination of orientation of the insert. *Bam*HI and *Bgl*II generate an identical 5' overhang but the fusion of *Bam*HI and *Bgl*II cleaved terminii creates a sequence that cannot be cleaved by either enzyme but can be cleaved by *Bst*Y1. DNA fragments inserted into the *Bgl*II site in this way can also be dropped out using the flanking *Eco*R1 restriction sites.

The transactivation assay requires that the GAL4-fusion protein localizes to the nucleus. The GAL4(1-147) polypeptide contains a nuclear localization signal and thus novel GAL4-fusion proteins will usually localize to the nucleus even when the fusion partner contains only a segment of the test protein. However, appropriate localization should be confirmed in an immunofluoresence assay. Confirmation that the intact GAL4-fusion protein is expressed should also be obtained by Western analysis. Specific immunological reagents recognizing the GAL4 DNA binding domain or the GAL4 activation domain are commercially available for these assays.

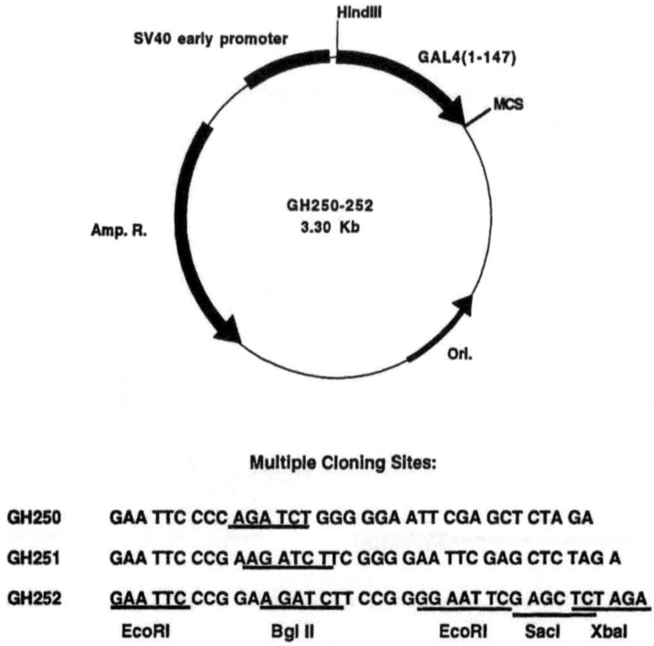


Fig. 3. Cloning vestors for Gal4 fusion proteins.

### 1.2. Activation Domain-Fusions for Protein-Protein Interaction Assays

In the protein-protein interaction assay (**Fig. 2**), one protein is expressed as a fusion with the GAL4 DNA binding domain and the second protein is expressed fused to an activation domain. The activation domain vector shown in **Fig. 4** expresses a fusion protein with an epitope from the influenza hemaglutinin (HA) protein added at the amino-terminus and the activation domain and nuclear localization signal from the EBV EBNA2 protein added at the carboxyterminus. The vector backbone is pSG5 (Stratagene) which utilizes the SV40 early promoter. The two versions of this plasmid, pJH181 and pJH180, have the *Bgl*II cloning site in reading frame 1 or frame 2, respectively. Expression of the HA-fusion-E2TANLS protein can be detected using commercially available immunological reagents that recognize either the amino-terminal HA epitope or the carboxy-terminal EBNA2 sequences. The addition of the EBNA2 nuclear localization signal also means that fusions containing only a segment of the test protein should be targeted to the nucleus.

### 1.3. Reporter Plasmids

The most commonly used reporter plasmids for assaying the function of GAL4-fusion proteins are those expressing the CAT or luciferase proteins. **Figure 5** illustrates the structure of two CAT reporter plasmids, 5xGal4E1bCAT and 5xGal4TKCAT. Each reporter has 5 tandem copies of the GAL4 binding site located in the upstream regula-

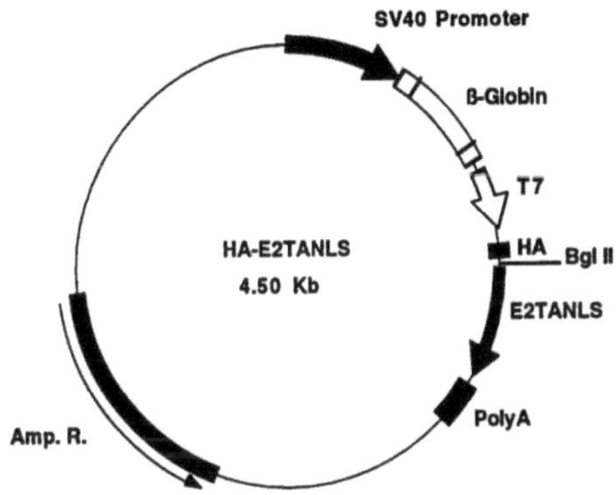


JH181 GAT CGA AGA TCT CCA ATA CAT GAA
Bgl II

JH180 TTG GGA GAT CTA CCA ATA CAT GAA
Bgl II

Fig. 4. Cloning vectors for E2TANLS fusion proteins.

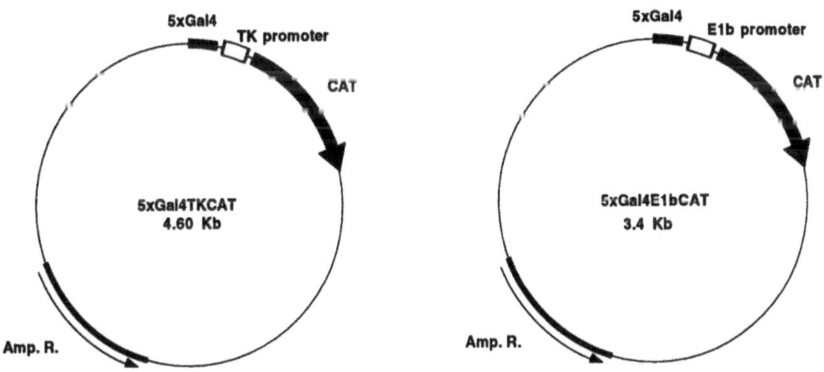


Fig. 5. Diagram of CAT reporters containing Gal4 binding sites.

tory sequences. The E1b promoter is derived from adenovirus and has very low basal activity. Thus, the 5xGal4E1bCAT reporter is most useful for assays measuring transcriptional activation. Detection of transcriptional repression requires that the reporter gene has sufficient basal activity to permit decreases in activity to be readily quantitated. The TK promoter is derived from herpes simplex virus and has an intermediate level of basal activity and 5xGal4TKCAT is well-suited for studies of transcriptional repression. To control for variations in transfection efficiency that might affect the interpretation of the results, a second reporter that lacks GAL4 binding sites should

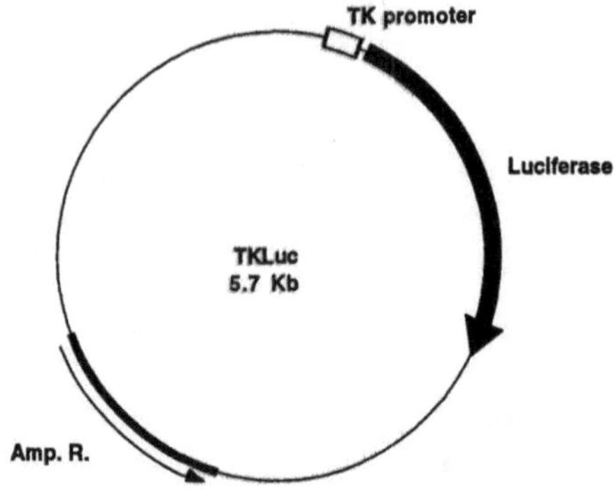


Fig. 6. Diagram of TKLuciferase reporter.

also be included in the assays. An example, TKLuc, is shown in **Fig. 6**. In this reporter plasmid the luciferase open reading frame is expressed from the herpes simplex TK promoter.

## 2. Materials

### 2.1. Plasmid DNAs (see Note 1)

1. Reporters: 5xGAL4E1bCAT or 5xGAL4TKCAT and TKLuc (pJH103).
2. Effectors: GAL4(1-147)-fusions (in pGH250–252).
3. Control: GAL4(1-147).

### 2.2. Tissue Culture

1. Incubators: 37°C with 5% $CO_2$ and 35°C with 2–4% $CO_2$.
2. Cell lines: HeLa or Vero (adherent cell lines), DG75 ( B cells) or Jurkatt (T cells) (*see* **Note 2**).
3. Tissue culture plates: 6-well and 24-well.
4. Complete tissue-culture media: Dulbecco's Modified Eagle's Medium (DMEM) with 4.5 g/L glucose plus L-glutamine or RPMI 1640 plus L-glutamine (suspension cells), plus 10% bovine serum (Fetalclone I from HyClone), plus penicillin/streptomycin (from a 100X stock, GibcoBRL).
5. 10X Phosphate-buffered saline (PBS): 1 L consists of 80 g NaCl, 2 g KCl, 14 g $Na_2HPO_4$ and 2 g $KH_2PO_4$. Adjust pH to 7.4 with HCl. Filter-sterilize through a 0.2-µm filter and store at 4°C.
6. Harvest buffer: 40 m*M* Tris-HCl, pH 7.5, 1 m*M* ethylenediaminetetraacetic acid (EDTA), 150 m*M* NaCl.

### 2.3. Transfection of Adherent Cells

1. 2.5 *M* $CaCl_2$: Filter-sterilize through a 0.2-µm filter and store at 4°C.
2. 2X BES-buffered saline (BBS): 50 m*M* BES (Calbiochem), 280 m*M* NaCl, and 1.5 m*M* $Na_2HPO_4$. Adjust pH to 6.95 with NaOH. Filter-sterilize through a 0.2-µm filter and store at 4°C.
3. Reporter and effector DNAs (*see* **Note 3**).

### 2.4. Transfection of Suspension Cells

1. CaTBS: 1 L consists of 0.1 g $MgCl_2 \cdot 6H_2O$, 0.1 g $CaCl_2$, 8 g NaCl, 0.38 g KCl, 0.1 g $Na_2HPO_4 \cdot 12H_2O$ and 3 g Tris base. Adjust pH to 7.5 with HCl. Filter-sterilize through a 0.2-µm filter and store at 4°C .
2. DEAE Buffer: 1 mg/mL DEAE-Dextran in CaTBS.
3. Reporter and effector DNAs (*see* **Note 3**).

### 2.5. CAT Assay

1. 0.25 *M* Tris-HCl, pH 7.9, sterilized.
2. BCA Kit (Pierce).
3. CAT assay solution: Make fresh. 100 µL consists of 70 µL 1 *M* Tris-HCl, pH 7.9, 27 µL distilled $H_2O$, 2 µL 40 m*M* acetyl-CoA (A2056, Sigma, stored at –20°C) and 1 µL 0.1 µCi/µL $^{14}C$-chloramphenicol.
4. Ethyl acetate.
5. Silica gel 60 $F_{254}$ precoated TLC plates (20 × 20 cm).
6. Whatman 3MM paper.
7. Thin-layer chromatography (TLC) developing tank.
8. Chloroform.
9. Methanol.
10. High vacuum grease (Dow Corning).
11. PhosphorImager (Molecular Dynamics).

### 2.6. Luciferase Assay

1. Luciferase reaction buffer: 25 m*M* glycylglycine, pH 7.8, 5 m*M* ATP, pH 7.5, 15 m*M* $MgSO_4$ and 4 m*M* EGTA, pH 8.0. Filter-sterilize and store at –20°C.
2. Sarstedt 5 mL tubes (#55.476).
3. Luciferin buffer: 1 m*M* luciferin (L5256, Sigma) in luciferase reaction buffer.
4. Luminometer: Lumat LB 9501(Berthold) or equivalent.

## 3. Methods

### 3.1. Preparation of Adherent Cells for Transfection

1. To split adherent tissue-culture cells wash cells with 1X PBS, incubate for 5 min at 37°C with 2 mL (for a 75-$cm^2$ flask) of 1X trypsin until cells lose adherence (*see* **Notes 2** and **4**).
2. Add approx 20 mL culture medium (per 75 $cm^2$ flask of adherent cells) generating a cell suspension.
3. Determine cell number using a hemacytometer.
4. Seed approximately 2–5 × $10^5$ adherent cells in 3 mL of complete tissue-culture medium into each well of a 6-well dish.
5. Culture cells approximately 24 h before transfecting with DNA (*see* **Note 5**).

### 3.2. DNA Transfection of Adherent Cells (BBS Method; *see* Note 6)

1. Replace culture medium 4–6 h before transfection with 2.5 mL of fresh complete tissue-culture medium.
2. Mix DNAs (up to 7 µg) (*see* **Notes 7–9**) with 12 µL of 2.5 *M* $CaCl_2$ and the appropriate amount of water to make up a 125 mL DNA-$CaCl_2$ mixture.
3. Add 125 µL of 2X BBS into the DNA-$CaCl_2$ mixture and thoroughly mix by pipetting up and down.

4. Incubate the resulting transfection mixture at room temperature for 20 min.
5. Add the mixture dropwise to the cells in each well and rock gently to allow complete mixing.
6. Incubate the dishes for 15–24 h at 35°C under 2–4% $CO_2$.
7. The next day, replace the medium with 3 mL of complete tissue-culture medium.
8. Harvest the cells 40–48 h after transfection.

### 3.3. Preparation of Suspension Cells for Transfection

1. Determine cell number using a hemacytometer.
2. Dilute cells to $5 \times 10^5$/mL with complete tissue-culture medium.
3. Culture cells overnight.

### 3.4. DNA Transfection of Suspension Cells (DEAE Method; *see* Note 6)

1. Prepare DNA by mixing DNA with 300 μL of CaTBS per transfection sample in an Eppendorf tube and leave on ice (*see* **Notes 8** and **9**).
2. Use $5 \times 10^6$ cells (approx 10 mL of culture) per sample.
3. Centrifuge the required volume of cell culture at 1,200*g* for 5 min at room temperature.
4. Resuspend cell pellets in an equal volume of CaTBS.
5. Repellet cells. Decant supernatant.
6. Resuspend cells in one hundredth volume of CaTBS (100 μL per transfection sample).
7. Add 300 μL of DEAE Buffer to the 300 μL DNA-CaTBS mixture and mix well.
8. Add 100 μL of cells in CaTBS to the 600 μL of DNA-CaTBS-DEAE and mix.
9. Incubate at 37°C for 1 h. Mix every 15 min by gently rocking.
10. Microcentrifuge at 800*g* for 3 min and aspirate off the supernatant.
11. Resuspend cells in 0.5 mL of 1X PBS.
12. Repellet cells at 800*g* for 3 min and aspirate off the supernatant.
13. Resuspend cells in 1.5 mL of complete tissue-culture medium.
14. Transfer the cell suspensions to a 24-well plate.
15. Incubate at 37°C under 5% $CO_2$ for approx 40 h.
16. Harvest cells for activity measurements.

### 3.5. Preparation of Cell Extract for Assays (Adherent Cells)

1. Aspirate off the culture medium.
2. Wash the cells with 2 mL of 1X PBS and aspirate off the supernatant.
3. Add 1.5 mL of pre-chilled harvest buffer.
4. Scrape the transfected cells off the dish into the harvest buffer with a rubber policeman and transfer the cells to an Eppendorf tube.
5. Pellet the cells by microcentrifugation at 14,000*g* for 30 s and remove the supernatant.
6. Resuspend the pellet in 100 μL of 0.25 *M* Tris-HCl, pH 7.9.
7. Immediately freeze by placing the tubes in a dry ice-ethanol bath for 5 min.
8. Quickly thaw by placing the tubes in a 37°C water bath.
9. Repeat freeze-thaw cycle two more times.
10. Microcentrifuge the cell extracts at 14,000*g* for 10 min at 4°C and collect the supernatants for assaying.
11. Determine the quantity of protein in each sample using a BCA kit (Pierce) and 10 μL of each supernatant (*see* **Note 10**).

### 3.6. Preparation of Cell Extract for Assays (Suspension Cells)

1. Transfer the transfected cells from the 24-well plates into Eppendorf tubes. Leave tubes on ice while completing the harvest.

2. Pellet the cells by microcentrifugation at 14,000*g* for 30 s and remove the supernatant.
3. Resuspend the cells in 1.5 mL of 1X PBS.
4. Pellet the cells by microcentrifugation at 14,000*g* for 30 s and remove the supernatant.
5. Go to **step 6** in **Subheading 3.5.** and continue through to **step 11**.

### 3.7. CAT Assay

1. Add 100 µL of CAT assay solution to each of the required number of tubes.
2. Add between 5 and 50 µL of the prepared cell extracts (*see* **Subheadings 3.5.** and **3.6.**) to the assay solution and mix (*see* **Note 11**).
3. Incubate in a 37°C water bath for 1–3 h (*see* **Note 11**).
4. Add 1 mL of ethyl acetate to each reaction and vortex vigorously for 30 s (*see* **Note 12**).
5. Microfuge at 14,000*g* for 1 min.
6. Transfer the supernatant to a new Eppendorf tube.
7. Punch holes in the cap of the Eppendorf tubes with a needle.
8. Vacuum-desiccate the samples.
9. Resuspend the samples in 17 µL of ethyl acetate.
10. Spot samples onto a 20 cm × 20 cm Silica gel 60 precoated plate for TLC (*see* **Note 13**).
11. Place a strip of Whatman 3MM paper on each side of a chromatography tank running from top to bottom to form a wick.
12. Pour the organic solvent developer containing 190 mL of chloroform and 10 mL of methanol into the tank.
13. Seal the tank by applying a layer of high vacuum grease (Dow Corning) between the lid and the mouth of the tank.
14. Leave for 15 min to allow the liquid and gaseous phases to equilibrate.
15. Place the chromatography plate into the tank with the samples at the bottom and facing the center of the tank.
16. Leave for 45–60 min until the solvent reaches 1 cm from the top of the plate.
17. Remove the plate, air-dry, and place against X-ray film to visualize the results. To quantitate the results scan the plates in a PhosphorImager (*see* **Notes 14** and **15**).

### 3.8. Luciferase Assay

1. Add 350 µL of luciferase reaction buffer to each Sarstedt 5-mL tube (75 × 12 mm).
2. Add 5–50 µL of cell extract (*see* **Subheadings 3.5.** and **3.6.**) to the reaction buffer and vortex to mix.
3. Inject 100 µL of luciferin buffer into each sample.
4. Measure light emission for 10-s intervals using a luminometer (*see* **Notes 14** and **15**).

## 4. Notes

1. Fusion constructions are generated by inserting cDNA fragments of the gene under investigation in frame into the cloning sites of the expression vectors ***(10)***. cDNA fragments are most conveniently obtained using the polymerase chain reaction (PCR) ***(11)*** with primers carrying the desired restriction enzyme sites. The maintenance of a continuous open reading frame across the fusion junction should be confirmed by DNA sequencing ***(12)***. Expression of the fusion-protein is determined by Western blotting ***(11)*** using anti-GAL4 polyclonal antibody (PAb) (Upstate Biotechnology Inc., New York), anti-HA monoclonal antibody (MAb) (Berkeley Antibody Co., Richmond, CA) or anti-EBNA2 MAb (Dako Corp., Carpinteria, CA). Cos cells express SV40 T-antigen and allow amplification of transfected plasmids containing the SV40 origin of replication. The increased

DNA copy number results in increased expression of the encoded proteins and Cos cells are therefore particularly useful for demonstrating expression and intracellular localization of GAL4-fusion proteins.

2. A variety of cell lines may be used. Adherent cell lines such as Hela and Vero are grown in DMEM medium plus 10% fetal bovine serum (FBS) and suspension cells such as DG75 B cells are cultured in RPMI with 10% FBS. Cells are incubated at 37°C with 5% $CO_2$. Hela, Vero, and DG75 cells are readily transfectable. Adherent cells are split when they become approx 90% confluent. Suspension cells are split when the cell number reaches $10^6$/mL.
3. DNA for transfection can be prepared using plasmid purification kits (Qiagen) or purified by CsCl gradient centrifugation ***(10)***.
4. Loss of adherence to the plastic can be checked using an inverted microscope.
5. Ideally, cells are transfected when they reach approx 70% confluence.
6. The BBS transfection method ***(13)*** is suitable for most adherent cells as is the DEAE transfection method ***(14)*** for most suspension cells. Alternative protocols ***(12)*** use Lipofectamine (GibcoBRL) for adherent cells and electroporation for suspension cells.
7. Transfection of excess DNA is toxic to the cells.
8. Performing the experiment in a dose-response format, in which the response to several different amounts of effector DNA is measured, is very informative and allows optimal responses to be determined.
9. The total amount of DNA transfected must be kept the same for all samples in the experiment. Use empty vector DNA to balance the total amount of DNA in control wells and in dose-response experiments.
10. An equal amount of protein is added to each assay reaction.
11. The amount of cell extract used and the incubation time are dependent on the transfection efficiency and the interaction between reporters and effectors.
12. This step stops the reaction and extracts the $^{14}$C-chloramphenicol into the organic phase.
13. Usually, 12 samples are placed 2 cm from the bottom of the plate and at fixed intervals across the plate.
14. If reporter activity is too high or low, parameters that can be modified include: changing the amount and ratios of the reporter and effector DNAs; increasing or decreasing the amount of cell extract assayed and altering the incubation time with the substrate.
15. If no reporter activity is detected, check that your fusion protein is expressed and localizes to the nucleus. If the luciferase reporter carrying the TK promoter but lacking the GAL4 binding sites is also inactive, then the problem may lie with the transfection efficiency. Different cell types, the growth condition of the cells, the amount and ratio of reporter and effector, the quality of the DNA, and the pH of the transfection buffer all affect transfection efficiency. The test protein may also be toxic to the cells at high levels of expression.

## References


1. Cohen, J. I. and Kieff, E. (1991) An Epstein-Barr virus nuclear protein 2 domain essential for transformation is a direct transcriptional activator. *J. Virol.* **65,** 5880–5885.
2. Ling, P. D., Ryon, J. J., and Hayward, S. D. (1993) EBNA-2 of herpesvirus papio is significantly diverged form the type A and type B EBNA-2 proteins of Epstein-Barr virus but retains a efficient transactivation domain with a conserved hydrophobic motif. *J. Virol.* **67,** 2990–3003.

3. Hsieh, J. J.-D. and Hayward, S. D. (1995) Masking of the CBF1/RBPJk transcriptional repression domain by Epstein-Barr virus EBNA2. *Science* **268,** 560–563.
4. Hsieh, J. J.-D., Henkel, T., Salmon, P., Robey, E., Peterson, M. G., and Hayward, S. D. (1996) Truncated mammalian Notch1 activates CBF1/RBPJk repressed genes by a mechanism resembling that of Epstein-Barr virus EBNA2. *Mol. Cell. Biol.* **16,** 952–959.
5. Sadowski, I., Ma, J., Triezenberg, S., and Ptashne, M. (1988) GAL4-VP16 is an unusually potent transcriptional activator. *Nature* **335,** 563–564.
6. Lillie, J. W. and Green, M. R. (1989) Transcription activation by the adenovirus E1a protein. *Nature* **338,** 39–44.
7. Gorman, C. M., Moffat, L. F., and Howard, B. H. (1982) Recombinant genomes which express chloramphenicol acetyltransferase in mammalian cells. *Mol. Cell. Biol.* **2,** 1044–1051.
8. de Wet, J. R., Wood, K. V., DeLuca, M., Helinski, D. R., and Subramani, S. (1987) Firefly luciferase gene: structure and expression in mammalian cells. *Mol. Cell Biol.* **7,** 725–737.
9. Durfee, T. Becherer, K., Chen, P. L., Yeh, S. H., Yang, Y., Kilburn, A. E., Lee, W. H., and Elledge, S. J. (1993) The retinoblastoma protein associates with the protein phosphatase type 1 catalytic subunit. *Genes Dev.* **7,** 555–569.
10. Sambrook, J., Fritsch, E. F., and T. Maniatis. (1989) *Molecular Cloning: A Laboratory Manual*, vol. 1. Cold Spring Harbor Laboratory Press, Cold Spring Harbor, NY.
11. Ausubel, F. M., Brent, R., Kingston, R. E., Moore, D. D., Seidman, J. G., Smith, J. A., and Struhl, K. (1995) *Current Protocols in Molecular Biology,* vol. 2. Wiley, New York, NY.
12. Ausubel, F. M., Brent, R., Kingston, R. E., Moore, D. D., Seidman, J. G., Smith, J. A., and Struhl, K. (1995) *Current Protocols in Molecular Biology,* vol. 1. Wiley, New York, NY.
13. Chen, C. and Okayama, H. (1987) High-efficiency transformation of mammalian cells by plasmid DNA. *Mol. Cell Biol.* **7,** 2745–2752.
14. Takada, K., Shimizu, N., Sakuma, S., and Ono, Y. (1986) *trans*-Activation of the latent Epstein-Barr virus (EBV) genome after transfection of the EBV DNA fragment. *J. Virol.* **57,** 1016–1022.

# 30

# Magnetic DNA Affinity Purification of a Cellular Transcription Factor

**Lothar J. Strobl and Ursula Zimber-Strobl**

## 1. Introduction

The Epstein-Barr viral nuclear antigen 2 (EBNA2) plays a key role during establishment and maintenance of B-cell immortalization after Epstein-Barr virus (EBV) infection *(1)*. EBNA2 acts as a transcriptional activator of cellular and viral genes *(2–8)* and is tethered to EBNA2 responsive promoter elements by interaction with a cellular DNA binding protein *(9,10)*. We purified this transcription factor by classical chromatographic methods, however, instead of the usual final DNA affinity column step, we applied a magnetic DNA affinity purification protocol. This increased the purity of the transcription factor from about 0.01% to almost homogeneity and allowed subsequent identification of the protein as RBP-Jκ *(11)*.

In this chapter we describe the preparation of magnetic DNA affinity beads and their use in the purification of RBP-Jκ. After optimization of conditions this method should be applicable for any high-affinity sequence-specific DNA-binding factor. All steps can be performed in small test tubes within a short time. **Figure 1** outlines the procedure: first the specific DNA-binding sequence for the transcription factor of interest has to be coupled to magnetic beads. This is achieved by incubation of previously 5' end-biotinylated double-stranded DNA with superparamagnetic polystyrene beads that have the biotin ligand, streptavidin, covalently attached to the bead surface. The biotin-streptavidin interaction is very strong *(12)* and resistant to high concentrations of urea and salt. For purification, a protein fraction containing the partially enriched DNA-binding protein is incubated with the DNA affinity beads. The ratio of specific protein to the immobilized DNA should be near saturation of the DNA binding sites. With a strong permanent magnet the specific protein bound to the magnetic DNA affinity beads can be separated in seconds from the majority of nonspecific proteins remaining in solution. To remove nonspecific proteins still binding to the immobilized DNA, the beads are washed a few times. By inclusion of excess competitor

From: *Methods in Molecular Biology, Vol. 174: Epstein-Barr Virus Protocols*
Edited by: J. B. Wilson and G. H. W. May © Humana Press Inc., Totowa, NJ

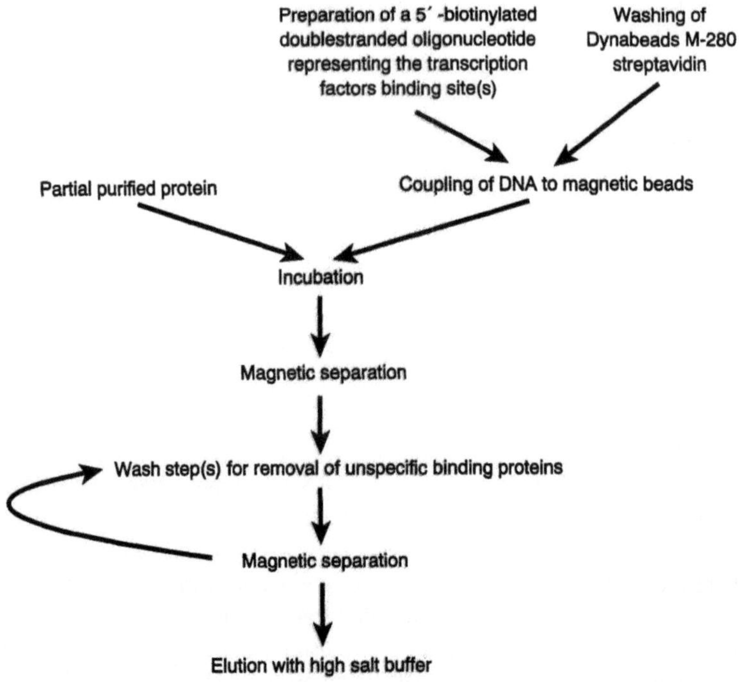


Fig. 1. Schematical overview of the described steps of the magnetic DNA affinity purification.

DNA in the washes the purity can be greatly improved. Finally the specific protein can be eluted from the DNA affinity beads by a buffer with high ionic strength. The beads are removed by magnetic separation, leaving the DNA-binding protein purified to near homogeneity.

## 2. Materials

1. Dynabeads M-280 streptavidin, 10 mg/mL (Dynal, Hamburg, Germany). Magnetic particle concentrator (MPC) as permanent magnet (Dynal, Hamburg).
2. Wash-buffer: 10 m*M* Tris-HCl, pH 7.5, 1 m*M* EDTA, 100 m*M* NaCl, 2 m*M* DTT, 0.1% bovine serum albumin (BSA).
3. Coupling buffer: 10 m*M* Tris-HCl, pH 8.0, 1 *M* NaCl, 1 m*M* ethylenediammetetraacetic acid (EDTA), 2 m*M* dithiothreitol (DTT), 0.1% BSA.
4. Custom synthesized oligonucleotides, only one strand of a double stranded DNA should be biotinylated at the 5' end (*see* **Note 1**).
5. Annealing buffer: 10 m*M* Tris-HCl, pH 7.5, 50 m*M* NaCl, 10 m*M* $MgCl_2$.
6. Klenow fragment of polynucleotide kinase, reaction buffers, and radioactively labeled dNTP, depending on procedure.
7. 4X Gel-shift buffer: 40 m*M* HEPES, pH 7.9, 400 m*M* KCl, 4 m*M* EDTA, 16% Ficoll. Add 4 m*M* DTT and 4 m*M* Pefabloc (Boehringer Mannheim) prior to use.
8. Gelshift mix: 5/9 volumes 4X gelshift buffer, 2/9 volumes poly [dI-dC] (1 mg/mL), 2/9 volumes BSA (10 mg/mL).

9. TBE buffer: 90 m*M* Tris-borate, pH 8.3, 1 m*M* EDTA.
10. Acrylamide and bisacrylamide.
11. Ammoniumpersulfate.
12. TEMED.
13. X-ray film.
14. TNE buffer: 10 m*M* Tris-HCl, pH 8.0, 100 m*M* NaCl, 1 m*M* EDTA.
15. 2X TGE: 40 m*M* Tris-HCl, pH 8.0, 20% glycerol, 4 m*M* EDTA, 0.02% Triton-X-100; add the appropriate concentration of NaCl and 2 m*M* DTT, 20 µg/mL insulin, and 1 m*M* Pefabloc (Boehringer Mannheim) prior to use.

## 3. Methods

### 3.1. Preparation of DNA Affinity Beads

#### 3.1.1. Washing the Dynabeads (*see* **Note 2**)

1. To wash the affinity beads, resuspend the Dynabeads M-280 Streptavidin by gently shaking the vial to get a homogenous suspension.
2. Transfer an appropriate amount of Dynabeads M-280 Streptavidin to a reaction tube (1 mg of Dynabeads M-280 Streptavidin binds up to 200 pmoles of a biotinylated single-stranded oligonucleotide and up to 100 pmoles of a double-stranded oligonucleotide).
3. Place the reaction tube in the Dynal MPC (magnetic particle concentrator) for at least 30 s.
4. Remove the supernatant carefully with a pipet while the reaction tube is still situated in the MPC.
5. Remove the tube from the MPC and add 500 µL of wash buffer along the inside of the tube where the magnetic beads are positioned. Resuspend gently.
6. Repeat **steps 3–5** three times. Finally resuspend the washed beads in an appropriate volume of coupling buffer (a concentration of 20–50 mg/mL Dynabeads M-280 Streptavidin is suitable for the following coupling reaction).

#### 3.1.2. Preparation of Biotinylated Double-Stranded DNA

1. Resuspend 2.5 nmoles of both single-stranded oligonucleotides (only one should be 5' end biotinylated, see **Note 1**) in one reaction tube with 100 µL annealing buffer.
2. Heat the tube for 3 min at 80°C.
3. Cool the tube to room temperature with a rate of –1°C/min to allow the oligonucleotides to anneal (*see* **Note 3**).

#### 3.1.3. Testing the Oligonucleotide for Protein Binding Activity by Gel-shift Assay

1. Radioactively label 1 pmol of annealed oligonucleotide with Klenow fragment or Polynucleotide kinase (***13*** and *see* Chapters 30 and 31).
2. Pipet into a reaction tube in the following order: $H_2O$ to a total volume of 20 µL, 9 µL of Gelshift buffer and 50–1000 ng (depending on the purity of the protein) of the protein fraction containing the partially enriched DNA-binding protein. Incubate at room temperature for 5 min (*see* **Note 4**).
3. Add 5–30 fmoles of labeled oligonucleotide and incubate at room temperature for 15 min.
4. Load a 1X TBE polyacrylamide gel (the concentration depends on the molecular weight of the oligonucleotide and on the extent of retardation by the protein) and run at room temperature at 6.5 V/cm until the unbound oligonucleotide has reached the bottom of the gel.
5. Dry the gel and expose it to X-ray film.

#### 3.1.4. Coupling the DNA to Magnetic Beads (*see* **Note 5**)

1. Mix annealed oligonucleotide and washed Dynabeads M-280 Streptavidin in a ratio of 20–50 pmol DNA/mg of Dynabeads in a reaction tube. Add coupling buffer to obtain a final bead concentration of 10–20 mg/mL.
2. Incubate at room temperature for 30 min using gentle rotation.
3. Separate the beads now coated with the biotinylated DNA from the reaction mixture using the MPC. Leave the tube in the MPC for at least 30 s.
4. Wash 3 times with coupling buffer using the MPC (as in **Subheading 3.1., steps 3–5**).
5. Resuspend to a bead concentration of 10 mg/mL with TNE buffer supplemented with 2 m*M* DTT and 20 µg/mL insulin.

### 3.2. Purification of Transcription Factor

#### 3.2.1. Optimizing the Conditions for Binding (*see* **Note 6**)

1. Add NaCl and $H_2O$ to 2X TGE buffer to give final concentrations of 100 m*M*, 150 m*M*, 200 m*M*, and 250 m*M*, respectively. Don't forget to add DTT, insulin, and Pefabloc.
2. Wash 100 µL (1 mg) of DNA-coupled magnetic beads with 500 µL of TGE containing 100 m*M* NaCl four times as described in **Subheading 3.1.1.**
3. Resuspend the beads in 400 µL TGE containing 100 m*M* NaCl and aliquot into four tubes.
4. Adjust the salt concentration to 100 m*M*, 150 m*M*, 200 m*M*, and 250 m*M* NaCl, respectively, by washing the beads once in TGE containing the corresponding salt concentration.
5. Remove the buffers by magnetic separation.
6. Adjust a nonsaturating amount of protein extract with TGE containing 100 m*M*, 150 m*M*, 200 m*M*, or 250 m*M* NaCl to a final volume between 100 µL and 200 µL and add to the equilibrated beads.
7. Incubate for 15 min at room temperature.
8. Remove the supernatants after magnetic separation and transfer them to new tubes.
9. Test the supernatants in a gel shift assay as described in **Subheading 3.1.3.**
10. Use the unadsorbed protein fraction as positive control.
11. Choose the binding buffer which leads to optimal removal of the protein of interest from the extract (*see* **Note 7**).

#### 3.2.2. Optimizing the Conditions for Elution

1. Add NaCl and $H_2O$ to 2X TGE buffer to obtain final concentrations of 200 m*M*, 400 m*M*, 600 m*M*, 800 m*M*, 1000 m*M*, 1500 m*M*, and 2000 m*M*. Don't forget to add DTT, insulin, and Pefabloc.
2. Wash 1.5 mg of DNA-coupled beads with 500 µL of optimized binding buffer 5 times.
3. Adsorb the protein to the magnetic beads using the binding conditions determined in **Subheading 3.2.1.**
4. Wash the beads three times with 500 µL of optimized binding buffer.
5. Resuspend the beads in 700 µL of binding buffer and aliquot into 7 tubes.
6. Remove the supernatant by magnetic separation and equilibrate the beads in 20 µL TGE buffer containing 200 m*M*, 400 m*M*, 600 m*M*, 800 m*M*, 1000 m*M*, 1500 m*M* and 2000 m*M* NaCl, respectively.
7. Remove the supernatant by magnetic separation.
8. Remove a small aliquot from the supernatants.
9. Adjust the salt concentration to acceptable limits allowing binding of your protein and perform a gel-shift assay as described in **Subheading 3.1.3.** Use the unadsorbed protein as a positive control.

10. Choose the salt concentration resulting in quantitative elution of the protein as your elution buffer (*see* **Note 8**).

### *3.2.3. Testing the Saturation of the Beads* (*see* **Note 9**)

1. Wash 1 mg of DNA-coupled magnetic beads five times with 500 µL of binding buffer as described in **Subheading 3.1.1.**
2. Resuspend the beads in 600 µL of binding buffer and aliquot them into 6 tubes (0.2 mg of beads/tube).
3. Remove the supernatant by magnetic separation.
4. Desalt the protein solution by dialysis if necessary.
5. Adjust the NaCl concentration of your protein solution to the conditions of your binding buffer.
6. Add increasing volumes of the protein solution to the beads (e.g., 40 µL, 80 µL, 160 µL, 320 µL, 640 µL) and incubate at the chosen binding conditions.
7. Remove all supernatants in order to test the DNA binding activities in gel shift assays.
8. Wash once with binding buffer.
9. Wash two times with binding buffer containing a 10-fold excess of competitor DNA (poly [dI-dC]).
10. Wash once with binding buffer to remove the competitor DNA
11. Remove the wash buffer completely.
12. Elute the protein with 30 µL of the optimized elution buffer.
13. Carry out gel shift analysis with an aliquot of all supernatants.
14. Determine the binding activities in the different eluted fractions.
15. Choose the protein concentration where nearly no binding activity can be detected in the supernatants after protein adsoption and washing procedures for further experiments.

### *3.2.4. Scaling Up the Procedure*

For preparative purposes the optimized procedure can be scaled up by: 1) repetitions of the analytical scale conditions, or 2) increasing the amounts of beads, DNA, and protein.

## 4. Notes

1. Biotinylated oligonucleotides are commercially available from a number of companies. Alternatively biotinylation can be achieved in the laboratory 1) by using biotin phosphoramidites on a DNA synthesizer or 2) by chemical incorporation of 5' end aminomodified oligonucleotides. In all cases some points of optimization should be considered: for reduction of steric hindrance, a spacer arm should connect the biotin with the oligonucleotide. For the same reason 5' end biotin labeling is preferable to internal incorporation into the oligonucleotide. Finally all excess biotin must be removed after biotinylation, because free biotin would compete with the biotinylated oligonucleotides for streptavidin binding sites on the magnetic beads. The use of double-stranded oligonucleotides with protruding 5' ends allows $^{32}$P-dNTP labeling of the DNA with the Klenow fragment of DNA Polymerase I. A labelled aliquot of the oligonucleotide makes it possible to control all subsequent manipulations.
2. The magnetic beads should be washed before coupling of the biotinylated DNA to remove the $NaN_3$ added as a preservative by the manufacturer.
3. To remove incompletely synthesized or remaining single stranded oligonucleotides from the preparation electrophoretic purification of the annealed oligonucleotide is advisable.

A detailed description can be found in ***(13)***. After purification the concentration of the double stranded oligonucleotide should be determined.

4. Depending on the protein of interest binding conditions have to be modified. It is possible that the KCl concentration has to be changed for optimal binding. The nonspecific DNA contained in the Gelshift buffer can be changed from poly[dI-dC] to poly[dA-dT]. With increasing protein purity the amount of nonspecific DNA should be reduced to avoid loss of the specific protein. Some proteins are unstable at room temperature. For these proteins, the binding reaction and electrophoresis should be performed at 4°C. Optimization of the gel-shift conditions is valuable for the establishment of the conditions for binding to magnetic DNA affinity beads.
5. The coupling reaction can be monitored by agarose gel electrophoresis of DNA samples taken before and after coupling.
6. The salt conditions for binding should be optimized. Too high salt concentrations may hamper the binding of the protein to DNA. If the salt concentration is too low nonspecific binding of proteins could be promoted. In finding the optimal conditions for binding of the protein to DNA, the salt concentration used in gel-shift analysis could be a lead. For example the optimal salt concentration for binding of RBP-Jκ in gel-shift analyses is 200 m*M* KCl. We have tested salt concentrations of 100 m*M*, 150 m*M*, 200 m*M*, and 250 m*M* NaCl. For adsorption, a salt concentration as high as possible should be used, where the protein is quantitatively bound to DNA and not detected in the supernatant.

   If the protein is very unstable the adsorption to the magnetic beads could be carried out on ice instead of room temperature. Because the kinetics of DNA binding are slightly slower on ice, it is possible that the incubation time has to be extended. For further information about this section, the reader is referred to ***(14)***.
7. For the binding of RBP-Jκ the optimal ionic strength was found to be 150 m*M* NaCl.
8. For RBP-Jκ this was found to be TGE containing 400 m*M* NaCl.
9. For protein adsorption we have used a protein extract precleared on a phosphocellulose and MonoQ column. The protein concentration of the MonoQ fraction used for protein adsorption was 0.5 mg/mL. Compared to the crude extract RBP-Jκ was enriched around 10-fold in the MonoQ fraction.

   In the second wash of the protein coupled beads we have added a 10-fold excess of competitor DNA in order to remove proteins nonspecifically bound to the magnetic beads. Poly [dA-dT] or DNA of a plasmid, which does not contain a protein binding site, can be used instead of poly [dI-dC].

## References

1. Kempkes, B., Spitkovsky, D., Jansen-Dürr, P., Ellwart, J. W., Kremmer, E., Delecluse, H. J., et al. (1995) B-cell proliferation and induction of early G1–regulating proteins by Epstein-Barr virus mutants conditional for EBNA2. *EMBO J.* **14,** 88–96.
2. Calender, A., Billaud, M., Aubry, J., Banchereau, J., Vuillaume, M., and Lenoir G. M. (1987) Epstein-Barr virus induces expression of B cell activation markers on in vitro infection of Epstein-Barr virus negative B lymphoma cells. *Proc. Natl. Acad. Sci. USA* **84,** 8060–8064.
3. Wang, F., Gregory, C. D., Rowe, M., Rickinson, A. B., Wang, D., Birkenbach, M., et al. (1987) Epstein-Barr virus nuclear antigen 2 specifically induces expression of the B-cell activation antigen CD23. *Proc. Natl. Acad. Sci. USA* **84,** 3452–3456.
4. Cordier, M., Calender, A., Billaud, M., Zimber, U., Rousselet, G., Pavlish, O., et al. (1990) Stable transfection of Epstein-Barr virus (EBV) nuclear antigen 2 in lymphoma cells con-

taining the EBV P3HR1 genome induces expression of B-cell activation molecules CD21 and CD23. *J. Virol.* **64,** 1002–1013.
5. Knutson, J. C. (1990) The level of c-fgr RNA is increased by EBNA-2, an Epstein-Barr virus gene required for B-cell immortalization. *J. Virol.* **64,** 2530–2536.
6. Fahraeus, R., Jansson, A., Ricksten, A., Sjoblom, A., and Rymo, L. (1990) Epstein-Barr virus-encoded nuclear antigen 2 activates the viral latent membrane protein promoter by modulating the activity of a negative regulatory element. *Proc. Natl. Acad. Sci. USA* **87,** 7390–7394.
7. Sung, N. S., Kenney, S., Gutsch, D., and Pagano, J. S. (1991) EBNA-2 transactivates a lymphoid-specific enhancer in the *Bam*HI C promoter of Epstein-Barr virus. *J. Virol.* **65,** 2164–2169.
8. Zimber-Strobl, U., Suentzenich, K. O., Laux, G., Eick, D., Cordier, M., Calender, A., et al. (1991) Epstein-Barr virus nuclear antigen 2 activates transcription of the terminal protein gene. *J. Virol.* **65,** 415–423.
9. Zimber-Strobl, U., Kremmer, E., Grasser, F., Marschall, G., Laux, G., and Bornkamm, G. W. (1993) The Epstein-Barr virus nuclear antigen 2 interacts with an EBNA2 responsive cis-element of the terminal protein 1 gene promoter. *EMBO J.* **12,** 167–175.
10. Ling, P. D., Rawlins, D. R., and Hayward, S. D. (1993) The Epstein-Barr virus immortalizing protein EBNA-2 is targeted to DNA by a cellular enhancer-binding protein. *Proc. Natl. Acad. Sci. USA* **90,** 9237–9241.
11. Zimber-Strobl, U., Strobl, L. J., Meitinger, C., Hinrichs, R., Sakai, T., Furukawa, T., et al. (1994) Epstein-Barr virus nuclear antigen 2 exerts its transactivating function through interaction with recombination signal binding protein RBP-J kappa, the homologue of Drosophila Suppressor of Hairless. *EMBO J.* **13,** 4973–4982.
12. Wilchek, M. and Bayer, E. A. (1988) The avidin-biotin complex in bioanalytical applications. *Anal. Biochem.* **171,** 1–32
13. Maniatis, T., Fritsch, E. F., and Sambrook, J. (1989) *Molecular Cloning: A Laboratory Manual,* 2nd ed. Cold Spring Harbor Laboratory Press, Cold Spring Harbor, NY.
14. Gabrielsen, O. S. and Huet, J. (1993) Magnetic DNA Affinity Purification of yeast transcription factor. *Methods Enzymol.* **218,** 508–525.

# 31

# Screening an Expression Library with a DNA Binding Site

**Qin Zhang and Eduardo A. Montalvo**

## 1. Introduction

The molecular cloning of a sequence-specific DNA binding protein using the recognition binding site as a probe was first described in 1988 *(1)*. An Epstein-Barr virus protein (EBNA 1) and its DNA binding site (oriP) were instrumental in the development of this cloning technique *(2)*. An oriP probe containing two high-affinity binding sites for EBNA1 was used to probe λEB, a λgt11 recombinant encoding a β-galactosidase fusion protein containing the DNA binding domain of EBNA 1 *(1)*. A similar pattern of plaques on nitrocellulose replica filters was recognized with the oriP probe and with anti-EBNA1 antibody probes confirming the specificity and sensitivity of the "binding site" screening procedure. The technique was subsequently used to isolate a cDNA encoding a protein with binding affinity for the major histocompatibility complex (MHC) class I enhancer *(1)*.

Within a year, three other studies described modifications that enhanced the detection of cDNAs encoding sequence-specific DNA binding proteins *(3–5)*. These modifications included 1) concatenating the single-site probe into multiple DNA binding sites, 2) using sonicated and denatured calf thymus DNA as a nonspecific competitor, and 3) denaturing and renaturing the bacterial fusion protein immobilized on the nitrocellulose replica filters.

Concatenated probes provide a high density of protein binding sites, presumably allowing a single DNA molecule to be tethered to multiple protein molecules immobilized on the membrane. This results in a stronger binding reaction that is less likely to be affected by washing conditions. It is possible to detect specific DNA binding with single-site probes but detection with DNA probes containing multiple binding sites is, in general, more sensitive. Thus, most expression library screenings are now routinely carried out with concatenated DNA probes.

The addition of excess nonspecific competitor in the probe solution is absolutely necessary to reduce background and the detection of nonspecific DNA binding proteins.

From: *Methods in Molecular Biology, Vol. 174: Epstein-Barr Virus Protocols*
Edited by: J. B. Wilson and G. H. W. May © Humana Press Inc., Totowa, NJ

The best results have been obtained when sonicated denatured calf thymus or salmon sperm DNA (ssDNA) are used as nonspecific competitors. DNA polymers such as poly (dI-dC)·poly (dI-dC) are frequently used as nonspecific competitors in other DNA binding assays (e.g., mobility shifts) but screening with these synthetic DNA molecules may result in the detection of fusion proteins that preferentially bind single-stranded DNA *(1)*.

Denaturing and renaturing of fusion proteins produced by bacteriophage-infected bacteria is thought to enhance the percentage of protein molecules with the proper DNA binding conformation. Using these modifications, as little as 1 pg of DNA binding fusion protein may be detected with a probe that has been radiolabeled to a specific activity exceeding $10^8$ cpm/µg *(6,7)*. Each bacteriophage plaque contains 50–100 pg of fusion protein but only a small fraction of the renatured protein binds DNA.

This chapter provides all of the steps necessary for screening an expression library. The procedures for preparation of a phage lysogen from a positive plaque and for preparation of a crude lysate from the lysogen, included in this chapter, are previously published techniques *(7)* with minor modifications. Once a crude lysate is prepared, specific binding can be tested by other DNA binding assays such as the mobility shift or DNase I footprinting. Also included in this chapter is a procedure for the isolation of λ DNA for subcloning of the cDNA insert. Procedures that describe the construction of a lambda library are described elsewhere *(8)*. However, many expression libraries are now commercially available or can be obtained from another laboratory that will save you the laborious task of having to construct your own library.

## 2. Materials

### 2.1. Preparation of Concatenated DNA

1. Complementary synthetic oligonucleotides of sequence of interest.
2. 10X kinase/ligase buffer: 500 m*M* Tris-HCl, pH 7.5, 100 m*M* $MgCl_2$, 50 m*M* dithiothreitol (DTT), 5 m*M* spermidine. Aliquot and store at –20°C.
3. 100 m*M* ATP: Dissolve 551 mg of ATP in 9 mL of water, adjust the pH to 7.0 with NaOH, and bring the volume to 10 mL. Aliquot and store at –20°C.
4. T4 polynucleotide kinase.
5. 1X TEN buffer: 10 m*M* Tris-HCl, pH 8.0, 100 m*M* NaCl, 1 m*M* ethylenediaminetetra-acetic acid (EDTA).
6. T4 DNA ligase.
7. Phenol, phenol/chloroform (1:1 in vol), and chloroform.
8. 3 *M* sodium acetate, pH 5.2: Dissolve 408 g sodium acetate × 3 $H_2O$ in 800 mL of water. Adjust pH to 5.2 with glacial acetic acid. Bring volume to 1 L.
9. Ethanol.
10. TE, pH 8.0: 10 m*M* Tris-HCl, pH 8.0, 1 m*M* EDTA.

### 2.2. Preparation of Radiolabeled Probe

1. Nick translation nucleotide mix: 100 µ*M* each of dTTP, dGTP and dATP.
2. Nick translation buffer (10X): 500 m*M* Tris-HCl, pH 7.2, 100 m*M* $MgSO_4$, 1 m*M* DTT. Aliquot and store at –20°C.
3. [α-$^{32}$P] - dCTP (3000 Ci/mmol, 10 µCi/µL).

4. Nick translation enzyme mix: *E. coli* DNA polymerase I (1 U/μL) and DNase I (0.2 ng/μL) in a 50% glycerol solution containing 50 m*M* Tris-HCl, pH 7.2, 10 m*M* $MgSO_4$, 0.1 m*M* DTT, and 0.5 m*M* nuclease-free BSA. This enzyme mix is available commercially from Promega, Madison, WI.
5. Nick translation stop solution: 0.25 *M* EDTA, pH 8.0.
6. Sephadex G-50 column. Available from several suppliers, e.g., Stratagene.

## 2.3. Preparation of Replicate Filters

1. Phage broth: In a 2 L beaker, mix 5 g NaCl, 5 g Bacto yeast extract, 10 g Bacto tryptone, 10 mL Tris-HCl, pH 7.5, 10 mL 1 *M* $MgSO_4$. Add water to bring volume to 1 L. Pour into 500-mL bottles and autoclave. Add fresh prior to using: 1:100 dilution of sterile 20% maltose in water (final concentration 0.2%) and 1:200 dilution of sterile 10 mg/mL solution of ampicillin (final concentration 50 μg/mL) when required.
2. *Escherichia coli* strains Y1090 and Y1089 (commercially available from Promega).
3. λgt11 cDNA library.
4. Top agarose: Prepare as phage broth and add 7 g agarose/L. Do not add maltose or ampicillin. Aliquot into 100-mL bottles and autoclave.
5. Phage plates: Prepare as phage broth and add 15 g agar/L. Do not add maltose or ampicillin. Autoclave. Cool to 60°C and pour 80 mL into 15 × 150-mm or 20 mL into 15 × 100-mm Petri dishes (Pour under sterile conditions).
6. 15 × 150-mm and 15 × 100-mm Petri plates.
7. Nitrocellulose filters (Schleicher & Schüll, 82 mm and 132 mm, type BA85. 0.45-μm pore size).
8. 10 m*M* IPTG (Isopropyl-β-D-thiogalactopyranoside) in water.
9. Whatman 3MM paper.
10. 15-mL plastic snap cap tubes.

## 2.4. Denaturation/Renaturation of Protein

1. 12 × 8 inch baking dishes.
2. Binding buffer (10X): 250 m*M* HEPES, pH 7.9, 30 m*M* $MgCl_2$, 400 m*M* KCl. Filter the 10X buffer and store at room temperature. To make 1X working solution, dilute 1:10 with $H_2O$, add DTT to a final concentration of 1 m*M*. Stock solutions of 1 *M* DTT in water should be stored at –20°C. DTT is unstable and should be added fresh from the frozen stock at the proper concentration immediately before use.
3. Guanidine hydrochloride.
4. Instant nonfat dry milk.

## 2.5. Screening Nitrocellulose Filters and Identification and Purification of Positive Clones

1. 10 mg/mL calf thymus DNA: Add 100 mL TE, pH 8.0 to 1 g calf thymus DNA. Mix and sonicate until all of the DNA is dissolved and sheared. The solution at this point should no longer be viscous. Aliquot and store at –20°C. Before use, denature the DNA by boiling for 10 min followed immediately by chilling in ice water.
2. Luminescent stickers (Stratagene, GlogosII autoradiogram alignment stickers).
3. Kodak XAR-5 film.
4. SM buffer: 5.8 g NaCl, 2 g $MgSO_4$, 50 mL Tris-HCl, pH 7.5, 5 mL of 2% gelatin. Bring up to 1 L volume with water. Aliquot into 100 mL bottles and autoclave.

### 2.6. Isolation of Recombinant Phage Lysogens and Preparation of Crude Cell Extracts

1. LB medium: 10 g Bacto tryptone, 5 g Bacto yeast extract, 5 g NaCl. Adjust to 1 L with $H_2O$. Adjust pH to 7.5. Autoclave. Add ampicillin to a concentration of 50 μL/mL when indicated.
2. 1 *M* $MgCl_2$.
3. LB agar plates: Prepare LB medium as above but add 15 g/L of agar. Autoclave and pour plates.
4. Cell extract buffer: 50 m*M* Tris-HCl, pH 7.5, 1 m*M* EDTA, 1 m*M* DTT, 1 m*M* PMSF.
5. Lysozyme.
6. 5 *M* NaCl.

### 2.7. Identification of cDNA Inserts in λ Phage DNA

1. Rnase A.
2. Dnase I.
3. Phage precipitation solution: 20% (w/v) polyethylene glycol (PEG) (MW 8000), 2 *M* NaCl in SM buffer.
4. 10% SDS.
5. 0.5 *M* EDTA, pH 8.0.
6. 3 *M* sodium acetate (*see* **Subheading 2.1.**).
7. 70% and 100% Ethanol.
8. Phenol, phenol/chloroform (1:1 in vol), and chloroform.

## 3. Methods

### 3.1. Preparation of Concatenated DNA

1. Anneal complementary synthetic oligonucleotides: To phosphorylate the end of each oligonucleotide, add in separate microfuge tubes 2 μg of each oligonucleotide, 5 μL of 10X kinase/ligase buffer, 5 μL of 10 m*M* ATP, 5 μL of T4 polynucleotide kinase (10 U/μL). Adjust volume to 50 μL with water. Incubate at 37°C for 1 h. After phosphorylation is complete, mix the two reactions. Incubate at 88°C for 5 min, 65°C for 15 min, 37°C for 15 min, at room temperature for 15 min and 0°C for 5 min (*see* **Note 1**).
2. Add 4 U T4 DNA ligase and 0.6 μL 100 m*M* ATP. Incubate overnight (> 8 h) at 16°C.
3. Extract the mixture with phenol/chloroform.
4. Precipitate DNA: Add 1/10 vol of 3 *M* sodium acetate and 2X vol of ethanol. Mix and centrifuge at full speed (≥ 14,000*g*) in a microfuge for 10 min. Remove the supernatant. Dry the pellet and resuspend in 20 μL of TE, pH 8.0.
5. Check the effectivity of the ligation reaction on an acrylamide or agarose gel (*see* **Note 2**). The DNA can be stored at –20°C until needed.

### 3.2. Preparation of Radiolabeled Probe (*see* Note 3)

1. Mix 10 μL of nick translation nucleotide mix, 5 μL 10X nick translation buffer, 1 μg DNA to be labeled, 7 μL [$\alpha$-$^{32}$P] dCTP (70 μCi at 3000 Ci/mmole and 10 mCi/mL), 5 μL nick translation enzyme mix. Adjust volume to 50 μL.
2. Incubate at 15°C for 60 min.
3. Add 5 μL of stop solution.
4. Separate free nucleotides from radiolabeled probe by chromatography on a Sephadex G-50 column. (You may use commercially available columns for this step.)

### 3.3. Preparation of Replicate Filters

1. Pipet 10 mL of phage broth into a 50-mL conical tube (remember to add maltose and ampicillin before use). Inoculate with *E. coli* strain Y1090 from a single colony or from a glycerol stock. Grow to saturation in a 37°C shaking incubator (6–12 h).
2. Dilute λgt11 cDNA library stock to $5 \times 10^5$ plaque forming units (pfu)/mL with SM buffer. The pfu of the library can be determined by serially diluting the stock and plating.
3. Melt top agarose in microwave oven (8 mL per 15 × 150 mm plate). Place in a 50°C water bath. Warm phage plates (15 × 150) in a 42°C incubator (*see* **Note 4**).
4. For each plate, pipet 0.3 mL of saturated *E. coli* (Y1090) into a 15-mL plastic snap cap tube. Add 100 µL of λgt11 library that has been diluted to a concentration of $5 \times 10^5$ pfu/mL (i.e., total amount of virus added per tube is $5 \times 10^4$ pfu). Mix briefly with mild vortexing and incubate at room temperature for 15 min.
5. Place tubes containing the phage-infected *E. coli* into a test tube rack in the 50°C water bath (3–4 at a time). Remove from the 42°C incubator 3–4 plates at a time. Add 8 mL, of prewarmed top agarose to the 15-mL tubes containing the phage-infected *E. coli*. Cap tube and invert 2–3 times to mix the solutions. Pour mixture onto the prewarmed phage plates. Rock to cover the entire surface of plate with top agarose solution. Allow to solidify at room temperature (approx 5 min).
6. Number each of the plates and incubate plates at 42°C until plaques are visible (3–4 h) (*see* **Note 5**).
7. Dip a 132-mm nitrocellulose filter into a freshly made aqueous solution of 10-m*M* IPTG. Blot on Whatman 3MM paper to drain off excess liquid. Overlay filter on each plate from **step 6** before filter dries (*see* **Note 6**).
8. With a pencil or pen, identify the filter by writing the number corresponding to the number on the plate. Mark filters while on plates by vertically sticking an india ink-dipped needle at three asymmetric locations around the periphery of the plate so that you can orient later. Make sure the needle is pressed completely through the agar to assure that the marks are visible from the bottom of the plate (*see* **Note 7**).
9. Incubate the plates at 42°C for 4–6 h (use an air-blowing incubator if possible).
10. Lift filters from plates with blunt end forceps and put on Whatman 3 MM paper with plaque-exposed side up. Dry filters on the lab bench for 15 min at room temperature.
11. Overlay each plate with a second IPTG-impregnated filter and mark each plate with india ink-dipped needle at the same location as the initial marks. Incubate plates for an additional 2 h (*see* **Note 8**).
12. Repeat **step 10**. Store plate at 4°C after the second filter is removed.

### 3.4. Denaturation/Renaturation of Protein

All steps should be carried out at 4°C.

1. Place filters in a 12 × 8 inch baking dish containing 200 mL of 6 *M* guanidine hydrochloride in 1X binding buffer. Shake gently for 5 min. Decant and repeat.
2. Pour off the second guanidine-HCl wash into a 500-mL graduated cylinder. Add an equivalent amount of 1X binding buffer (i.e., make a 1:2 dilution of the denaturing solution with 1X binding buffer). Pour into another baking dish and transfer filters to the solution one at a time. Make sure each filter is exposed to diluted solution. Shake gently for 5 min.
3. Repeat **step 2** four more times diluting the solution 1:2 each time so that at the final step the denaturing solution has been diluted 1:32.

4. Rinse filters two more times with 1X binding buffer
5. Place filters into 1X binding buffer containing 5% instant nonfat dry milk. Shake gently for 30 min.
6. Rinse filters in 1X binding buffer containing 0.25% nonfat dry milk.

### 3.5. Screening Nitrocellulose Filters

All steps should be carried out at 4°C.

1. Add $^{32}P$-labeled concatenated DNA probe to 1X binding buffer containing 0.25% nonfat dry milk and 5 µg/mL sonicated and denatured calf thymus DNA. A minimum concentration of probe should be $1 \times 10^6$ cpm/mL. There should be approx 250 ng probe DNA or a total of $5 \times 10^7$ cpm per 50 mL binding buffer. Make sure the amount of binding solution is sufficient to allow the free movement of each filter in solution during the gentle shaking step.
2. Incubate at 4°C for 2–12 h with gentle shaking.
3. Wash each filter 3 times, each for 5 min, at 4°C with 1X binding buffer containing 0.25% nonfat dry milk with gentle shaking.
4. Blot filters on Whatman 3MM paper to drain off excess liquid. Tape filters on Whatman paper or old used films wrapped with plastic food wrap (e.g., Saran wrap). Place 3–4 luminescent stickers on the Whatman paper or film. Wrap with another layer of plastic wrap and autoradiograph at –70°C for 24–48 h using Kodak XAR-5 film and an intensifying screen.

### 3.6. Identification and Purification of Positive Clones

1. Carefully align the developed film with the filter on Whatman paper according to the images of luminescent stickers. Once aligned, mark on the film the corresponding filter number and the three previously placed asymmetric marks on each filter. Identify, mark, and number possible positive clones on the film (*see* **Note 9**).
2. Identify positive plaques by aligning the plate with the numerically corresponding filter at the three asymmetric marks. Isolate positive plaques by carefully picking up the agarose containing the plaque. This can be done with the open end of a P-200 micropipet tip. Place the agarose plug in 1 mL SM buffer. Add approx 25 µL chloroform to inhibit bacterial growth and store phage at 4°C. These are your secondary phage stocks. Allow the phage to diffuse out of the agarose for at least 4 h before using it for subsequent infections.
3. Grow an overnight culture of *E. coli* Y1090 in phage broth containing 0.2% maltose and 50 µg/mL ampicillin. Infect 150 µL of overnight culture with appropriately diluted secondary phage stocks (approx $2.5 \times 10^4$ pfu).
4. Repeat **steps 5–12** in **Subheading 3.3.** using 82-mm nitrocellulose filters and 100-mm plates.
5. Screen secondary filters with the wild-type probe and a negative control probe (this may be either a totally unrelated sequence or a mutant of the wild-type sequence that is not bound by DNA binding protein).
6. Repeat **steps 3–5** between 1 and 3 times. This is usually necessary to obtain pure plaques.
7. Plaque purify the phage that binds specifically to wild-type probe (*see* **Note 10**).

### 3.7. Isolation of Recombinant Phage Lysogens

1. Grow *E. coli* Y1089 to saturation in phage broth containing 0.2% maltose and 50 µg/mL ampicillin at 37°C.
2. Dilute the saturated culture 1:100 in LB media containing 10 m*M* $MgCl_2$.

3. Mix 100 µL of diluted culture with 5 µL of phage stock and incubate for 20 min at 32°C.
4. Dilute this mix 1:1000 in LB medium and plate 100 µL aliquots onto 100-mm LB agar plates containing 50 µg/mL ampicillin (LB/Amp plates).
5. Incubate plates at 32°C overnight.
6. Pick colonies and streak each in the same position onto two LB/Amp plates. Incubate one at 32°C and the other at 42°C. Lysogens will grow at 32°C but not at 42°C.

### 3.8. Preparation of Crude Cell Extracts from Recombinant Phage Lysogens

1. Grow overnight cultures of recombinant lysogens in LB medium containing 50 µg/mL ampicillin (LB-AMP) at 32°C.
2. Add 20 µL of overnight culture to 2 mL LB-AMP and grow at 32°C until $OD_{600} = 0.5$ (this will take approx 3 h).
3. Shift to 44°C for 20 min.
4. Add IPTG to a final concentration of 10 m*M* to induce the expression of fusion protein and grow at 37°C for 1 h.
5. Pellet 1 mL of cells in a microfuge for 1 min at maximum speed.
6. Discard supernatant and resuspend the pellet in 100 µL of cell extract buffer.
7. Freeze cell suspension in liquid nitrogen, thaw, and add lysozyme to a final concentration of 500 µg/mL. Incubate 15 min on ice.
8. Adjust suspension to 1 *M* NaCl, mix and incubate in rotator for 15 min at 4°C.
9. Centrifuge in microfuge for 30 min at 4°C at 14,000*g*.
10. Dialyze the supernatant against 100 mL cell extract buffer for 60 min at 4°C (*see* **Note 11**).
11. Snap freeze in liquid nitrogen and store at –70°C until needed (*see* **Note 12**).

### 3.9. Identification of cDNA Insert in λ Phage DNA

1. Infect 150 µL of an overnight culture of *E. coli* Y1090 with $10^5$ phage. Mix with 4 mL top agarose and pour onto 15 × 100-mm phage plate containing agarose (instead of agar, see **Note 13**). Invert the plate and incubate at 37°C for 9–14 h until the plaques cover almost the entire surface of the plate.
2. Add 7 mL of SM buffer directly onto the plate and allow the bacteriophage to elute by shaking gently at room temperature for at least 1–2 h. Transfer the top SM to a centrifuge tube and remove the bacterial debris by centrifugation at 8000*g* for 10 min at 4°C.
3. Transfer the supernatant to a new tube. Add Rnase A and Dnase I, each to a final concentration of 1 µg/mL. Incubate for 30 min at 37°C. Add an equal volume of ice-cold phage precipitation solution and incubate for 1 hour at 0°C (in ice water). Recover the phage particles by centrifugation at 10,000*g* for 20 min at 4°C
4. Remove the supernatant by careful aspiration. Stand the tube in an inverted position on a paper towel to allow all of the fluid to drain. Wipe-dry inside of the tube if necessary. Add 0.5 mL SM buffer to resuspend the bacteriophage. Assist the resuspension by pipetting or vortexing. Transfer the suspension to an Eppendorf tube and centrifuge at 8000*g* for 2 min at 4°C to remove any bacteria or agarose debris.
5. Pipet the supernatant to a new Eppendorf tube. To break the bacteriophage particle, add 5 µL of 10% SDS and 5 µL of 0.5 *M* EDTA, pH 8.0. Incubate at 68°C for 15 min. Extract the phage solution with an equal volume of phenol once, phenol/chloroform once and chloroform once. Vortex vigorously while extracting.
6. To the final aqueous phase, add 0.1 volume of 3 *M* sodium acetate, pH 5.2, and 2.5–3.0 volumes of ethanol. Store at –70°C for at least 15 min. Thaw and centrifuge at 14,000*g*

for 15 min at 4°C. Carefully pour out the supernatant without losing the pellet. Wash the pellet by adding 0.5 mL 70% ethanol, vortexing and centrifuging 5 min at room temperature. Pour off the supernatant. Wash one more time. Dry pellet by air-drying or by SpeedVac. Resuspend the pellet in 50 µL TE, pH 8.0.

7. Digest 10 µL of above DNA preparation in 20 µL volume with appropriate buffer and restriction enzyme for 3–4 h. Observe the insert by gel electrophoresis. Insert can be recovered from the gel for subcloning (*see* **Note 14**).

## 4. Notes

1. The five temperature stepwise annealling process can be replaced by heating the mixed oligonucleotides in 0.5X TEN at 75°C for 15 min in a heating block. Turn the heating switch off and allow the heating block to cool to room temperature (approx 4 h).
2. If effective ligation has occurred, you will see a ladder of DNA corresponding to different numbers of copies of your DNA binding site. Ideally, you should isolate the larger fragments and subclone these into a pUC based vector.
3. If you do not wish to prepare all of the reagents individually needed for nick translation of DNA, kits for labeling DNA by nick translation are commercially available.
4. Usually you will need to screen approx $10^6$ plaques to make sure that your cDNA of interest is included in the screen. Each plate contains $5 \times 10^4$ phage, therefore 20 plates are needed. The number of plaques that produce the fusion protein of interest depends on the abundance of the message and the success of cloning the corresponding cDNA in frame. If the mRNA is rare in the cells used to construct the cDNA library, more plaques may need to be screened.
5. It is important to minimize the amount of condensation on the plate lids. If an air-blowing incubator is available in the laboratory, use it. Otherwise, make sure to remove condensation.
6. To avoid trapping bubbles between the filter and the agarose, hold the edge of the filter with two gloved hands. Put the center of the filter onto the agar first and then gradually extend contact between the agar and the filter.
7. If india ink is not available, an 18-gauge needle will make the holes sufficiently large to visualize at later times.
8. Duplicate filters are necessary to make the proper identification of positive clones and eliminate false-positives. At the identification step, the positive should be present in both filters with a stronger signal seen in the first lift.
9. A true positive signal almost always has a tail owing to the lifting of the filter. Perfectly round images on the filter are generally false-positives. In addition, the positive signal should be in exactly the same place in duplicate filters although in some cases they may be very faint in the second lift.
10. Obtaining a pure positive plaque requires that the plaques on the plate are sufficiently separated for easy isolation. Depending on the purity of the plaque isolated from the previous screen, the amount of phage used for subsequent screening should be reduced accordingly. It may be useful to plate out serial dilutions of phage if contamination is suspected. Once you are reasonably sure that your phage is pure, set up one last screening. If almost all of the phage plaques are positive with a wild-type probe and negative with either a mutant probe or unrelated probe in your final screen, you have a pure clone.
11. Use Type VS millipore filters, 0.025-µm pore size for dialysis. To dialyze, place the dialysis solution in a 150-mm Petri dish. Float the millipore filter on the dialysis solution and gently drop the extract on the filter.

12. The extract can now be used to carry out DNA binding studies. The DNA binding specificity of your cloned protein can be determined either by DNase I footprinting or mobility shift assays.
13. Agarose must be used instead of agar in both layers of the plate to insure clean DNA preparation for restriction digestions. Agar frequently interferes with the restriction endonucleases and prevents efficient digestion of DNA.
14. Inclusion of 2–3 m*M* spermidine and 20 µg/mL RNase A in the reaction will improve the restriction digestion. Bacteriophage DNA prepared in this manner can also be used in any PCR application.

## References


1. Singh, H., LeBowitz, J. H., Baldwin, A. S. J., and Sharp, P. A. (1988) Molecular cloning of an enhancer binding protein: isolation by screening of an expression library with a recognition site DNA. *Cell* **52,** 415–423.
2. Rawlins, D. R., Milman, G., Hayward, S. D., and Hayward, G. S. (1985) Sequence-specific DNA binding of the Epstein-Barr viral nuclear antigen (EBNA-1) to clustered sites in the plasmid maintenance region. *Cell* **42,** 859–868.
3. Clerc, R. G., Corcoran, L. M., Lebowitz, J. H., Baltimore, D., and Sharp, P. A. (1988) The B-cell specific Oct-2 protein contains Pou box and homeo box-type domains. *Genes Dev.* **2,** 1570–1581.
4. Staudt, L. M., Clerc, R. G., Singh, H., LeBowitz, J. H., Sharp, P. A., and Baltimore, D. (1988) Cloning of a lymphoid specific cDNA encoding a protein binding the regulatory octamer DNA motif. *Science* **241,** 577–580.
5. Vinson, C. R., LaMarco, K. L., Johnson, P. F., Landschulz, W. H., and McKnight, S. L. (1988) In situ detection of sequence-specific DNA binding activity specified by a recombinant bacteriophage. *Genes Dev.* **2,** 801–806.
6. Sambrook, J., Fritsch, E. F., and Maniatis, T. (1989) Screening cDNA libraries constructed in bacteriophage λ expression vectors with synthetic oligonucleotides, in *Molecular Cloning: A Laboratory Manual,* 2nd ed. (Nolan, C. ed.), Cold Spring Harbor Laboratory Press, Cold Spring Harbor, NY, pp. 12.30–12.40.
7. Singh, H.,Clerc, R. G., and Lebowitz, J. H. (1989) Molecular cloning of sequence-specific DNA binding proteins using recognition site probes. *BioTechniques* **7,** 252–261.
8. Siedman, J. G. (1995) Construction of recombinant DNA libraries, in *Current Protocols in Molecular Biology,* vol. 1. (Ausubel, F. M., Brent, R., Kingston, R. E., et al., eds.), Wiley, New York, NY, pp. 5.01–5.11.

32

# Analysis of DNA Binding Proteins by Mobility Shift Assay

**Yi-Chun James Wang and Eduardo A. Montalvo**

## 1. Introduction

DNA binding proteins are involved in replication, repair, recombination, and transcription. In recent years, the heightened interest in transcriptional regulation has led to the development of several distinct techniques for the study of DNA binding proteins. These include the gel mobility shift assay *(1,2)*, DNase I footprinting analyses *(3)*, and the methylation-interference assay *(4,5)*. Although each technique can be used to obtain valuable information regarding DNA/protein interactions, each method has its limitations and technical difficulties. Taken together, these methods can be used to identify important regulatory elements in mammalian and viral gene promoters, to characterize the DNA binding activity of the proteins that bind to these elements and to identify protein(s) that bind to these sites.

The mobility shift assay is a relatively simple and very sensitive technique. This assay is based on the principle that binding of a protein to a radiolabeled DNA fragment will alter or retard the mobility of the DNA fragment during electrophoresis through a nondenaturing polyacrylamide gel. The stability of the DNA/protein complex during electrophoresis is dependent on the low ionic strength of the buffer and the gel matrix, which provides a "caging effect" to prevent diffusion of proteins *(1,2)*.

Mobility shift assays can be used to assess several properties of a DNA binding protein including 1) binding affinity and specificity; 2) abundance in a nuclear or cytoplasmic extract; 3) association/dissociation rate of binding; and 4) identification of the bound protein. Ideally, the mobility shift assay should be used in combination with other DNA binding assays (e.g., DNase I footprinting, methylation interference assays) that can be used to identify a relatively small region as the protein binding site. Once the binding site has been identified, synthetic oligonucleotides corresponding to the footprinted region can be made and used to study and characterize DNA/protein interactions with the mobility shift assay. This technique has been used successfully to

From: *Methods in Molecular Biology, Vol. 174: Epstein-Barr Virus Protocols*
Edited by: J. B. Wilson and G. H. W. May © Humana Press Inc., Totowa, NJ

identify protein binding sites in the Epstein-Barr virus (EBV) genome necessary for viral replication *(6–8)* and to study transcription factor binding sites that are cis-acting regulatory elements in EBV latent *(9)* and lytic promoters *(10–12)*. A major advantage of this assay is that it is relatively simple and rapid. For example, the presence of specific DNA binding proteins in different EBV-infected cell types can be easily compared with this technique *(12)*. Comparisons can also be made, within the same cell line, between latently infected cells and cells induced into lytic replication *(12)*. Furthermore, in cases where various members of a protein family (e.g., CREB/ATF family) bind the same site, specific antibodies can be used in the mobility shift assay to identify the specific protein(s) in a DNA/protein complex *(12)*.

The basic mobility shift experiment requires the preparation of 1) a nuclear extract or purified protein, 2) an end-labeled radioactive probe, and 3) a low ionic strength nondenaturing polyacrylamide gel. After these components are prepared, the binding reaction is carried out by a short incubation of the radiolabeled DNA probe with the nuclear extract. The components of the binding reaction are then electrophoresed through a nondenaturing gel, which is subsequently dried and exposed to film. The migration of the DNA probe in the absence (free probe) and presence of protein (bound probe) can easily be visualized once the film is developed.

An unlabeled nonspecific competitor DNA is added to the binding reaction to inhibit the formation of nonspecific DNA/protein complexes. However, in some cases it is difficult to determine whether the complex is specific even in the presence of excess nonspecific competitor. To circumvent this problem, it is best to compare DNA/protein complex formation in the absence and presence of an unlabeled specific competitor *(13,14)* (i.e., competitive binding). Generally, different increasing concentrations of competitor are added (e.g., 5-fold, 25-fold, and 100-fold molar excess) to the binding reaction. If the competitor DNA has an unrelated sequence (nonspecific competitor), the amount of DNA/protein complex is unaffected because the affinity of protein for a specific sequence is greater than for the nonspecific competitor fragment. However, if the competitor and probe contain the identical DNA sequence (homologous competitor), the retarded DNA protein complex will be reduced or abolished, depending on the molar excess of competitor. The protein affinity for a related sequence can also be analyzed by using a heterologous competitor. By adding increasing increments of excess heterologous competitor, the relative affinity of protein for similar sequences can be determined by comparing complex formation in the presence of homologous vs heterologous competitor. Thus, comparisons can easily be made between different binding sites.

The protein(s) present in a particular DNA/protein complex can be identified by adding specific antibodies to the binding reaction *(15)*. If the antibody added to the binding reaction is specific for a protein present in the complex, the mobility of the complex will either be further retarded (i.e., supershift) or abolished entirely. By comparing the mobility of the DNA/protein complex in the absence and presence of antibody, specific proteins in a complex can be identified.

The protocol in this chapter includes the use of a specific competitor in the binding reaction. If you suspect that a certain protein is binding your sequence of interest, the use of a specific antibody for identification purposes is listed in the Notes section of this chapter. In addition, a scaled-down method for the preparation of cytoplasmic/nuclear extract is given that can be used when only small amounts of cells are available for your analyses.

## 2. Materials

### 2.1. Nuclear Extract

1. PBS: 0.8% NaCl, 0.02% KCl, 0.14% $Na_2HPO_4$, 0.02% $KH_2PO_4$, pH 7.0.
2. Dignam A buffer: 10 m*M* N-2-hydroxyethylpiperazine-N'-ethane-sulfonic acid (HEPES), pH 7.9, 1.5 m*M* $MgCl_2$, 10 m*M* KCl and 0.5 m*M* dithiothreitol (DTT), 1 m*M* Phenylmethylsulfonyl fluoride (PMSF), 1 m*M* Benzamidine-HCl, 0.5 µg/mL Leupeptin, 0.4 µg/mL Aprotinin, and 0.7 µg/mL Pepstatin (*see* **Notes 1** and **2**).
3. Dignam C buffer: 20 m*M* HEPES, pH 7.9, 0.6 *M* KCl, 1.5 m*M* $MgCl_2$, 0.2 m*M* ethylenediaminetetraacetic acid (EDTA), 0.5 m*M* DTT, 25% glycerol (v/v), 1 m*M* PMSF, 1 m*M* Benzamidine-HCl, 0.5 µg/mL Leupeptin, 0.4 µg/mL Aprotinin, and 0.7 µg/mL Pepstatin.
4. Dignam D buffer: 20 m*M* HEPES, pH 7.9, 0.1 *M* KCl, 0.2 m*M* EDTA, 0.5 m*M* PMSF, 0.5 m*M* DTT, 20% glycerol (v/v), 1 m*M* Phenylmethylsulfonyl fluoride (PMSF), 1 m*M* Benzamidine-HCl, 0.5 µg/mL Leupeptin, 0.4 µg/mL Aprotinin, and 0.7 µg/mL Pepstatin.
5. Dounce homogenizer with a loose pestle.
6. Labquack™ test tube shaker.
7. Microdialyzer.
8. Liquid nitrogen.
9. Triton lysis buffer: 10 m*M* Tris-HCl, pH 8.0, 150 m*M* NaCl, 1 m*M* $MgCl_2$, 0.08% Triton X-100, 1 m*M* DTT, 1 m*M* PMSF, 1 m*M* Benzamidine-HCl, 0.5 µg/mL Leupeptin, 0.4 µg/mL Aprotinin, and 0.7 µg/mL Pepstatin.

### 2.2. End-Labeled Probe

1. 1 m*M* solution of each synthetic oligonucleotide with one base overhang (preferably the same base overhang on each strand), for example: 5'-TAATCATCAGCGG-3' and 5'-TCCGCTGATGATT-3'
2. TEN buffer: 10 m*M* Tris-HCl, pH 8.0, 100 m*M* NaCl and 1 m*M* EDTA.
3. $\alpha$-[$^{32}$P] dNTP and unlabeled 10 m*M* dNTP solution (N represents nucleotide complementary to the single base overhang, e.g., dATP).
4. Exo (–) Klenow and reaction buffer (New England Biolab, 5 units/µL).
5. Nuctrap® push column (Stratagene) (*see* **Note 3**).

### 2.3. Binding Reaction

1. 2X binding buffer: HEPES, pH 7.9, 10% (v/v) glycerol, 10 m*M* $MgCl_2$, 60 m*M* KCl, 2 m*M* DTT, 50 µg/mL bovine serum albumin (BSA), 0.1 m*M* EDTA, 0.1% nonidet-P40 (NP40) (*see* **Note 4**).
2. Poly (dI-dC) · poly(dI-dC): 1 mg/mL in $H_2O$ (Pharmacia, see **Note 5**).
3. Radiolabeled probe.
4. Unlabeled competitor DNA (*see* **Note 6**).
5. Nuclear extract (freshly diluted to 1 mg/mL in Dignam D).
6. Sterile deionized water.

### 2.4. Nondenaturing Gel Electrophoresis Autoradiography

1. 20% acrylamide: 19:1 acrylamide:bisacrylamide mix.
2. TBE buffer: 89 m*M* Tris-HCl, 89 m*M* boric acid, 2 m*M* EDTA.
3. Ammonium persulfate.
4. TEMED (N,N,N',N'-tetramethylethylenediamine).
5. Vertical gel electrophoresis apparatus.
6. 10X Bromophenol blue dye: 0.25% bromophenol blue, 20% Ficoll.
7. Gel dryer.
8. X-ray film (e.g., Kodak XAR-5 film).
9. Film cassette for autoradiography.
10. Whatman 3MM paper.

## 3. Methods

### 3.1. Preparation of Nuclear Extract (Maxiprep)

1. Pellet approx $10^9$ cells in a centrifuge at 1850*g* for 10 min at 4°C. Resuspend the pellet and wash once with PBS, pellet the cells again (*see* **Note 7**).
2. Resuspend pellet in 5X packed cell volume (PCV) of ice-cold Dignam A buffer, then pellet the cells again.
3. Resuspend cell pellet with ice-cold Dignam A to a final volume of 3X original PCV, incubate 10 min on ice, then Dounce homogenize with 10 up-and-down strokes.
4. Centrifuge at 4°C for 15 min at 3300*g*. Remove supernatant carefully.
5. Resuspend pellet (crude nuclei) in 1X packed nuclei volume of ice-cold Dignam C buffer containing 0.6 *M* KCl (*see* **Note 8**).
6. Rock at 4°C for 30 min.
7. Centrifuge at 15,000*g* for 30 min at 4°C.
8. Carefully recover supernatant and microdialyze for 5 h at 4°C vs 50 vol of Dignam D buffer.
9. Take 2 µL of extract and determine protein concentration (*see* **Note 9**).
10. Aliquot the extract in microfuge tubes at 20–30 µL per tube (precool microfuge tube on ice prior to aliquoting the sample). Snap-freeze in liquid nitrogen and store frozen nuclear extracts at –70°C.

### 3.2. Minipreparation of Nuclear Extract

1. Pellet approx $5 \times 10^6$ cells and wash them twice with PBS.
2. Resuspend the washed cell pellet in 50 µL of Triton lysis buffer, incubate on ice for 5 min.
3. Pellet the nuclei in a microcentrifuge at 800*g* for 5 min at 4°C.
4. Carefully remove the cytoplasmic fraction from the nuclear pellet and resuspend the pellet in approx 20 µL Dignam C buffer containing 0.6 *M* KCl.
5. Incubate on ice for 1 h.
6. Spin the nuclear extract in a microfuge at 16,000*g* for 20 min at 4°C.
7. Collect the supernatant and snap-freeze in liquid nitrogen, store at –80°C (*see* **Note 10**).

### 3.3. Preparation of Radiolabeled Probe

1. Once you have determined the concentration of each synthetic oligonucleotide, prepare a 10 µ*M* working solution of each oligonucleotide.
2. In a microfuge tube, add 1 µL of each oligonucleotide, 5 µL of sterile water. Heat to 75°C for 15 min and allow to cool slowly to room temperature (*see* **Note 11**).

**Table 1**
**Pipetting Scheme for DNA Binding Reactions**

| Tube number | 2X Binding buffer | Poly dI-dC | 100X Competitor | Probe | Water | Protein extract | Total |
|---|---|---|---|---|---|---|---|
| 1 | 6 µL | 1 µL | None | 1 µL | 4 µL | None | 12 µL |
| 2 | 6 µL | 1 µL | None | 1 µL | 3 µL | 1 µL | 12 µL |
| 3 | 6 µL | 1 µL | 1 µL | 1 µL | 2 µL | 1 µL | 12 µL |
| 4 | 6 µL | 1 µL | 1 µL | 1 µL | 2 µL | 1 µL | 12 µL |

3. Once the mix has been cooled to ambient temperature, add 2 µL 10X Klenow buffer, 10 µL of [α-$^{32}$P]-dNTP (3000 Ci/mmol) and 1 µL of Klenow enzyme. Incubate at room temperature for 30 min. Add 80 µL TEN buffer to stop the reaction.
4. Save 1 µL aliquot of the reaction mix to determine the labeling efficiency by TCA precipitation (*see* **Note 12**).
5. Separate free dNTPs from radiolabeled probe by passing the labeling reaction mix through a push column.
6. Wash the column with another 100 µL of TEN buffer, combine both flow fractions. Determine volume of flow through. This should be about 200 µL. If the volume is less than 200 µL, add sufficient water to bring to appropriate volume.
7. Determine the radioactive incorporation and the final probe concentration (*see* **Note 13**).

### 3.4. Preparation of Specific Cold Competitor DNA

1. Mix 10 µL of each 10 µ*M* single-strand oligonucleotide in a microfuge tube.
2. Heat the mixture to 75°C for 15 min, then gradually cool it down to room temperature through a minimum 30-min period.
3. Add 5 µL of 10X Klenow buffer, 1 µL of 10 m*M* cold nucleotide solution, 21 µL of dd$H_2O$, and 3 µL of Klenow enzyme. Mix well, then incubate at room temperature for 30 min.
4. Store the final 1 µ*M* double-strand DNA solution at –20°C. This is 100-fold molar excess competitor (*see* **Note 13**).

### 3.5. Preparation of Nondenaturing Gel

1. Assemble glass plates and spacers making sure the bottom and sides of the glass plates are well sealed.
2. Mix 20 mL of 20% acrylamide, 25 mL of TBE buffer and 55 mL of deionized water (*see* **Note 14**).
3. Add 0.1 g of ammonium persulfate. Mix thoroughly until the ammonium persulfate has gone into solution. Add 30 µL of TEMED, mix and quickly pour the polyacrylamide solution between the glass plates. Insert comb and allow to polymerize for at least 30 min.

### 3.6. Binding Reaction

1. In an ice-cold microfuge tube, dilute nuclear extract with Dignam D buffer (with DTT and protease inhibitors) to 1 mg/mL.
2. In four separate microfuge tubes, add 1 µL of poly(dI-dC) · poly(dI-dC), 6 µL of 2X binding buffer, and 1 µL probe (5–10 × $10^4$ cpm) to each tube (*see* **Table 1** and **Note 13**).
3. Add 1 µL of competitor to tubes 3 and 4.
4. Add 4 µL water to tube 1, 3 µL to tube 2, and 2 µL to tubes 3 and 4.

**Table 2**
**Protease Inhibitors and Their Uses**

| Inhibitors | Protease inhibited | Stock solution | Storage | Working conc. |
|---|---|---|---|---|
| Aprotinin | Serine (Trypsin) | 2 mg/mL in $H_2O$ | 4°C | 0.4 µg/mL |
| Benzamidine-HCl | Serine (Trypsin) | 100 m*M* in methanol | 4°C | 1 m*M* |
| Leupeptin | Serine and thiol | 5 mg/mL in $H_2O$ | –20°C | 0.5 µg/mL |
| Pepstatin | Acid | 0.7 mg/mL in methanol | –20°C | 0.7 µg/mL |
| PMSF | Serine and thiol | 100 m*M* in isopropanol | 4°C | 1 m*M* |

5. Add 1 µL diluted nuclear extract (1 mg/ mL) to tubes 2–4.
6. Incubate mix at room temperature for 20–30 min (*see* **Note 15**).
7. Load each mix into separate lanes in the assembled gel apparatus.
8. In a separate lane, load 5 µL of 1X bromophenol blue dye.
9. Electrophorese at 10–15 V/cm.
10. When the bromophenol blue is 2–3 cm from the bottom of the gel, turn off the current. Carefully, separate the plates from each other. The gel should remain on the bottom plate. Place a moistened piece of Whatman 3MM paper on the gel. Press the paper gently against the gel and carefully lift the paper from the glass plate beginning at one end. The gel will be attached to the paper at this point. Place plastic wrap on gel surface.
11. Dry the gel at 80°C under vacuum for 30–60 min.
12. Expose dried gel to Kodak XAR-5 film.

## 4. Notes

1. All buffers should be stored at 4°C. Dithiothreitol is unstable and should be freshly added from a 0.5–1.0 *M* stock solution, aliquots at –20°C.
2. All protease inhibitors should be added fresh, immediately before using the solution. Some general protease inhibitors and their uses are listed in **Table 2**.
3. Commercially available columns for the separation of unincorporated nucleotides from radiolabeled DNA are available from several manufacturers. The protocol listed is modified from Nuctrap push columns (Stratagene) but other columns can be used provided the exclusion volume is appropriate for the size of probe prepared.
4. The binding buffer given in this protocol is generally a good starting point because most DNA binding proteins will bind in a buffer containing 50 m*M* KCl and 2 m*M* $MgCl_2$. However, it may be necessary to alter the salt and magnesium concentration for other DNA binding proteins. If no binding is observed with the binding buffer given in this protocol, try using a range of 0–150 m*M* KCl and 0–4 m*M* $MgCl_2$.
5. poly(dI-dC) · poly(dI-dC) is a DNA polymer that is commonly used as a nonspecific competitor in binding reactions to prevent binding by nonspecific DNA binding proteins present in the nuclear extract. In some situations, it may be necessary to use a different competitor such as poly (dA-dT) · poly(dA-dT).
6. Homologous competitor DNA (same DNA sequence as probe) is added in molar excess in some of the binding reactions to determine the specificity of the DNA/protein complex. Although nonspecific competitor is present in the binding reaction, some nonspecific DNA binding proteins may not be effectively competed by nonspecific DNA

sequences. Cold competitor DNA containing the exact DNA sequence as the radioactive probe, added in molar excess, will effectively compete for the same DNA binding protein resulting in either a reduction or the elimination of the complex. To compare whether identical or similar binding sequences can compete prepare 5-fold, 25-fold, and 100-fold molar excess of competitor DNA. If you wish to determine which bases are essential for DNA/protein complex formation, specific point mutations can be introduced into either the DNA used as probe or the cold competitor. If bases necessary for protein/DNA interaction are mutated in the probe, you will see the disappearance of the DNA/protein complex. If similar mutations are made in the cold competitor, the mutant competitor will not effectively compete against DNA/protein complexes seen with the wild-type probe.

7. It will be easier to determine the packed cell volume at the next step if you transfer the cell suspension to a conical tube at this point.
8. Sometimes it is difficult to resuspend the packed nuclei to homogeneity. However, nuclei can be homogenized with 2–5 up-and-down strokes in a Dounce homogenizer (loose pestle).
9. Normally at this point the protein concentration should be between 6–10 mg/ mL.
10. The nuclear extract made by the minipreparation protocol contains high salt. Therefore, it is necessary to dilute the extract with salt-free Dignam D buffer before use.
11. It is convenient to mix 100 µL of each 10 µ*M* oligonucleotide stock to anneal them at once to make a 5 µ*M* double-stranded DNA stock and store it at –20°C for later labeling reactions.
12. Dilute the 1 µL reaction mix into 199 µL of TE buffer (10 m*M* Tris-HCl, pH 8.0, 1 m*M* EDTA) containing 100 µg of carrier yeast tRNA. Mix 100 µL of this dilution with aqueous counting fluid and determine the total amount of radioactive nucleotide in the sample by a scintillation counter. Add the remaining 100 µL to 2 mL ice-cold 10% trichloracetic acid (TCA), vortex briefly, and incubate on ice bath for 10 min. Collect the precipitated material by vacuum filtration through a Whatman GF/C glass fiber filter (prewet with TCA solution). Wash the tube once with another 2 mL of 10% TCA solution and pass the washes through the filter. Repeat the wash twice more with 2 mL 95% ethanol. Immerse the filter in aqueous counting fluid and count to determine the amount of radioactive nucleotide incorporated into probe. The ratio of cpm on the filter to total cpm is the labeling efficiency. It is usually greater than 50%.
13. If efficient labeling is achieved, your probe should be between 3–5 × $10^5$ cpm/µL. At this point the concentration of the probe is 50 nM (i.e., 50 femptomoles per µL). For gel mobility shift assay, usually 5–10 × $10^4$ cpm is used for each binding reaction. Therefore, the final probe concentration in each reaction is about 10 femptomoles.
14. The ratio of bis:acrylamide given is for smaller probes in the range of 15–100 bases. For probes of less than 100 bp, a ratio of 19 acrylamide:1 bisacrylamide should be used. For probes longer than 100 bp, use a 59 acrylamide:1 bisacrylamide ratio.
15. Antibodies can be used to identify proteins in specific DNA/protein complexes. The antibodies (usually 1 µg per reaction) are added after the 20–30 min binding reaction and the mixture is incubated for an additional 15–20 min before loading onto the gel.

## References

1. Fried, M. and Crothers, D. M. (1981) Equilibria and kinetics of *lac* repressor-operator interactions by polyacrylamide gel electrophoresis. *Nucleic Acids Res.* **9,** 6505–6525.
2. Garner, M. M. and Revzin, A. (1981) A gel electrophoresis method for quantifying the binding of proteins to specific DNA regions: application to components of the *Escherichia coli* lactose operon regulatory system. *Nucleic Acids Res.* **9,** 3047–3060.

3. Galas, D. and Schmitz, A. (1978) DNase footprinting: A simple method for the detection of protein-DNA binding specificity. *Nucleic Acids Res.* **5,** 3157–3170.
4. Baldwin, A. S. (1988) Methylation interference assay for analysis of DNA-protein interactions, in *Current Protocols in Molecular Biology,* vol. 2. (Ausubel, F. M., Brent, R., Kingston, R. E., et al., eds.), Wiley, New York, NY, pp. 12.3.1–12.3.6.
5. Siebenlist, U. and Gilbert, W. (1980) Contacts between *E. coli* RNA polymerase and an early promoter of phage T7. *Proc. Natl. Acad. Sci. USA* **77,** 122–126.
6. Ambinder, R. F., Shah, W. A., Rawlins, D. R., Hayward, G. S., and Hayward, S. D. (1990) Definition of the sequence requirements for binding of the EBNA-1 protein to its palindromic target sites in Epstein-Barr virus DNA. *J. Virol.* **64,** 2369–2379.
7. Jones, C. H., Hayward, S. D., and Rawlins, D. R. (1989) Interaction of the lymphocyte-derived Epstein-Barr virus nuclear antigen EBNA-1 with its DNA-binding sites. *J. Virol.* **63,** 101–110.
8. Summers, H., Barwell, J. A., Pfuetzner, R. A., Edwards, A. M., and Frappier, L. (1996) Cooperative assembly of EBNA1 on the Epstein-Barr virus latent origin of replication. *J. Virol.* **70,** 1228–1231.
9. Zimber, S. U., Kremmer, E., Grasser, F., Marschall, G., Laux, G., and Bornkamm, G. W. (1993) The Epstein-Barr virus nuclear antigen 2 interacts with an EBNA2 responsive cis-element of the terminal protein 1 gene promoter. *EMBO J.* **12,** 167–175.
10. Borras, A. M., Strominger. J. L., and Speck, S. H. (1996) Characterization of the ZI domains in the Epstein-Barr virus BZLF1 gene promoter: role in phorbol ester induction. *J. Virol.* **70,** 3894–3901.
11. Schwarzmann, F., Prang, N., Reichelt, B., Rinkes, B., Haist, S., Marschall, M., and Wolf, H. (1994) Negatively cis-acting elements in the distal part of the promoter of Epstein-Barr virus trans-activator gene BZLF1. *J. Gen. Virol.* **75,** 1999–2006.
12. Wang, Y-C. J., Huang, J.-M., and Montalvo, E. A. (1997) Characterization of proteins binding to the ZII element in the Epstein-Barr virus BZLF1 promoter: transactivation by ATF1. *Virology* **227,** 323–330.
13. Carthew, R. W., Chodosh, L. A., and Sharp. P. A. (1986) An RNA polymerase II transcription factor binds to an upstream element in the adenovirus major late promoter. *Cell* **43,** 439–448.
14. Singh, H., Sen, R., Baltimore, D., and Sharp, P. A. (1986) A nuclear factor that binds to a conserved sequence motif in transcriptional control elements of immunoglobulin genes. *Nature* **319,** 154–158.
15. Kristie, T. M. and B. Roizman (1986) α4, the major regulatory protein of herpes simplex virus type 1, is stably and specifically associated with promoter-regulatory domains of a genes and/or selected viral genes. *Proc. Natl. Acad. Sci. USA* **83,** 3218–3222.

33

# Analysis of RNA-Protein Interactions of the EBV-Encoded Small RNAs, the EBERs

## *In Vitro Assays*

**Kenneth G. Laing, Androulla Elia, Ian W. Jeffrey, and Michael J. Clemens**

## 1. Introduction

As indicated in Chapter 5, in spite of the fact that the two small virally encoded RNA species, EBER-1 and EBER-2, are abundantly expressed in almost all Epstein-Barr virus (EBV)-infected cell types, their functions remain to be elucidated. Because these RNAs do not code for any proteins themselves, it is likely that their mode of action involves their association with cellular or viral proteins in vivo. The properties of such proteins may be modified by binding of the EBERs.

The small EBV RNAs can bind to at least three distinct proteins: the La antigen; ribosomal protein L22 (also known as EAP); and the interferon-inducible, double-stranded RNA-activated protein kinase (PKR) *(1)*. In this chapter we describe techniques for the in vitro analysis of RNA-protein interactions involving the EBERs, with specific reference to the example of PKR.

### *1.1. In Vitro transcription*

An essential requirement in many of the in vitro assays described in this section, including the inhibition and rescue of protein synthesis in the reticulocyte lysate by the small RNAs such as the EBERs, is the ability to synthesize large amounts of homogeneous transcripts from cloned sequences. Furthermore, for northern blotting, UV crosslinking and filter binding, it is necessary to be able to synthesize RNAs labeled to a high-specific activity from these same clones. The ability to do so stems from the development in the 1980s of the technique of in vitro transcription, utilizing RNA polymerases from bacteriophages such as T7, SP6, and T3 *(2,3)*. Since its original development, the technique has been refined, enabling it to be carried out on a truly preparative scale. Most RNAs made in this way have been cloned into one of the many

From: *Methods in Molecular Biology, Vol. 174: Epstein-Barr Virus Protocols*
Edited by: J. B. Wilson and G. H. W. May © Humana Press Inc., Totowa, NJ

commercial vectors readily available by placing the sequence of interest adjacent to the polymerase promoter. Transcription is then normally carried out on the linearized template. This strategy has the disadvantage that intervening sequences derived from the multicloning site either 5' or 3' to the sequence are often also transcribed, yielding a chimaeric RNA. The effect of these sequences must always be considered, especially in assays where structure may influence RNA function. An alternative strategy is to introduce a promoter immediately upstream and a convenient restriction site immediately distal to the cloned sequence either by means of mutagenesis or polymerase chain reaction (PCR). However, utilizing bacteriophage promoters may necessarily require the alteration of the 5' sequence of a gene of interest since the +1–5 positions of such promoters affect their activity *(4,5)*. Where the sequences are relatively short it is also possible to transcribe from synthetic DNA oligonucleotides (reviewed in **ref. *6***). The T7 and SP6 polymerases differ in a number of ways; whereas the yield from transcription with SP6 is little affected by template length, the yield from a T7 promoter is roughly proportional to length of the template. In addition, SP6 has a higher requirement for $Mg^{2+}$ (approx 4 m*M* above the sum of rNTP concentrations, whereas the optimum for T7 is equal to the sum of the rNTPs *[7]*). Recent reports have also shown that inorganic pyrophosphatase enhances the transcription of short templates by bacteriophage polymerases *(8,9)* and reduces the dependence on $Mg^{2+}$ for both T7 and T3 polymerase. Similarly pyrophosphatase appears to reduce the rNTP concentration optimum for SP6 and T3 polymerases but not for T7. However, the yield from standard reactions is normally sufficient for the synthesis of the amount and quality of RNA necessary for the assays described here, and readers are referred to the aforementioned references if they wish to include pyrophosphatase in preparative reactions. One of the other major factors influencing the yield of RNA in preparative synthesis is the acidification of the reaction upon polymerization. Therefore, a necessary consideration is the capacity of the buffer used and this is an important change from the original protocols described *(2,3)*.

When radioactively labeling RNA to a high-specific activity, as required for northern blotting, filter-binding, or UV crosslinking, the primary consideration is no longer one of yield, but one of the maximal incorporation of the radiolabel, while maintaining the proportion of full-length transcript produced. Because these are opposing factors determined by the reaction conditions, a compromise is usually adopted where the specific activity of the labeled rNTP is maximized while maintaining its concentration above 12–24 µ*M*. Below this concentration, premature termination becomes an increasing problem as the availability of the rNTP becomes rate-limiting and this results in pausing and termination by the RNA polymerase.

### 1.2. UV Crosslinking of the EBV-Encoded Small RNAs EBER-1 and EBER-2 to the Double-Stranded RNA-Activated Protein Kinase (PKR)

Many nucleic acids function through the formation of complexes with proteins via specific intermolecular interactions. Following a variety of treatments the noncovalent interactions between the components of such macromolecules that are in direct contact can be converted into covalent bonds and the formation of such bonds can therefore be used in the experimental identification of the interacting components. Induced formation of covalent crosslinks may involve heavy metal, chemical, or photochemical activation of interacting components *(10,11)*.

Direct excitation of nucleotides or amino acids with short-wavelength UV light can generate chemically reactive species and the formation of covalent bonds between these species upon UV irradiation can be used to investigate the interaction between DNA/RNA and proteins. Most methods describing UV crosslinking are based on the conditions required to obtain the maximum specificity of crosslinking. Noncovalent interactions are determined by the chemical and hence the electronic structure of intact components. Activation leads to an alteration of the electronic structure of the component, resulting in disappearance of contacts existing prior to activation and the occurrence of new contacts. The principle factor determining the specificity of crosslink formation is the life time of the activated state. Radiational methods can lead to activated states of macromolecular components with lifetimes sufficiently short to permit formation of specific crosslinks. Using UV crosslinking, EBER-1 and -2 have been shown to interact with PKR. As with several methods involving photoreactive UV crosslinking, identification of proteins crosslinked with polynucleotides can be achieved by immunochemical methods. To aid analysis, radiolabeling of the DNA/RNA is often included because this can allow some degree of quantification of binding. Crosslinked complexes can also be resolved by sodium dodecyl sulfate-polyacrylamide gel electrophoresis (SDS-PAGE) *(12)* and the proteins covalently crosslinked to RNA then detected by autoradiography or phosphorimaging.

### 1.3. Filter Binding of the EBV-Encoded Small RNAs EBER-1 and EBER-2 to the Double-Stranded RNA-Activated Protein Kinase (PKR)

In the previous section, UV crosslinking was described as a method for investigating protein-RNA interactions, such as between the EBERs and PKR. Here a more quantitative method for analyzing this interaction is described *(13,14)*. Filter-binding assays have been widely used for assessing the binding of ligands to proteins, including small RNAs such as EBER-1 and EBER-2, the adenovirus-encoded $VA_I$ RNA and the human immunodeficiency virus-encoded transactivation-responsive region (TAR) RNA *(15–17)*. This method can be used to investigate the specificity of RNA-protein interactions, to demonstrate competition for binding between different RNA ligands, and to determine the dissociation constants of complexes by Scatchard analysis *(15–17)*.

Nitrocellulose filters are able to bind both protein and DNA under certain conditions. The binding properties of different types of membrane have allowed for the retention of proteins on such materials to be used as the basis for the aforementioned types of assays. Whereas RNA alone will not be retained by nitrocellulose based filters, when RNA-protein complexes are passed through such filters proteins retained on the membrane will form a bridge between the membrane and bound RNA *(18)*. By radioactively labeling the RNA prior to binding to a purified protein the interaction can be quantitated by scintillation counting. The background owing to unbound RNA is very low.

The specificity and competitiveness of binding can be investigated by incubation of a small excess of labeled RNA ligand with the protein in the presence of increasing amounts of unlabeled competitor RNA. In this way, the binding of different RNA ligands to identical or overlapping sites in a protein can be investigated. Conversely, Scatchard analysis may be carried out by incubating a limiting fixed amount of protein with increasing concentrations of labeled RNA. After subtraction of nonspecific background binding (measured in the presence of an excess of the respective unlabeled RNA) the data can be used to calculate dissociation constants for the RNA-protein complexes, by plotting bound/free against bound radioactivity and measuring the slope of the plot *(15)*.

### 1.4. PKR Autophosphorylation Assay

PKR is activated when it is incubated with low concentrations of dsRNA, e.g., 0.1–1 μg/mL poly(I):poly(C), and the active kinase can then phosphorylate the α subunit of eukaryotic protein synthesis initiation factor eIF2 and possibly other substrates (reviewed in **ref.** *19*). The activation process itself is independent of substrate, but requires an autophosphorylation step that involves at least seven different serine and threonine residues in PKR. Several species of virally encoded RNAs are known to inhibit the kinase (reviewed in **refs.** *20* and *21*) including the EBV gene product EBER-1 (reviewed in **ref.** *22*). The precise mechanism by which these RNAs inhibit PKR is not fully understood, but the autophosphorylation assay described here can help us analyze this process further.

### 1.5. Effects of EBER RNA on Protein Synthesis in the Reticulocyte Lysate System

The rabbit reticulocyte lysate system has been used extensively to study the regulation of initiation of protein synthesis *(23)*. Reticulocyte lysates contain endogenous mRNAs, coding mainly for α and β globin, which under suitable conditions may be translated. The system may also be used to translate exogenous mRNAs by treating lysates with micrococcal nuclease, although this will not be considered here *(23)*. Early studies on the regulation of protein synthesis identified phosphorylation of the α subunit of initiation factor eIF2 as a major control point *(24)*. Two protein kinases involved in this phosphorylation are present in reticulocyte lysates. One called HCR (heme-controlled repressor) becomes active if hemin is absent during the incubation at 30°C (*see* **Note 1**); however the second, PKR, is more relevant here since this renders the reticulocyte lysate extremely sensitive to RNA with a high degree of secondary structure *(19)*. The synthetic dsRNA poly (I):poly (C) activates PKR at low concentrations but inhibits the enzyme at high concentrations, resulting in the characteristic bell-shaped curve that defines PKR activity. Several small viral RNAs such as EBER-1, $VA_I$, and TAR have been shown to prevent the activation of PKR and so the inhibition of protein synthesis observed in the presence of dsRNA *(21,25,26)*. The reticulocyte lysate is therefore an excellent eukaryotic system to characterize the regulation of protein synthesis by small RNAs such as the EBERs.

## 2. Materials

### 2.1. In Vitro Transcription

1. 2X reaction buffer (*see* **Note 2**):
   For T7 polymerase: 400 m*M* HEPES-KOH, pH 7.6, 14 m*M* of each rNTP (*see* **Note 3**), 56 m*M* $MgCl_2$, 4 m*M* spermidine, 80 m*M* dithiothreitol (DTT).

For SP6 polymerase: 240 m*M* HEPES-KOH, pH 7.6, 10 m*M* of each rNTP (*see* **Note 3**), 48 m*M* $MgCl_2$, 4 m*M* spermidine, 80 m*M* DTT.

For T3 polymerase: 600 m*M* HEPES-KOH, pH 7.6, 14 m*M* of each rNTP (*see* **Note 3**), 64 m*M* $MgCl_2$, 4 m*M* spermidine, 80 m*M* DTT.

2. 100 mg/mL acetylated bovine serum albumin (BSA) (*see* **Note 4**).
3. RNase inhibitor (*see* **Note 5**).
4. Linearized template: 1 mg/mL DNA (*see* **Note 6**).
5. Bacteriophage RNA polymerase (100,000 U/mL).
6. Labeled rNTP (*see* Notes 3 and 7).
7. RNase-free DNase I (10,000 U/mL).
8. 0.5 *M* EDTA.
9. 3 *M* sodium acetate, pH 5.2.
10. 20 mg/mL glycogen (molecular biology grade).
11. Isopropanol.
12. Ethanol.
13. Diethyl pyrocarbonate (DEPC)-treated water.

## 2.2. UV Crosslinking of RNA-Protein Complexes

1. $^{32}P$-labeled RNA (*see* **Note 8**).
2. 1 *M* KCl.
3. 100 m*M* Tris-HCl, pH 7.5.
4. Test protein (*see* **Note 9**).
5. Source of UV radiation such as an 8 W germicidal lamp of 254-nm wavelength (Steril-Air G-9) or similar.
6. 24-well plate (2 $cm^2$ wells, Nunc).
7. 10% (w/v) N-laurylsarcosine.
8. 10 Kunze U/µL RNase T1, 10 mg/mL RNase A.

## 2.3. Filter Binding

1. $^{32}P$-labeled RNA (*see* **Note 8**).
2. 2.5 *M* KCl.
3. 100 m*M* Tris-HCl, pH 7.6.
4. 1 *M* magnesium acetate.
5. Test protein (*see* **Note 10**).
6. Wash buffer: 10 m*M* Tris-HCl, pH 7.6, 75 m*M* KCl, 0.8 m*M* magnesium acetate.
7. 0.45 µm HATF nitrocellulose filters or a Millititre HA™ 96-well filtration plate (Millipore).
8. Millipore filtration unit.
9. Millipore punch unit (*see* **Note 11**).
10. Organic scintillation fluid.
11. Beta scintillation counter.

## 2.4. PKR Autophosphorylation Assay

1. Purified PKR is prepared in PKR buffer: 20 m*M* Tris-HCl, pH 7.6, 10 m*M* 2-mercapto-ethanol, 10% (v/v) glycerol, 0.1 m*M* EGTA, 0.1 m*M* EDTA, 200 m*M* KCl. PKR can be purified from a number of different sources such as ribosomal salt wash from reticulocytes *(26)*, liver *(15,27)*, or interferon-treated HeLa cells *(28,29)*.

2. Biorad Mini-Protean™ II gel electrophoresis apparatus or equivalent. For materials and methods for SDS-PAGE, *see* Chapter 24.
3. 5X Incubation buffer: 50 m*M* Tris-HCl, pH 7.6, 50% (v/v) glycerol, 250 µ*M* EDTA, 10 m*M* $MgCl_2$, 10 m*M* $MnCl_2$ , 250 m*M* NaF. This buffer can be made in advance, frozen, and stored at –20°C.
4. 4X Incubation buffer (made fresh on the day): Take 95 µL of the above 5X incubation buffer, add 5 µL of 500 µ*M* ATP, then take 20 µL of this and add 5 µL of $\gamma^{32}$P-ATP (4500 Ci/mmol, 10 µCi/µL) (*see* **Note 7**).
5. Radiolabeled molecular weight markers.
6. Whatman 3 MM paper.
7. Gel dryer.

### 2.5. Reticulocyte Lysate Protein Synthesis Assay

1. Reticulocyte lysates can be prepared from reticulocytes isolated from rabbits made anemic with acetylphenylhydrazine (*see* **Notes 1**, **12**, and **13**).
2. 5X Salts-amino acids-energy mix: 0.375 *M* KCl, 15 m*M* glucose, 5 m*M* ATP, 50 m*M* Tris-HCl, pH 7.6, 10 m*M* Mg acetate, 0.25–1.0 m*M* amino acids (*see* **Note 14**), 1 m*M* GTP, 20 µCi/mL [$^{14}$C] leucine (20–30 mCi/mmol), or up to 2.5 mCi/mL [$^{35}$S] methionine (ca. 1200 Ci/mmol). This can be made up in advance, frozen, and stored at –20°C; however, one must bear in mind that the half-life of [$^{35}$S]-methionine is 3 mo (*see* **Note 15**).
3. 10X Creatine phosphate-creatine phosphokinase: 70 m*M* creatine phosphate, 10 mg/mL creatine phosphokinase (*see* **Note 16**).
4. Hemin stock solution: Dissolve 6.5 mg of hemin in 0.25 mL of 1 *M* KOH. Add in order, mixing after each addition: 0.5 mL of 0.2 *M* Tris-HCl, pH 7.8, 8.9 mL of ethylene glycol, 0.25 mL of 1 *M* HCl. Store at –20°C. The final concentration of hemin is 1 m*M*.
5. Whatman No. 1 filter paper discs of 2.5 cm diameter.
6. TCA: 10% and 5% (w/v) Trichloroacetic acid in aqueous solutions.
7. Absolute ethanol.
8. Acetone.
9. Aluminium foil.
10. Toluene-based scintillation fluid.
11. A constant temperature bath or heating block for incubating the translation reactions at 30°C.

## 3. Methods

### 3.1. In Vitro Transcription

#### 3.1.1. Preparative Transcription

1. At room temperature add the following, in the order given, to a microcentrifuge tube containing a 50 µL aliquot of the appropriate 2X reaction buffer: $H_2O$ sufficient for the final volume to reach 100 µL, acetylated BSA to 100 µg/mL, RNase inhibitor to 200 U/mL (*see* **Note 15**).
2. Add the linearized template (*see* **Note 6**) to a final concentration of 3–30 µg/mL (for SP6 or T3 RNA polymerases) or 10–50 µg/mL (for T7 RNA polymerase), i.e., 0.2–3 µL (*see* **Note 17**).
3. Warm to 37 °C and add the polymerase to a final concentration of 1000 U/mL (*see* **Note 17**) and incubate at 37°C (*see* **Note 18**) for 2 h.
4. Add 5 µL (50 U) of DNase I and incubate at 37°C for a further 30 min.

5. Add 5 µL of 0.5 *M* EDTA, 10 µL of 3 *M* sodium acetate, pH 5.2, 1 µL of 20 mg/mL glycogen, mix, and then add 70 µL of isopropanol. Leave at room temperature for 20 min and then centrifuge at 15,000*g* for 20 min at 4°C.
6. Remove the supernatant and carefully add 500 µL of 70% (v/v) cold ethanol and re-centrifuge as mentioned.
7. Remove the supernatant and resuspend the pellet in 50 µL of DEPC-treated $H_2O$.

### *3.1.2. Transcription of Labeled RNA*

1. At room temperature add the following, in the order given, to a microcentrifuge tube containing a 10 µL aliquot of the appropriate 2X reaction buffer containing an appropriate radiolabeled rNTP, e.g., [$\alpha^{32}$P]UTP, for a labeling reaction: $H_2O$ sufficient for the final volume to be 20 µL, acetylated BSA to 100 µg/mL, RNase inhibitor to 200 U/mL (*see* **Note 15**).
2. Add the linearized template to a final concentration of 3–30 µg/mL (for SP6 or T3 RNA polymerases) or 10–50 µg/mL (for T7 RNA polymerase), i.e., 0.2–3 µL (*see* **Note 17**).
3. Warm to 37°C and add the polymerase to a final concentration of 1000 U/mL (*see* **Note 17**) and incubate at 37°C (*see* **Note 18**) for 1 h.
4. Add 5 µL (50 U) of DNase I and incubate at 37°C for a further 30 min.
5. Add 5 µL of 0.5 *M* EDTA, 10 µL of 3 *M* sodium acetate, pH 5.2, 1 µL of 20 mg/mL glycogen, mix, and then add 70 µL of isopropanol. Leave at room temperature for 20 min and then centrifuge at 15,000*g* for 20 min at 4°C.
6. Remove the supernatant and carefully add 500 µL of 70% (v/v) cold ethanol and re-centrifuge as noted.
7. Remove the supernatant and resuspend the pellet in 50 µL or an appropriate volume of DEPC-treated $H_2O$.

## *3.2. UV Crosslinking*

1. To a 0.5-mL Eppendorf tube add $10^5$cpm of $^{32}$P-labeled RNA, 80–100 m*M* KCl (*see* **Note 19**), 10 m*M* Tris-HCl, pH 7.5, and the appropriate amount of PKR (*see* **Note 9**), in a final volume of 25 µL.
2. Incubate at 30°C for 30 min.
3. While the reaction is incubating, prepare an ice bucket containing a heaped amount of ice and cover with aluminium foil, such that the foil is in contact with the ice.
4. On top of the foil pre-chill a 24-well multiwell plate.
5. Transfer the reaction to one of the wells (*see* **Note 20**).
6. Crosslink the RNA to the protein by irradiating the reaction at 254 nm using an 8 W germicidal lamp for 5 min (*see* **Note 21**), at a distance of 4 cm (*see* **Note 22**).
7. Transfer the crosslinked samples into 0.5-mL Eppendorf tubes and add N-laurylsarcosine to a final concentration of 0.5% (w/v) (*see* **Note 23**).
8. Add 20 U of RNase T1 and 10 µg of RNase A and digest for 1 h at 37°C (*see* **Notes 24** and **25**).
9. Add 25 µL of 2X electrophoresis buffer to each sample and resolve the crosslinked complexes by electrophoresis on a 12.5% SDS polyacrylamide gel (for SDS-PAGE see Chapter 26).
10. Detect proteins covalently crosslinked to RNA by autoradiography or phosphorimaging.

## *3.3. Filter Binding Assay*

1. Add the test protein in 10 m*M* Tris-HCl, pH 7.6, 100–150 m*M* KCl, 0.8 m*M* magnesium acetate to the appropriate RNA ($10^5$ cpm). Water is used to bring the final volume to 25 µL.

2. Incubate the reaction for 15 min at 30°C (*see* **Note 26**).
3. Pipet 20 µL of each sample on to 0.45 µm HATF nitrocellulose filters or a Millititre HA 96-well filtration plate™ (Millipore) that has been pre-washed with 75 µL of wash buffer.
4. Filter the samples under vacuum (*see* **Note 27**).
5. Wash each filter three times with 300 µL of wash buffer.
6. Remove the Millititre plate from the vacuum apparatus and allow to dry.
7. Punch out each disc from the plate into a scintillation vial and add 3 mL of organic scintillation fluid to each (*see* **Note 28**).
8. Determine the bound radioactivity in a beta scintillation counter.

### 3.4. PKR Autophosphorylation Assay

1. Set up a 12.5% (w/v) polyacrylamide gel (*see* **Note 29** and Chapter 26) in a Bio-Rad Mini-protean™ II apparatus using 0.75-mm spacers. Pour a stacking gel about 1 h before loading the samples from the autophosphorylation assay. Wash the wells out thoroughly with running buffer before loading the samples.
2. For each incubation (final volume 20 µL) mix the following components on ice in a sterile microfuge tube (*see* **Note 30**): 10 µL of purified PKR (*see* **Note 31**), 5 µL of 4X incubation buffer, 5 µL of water, and/or dsRNA and/or test RNA (*see* **Note 32**).
3. Incubate this mix at 30°C for 20 min.
4. Add 20 µL of 2X SDS sample buffer to stop the reaction.
5. Heat the samples for 2 min at 95°C.
6. Load 10–15 µL onto a 12.5% (w/v) SDS gel (*see* **Note 32**).
7. Run the gel at 100 volts until the bromophenol blue dye has just run off the bottom.
8. Carefully remove the glass plates from the gel, place a piece of Whatman 3MM paper (cut to cover the gel) on one side of the gel and a piece of Saran wrap on the other.
9. Dry the gel in a gel dryer.
10. Place the dried gel into a cassette with X-ray film or a screen for autoradiography or phosphorimaging, respectively (*see* **Note 33**).

### 3.5. Reticulocyte Lysate Protein Synthesis Assay

1. For each incubation (final volume 100 µL), mix the following components carefully on ice in a sterile microfuge tube: 50 µL of reticulocyte lysate (*see* **Notes 12** and **13**), 20 µL of 5X salts-amino acids-energy mix, 10 µL of 10X creatine phosphate-creatine phosphokinase, 20 µL of water, hemin stock solution, dsRNA, and/or test RNA (*see* **Note 34**).
2. Incubate reaction mix at 30°C.
3. Pipet 10 µL aliquots from the reaction mix on to Whatman No. 1 filter paper discs after 0, 5, 10, 20, 30, 45, and 60 min (*see* **Note 35**).
4. Place the discs into a beaker containing 200 mL of 10% (w/v) TCA and wash them by swirling gently for 15 min.
5. Transfer the discs to 200 mL of 5% (w/v) TCA at 90°C and incubate at this temperature for 15 min (*see* **Note 36**).
6. Transfer the discs to fresh 5% (w/v) TCA at room temperature and wash them by swirling gently.
7. Wash the discs successively in excess absolute ethanol and then acetone with gentle swirling, each for about 1 min.
8. Allow the discs to dry at room temperature on aluminium foil.
9. Place each disc in a vial or vial insert and determine the radioactivity using toluene-based scintillation fluid.

## 4. Notes

1. The incorporation of radiolabeled amino acid into protein should show linear kinetics for up to 60 min when 10–20 μ*M* hemin is present in the reaction. The concentration of poly(I):poly(C) which causes maximum inhibition of protein synthesis (usually 0.1–1 μg/mL) in the presence of the optimal hemin concentration should also be determined when regulation of PKR activity is being studied.
2. Stocks of 2X buffer can be made in advance and stored as aliquots at –20°C.
3. When preparing buffers for labeling reactions the concentration of the labeled rNTP must be significantly reduced from that stated for preparative transcriptions. Because the specific activity of an RNA made by in vitro transcription is proportional to the specific activity of the labeled ribonucleotide in the reaction, usually UTP, this is maximized by reducing the concentration of the unlabeled UTP present. However, the yield of full-length transcript decreases drastically as the concentration of any one nucleotide becomes rate-limiting, normally around 12–24 μ*M*. As it is usual to add 50–60 μCi of $\alpha^{32}$P-labeled UTP to a 20 μL reaction volume, it is necessary to supplement the labeled ribonucleotide with unlabeled UTP in the reaction buffer. Because 50 μCi of UTP with a specific activity of 3000 Ci/mmol added to a 20 μL reaction volume gives a concentration of 0.8 μ*M*, the 2X buffer used for the transcription should contain 24–48 μ*M* unlabeled UTP and a minimum of 2.5–3 m*M* for all other rNTPs. It is therefore recommended that the specific activity of the label is borne in mind when determining the composition of the 2X buffer used. An alternative is to omit the UTP altogether from the reaction buffer and use a low specific activity label such as 100 μCi at 400 Ci/mmol.
4. BSA was shown by Melton et al. *(3)* to increase the activity of SP6 polymerase more than twofold. However the advantage of including BSA under the different conditions used here has not been tested. We do not find it necessary routinely to include acetylated BSA in transcriptions.
5. RNase inhibitors can also be routinely included in transcription reactions but are rarely necessary providing care is taken in handling stock solutions, enzymes, etc. Another precautionary measure taken in the preparation of buffers and solutions is DEPC treatment wherever possible. DEPC treatment of buffers can be carried out by the addition of DEPC to 0.1% (v/v). However, Tris-HCl buffers are not compatible with DEPC, nor are heat-labile compounds, because it is necessary subsequently to autoclave a solution following the addition of DEPC. The treated solution should be vigorously mixed, allowed to stand at room temperature for longer than 12 h and then autoclaved. Compounds incompatible with DEPC should be made up with DEPC-treated water.
6. Templates should be linearized with an appropriate restriction enzyme, the product checked to ensure complete digestion, and the reaction stopped. It is advisable that the DNA is cleaned up by phenol/chloroform extraction, precipitated and resuspended at 1 mg/mL in 10 m*M* Tris-HCl, pH 8.0, 1 m*M* EDTA. Enzymes leaving 3' overhangs should be avoided wherever possible because they tend to cause nontemplate-dependent 3' additions to the transcribed RNA *(3)*. Where these cannot be avoided, it may be advisable to blunt-end the DNA prior to transcription. If a stock of the linearized DNA is to be retained it should be heat-denatured and rapidly cooled from time to time to prevent re-annealing of sticky ends upon repeated freeze thawing.
7. All radioactivity should be handled using safe practice and disposed of in accordance with local health and safety regulations.
8. EBER-1 is synthesized in vitro by transcription of linearized plasmid with T7 RNA polymerase *(15,25,26)* in the presence of [$\alpha^{32}$P]UTP using standard transcription conditions

(*see* **Subheading 1.1.**). For crosslinking purposes RNA must be labeled to a high specific activity (ca. $10^4$ cpm/ng RNA; $10^5$ cpm per reaction).

9. The amount of protein to be used will be determined by the purity of the preparation and the source; for example, around 60 µg of reticulocyte lysate can be used as an enriched source of PKR. It is always essential that a concentration range of PKR is used in crosslinking in order to establish optimum binding. In competition assays the molar concentration of PKR must be kept less than that of the labeled ligand such that any addition of unlabeled ligand will result in competition for binding to the target protein.
10. The amount of protein to be used will be determined by the purity of the preparation and the source. The preparation should not contain other proteins that will also bind the ligand. (*See* **Note 9** concerning competition assays.)
11. Punching out the filters can also be done manually using a cork borer.
12. Reticulocyte lysates are commercially available (e.g., from Ambion Inc. Austin, Texas or Promega Corp., Madison). However they are prohibitively expensive for use in large quantities. Each batch of lysate should be characterized for its response to hemin and dsRNA (*see* **Subheading 1.5.**). Some commercial lysates may contain additives which prevent inhibition by dsRNA.
13. Repeated freeze thawing reduces the translational activity of reticulocyte lysates; therefore, lysates should be frozen in small aliquots and stored in liquid nitrogen where they will remain active for at least 2 yr.
14. An amino acid mixture (50X stock) that reflects the composition of globin is prepared in advance as follows: Mix 0.38 mL of 20 m*M* Ala, 0.09 mL of 20 m*M* Arg, 0.07 mL of 100 m*M* Asn, 0.54 mL of 20 m*M* Asp, 0.2 mL of 100 m*M* Gly, 0.07 mL of 100 m*M* Gln, 0.34 mL of 20 m*M* Glu, 0.44 mL of 20 m*M* His, 0.06 mL of 20 m*M* Ile, 0.75 mL of 20 m*M* Leu, 0.27 mL of 20 m*M* Lys, 0.06 mL of 20 m*M* Met, 0.3 mL of 20 m*M* Phe, 0.26 mL of 20 m*M* Pro, 0.32 mL of 20 m*M* Ser, 0.32 mL of Thr, 0.05 mL of 20 m*M* Trp, 0.15 mL of 20 m*M* Tyr, and 0.58 mL of 20 m*M* Val. Then add water to make a final volume of 5 mL. This is diluted 10-fold into the 5X salts-amino acids-energy mix.
15. Before use check that components of the reaction buffer have not precipitated out of solution; spermidine and DTT are particularly prone to this upon storage of the stock at –20°C. DNA is also prone to precipitation in the presence of spermidine upon addition to the reaction, especially if the components are added while on ice or in the wrong order.
16. It is sufficient to add a few crystals of creatine phosphokinase to 1 mL of 70 m*M* creatine phosphate in water.
17. DNA concentrations for normal transcription conditions are 3–30 µg/mL (for SP6 or T3 RNA polymerases) or 10–50 µg/mL (for T7 RNA polymerase). In practice a concentration of 10–30 µg/mL of template is used irrespective of the polymerase, depending on the size of the vector and the transcription unit. This amount can be increased to as much as 50 µg/mL when higher amounts of enzyme (1500 U/mL) are added to maximize yield. For most purposes however, the small increase in yield obtained by increasing the enzyme concentration does not normally warrant the use of additional polymerase.
18. Krieg ***(30)*** has suggested that lowering the temperature leads to a decrease in premature termination in T7, T3, and SP6 labeling reactions. However this work adopted the traditional Tris-HCl-buffered conditions and very low concentrations of UTP (5 µ*M*). Since the concentration recommended in the labeling reaction described earlier is at least 12–24 µ*M* UTP (*see* **Note 3**), premature termination should not normally be a problem and the lowering of the temperature should therefore not be necessary. Although Gurevich et al. *(7)* found that a decrease in the temperature to 30°C had little effect on yield, in preparative

scale reactions a further decrease to 25°C decreased the yield by twofold and it is therefore not recommended to reduce the temperature in preparative scale reactions. Indeed Pokrovskaya and Gurevich *(9)* found that within a narrow range of temperatures (37–42°C) T7 and T3 polymerases show little effect on preparative yield at different rNTP concentrations. However, the yield from SP6 polymerase is greatest at 41°C for the higher concentration of rNTPs used in the preparative reaction conditions. Under the conditions described for preparative transcription the rate of RNA synthesis falls by approx half in each subsequent hour.

19. Remember to take into account the amount of KCl in the protein source when calculating the final KCl concentration in the reaction.
20. Take care to pipet the entire volume in one drop. Spreading the drop out makes recovery of the sample more difficult and subject to greater losses in the well. By keeping the sample in one drop, this problem is reduced.
21. It is always a good idea to do a time course of UV irradiation to determine optimal time for crosslinking to occur. Excessive periods of UV irradiation result in many breakdown products and artifactual crosslinks.
22. This distance may be achieved by directly balancing the outer casing surrounding the lamp on the outside of the multiwell plate, taking care not to disturb the samples in any of the wells.
23. N-laurylsarcosine is a detergent used to reduce aggregate formation in the reaction. Owing to its presence too vigorous mixing of the sample results in unnecessary bubbles; such bubbles can be removed by placing the tube at –70°C momentarily (until frozen) and then thawing the sample at 37°C.
24. Treatment of the crosslinked fragments with these RNases removes non-crosslinked RNA sequences.
25. At this stage, proteins in RNA-protein complexes may be identified via immunoprecipitation if appropriate antibodies are available *(26)*.
26. While reactions are incubating the Millititre HA 96-well filtration plate may be prepared by washing the filters with wash buffer under suction.
27. A tap-operated pump may not provide sufficient suction. In our laboratory, a GeneVac CVP rotary pump is used for this purpose.
28. Punching out the filters can be time-consuming as it requires precision and accuracy.
29. The 12.5% resolving gel can be made in advance, wrapped in Saran wrap, and stored in the fridge for several days.
30. The volume of purified PKR required in an assay will depend on the concentration and activity of the enzyme and will vary between preparations.
31. When less than 10 µL is necessary, PKR buffer should be added so that the concentrations of the components in the assay remain unchanged. The final concentrations in the assay are: 20 m*M* Tris-HCl, pH 7.6, 100 m*M* KCl, 15% glycerol, 2 m*M* $MgCl_2$, 2 m*M* $MnCl_2$, 0.1 m*M* EDTA, 50 µ*M* EGTA, 5 µ*M* $\gamma^{32}$P-ATP (50 µCi), 50 m*M* NaF, and 5 m*M* 2-mercaptoethanol.
32. PKR autophosphorylation should be totally dependent on dsRNA and the concentration of poly(I):poly(C) that gives maximum activation should be determined for each PKR preparation. Any test RNA that inhibits this activation, such as EBER-1, can then be studied. The stock test RNA and the synthetic dsRNA poly(I):poly(C) should be dissolved and stored in 50 m*M* KCl so that their secondary structure is maintained. It is also advisable to include a lane of radiolabeled molecular weight markers on each gel to confirm that the phosphorylated band runs at approx 68 kDa.

33. The use of a phosphorimager is highly recommended where possible because this provides a more rapid and sensitive method than autoradiography for detecting phosphorylated protein bands on dried gels. Phosphorimaging also permits more quantitative determination of the protein kinase activity of PKR. Autophosphorylation of PKR gives a labeled band that runs at approx 68 kDa on SDS gels. The phosphorylation of other PKR substrates, notably eIF2α (38 kDa), can also be assayed by the same approach.
34. Each time a protein synthesis experiment is carried out at least one incubation should serve as a control with no test RNA present, only its solvent, e.g., 50 m*M* KCl. The reticulocyte lysate should be thawed quickly in the hand or in a 30°C water bath. As soon as the lysate is thawed it should be kept on ice with the other components of the translational assay to avoid activating the eIF2α kinase HCR (*see* **Subheading 1.5.**). The 5X salts-amino acids-energy mix and the 10X creatine phosphate-creatine phosphokinase should be added to the lysate followed by the hemin (final concentration of 10–20 μ*M*), dsRNA, and/or the test RNA (or 50 m*M* KCl). It is worth noting that the lysate is viscous and so the components of the translation reaction should be mixed carefully. Air bubbles may impair mixing and can be removed by spinning the tubes for a few seconds in a microfuge. The stock test RNA and the synthetic dsRNA, poly(I):poly(C), should be dissolved and stored at –20°C in 50 m*M* KCl so that their secondary structure is maintained.
35. Pre-label 2.5-cm diameter Whatman No.1 filter paper discs with a pencil (not a pen).
36. Charged tRNA is hydrolyzed by placing the filter papers in a beaker containing 200 mL of hot 5% (w/v) TCA and then boiling this for 15 min. This procedure is hazardous and should be done on a hot plate in a fume cupboard.

## Acknowledgments

Research in this laboratory was funded by the Cancer Research Campaign, the Leukaemia Research Fund, the Wellcome Trust, and the Sylvia Reed Fund.

## References


1. Clemens, M. J. (1993) The small RNAs of Epstein-Barr virus. *Mol. Biol. Reports* **17,** 81–92.
2. Butler, E. T. and Chamberlin, M. J. (1982) Bacteriophage SP6-specific RNA polymerase. I. Isolation and characterisation of the enzyme. *J. Biol. Chem.* **257,** 5772–5778.
3. Melton, D. A., Krieg, P. A., Rebagliati, M. R., Maniatis, T., Zinn, K., and Green, M. R. (1984) Efficient in vitro synthesis of biologically active RNA and RNA hybridisation probes from plasmids containing a bacteriophage SP6 promoter. *Nucleic Acids Res.* **12,** 7035–7055.
4. Ikeda, R. A. Lin, A. C., and Clarke, J. (1992) Initiation by T7 RNA polymerase at its natural promoters. *J. Biol. Chem.* **267,** 2640–2649.
5. Kang, C., and Wu, C. W. (1987) Studies on SP6 promoter using a new plasmid vector that allows gene insertion at the transcription initiation site. *Nucleic Acids Res.* **15,** 2279–2294.
6. Milligan, J. F. and Uhlenbeck, O. C. (1989) Synthesis of small RNAs using T7 RNA polymerase. *Methods Enzymol.* **180,** 51–62.
7. Gurevich, V. V., Pokrovskaya, I. D., Obukhova, T. A., and Zozulya, S. A. (1991) Preparative in vitro mRNA synthesis using SP6 and T7 RNA polymerases. *Anal. Biochem.* **195,** 207–213.
8. Cunningham, P. R. and Ofengand, J. (1990) Use of inorganic pyrophosphatase to improve the yield of *in vitro* transcription reactions catalysed by T7 RNA polymerase. *Biotechniques* **9,** 713–714.

9. Pokrovskaya, I. D. and Gurevich, V. V. (1994) *In vitro* transcription: preparative RNA yields in analytical scale reactions. *Anal. Biochem.* **220,** 420–423.
10. Budowsky, E. I. and Abdurashidova, G. G. (1989) Polynucleotide-protein cross-links induced by ultraviolet light and their use for structural investigation of nucleoproteins. *Prog. Nucleic Acids Res.* **37,** 1–65.
11. Hanna, M. (1989) Photoaffinity cross-linking of RNA protein. *Methods Enzymol.* **180,** 383–409.
12. Laemmli, U. K. (1970) Cleavage of structural proteins during the assembly of the head of bacteriophage T4. *Nature* **227,** 680–685.
13. Gopalakrishna, R., Chen, Z. H., Gundimeda, U., Wilson, J. C, and Anderson, W. B., (1992) Rapid filtration assays for protein kinase C activity and phorbol ester binding using multiwell plates with fitted filtration disc. *Anal. Biochem.* **206,** 24–35.
14. Gopalakrishna, R., Gundimeda, U., Wilson, J. C, and Chen, Z. H., (1993) Multiwell filtration assay for rapid determination of protein phosphatase activity. *Anal. Biochem.* **212,** 296–299.
15. Sharp, T. V., Schwemmle, M., Jeffrey, I., Laing, K., Mellor, H., Proud, C. G., Hilse, and Clemens, M. J., (1993) Comparative analysis of the regulation of the interferon-inducible protein kinase PKR by Epstein-Barr virus RNAs EBER-I and EBER-II and adenovirus $VA_I$ RNA. *Nucleic Acids Res.* **21,** 4483–4490.
16. McCormack, S. J. and Samuel, C. E, (1995) Mechanism of interferon action: RNA-binding activity of full length and R domain forms of the RNA-dependent protein kinase PKR-determination of KD values for $VA_I$ and TAR RNAs. *Virology* **206,** 511–519.
17. Dingwall, C., Ernberg, I., Gait, M. R., Green, S. M., Heaphy, S., Karn, J., Lowe, A. D., Singh, M., Skinner, M. A., and Valerio, R. (1989) Human immunodeficiency virus 1 tat protein binds trans-activation-responsive region (TAR) RNA *in vitro. Proc. Natl. Acad. Sci.* **86,** 6925–6929.
18. Freifelder, D. (1982) Membrane filtration and dialysis, in *Physical Biochemistery: Applications to Biochemistry and Molecular Biology,* 2nd ed., WH Freeman and Co., San Francisco, pp. 193–203.
19. Clemens, M. J. and Elia, A. (1997) The Double-stranded RNA-dependent Protein kinase PKR: Structure and Function. *J. Interferon Cytokine Res.* **17,** 503–524.
20. Mathews, M. B. and Shenk, T. (1991) Adenovirus-associated RNA and translational control. *J. Virol.* **65,** 5657–5662.
21. Katze, M. G. (1992) The war against the interferon-induced dsRNA-activated protein kinase: Can viruses win? *J. Interferon Res.* **12,** 241–248.
22. Clemens, M. J., Laing, K., Jeffrey, I. W., Schofield, A., Sharp, T. V., Elia, A., et al. (1994) Regulation of the interferon-inducible eIF-2$\alpha$ protein kinase by small RNAs. *Biochimie* **76,** 770–778.
23. Clemens, M. J. (1984) Translation in Eukaryotic Messenger RNA in Cell-free extracts, in *Transcription and Translation: A Practical Approach.* (Hames, B.D. and Higgins, S. J., eds.), IRL Press, Oxford and Washington DC, pp. 231–270.
24. Farrell, P., Balkow, K., Hunt, T., Jackson, R., Trachsel, H., (1977) Phosphorylation of initiation factor eIF-2 and the control of reticulocyte protein synthesis. *Cell* **11,** 187–200.
25. Clarke, P. A., Sharp, N. A., and Clemens, M. J., (1990) Translational control by the Epstein-Barr virus small RNA EBER-1. *Eur. J. Biochem.* **193,** 635–641.
26. Clarke, P. A., Schwemmle, M., Schickinger, J., Hilse, K., and Clemens, M. J., (1991) Binding of Epstein-Barr virus small RNA EBER-1 to the double stranded RNA-activated protein kinase DAI. *Nucleic Acids Res.* **19,** 243–248.

27. Colthurst, D. R., Campbell, D. G. and Proud, C. G., (1987) Structure and regulation of eukaryotic initiation factor eIF-2. Sequence of the site in the alpha subunit phosphorylated by the haem-controlled repressor and by the double-stranded RNA-activated inhibitor. *Eur J. Biochem.* **166,** 357–363.
28. Kostura, M. and Mathews, M. B., (1989) Purification and activation of the double-stranded RNA-dependent eIF-2 kinase DAI. *Mol. Cell. Biol.* **9,** 1576–1586.
29. Elia, A., Laing, K. G., Schofield, A., Tilleray, V. J. and Clemens, M. J., (1996) Regulation of the double-stranded RNA-dependent protein kinase PKR by RNAs encoded by a repeated sequence in the Epstein-Barr virus genome. *Nucleic Acids Res.* **24,** 4471–4478.
30. Krieg, P. A. (1990) Improved synthesis of full-length RNA probe at reduced incubation temperatures. *Nucleic Acids Res.* **18,** 6463.

# VII

# Protein Activity Assays

# 34

## Chimeric and Mutated Variants of LMP1

### *A Helpful Tool to Analyze the Structure-Function Relationship of a Pseudoreceptor*

**Olivier Gires, Marius Ueffing, and Wolfgang Hammerschmidt**

### 1. Introduction

Epstein Barr virus (EBV) efficiently immortalizes human B cells in vitro generating lymphoblastoid cell lines (LCL) with indefinite lifespan. Latent membrane protein 1 (LMP1) belongs to a set of nine viral proteins expressed in vitro, five of which appear to be essential for B-cell immortalization (for review, *see* **ref.** ***1***). LMP1 is a membrane protein composed of a short cytoplasmic aminoterminus (24 residues), a transmembrane domain with six membrane-spanning segments separated by short reverse turns and a long cytoplasmic carboxy terminus (200 residues; *see* **Fig. 1**) ***(2–4)***. Genetic analysis has shown that LMP1 is indispensable but not sufficient for B-cell immortalization ***(5–7)***. In the last years the hypothesis was raised that LMP1 might act as a constitutively active receptor because it integrates into the plasma membrane and patches as an oligomer ***(3,8)***. This idea was further supported by LMP1's ability to bind molecules involved in the signaling cascade of the TNF-receptor family members ***(9–12)***. In analogy to known receptors such as CD40 or TNF-R2, LMP1 activates cellular transcription factors of the NFκB and AP-1 family ***(13–15)***. Transcriptional activation of target genes is supposed to play a key role in EBV-mediated immortalization as well as LMP1-mediated oncogenicity.

So far neither a ligand nor a ligand binding-site has been identified in LMP1, which is in line with the observation that LMP1 patches and signals in a constitutive fashion as an integral plasma membrane protein. The receptor hypothesis stated earlier was difficult to prove in a convincing experimental setting because LMP1 signaling seems to be constitutive. Furthermore, the contribution of different structural domains of LMP1 could only be studied by deletion and not by gain of function mutants. Several strategies have been adopted recently to overcome these obstacles. "One finger

From: *Methods in Molecular Biology, Vol. 174: Epstein-Barr Virus Protocols*
Edited by: J. B. Wilson and G. H. W. May © Humana Press Inc., Totowa, NJ

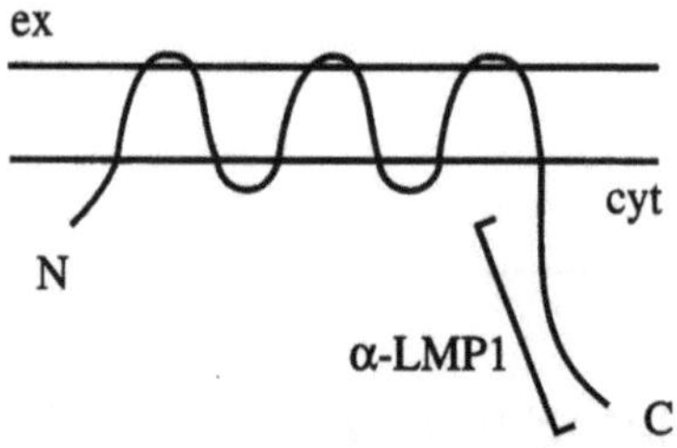


Fig. 1. Schematic representation of the wild-type LMP1 molecule. LMP1wt consists of a short amino terminus (24 AA), six transmembrane segments separated by short reverse turns and a long carboxy terminus (200 AA). Recognition site for the S12 αLMP1 antibody within the LMP1 molecule is annotated (αLMP1).

mutants" of LMP1 (**Fig. 2A**), which lack four of the six transmembrane segments and are defective in signaling, have been developed as epitope-tagged variants *(16)*. "One finger"-HA is a LMP1 variant that carries the hemaglutinin epitope between the fifth and sixth transmembrane segments such that it can be crosslinked from the outside of the cell using antibodies (**Fig. 2B**). "One finger"-3xFKBP12 includes a trimer of FKBP12 *(17)* at the C-terminus of "one finger LMP1" in order to crosslink it from within the cell with the aid of the dimerizing compound AP1510 (ARIAD Pharmaceuticals) (**Fig. 2C**). The signaling potential of these molecules can be assessed in crosslinking experiments after transient transfection or in stably transfected cell lines. Both crosslinkable variants clearly demonstrated that LMP1 needs to aggregate in the plasma membrane in order to transduce signals efficiently *(13,16)*. A second strategy that was useful to study the function of the transmembrane domain and the C-terminus of LMP1 separately was to construct chimeric receptors that fuse LMP1s functional domains with corresponding domains of cellular receptors in a combinatorial fashion. With this approach we generated hybrid molecules consisting of the cytoplasmic or transmembrane domain of LMP1 and the extracellular or cytoplasmic portion of heterologous receptors to obtain chimeric receptors (**Fig. 3A**). We could show that CD40 and TNF-R2 become constitutively activated receptors when their intracellular signaling domains were fused to the six transmembrane domains of LMP1 as in LMP1:CD40 and LMP1:TNF-R2 (**Fig. 3B**). In addition, co-immunoprecipitation studies with FLAG-tagged transmembrane domains of LMP1 (**Fig. 3C**) clearly demonstrated that aggregation is the function of the transmembrane part of the protein. On the other hand, hybrid molecules containing the C-terminus of LMP1 fused to the transmembrane and extracellular part of different cellular receptors (i.e., CD2, CD4, or NGF-R; **Fig. 3A**) behave like ligand-dependent, inducible receptors that signal after ligand induced crosslinking *(16)*.

Conditional LMP1 chimeras provide an important tool for the study of this pseudoreceptor. It is now technically feasible to investigate the signaling capacities of LMP1 in a conditional fashion with rapid activation kinetics for different cellular readouts. Materials and methods for the study of such chimeric molecules with specific focus on cellular and biochemical assays employing transient and stable gene expression of LMP1 mutants in two cell lines shall be described in the present chapter.

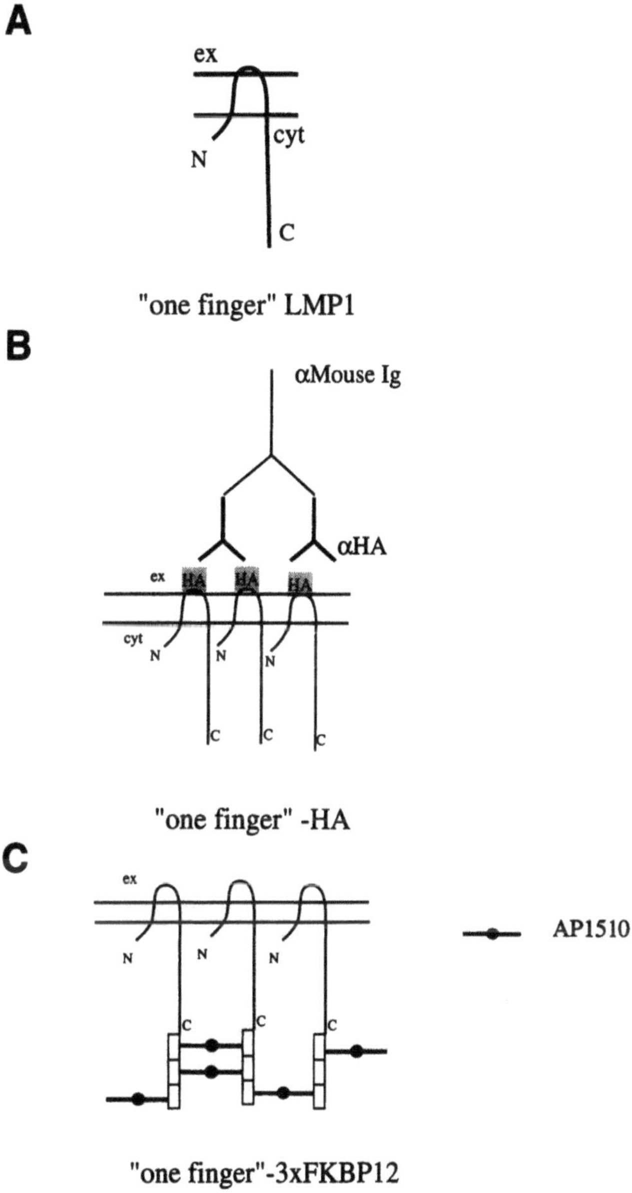


Fig. 2. Schematic representation of "one finger" LMP1 and its crosslinkable variants. (**A**) "one finger" LMP1 lacks transmembrane segments one to four of LMP1wt. (**B**) "One finger" LMP1-HA carries an additional hemaglutinin epitope between the fifth and sixth transmembrane segments, which protrudes into the extracellular space. "One finger"-HA can be crosslinked by the addition of αHA and secondary antibody into the culture medium. (**C**) "One finger"-3xFKBP12 is a fusion of a trimer of FKBP12 *(17)* at the carboxy terminus of "one finger" LMP1. Cross-linking of "one finger"-3xFKBP12 is achieved by the incubation of the transfected cells with the dimerizing compound AP1510.

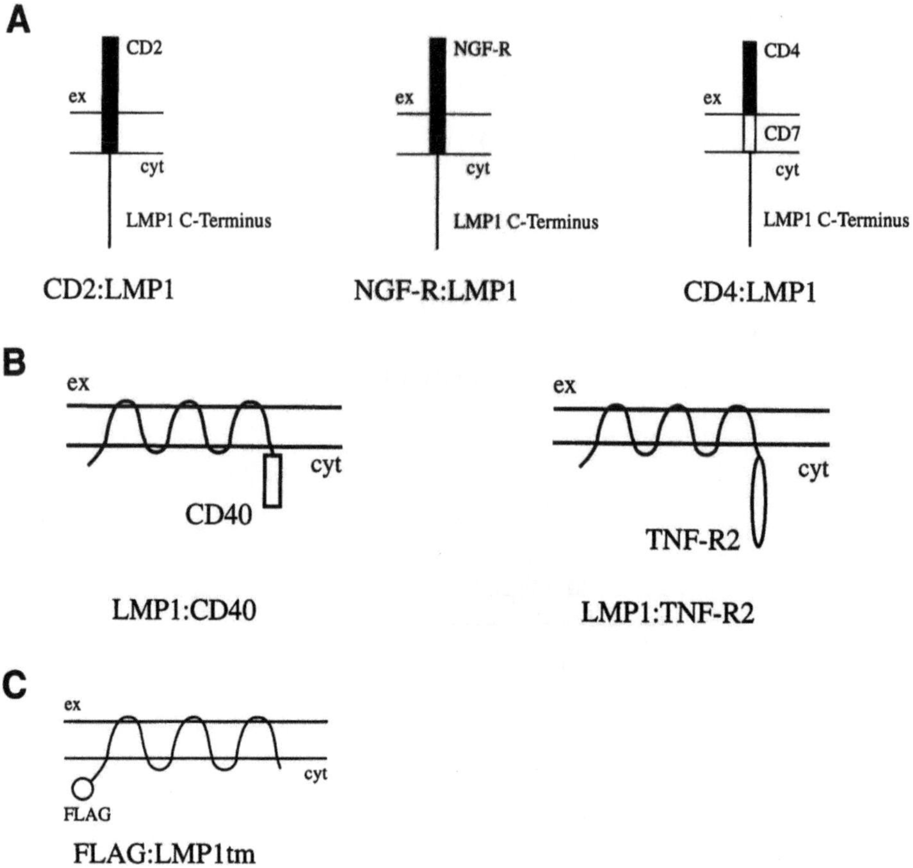


Fig. 3. Schematic representation of chimeric and tagged LMP1 molecules. **(A)** Chimera containing the signalling carboxyterminus of LMP1 fused to the extracellular and transmembrane domain of CD2, CD4:CD7 or NGF-R are depicted in the plasma membrane. These molecules can be crosslinked by incubation of the transfected cells with antibodies directed against the extracellular domain together with secondary antibody. **(B)** Hybrids containing the transmembrane domain of LMP1 fused to the signalling carboxyterminus of CD40 or TNF-R2 are depicted in the plasma membrane. Both LMP1:CD40 and LMP1:TNF-R2 are constitutively active receptors. **(C)** FLAG:LMP1tm lacks the entire carboxyterminus but carries an additional FLAG epitope at the aminoterminus. FLAG:LMP1tm can be immunoprecipitated using immobilized αFLAG antibodies.

## 2. Materials

### 2.1. Cell lines and Culture

1. Cell lines: EREB2-5 *(18)* is an EBV-immortalized B-cell line carrying a conditional EBNA2 gene. 293 cells are human embryonic kidney derived cells with an epitheloid phenotype *(19)*.

2. Supplemented RPMI: RPMI medium (GibcoBRL) supplemented with 10% fetal calf serum (FCS; Gibco BRL) and supplemented with 1 μ*M* of estrogen (Boehringer) for EREB2-5 cells only.
3. Dishes: 6-well plates, 96-well plates, 90-mm dishes.

### 2.2. Transfection Material, Plasmids, and Crosslinking Reagents

1. Lipofectamin (Gibco BRL).
2. Optimem 1 (Life Technologies, Gibco BRL).
3. Gene pulser (Biorad) or equivalent.
4. 4-mm electroporation cuvets.
5. Carrier DNA: Salmon testes DNA (Sigma).
6. Plasmid DNAs. a) Reporter gene plasmids: NFκB reporter *(15,16)* and AP1 reporter *(13)* plasmids. b) Expression vectors: LMP1wt (**Fig. 1**), "one finger LMP1" (**Fig 2A**; lacks the segments 1 to 4 of the transmembrane domain), "one finger"-HA (**Fig. 2B**; a variant of "one finger" carrying an HA epitope between the fifth and sixth transmembrane segment), "one finger"-3xFKBP12 (**Fig. 2C**; a trimer of FKBP12 fused to "one finger" LMP1 at its C-terminus), CD2:LMP1, CD4:CD7:LMP1, and NGF-R:LMP1 (chimera composed of the extracellular/transmembrane domains of CD2, CD4:CD7 or NGF-R fused to the carboxyterminus of LMP1; **Fig. 3A**), LMP1:CD40 (the amino/transmembrane domain of LMP1 fused to the carboxyterminus of CD40; **Fig. 3B**), LMP1:TNF-R2 (the amino/transmembrane domain of LMP1 fused to the carboxyterminus of TNF-R2; **Fig. 3B**), FLAG:LMP1tm (the amino and transmembrane domains of LMP1; **Fig. 3C**), Membrane anchor (based on the plasmid pCMF2E (ARIAD Pharmaceuticals), which was linearized with *Spe*I. A third FKBP12 unit was cloned into pCMF2E to obtain a trimer of FKBP12; **Fig. 4**), 3xFKBP12-LMP1 (a trimer of FKBP12 fused N-terminally to the carboxyterminus of LMP1; **Fig. 4A**), LMP1-3xFKBP12 (the carboxyterminus of LMP1 fused C-terminally to a trimer of FKBP12; **Fig. 4B**). All plasmid expression vectors are based on the episomal vector pHEBo which carries the Epstein-Barr Virus Nuclear Antigen 1 (EBNA1) that confers stable presence of the plasmid in primate cells *(20)*, except when mentioned otherwise.
7. Primary antibodies: murine αHA (Boehringer), αCD2, αCD4, and αNGF-R antibodies.
8. Secondary antibodies: αMouse Ig (Dianova).
9. Phosphate-buffered saline (PBS): 0.137 *M* NaCl, 2.7 m*M* KCl, 5.4 m*M* $Na_2HPO_4$, 1.8 m*M* $KH_2PO_4$. Adjust pH to 7.4 and filter through a 0.2-μ filter.
10. AP1510 dimerizer (ARIAD Pharmaceuticals).
11. Hygromycin.

### 2.3. Luciferase and MTT Assays

1. Lysis buffer: 100 m*M* $K_2HPO_4$, 1 m*M* DTT, 1% Triton X-100.
2. Test buffer: 25 m*M* glycylglycin, pH 7.8, 5 m*M* rATP, 15 m*M* $MgSO_4$.
3. d-Luciferin (USB).
4. MicroLumat (EG&G Berthold) or equivalent luminometer.
5. 96-well plates or test tubes adequate for the luminometer in use.
6. MTT reagent: 3-[4,5-Dimethylthiazol-2-yl]-2,5-diphenyltetrazolium bromide, EEC No. 206-069-5.
7. Superoxide dismutase (Sigma, cat # S2515).

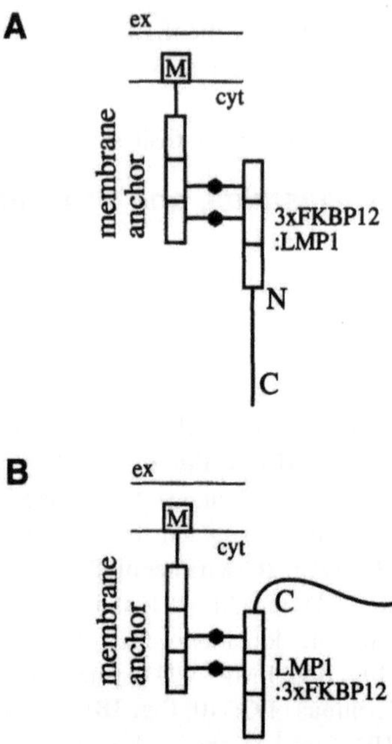


Fig. 4. Membrane targeting of the carboxyterminus of LMP1 using a myristoylated trimer of FKBP12. A myristoylated sequence carrying a trimer of FKBP12 can be used as an anchor for membrane targeting of proteins. Membrane targeting of either 3xFKBP12:LMP1 (**A**) or LMP1:3xFKBP12 (**B**) is induced by the addition of the dimerizing compound AP1510.

### 2.4. Immunoprecipitation of FLAG-Tagged LMP1

1. Buffer I (IP): 10 m*M* HEPES, pH 7.9, 10 m*M* KCl, 1.5 m*M* $MgCl_2$, 0.1 m*M* EGTA, 0.5 m*M* DTT, filter the buffer and add 0.5 m*M* PMSF fresh from 100X stock.
2. Gauge $27G^{3/4}$ needles and syringes.
3. NP40.
4. IP lysis buffer: PBS, 0.5% NP40, 0.5 m*M* PMSF.
5. αFLAG M2 Affinity Gel (Scientific Imaging Systems Kodak, cat. # IB13020).
6. RIPA buffer: 150 m*M* NaCl, 20 m*M* Tris-HCl, pH 7.5, 1% Triton-X100, 1% NP40, 0.1% SDS, 0.5% deoxycholate, 0.5 m*M* PMSF.
7. 20X Tris-buffered saline (TBS): 100 mL 1 *M* Tris-HCl, pH 7.4, 150 mL 5 *M* NaCl, 20 mL EDTA, pH 8.0, add water to 500 mL.
8. Equipment and materials for SDS-PAGE and Western blotting (*see* Chapter 26).
9. Hybond C membrane (Amersham) or PVDF membrane (Millipore cat. No. IPUH 00010) or equivalent.
10. 20X TBS-T (Tris-buffered saline-Tween): 100 mL 1 *M* Tris-HCl, pH 7.4, 150 mL 5 *M* NaCl, 20 mL EDTA, pH 8.0, 10 mL Tween-20, add water to 500 mL.
11. Blocking buffer: 1% BSA in TBS-T.
12. αLMP1 Antibody: S12 biotinylated (DAKO).
13. Streptavidin-HRP (Amersham Life Science).
14. ECL system (Amersham Life Science).

## 3. Methods

### 3.1. Transient Transfection and Activation of Conditional Crosslinkable LMP1 Variants or Constitutively Active Chimera in 293 Cells

1. Seed 1–3 × $10^5$ cells in 6-well plates 1 d before transfection in supplemented RPMI. Cells should reach approx 50–70% confluency for transfection.
2. Remove the medium completely and replace with 1 mL of Optimem 1. Incubate for 2 h at 37°C.
3. Dilute the expression plasmid (for either inducible or crosslinkable LMP1 variant, or LMP1:CD40, LMP1:TNF-R2, maximally 0.5–1 µg) together with a reporter gene plasmid (50 ng) in 100 µL of Optimem 1. For comparative assays, equalize the total amount of DNA/Lipofectamin mixtures by adding carrier DNA, in order to avoid differences in transfection efficiencies (*see* **Notes 1** and **2**).
4. Dilute an adequate volume of Lipofectamin (with a ratio of 6 µL of Lipofectamin to 1 µg of DNA) in 100 µL Optimem 1. Mix both and allow micelle formation for 45 min. Carefully add the DNA mix dropwise into the well. Maintain the cells in Optimem 1 with the DNA mix for 4 h at 37°C before adding 2 mL of supplemented RPMI.
5. Cross-link LMP1 mutants 6–16 h after transfection: Add 1 µg of the primary antibody (αHA, αCD2, αCD4, or αNGF-R) in 2 mL of supplemented RPMI and mix well. Then add the secondary antibody (5 µg/2 mL of medium) into the well (*see* **Note 3**). For FKBP12 variants add 50 nM AP1510 dimerizer. LMP1:CD40 and LMP1:TNF-R2 hybrids are constitutively active (for details, *see* **Note 4**). Maintain the cells with the crosslinking agents for at least 6 h prior to harvesting.
6. Aspirate off the culture medium and suspend cells in PBS (1 mL/well) by pipetting the solution up and down, thereby removing the loosely adherent cells after transfection (*see* **Note 5**). Centrifuge cells at 1000*g* for 10 min.
7. Lyse the pelleted cells in 100 µL of lysis buffer, keep on ice.
8. Pellet membranes, nuclei, and cellular debris at 10,000–18,320*g* for 10 min.
9. Aliquot 10 µL of each sample in duplicate into a 96-well plate (for the MicroLumat) or a disposable test tube (other types of luminometers) and add 150 µL of Test buffer. Measure luciferase activity as a correlate for NFκB or AP-1 activity in a luminometer by adding 50 µL of d-Luciferine to each sample. Compare the induction ratio with mock transfected cells or cells that have been transfected with a corresponding control reporter plasmid lacking the transcription factor specific sites on its promoter ***(15)***.

### 3.2. Immunoprecipitation Assays Using Epitope-Tagged LMP1 Variants

1. Seed 1–3 × $10^6$ 293 cells into 90 mm culture dishes 1 d before transfection. Cells should reach approx 50–70% confluency for transfection. Remove the medium completely and culture the cells for 2 h with 6 mL of Optimem 1 medium at 37°C.
2. Dilute the expression plasmid for FLAG:LMP1 and LMP1wt or "one finger" mutant at 5 µg each in desired combinations in 100 µL of Optimem1. Dilute Lipofectamin (6 µL per 1 µg DNA) in 100 µL of Optimem I. Mix both and allow micelle formation for 45 min. Carefully add the DNA mix dropwise into the dishes. Culture the cells in Optimem 1 together with the DNA mix for 4 h before adding 10 mL of supplemented RPMI medium.
3. Aspirate off the culture medium and suspend cells in 5 mL of PBS by pipetting the solution up and down and thereby removing the loosely adherent cells 1 d after transfection (*see* **Note 5**). Centrifuge at 1000*g* for 10 min.
4. Incubate cells in 3–4 volumes (approx 250-400 µL) of Buffer I (IP) for 30 min (*see* **Note 6**).

5. Gently break the cells with 10 strokes using a $27G^{3/4}$ needle. Centrifuge at 3000*g* for 10 min at 4°C.
6. Transfer the supernatant (which represents the cytoplasmic fraction) to new tubes and adjusts the NP40 concentration to 0.5%. Store this fraction at –20°C for further analysis.
7. Resuspend the pellet in 3–4 vol (approx. 150 µL) of IP lysis buffer and keep on ice for 30 min. Centrifuge at 3000*g* for 10 min at 4°C. The supernatant of this spin represents the detergent soluble, particulate fraction. Repeat the procedure and mix the supernatants. Save an aliquot of this fraction for Western blot analysis (1/10 of final volume).
8. Incubate the detergent soluble, particulate fraction of the cell lysate with 10 µL Anti-FLAG M2 Affinity Gel (Kodak) over night at 4°C in a tube roller/mixer.
9. Wash the beads three times in 0.5–1 mL of RIPA buffer and one time in TBS (*see* **Note 7**). Add 50 µL of SDS loading buffer to the beads, sonicate and boil the samples for 10 min. Centrifuge samples at 18320*g* for 5 min.
10. Load 10 µL of each sample onto a 10% SDS-PAGE. Run the gel at 30 mA, 150 V, for approx 2 h. Transfer the separated proteins by Western blotting onto a Hybond C membrane or equivalent (*see* Chapter 26).
11. Block nonspecific binding by incubation in blocking buffer for at least 1 h.
12. Incubate membrane in αLMP1 S12-biotin antibody (1:1000 in TBS) overnight at 4°C.
13. Wash the membrane extensively in TBS-T. Incubate the membrane in Streptavidin-HRP (1:500 in TBS) for 2 h. Wash extensively in TBS-T.
14. Detect HRP activity using the ECL system (Amersham).

### 3.3. Membrane Targeting of the LMP1 C-Terminus (*see* Note 8)

1. *See* **Subheading 3.1., step 1**.
2. Dilute 1 µg of each expression plasmid (3xFKBP12-LMP1 or LMP1-3xFKBP12) and 50 ng of a given reporter gene in 100 µL Optimem 1. Mix the DNA with Lipofectamin (6 µL per 1 µg DNA) diluted in 100 µL of Optimem 1. Allow micelle formation for 45 min and carefully add the mix dropwise to the wells. Incubate for 4 h at 37°C, then add 2 mL of supplemented RPMI.
3. 16 h after transfection incubate the cells with 300 nM AP1510 dimerizing compound.
4. 40 h after transfection resuspend the cells in 1 mL of PBS (*see* **Subheading 3.1., step 6**) and centrifuge them at 1000*g* for 10 min (*see* **Note 5**).
5. Lyse the cell pellet in 100 µL of lysis buffer, keep on ice.
6. Centrifuge membranes, nuclei, and cellular debris at 18,320*g* for 10 min.
7. *See* **Subheading 3.1., step 9**.

### 3.4. Analysis of LMP1 Functions in Stably Transfected B Cells (*see* Notes 1 and 9)

1. Concentrate $1 \times 10^7$ EREB2-5 cells in 250 µL of supplemented RPMI medium. Cell viability should be greater than 90%. Aliquot 10 µg each of CD2:LMP1, CD4:LMP1 or NGF-R:LMP1 expression plasmid into 4-mm cuvets. Add cells at $1 \times 10^7$/250 µL to the cuvet and electroporate at 230 V peak discharge (setting), 960 µF. The pulse time (t) should be at approx 40 ms. Add 250 µL of FCS immediately after pulsing.
2. Resuspend the cells in 10 mL of supplemented RPMI medium and seed 100 µL of this dilution into 96-well plates.
3. Select transfected cells on the basis of hygromycin resistance, starting with initial concentrations of 50 µg/mL hygromycin reaching a final concentration of 150 µg/mL after 2 wk.

4. Seed selected clones at $3 \times 10^4$ cells/100 µL/well into 96-well plates. For analysis of conditional LMP1 mutants with respect to their impact on cell survival and proliferation incubate the cells under the following conditions:
   a. with 1 µ*M* estrogen in the culture medium;
   b. without estrogen in the culture medium;
   c. without estrogen in the culture medium; but with addition of the 1st and 2nd antibodies crosslinking the extracellular domain of CD2:LMP1, CD4:LMP1, NGF-R:LMP1 (*see* **Subheading 3.1.**, **step 5**); and
   d. without estrogen in the culture medium; with the 2nd antibody only as a control. Antibody treatment should be repeated every 3 d.
5. Add 10 µL of MTT mix each at day 1, 3, 5, and 6.
6. Resuspend crystals after 4 h in HCl/isopropanol (1:24). Measure optical density (OD) at 550 nm (reference at 690 nm). MTT conversion is directly proportional to cell survival and should be compared to values at d 1.

## 4. Notes

1. Transfect maximally 0.5–1 µg of the LMP expression plasmid to avoid spontaneous aggregation of the molecules owing to overexpression. It may be necessary to titrate DNA amounts for LMP1 variants (0.1–1 µg for 6-well). Transfect equal amounts of DNA by adding carrier DNA.
2. Transfection efficiency in 293 cells can be easily monitored by co-transfection of 0.5 µg of green fluorescence protein expression plasmid (peGFP-C1, Clontech). Transfection efficiency should not be below 20% in order to achieve correct expression and efficient crosslinking of the chimeric molecules.
3. Crosslinking of "one finger" variants as well as chimeric LMP1 molecules has to be done sequentially; add the primary antibody alone for 5 min before adding the secondary antibody. This procedure prevents the formation of antibody aggregates in solution. Crosslinking as well as transfection efficiency may vary from one experiment to another. Therefore results should be given as a mean of 3–5 experiments. Variation in total protein levels are usually not significant.
4. Induction of transcription factor activity (i.e., NFκB or AP-1) by LMP1:CD40 can be compared to wild-type CD40 receptor. Transfection of 0.5 µg of CD40 expression plasmid together with 0.5 µg of a reporter plasmid usually leads to a 5–10-fold activation. For example coculture of CD40 transfected cells with CD40-L bearing cells ***(21)*** activates the CD40 receptor and results in a strong induction of NFκB. Both LMP1:CD40 and activated CD40 display comparable activation patterns. Activation of the TNF-2 receptor by the addition of TNF-α is not informative since 293 cells express the TNF-1 receptor endogenously.
5. The use of trypsin to harvest 293 cells might affect the stability of receptor proteins and should therefore be avoided.
6. Alternatively to **steps 4** and **5**, one may lyse the cell pellet in 250 µL of RIPA buffer, sonicate the cell lysate and centrifuge at 18,320*g* for 10 min before continuing with **step 6**.
7. Non-specific binding to agarose beads represent a serious problem for immunoprecipitation of a FLAG-tagged LMP1 transmembrane domain. Stringent and repetitive washing of the beads after immunoprecipitation helps to overcome such problems. Washing can be carried out with TBS-T in case RIPA leads to a complete loss of immunoprecipitated products. Therefore, efficiency of immunoprecipitation should be controlled in each experiment. Use a M2 αFLAG antibody in its biotinylated version in stead of the αLMP1

S12-biotin antibody together with Streptavidin-HRP. Using a biotinylated αFLAG antibody will avoid the appearance of immunoglobulin chains from the immunoprecipitating antibodies on western blots.

8. Membrane targeting of the carboxyterminus of LMP1 in the correct orientation (namely using 3xFKBP12:LMP1) is a prerequisite for efficient signaling. LMP1:3xFKBP12 had no effect on NFκB activity in transient transfections.
9. Surface expression of chimeric LMP1 molecules in the cell line EREB2-5 is not indefinitely stable. After a period of 6–10 wk surface expression is drastically decreased as observed in flow cytometry analysis (FACS), although hygromycin resistance persists. Assays should be carried out within this period and surface expression controlled by FACS. The measurement/detection of crosslinking effects directly correlates with the density of surface expression of NFG-R:LMP1 and are not measurable below 15% surface expression (FACS measurement).

## References

1. Farrell, P. J. (1995) Epstein-Barr virus immortalizing genes. *Trends Microbiol* **3,** 105–109.
2. Fennewald, S., van Santen, V., and Kieff, E. (1984) Nucleotide sequence of an mRNA transcribed in latent growth-transforming virus infection indicates that it may encode a membrane protein. *J. Virol.* **51,** 411–419.
3. Hennessy, K., Fennewald, S., Hummel, M., Cole, T., and Kieff, E. (1984) A membrane protein encoded by Epstein-Barr virus in latent growth- transforming infection. *Proc. Natl. Acad. Sci. USA* **81,** 7207–7211.
4. Liebowitz, D., Wang, D., and Kieff, E. (1986) Orientation and patching of the latent infection membrane protein encoded by Epstein-Barr virus. *J. Virol.* **58,** 233–237.
5. Zimber-Strobl, U., Kempkes, B., Marschall, G., Zeidler, R., Van Kooten, C., Banchereau, J., et al. (1996) Epstein-Barr virus latent membrane protein (LMP1) is not sufficient to maintain proliferation of B cells but both it and activated CD40 can prolong their survival. *EMBO J.* **15,** 7070–7078.
6. Kilger, E., Kieser, A., Baumann, M., and Hammerschmidt, W. (1998) Epstein-Barr virus-mediated B-cell proliferation is dependent upon latent membrane protein 1, which simulates an activated CD40 receptor. *EMBO J.* **17,** 1700–1709.
7. Kaye, K. M., Izumi, K. M., and Kieff, E. (1993) Epstein-Barr virus latent membrane protein 1 is essential for B-lymphocyte growth transformation. *Proc. Natl. Acad. Sci. USA* **90,** 9150–9154.
8. Martin, J. and Sugden, B. (1991) The latent membrane protein oncoprotein resembles growth factor receptors in the properties of its turnover. *Cell Growth Differ.* **2,** 653–600.
9. Izumi, K. M. and Kieff, E. D. (1997) The Epstein-Barr virus oncogene product latent membrane protein 1 engages the tumor necrosis factor receptor-associated death domain protein to mediate B lymphocyte growth transformation and activate NF- kappaB. *Proc. Natl. Acad. Sci. USA* **94,** 12592–12597.
10. Mosialos, G., Birkenbach, M., Yalamanchili, R., VanArsdale, T., Ware, C., and Kieff, E. (1995) The Epstein-Barr virus transforming protein LMP1 engages signaling proteins for the tumor necrosis factor receptor family. *Cell* **80,** 389–399.
11. Sandberg, M., Hammerschmidt, W., and Sugden, B. (1997) Characterization of LMP-1's association with TRAF1, TRAF2, and TRAF3. *J. Virol.* **71,** 4649–4656.
12. Devergne, O., Hatzivassiliou, E., Izumi, K. M., Kaye, K. M., Kleijnen, M. F., Kieff, E., and Mosialos, G. (1996) Association of TRAF1, TRAF2, and TRAF3 with an Epstein-

Barr virus LMP1 domain important for B-lymphocyte transformation: role in NF-κB activation. *Mol. Cell. Biol.* **16,** 7098–7108.

13. Kieser, A., Kilger, E., Gires, O., Ueffing, M., Kolch, W., and Hammerschmidt, W. (1997) Epstein-Barr virus latent membrane protein-1 triggers AP-1 activity via the c-Jun N-terminal kinase cascade. *EMBO J.* **16,** 6478–6485.
14. Hammarskjold, M. L. and Simurda, M. C. (1992) Epstein-Barr virus latent membrane protein transactivates the human immunodeficiency virus type 1 long terminal repeat through induction of NF-kappa B activity. *J. Virol.* **66,** 6496–6501.
15. Mitchell, T. and Sugden, B. (1995) Stimulation of NF-kappa B-mediated transcription by mutant derivatives of the latent membrane protein of Epstein-Barr virus. *J. Virol.* **69,** 2968–2976.
16. Gires, O., Zimber-Strobl, U., Gonnella, R., Ueffing, M., Marschall, G., Zeidler, R., et al. (1997) Latent membrane protein 1 of Epstein-Barr virus mimics a constitutively active receptor molecule. *EMBO J.* **16,** 6131–6140.
17. Spencer, D. M., Graef, I., Austin, D. J., Schreiber, S. L., and Crabtree, G. R. (1995) A general strategy for producing conditional alleles of Src-like tyrosine kinases. *Proc. Natl. Acad. Sci. USA* **92,** 9805–9809.
18. Kempkes, B., Spitkovsky, D., Jansen-Durr, P., Ellwart, J. W., Kremmer, E., Delecluse, H. J., et al. (1995) B-cell proliferation and induction of early G1–regulating proteins by Epstein-Barr virus mutants conditional for EBNA2. *EMBO J.* **14,** 88–96.
19. Graham, F. L., Smiley, J., Russell, W. C., and Nairn, R. (1977) Characteristics of a human cell line transformed by DNA from human adenovirus type 5. *J. Gen. Virol.* **36,** 59–74.
20. Sugden, B., Marsh, K., and Yates, J. (1985) A vector that replicates as a plasmid and can be efficiently selected in B-lymphoblasts transformed by Epstein-Barr virus. *Mol. Cell. Biol.* **5,** 410–413.
21. Galibert, L., Burdin, N., de Saint-Vis, B., Garrone, P., Van Kooten, C., Banchereau, J., and Rousset, F. (1996) CD40 and B cell antigen receptor dual triggering of resting B lymphocytes turns on a partial germinal center phenotype. *J. Exp. Med.* **183,** 77–85.

# 35

## Assaying the Activity of Kinases Regulated by LMP1

**Arnd Kieser**

### 1. Introduction

Latent infection of B lymphocytes by Epstein-Barr virus (EBV) results in the immortalization of the infected cells *(1,2)*. In vitro, expression of latent membrane protein 1 (LMP1) is essential for the proliferation of EBV-immortalized B cells in that LMP1 simulates an activated CD40 receptor *(3)*. LMP1 exerts its effects by initiating both anti-apoptotic and proliferative, growth factor-like signals in the cell *(4)*. Special interest has focused on the molecular basis of LMP1 function because LMP1 is the only EBV protein that also has an oncogenic potential in non-B cells. LMP1 transforms rodent fibroblasts in vitro, proving it to be a true viral oncogene *(5,6)*. As such the signaling pathways impacted by LMP1 are likely to play important roles in the regulation of proliferation and transformation of the target cell.

LMP1 is a transmembrane protein consisting of 386 amino acids that acts like a constitutively active receptor independently of the binding of a ligand *(7)* (*see* also Chapter 31, Chimeric and Mutated Variants of LMP1). Six transmembrane domains (162 amino acids) connect a short N-terminal stretch of 24 amino acids to a long C-terminal domain (200 amino acids), both of which are located in the cytoplasm *(2,8)*. Signaling events are thought to be initiated at the C-terminus of LMP1 (**Fig. 1**). LMP1 induces the expression of the anti-apoptotic genes bcl-2 *(9)* and A20, the latter via induction of the transcription factor NF-κB *(10)*. Deletion analysis revealed that two signaling domains in the LMP1 C-terminus are responsible for NF-κB activation, the C-terminal activator regions 1 (CTAR1, amino acids 194 to 232) and 2 (CTAR2, amino acids 331 to 386) *(4,11–15)*. Similar to receptors of the tumor necrosis factor-receptor (TNF-R) family LMP1 has been shown to bind TNF-R-associated factors (TRAFs) via a consensus motif in CTAR1 *(13,15,16)* and the TNF-R-associated death domain protein (TRADD) via a short motif in CTAR2 *(17)*. NF-κB induction by LMP1 is dependent on TRAF2 *(13,18)*.

Searching for new LMP1-triggered signaling pathways that could explain the proliferative and growth factor-like effects of LMP1, we have recently identified the

From: *Methods in Molecular Biology, Vol. 174: Epstein-Barr Virus Protocols*
Edited by: J. B. Wilson and G. H. W. May © Humana Press Inc., Totowa, NJ

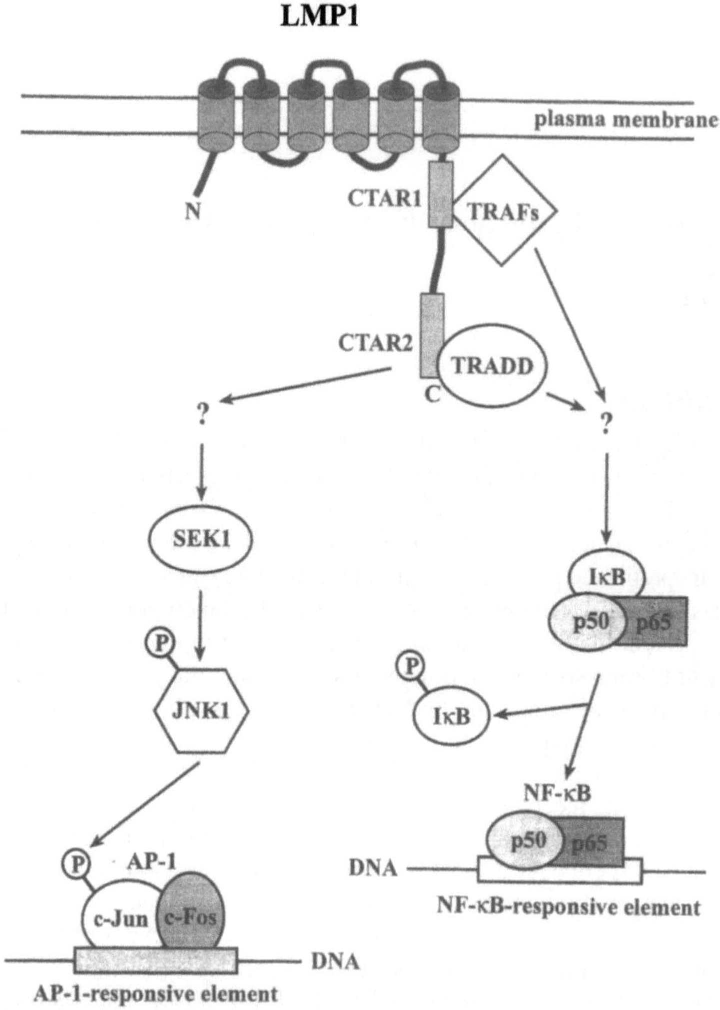


Fig. 1. Signal transduction by LMP1.

AP-1 transcription factor as a new target of LMP1 signal transduction *(19)*. AP-1 is a dimer of Jun/Jun or Jun/Fos family proteins *(20)*. AP-1 is induced by, and is necessary for the action of a wide variety of growth factors, mitogens, and oncogenes *(21)*. Moreover, the activated forms of c-jun and c-fos, v-jun and v-fos, have both been described as potent oncogenes *(21)*. Therefore, AP-1 is a very good candidate for mediating LMP1's proliferative and transforming activity. LMP1 induces the AP-1 transcription factor via induction of the c-Jun N-terminal kinase 1 (JNK1) signaling cascade *(19)*. Activated JNK1 phosphorylates the N-terminal transcriptional transactivation domain of c-Jun at serines 63 and 73, thereby leading to the activation of c-Jun/AP-1-dependent transcription *(22,23)*. LMP1 triggers the JNK1 -> c-Jun/ AP-1 pathway via its CTAR2 domain *(19,24)*. So far, JNK1 has been the only kinase described as being activated by LMP1.

Originally, JNKs were identified as kinases that are induced after exposure of cells to environmental stress such as UV-irradiation, osmotic shock, or treatment with genotoxic agents *(22,23,25–27)*. In addition, JNKs are activated by crosslinking of the CD40 receptor *(28,29)* and by stimulation of cells with proinflammatory cytokines such as TNF-α or interleukins 1 and 3 (IL-1, IL-2) *(25,26,30)*. So far, the physiological consequences of JNK1 activation in the cell are poorly defined. On one hand, JNK1 activation has been linked to the induction of apoptosis caused by cell stress or TNF-α, although JNK1 appears not to be the direct trigger for apoptosis *(27,31,32)*. On the other hand, JNK1 is also involved in noncytotoxic signaling events triggered by the TNF-R 1 or the CD40 receptor *(3,33,34)*. More recently, JNK1 has been demonstrated to mediate the proliferative response of pre-B-cells after stimulation with IL-3 *(35)*. We have shown that LMP1 induces proliferation paralleled by a strong increase in JNK1 activity in mini-EBV-immortalized B cells *(3,19)*. Hence, JNK1 appears to be involved in both processes, proliferation and apoptosis, induced by various stimuli. Cell fate after induction of JNKs might be defined by the time course of JNK induction or by induction of different costimulatory, e.g., anti-apoptotic, pathways.

This chapter describes protocols to assay the activity of LMP1-induced kinases, especially of JNK1 (**Subheadings 3.2.** and **3.3.**), and the purification of specific substrates necessary to conduct in vitro kinase reactions (**Subheading 3.1.**). Transient JNK1 assays in 293 human kidney cells comprise two major steps (**Subheading 3.2.**). First, 293 cells are transiently transfected with an LMP1 expression vector together with an expression vector for hemagglutinin-tagged JNK1 (HA-JNK1) (**Subheading 3.2.1.**). LMP1 will induce HA-JNK1 activity via the stress-enhanced kinase 1 (SEK1)-dependent signaling pathway (**Fig. 1**) *(19)*. SEK1 directly phosphorylates and thereby activates JNK1 *(36)* and, hence, the cotransfected HA-JNK1. Because the phosphorylation is a covalent modification, the activation status of HA-JNK1 can be conserved by lysis of the cells in the presence of phosphatase-inhibitors. In a second step, HA-JNK1 is immunoprecipitated via its HA-tag from total cell lysates (**Subheading 3.2.2.**). Subsequently in vitro kinase reactions are performed with the precipitated HA-JNK1 using purified glutathione-S-transferase (GST)-tagged c-Jun (GST-c-Jun) as a substrate. Cotransfection and subsequent immunoprecipitation of HA-JNK1 guarantees that only transfected cells are monitored in the kinase assays. This experimental set-up allows for the cotransfection of dominant-negative mutants of signal transducers of interest and hence, the evaluation of LMP1-dependent signaling pathways leading to JNK1 induction. In principle, by applying this method the LMP1-dependent regulation of any kinase can be studied as long as an expression vector for the tagged kinase of interest and a purified corresponding substrate are available. Another interesting aspect of this set-up is that a combination of inducible LMP1 mutants *(7,19)* (*see* also Chapter 31; Chimeric and Mutated Variants of LMP1) with the very fast JNK1 readout of LMP1 activity allows studies of time-dependent short-term effects of LMP1 induction *(19)*. In contrast to reporter gene readouts, JNK1 induction by LMP1 is independent of a transcriptional and translational step and thus, can be detected within a few minutes after triggering of LMP1 activity. **Subheading 3.3.** describes a protocol to assay endogenous JNK1 activity in cultured cells regulated by LMP1.

## 2. Materials

### *2.1. Purification and Analysis of GST-Tagged Kinase Substrates Produced in* Escherichia Coli

1. Bacterial expression vector for the specific substrate cloned into a glutathione-S-transferase (GST) vector (e.g., pGEX vectors from Pharmacia), from which the substrate is expressed as a GST fusion protein. Here we will refer to GST-c-Jun as the specific substrate for JNK1.
2. *E. coli* strain suitable to express the GST fusion protein, e.g., DH5α, BL21, or M15.
3. Buffers necessary to prepare transformation-competent *E. coli* according to Sambrook et al. *(37)*.
4. Luria-Bertani (LB)-medium containing the appropriate antibiotics (depending on the expression vector used) to grow *E. coli* according to Sambrook et al. *(37)*.
5. IPTG: 0.2 *M* isopropyl β-D-thiogalactopyranoside (IPTG) stock solution in $H_2O$, store at –20°C.
6. GST-lysis buffer: PBS (*see* **Subheading 2.2.**) containing 1% Triton X-100. Add fresh: 10 m*M* dithiothreitol (DTT), 1 m*M* phenylmethylsulfonylfluoride (PMSF), some mg of lysozyme.
7. Sonicator.
8. GST-elution buffer: 50 m*M* Tris-HCl, pH 8.0, 1% Triton X-100. Add fresh: 10 m*M* glutathione. Prepare a 1 *M* glutathione stock solution in $H_2O$, aliquot, and freeze at –80°C until use to prevent oxidation.
9. Glutathione-sepharose beads (e.g., Pharmacia). Suspend according to manufacturer's guidelines.
10. TBS buffer: 20 m*M* Tris-HCl, pH 7.4, 150 m*M* NaCl, 1 m*M* EDTA.
11. Materials and apparatus to perform sodium dodecyl sulfate-polyacrylamide gel electrophoresis (SDS-PAGE): We generally use the Hoefer-mighty-small gel chambers (Pharmacia). 12.5% separating gels: 35.4 mL of $H_2O$, 24 mL of acrylamide (30%)/bisacrylamide (0.8%) solution, 12 mL of Tris buffer (2 *M*), pH 8.9, 0.5 mL of EDTA solution (0.5 *M*). Add immediately before pouring the gels: 400 µL ammoniumpersulfate solution (10%) and 40 µL N,N,N',N'-tetramethylethylenediamine (TEMED). Stacking gels: 7.7 mL $H_2O$, 1.5 mL of acrylamide (30%)/bisacrylamide (0.8%) solution, 625 µL Tris-HCl buffer (2 *M*), pH 6.8, 50 µL SDS-solution (20%), 100 µL of EDTA solution (0.5 *M*). Add immediately before pouring the gels: 15 µL of ammoniumpersulfate solution (10%), and 2 µL TEMED/mL of gel. 10X SDS-running buffer (1 L): 30 g Tris, 144 g glycine, 10 g SDS.
12. Protein standard: 50 ng/µL of bovine serum albumin (BSA).
13. 4X SDS-loading buffer: 200 m*M* Tris-HCl, pH 6.8, 4 m*M* EDTA, 100 m*M* DTT, 40% glycerine, 8% SDS. Add bromophenol blue until buffer is dark blue.
14. SDS-molecular weight standard.
15. Coomassie-staining solution: 2.5 g/L coomassie brilliant blue, 10% acetic acid, 50% methanol.
16. Destaining solution: 7% acetic acid, 40% methanol.
17. Sorvall centrifuge (or equivalent) and appropriate bottles and 15-mL conical bottom tubes.
18. Microfuge and microfuge tubes.

### 2.2. Transient HA-JNK1 Assays in 293 Cells

1. 293 human kidney cells, grown in standard complete cell culture medium such as Dulbecco's Modified Eagle Medium (DMEM, GIBCO BRL) supplemented with 10% fetal calf serum (GIBCO BRL) and 2 m*M* L-glutamine. Cells are cultured in 6-well (1.5-cm/well) tissue-culture dishes and incubated in a humid incubator at 37°C and 5% $CO_2$.
2. Lipofectamine reagent and Optimem1 reduced serum medium (both: GIBCO BRL) for liposome-based transfection. For a detailed description of the reagents see the product data sheets supplied by the manufacturer.
3. Plasmids for transfection: SRα-HA-JNK1 ***(19,38)*** expressing HA-JNK1. LMP1 wildtype or mutant expression vectors. We use pSV-LMP1 and pSV-LMP1-based LMP1 mutans ***(19)*** and the inducible LMP1 mutant LMP-1:3xFKBP12 (also referred to as one-finger-3xFKBP12 (*see* Chapter 31, Chimeric and Mutated Variants of LMP1) ***(7,19)***. Empty vector as a control. Purify all plasmids from *E. coli* using the Qiagen Maxi-preparations system (Qiagen), or similar.
4. Salmon testes DNA solution in $H_2O$ as a carrier DNA for transfections.
5. PBS buffer (1 L): 8 g NaCl, 0.2 g KCl, 1.44 g $Na_2HPO_4$, 0.24 g $KH_2PO_4$, pH 7.4.
6. TBST: 20 m*M* Tris-HCl, pH 7.5, 150 m*M* NaCl, 1 m*M* EDTA, 1% Triton X-100. Add fresh: 1 m*M* PMSF and the following inhibitors of phosphatases: 0.5 m*M* β-glycerophosphate, 0.5 m*M* sodiumpyrophosphate, 0.5 m*M* NaF, 0.5 m*M* sodium-molybdate, and 0.5 m*M* sodiumorthovanadate. For preparation of a 0.5 *M* sodium-orthovanadate stock solution boil sodiumorthovanadate in 100 m*M* Tris, pH 9.0, buffer until the sodiumorthovanadate has dissolved. Titrate pH to 9.0 using concentrated HCl (color turns to yellow). Boil until color disappears. Aliquot and freeze at –20°C until use.
7. Protein-G-sepharose beads (e.g., gammabind plus sepharose from Pharmacia). Suspend according to manufacturer's guidelines.
8. Anti-HA-epitope antibody 12CA5 (Boehringer Mannheim).
9. PBS buffer containing 4% sucrose and 0.02% sodiumazide.
10. Kinase reaction buffer: 20 m*M* Tris-HCl, pH 7.4, 20 m*M* NaCl, 10 m*M* $MgCl_2$, 1 μ*M* DTT, 2 μ*M* adenosinc-5'-triphosphate (ATP).
11. Purified GST-c-Jun (*see* **Subheadings 2.1.** and **3.1.**).
12. $\gamma$-$^{32}$P-ATP, 3000 Ci/mmol, 10 mCi/mL.
13. 4X stop buffer: 200 m*M* Tris-HCl, pH 6.8, 4 m*M* EDTA, 100 m*M* DTT, 40% glycerine, 8% SDS, add bromophenol blue until buffer is dark blue.
14. Materials to perform SDS-PAGE (*see* **Subheading 2.1.**).
15. Blotting chamber for SDS-gels.
16. 10X blotting buffer (1 L): 30 g Tris-base, 95 g glycine.
17. Blotting membrane for proteins (e.g., Hybond-C membranes from Amersham).
18. Phosphoimager to quantify phosphorylation signals (optional).
19. Microfuge and microfuge tubes.

### 2.3. Assaying Endogenous JNK1 Activity

The materials necessary for assaying endogenous JNK1 activity are basically the same as described in **Subheading 2.2.**, except for an JNK1-specific antibody to precipitate endogenous JNK1 (instead of an anti-HA-epitope antibody). In our hands the anti-JNK1 antibody C-17 (rabbit polyclonal from Santa Cruz Biotech.) has proved to yield good results in the precipitation of JNK1 of human sources ***(3,19)***. Depending on the chosen experimental set-up and the used cell lines, transfection might not be necessary and/or another cell culture media might be required.

## 3. Methods

### 3.1. Purification of the JNK1 Substrate GST-c-Jun via Glutathione Beads (*see* Note 1)

It is important to conduct **steps 5–11** on ice or at 4°C.

1. Prepare competent *E. coli* according to the protocol described in Sambrook et al. *(37)*. Subsequently transform competent *E. coli* with the bacterial GST-c-Jun expression vector. Generally, any protocol to yield *E. coli* transformed with the bacterial GST-c-Jun expression vector can be applied.
2. Set up a 50-mL culture of the transformed *E. coli* in LB-medium containing the appropriate antibiotics (according to the GST-expression vector used) and incubate overnight at 37°C shaking.
3. The next day dilute the 50 mL overnight culture from **step 2** 1:20 with 1 L LB-medium and incubate for 3 h at 37°C. Add IPTG to 0.2 m*M* to induce the expression of GST-c-Jun and incubate for a further 4 h at 30°C.
4. Precipitate *E. coli* at 2000*g* for 10 min in a Sorvall centrifuge (or equivalent). Discard supernatant.
5. Resuspend the bacterial pellet in 20 mL of GST-lysis buffer, transfer the suspension to a 50-mL tube and incubate on ice for 10 min.
6. Sonicate the suspension 3 times for 10 s each at 30 Watts. Cool the sample on ice between the single sonication steps.
7. Centrifuge for 10 min at 17,000*g* in a Sorvall centrifuge (or equivalent). Transfer the supernatant containing the GST-c-Jun to two 15-mL tubes with conical bottom.
8. Add 700 µL of resuspended glutathione-sepharose beads per 10 mL of supernatant and rotate for 30 min.
9. Precipitate the GST-c-Jun bound to glutathione-sepharose beads by centrifugation for 1 min at 500*g* and remove the supernatant carefully.
10. Wash pellets 4 times with 10 mL each of GST-lysis buffer and subsequently 2 times with 10 mL each of TBS. For the washing steps resuspend the beads in GST-lysis buffer or TBS, respectively, and precipitate them by centrifugation for 1 min at 500*g*.
11. To elute GST-c-Jun from the glutathione-sepharose beads resuspend each pellet of beads in 300 µL of GST-elution buffer and transfer the suspension to an 1.5-mL tube. Elute GST-c-Jun by rotating tubes for 30 min. Precipitate the beads by centrifugation at 15,000*g* for 30 s. Transfer the supernatant containing the eluted GST-c-Jun to a new 1.5-mL tube. Repeat elution from the beads another two times and pool the supernatants (900 µL in total). This solution contains the GST-tagged kinase substrate to be used in the in vitro kinase assays described below. Evaluate the substrate concentration (*see* **step 12**), aliquot, and store at –20°C until use. The GST-c-Jun solution can be stored at –20°C for several months.
12. To evaluate the quality and protein concentration of the GST-c-Jun solution, analysis of the protein preparation should be performed by SDS-PAGE (*see* **Note 2**). Pour a 12.5% SDS gel and overlay with a stacking gel. Load different volumes of the GST-c-Jun preparation (1–20 µL is recommended), different amounts of BSA standard (5, 100, 500 ng BSA), and a SDS molecular weight standard. For preparation of the samples add 4X SDS

loading buffer to the protein solutions (final concentration: 1X), heat at 95°C for 5 min, and place on ice for 2 min. Run the gel in 1X SDS-running buffer (further details on SDS-PAGE are given in Chapter 22).

13. For blue-staining of the separated proteins incubate the SDS-gel in coomassie-staining solution for 1 h at room temperature and subsequently destain the gel in destaining solution until the protein bands are clearly visible. Change the destaining solution several times during the destaining process.
14. Evaluate the concentration of the kinase substrate by comparing the GST-c-Jun bands with the BSA standards. Use approx 200 ng of GST-c-Jun per kinase reaction.

### 3.2. Transient HA-JNK1 Assays in 293 Cells (*see* Note 3)

#### 3.2.1. Transient Transfection of 293 Cells (*see* **Note 4**)

1. Plate 293 human kidney cells in 6-well-plates in 3 mL of standard complete cell-culture medium the day before transfection. 293 cells should reach a confluence of about 50% at the moment of transfection (*see* **Note 5**).
2. The next day carefully remove the medium and overlay cells with 1.5-mL of prewarmed (37°C) Optimem1. Incubate the cells at 37°C during the preparation of the DNA-lipid complexes.
3. To prepare the DNA-lipid complexes set up the following solutions under sterile conditions. Solution A: to 100 µL Optimem1 add 1 mg of SRα-HA-JNK1 and 1 µg of pSV2-LMP1 or 1 µg of empty vector for a mock-transfected control. Solution B: to 100 µL Optimem1 add 4 µL of Lipofectamine reagent (*see* **Note 6**). Mix solutions A and B, incubate for 15 to 30 min at room temperature, and finally add 800 µL of prewarmed Optimem1.
4. Remove medium from the cells and carefully overlay them with the DNA-lipid solutions from **step 3**. Incubate at 37°C and 5% $CO_2$ for 4 h.
5. Remove Optimem1 containing the DNA-lipid complexes and overlay cells with 3 mL of standard complete cell culture medium (*see* **Note 7**). Incubate for about 20 h at 37°C and 5% $CO_2$.

#### 3.2.2. Immobilization of Anti-HA-Epitope Antibodies to Protein-G-Sepharose Beads, Immunoprecipitation of HA-JNK1, and In Vitro Kinase Reactions

1. Prepare the anti-HA-epitope antibodies 12CA5 immobilized to protein-G-sepharose beads (**steps 1–3**) ahead of time so that it is available when the transfected cells are lysed. Transfer 80 µL of resuspended protein-G-sepharose beads to an 1.5-mL tube. To wash the beads add 700 µL of TBST, resuspend the pellet by repeatedly inverting the tube, and subsequently centrifuge for 30 s at 15,000*g*. Discard the supernatant and wash the beads a second time with TBST.
2. Dissolve 200 µg of 12CA5 antibody in 500 µL of PBS containing 4% sucrose and 0.02% sodiumazide and incubate on ice for 15 min. Add the antibody to the washed protein-G-sepharose beads (**step 1**). Rotate for 2 h at 4°C. At this step the 12CA5 antibody binds to the protein G that is covalently bound to the sepharose beads.
3. Precipitate the beads by centrifugation at 15,000*g* for 30 s and wash three times with 700 µL of TBST (as in **step 1**). Finally resuspend the protein-G-sepharose beads binding the 12CA5 antibody in 1.2 mL of PBS containing 4% sucrose and 0.02% sodiumazide. Store at 4°C until use. Use 12 µL of 12CA5-beads per immunoprecipitation.
4. Using transfected cells (as described in **Subheading 3.2.**), remove the medium 24 h after transfection and wash the cells once with cold PBS. Carefully remove residual PBS. Lyse

the cells on the plate by adding 400 μL of TBST per well and incubate for 2 min on ice. Remove the cells using a cell scraper and transfer the lysates to 1.5-mL tubes. For all following steps keep the samples on ice or at 4°C until starting the kinase reactions (*see* **Note 8**).

5. Centrifuge at 15,000*g* for 5 min. Transfer the supernatant to a new 1.5-mL tube and add 12 μL of 12CA5-beads (**step 3**) for immunoprecipitation of HA-JNK1. Agitate the tube containing the 12CA5-beads (to resuspend the beads) each time before the transfer of beads to another tube.
6. Rotate samples overnight at 4°C.
7. Precipitate the 12CA5-beads binding HA-JNK1 by centrifugation at 15,000*g* for 30 s. Remove the supernatant except for the last 30–40 μL. Since the beads are hardly visible at the bottom of the tube be careful not to remove the beads together with the supernatant. Transfer the supernatant to a new 1.5-mL tube for further analysis (*see* **Note 9**) and proceed with the pellet.
8. Wash the beads two times with TBST (as described in **step 1**) and subsequently two times with kinase reaction buffer, leaving residual buffer in the tube each time. For washing, the kinase reaction buffer should not contain GST-c-Jun and $\gamma$-$^{32}$P-ATP. After the last washing step adjust the volumes of all samples to approx 25 μL. To avoid the loss of beads, the volumes should be adjusted by comparing the test tubes with a reference tube containing 25 μL of liquid.
9. Prepare the kinase reaction mix. Per reaction use 200 ng of GST-c-Jun (*see* **Subheading 3.1., step 11**), 1 μL of $\gamma$-$^{32}$P-ATP (equivalent to 10 μCi) and adjust the total volume to 10 μL/sample with kinase reaction buffer.
10. Start the kinase reaction by adding 10 μL of kinase reaction mix (**step 9**) to the precipitated HA-JNK1 (**step 8**), mix gently, and incubate for 25 min at 24–26°C. Depending on its activity, the precipitated HA-JNK1 will now transfer the $\gamma$-$^{32}$P-phosphate from $\gamma$-$^{32}$P-ATP to the substrate GST-c-Jun.
11. Stop the kinase reaction by adding 12 μL of 4X stop buffer per sample and place the reactions on ice for at least 2 min.
12. Heat samples at 95°C for 5 min and subsequently place them on ice for another 2 min.
13. Electrophorese the kinase reactions on a 12.5% SDS-gel (*see* **Subheading 3.1.**). Load 15 μL of each kinase reaction. Include an SDS-molecular weight standard. Stop the electrophoresis before the blue dye front runs out of the gel to avoid radioactive contamination of the gel chamber (residual $\gamma$-$^{32}$P-ATP runs approx with the blue front).
14. Electroblot the gel onto a Hybond-N membrane in 1X blotting buffer at 70 Vh (details on SDS gel electroblotting are given in Chapter 26).
15. Expose the blot to an X-ray film and quantify the signals using a Phosphoimager. The phosphorylated GST-c-Jun is visible as a double band corresponding to the mono- and biphosphorylated forms of GST-c-Jun.
16. It is necessary to show that the amounts of precipitated HA-JNK1 are approximately equal between the single kinase reactions and do not vary corresponding to the phosphorylation signals. Evaluate the amounts of precipitated HA-JNK1 by immunostaining of the kinase assay blot using a JNK1-specific primary antibody (Western protocols are described in Chapter 22).

### 3.3. Assaying Endogenous JNK1 Activity Regulated by LMP1

For some experimental systems it is necessary to assay endogenous JNK1 activity instead of a transfected HA-JNK1. This is especially the case when LMP1-regulated

JNK1 activity is assayed in cell lines that stably express LMP1 or LMP1 mutants that carry an inducible LMP1 allele *(3,19)* (*see* also Chapter 3, Genetic Analysis and Gene Expression with Mini-EBV Plasmids). The protocol to assay endogenous JNK1 activity is very similar to that already described earlier for transient HA-JNK1 assays (*see* **Subheading 3.2.**). The major difference is that endogenous JNK1 is precipitated by a JNK1-specific antibody. To immobilize the anti-JNK1 antibody to protein-G-sepharose, follow the procedure already described for the anti-HA-epitope antibody 12CA5 (*see* **Subheading 3.2.2.** and **Note 10**). Proceed with the kinase assays as described in **Subheading 3.2.2.**

## 4. Notes

1. The JNK1 substrate c-Jun is expressed as a GST-fusion protein in *E. coli* and is subsequently purified via glutathione-coupled sepharose beads. This protocol describes the preparation of GST-c-Jun but can be used for other GST-tagged kinase substrates or proteins as well. To yield higher levels of the purified GST-tagged protein a variation of the *E. coli* strain used to produce the substrate might be required (*see* **Subheading 2.1.**, *E. coli* Strains). Another option to increase the yield of tagged protein is to incubate the bacteria for up to 24 h at 30°C after IPTG-stimulation to allow sufficient expression of the tagged substrate.
2. In some cases the GST-fusion protein preparation might contain contaminations of bacterial proteins that unspecifically bind to the glutathione-sepharose beads. Although these co-purifying proteins usually do not influence the kinase reactions, they disturb the evaluation of the actual substrate concentration in protein assays such as the Bradford assay. In addition, the purified GST-fusion protein might be degraded partially. Therefore it is recommended to evaluate the actual substrate concentration, the purity, and quality of the preparation by SDS-PAGE.
3. The advantage of transient HA-JNK1 assays is that expression vectors coding for LMP1 mutants *(19)*, inducible LMP1 mutants *(7,19)* (*see* also Chapter 34, Chimeric and Mutated Variants of LMP1), or dominant-negative mutants of signal transducers of interest *(19)* can easily be transfected or cotransfected, respectively. Stable transfections requiring a time-consuming selection process, analysis of resulting cell clones, and a possible creation of artifacts owing to clonal variations can be avoided. Moreover, stable ectopic expression of some genes, e.g., some dominant-negative mutants, is toxic for the target cell. In many cases biological effects of such genes can be studied in transient but not in stable assays. For interpretation of the resulting data, however, one should bear in mind that the experimental set-up of transient HA-JNK1 assays in 293 cells represents a rather artificial system to analyze LMP1-dependent signaling, so far with no practicable alternative. Nevertheless, transient reporter gene and HA-JNK1 assays in 293 cells have delivered important contributions to our current understanding of LMP1-induced signal transduction.
4. In this chapter a transfection protocol using the Lipofectamine reagent (GIBCO BRL) to perform liposome-based transfection of 293 cells is described. In our hands this system yields transfection efficiencies of about 40–70% as monitored by transfection of a green fluorescent protein (GFP) expression vector. Generally, all transfection protocols can be applied as long as high enough transfection efficiencies are achieved. According to our experience transfection efficiencies of about 20% still suffice to yield satisfying results in the kinase assays. In addition, it is important to make sure that the applied transfection

procedure itself does not induce JNK1 activity by generating general cell stress. An alternative transfection method is, e.g., the classical calciumphosphate precipitation technique first described by Chen and Okayama *(39,40)*. This technique yields good results (in our hands transfection efficiencies in 293 cells up to 40%) at rather low costs. For 293 cells, transfect 2–3 µg of DNA per well of a 6-well-plate.

5. Although 293 is an adherent cell line, the cells detach easily when medium is removed or overlaid. To promote better adherence of the cells, let them grow overnight before transfection. When changing the medium, do not let the medium drop directly onto the cells. It is also very important that 293 cells are not confluent at the moment of transfection.
6. Transfect 2–3 µg of DNA per well of a 6-well-plate using 4 µL of Lipofectamine reagent. The amounts of transfected expression vectors should be optimized according to the experimental needs. Adjust the total amounts of transfected DNAs using salmon testes DNA.
7. If the kinase of interest is induced by serum stimulation, feed the cells with DMEM containing 1% fetal calf serum (FCS) (low serum conditions) to reduce the background level of kinase activity to a minimum.
8. For analysis of nonadherent cells growing in suspension lyse approx $5\times 10^5$ to $1\times 10^6$ cells in 500 µL TBST.
9. The supernatants of the immunoprecipitations represent the total cell lysates minus the precipitated HA-JNK1. Therefore, the supernatants can be analyzed further by immunoblotting, e.g., for the expression of the transfected LMP1 or a cotransfected dominant-negative kinase mutant.
10. Many IgG subtypes bind to protein G and hence can be precipitated via protein-G-sepharose beads, e.g., mouse IgG subtypes 1 and 3, rat IgG subtypes 1, 2a, 2b, 2c, and most rabbit polyclonal antibodies. The antibodies described in this chapter bind to protein G. However, note that antibodies from other host species or IgG subtypes might not bind to protein G. An alternative is to use protein-A- instead of protein-G-sepharose. For further information contact the supplier of the antibody.

## References

1. Farrell, P. J. (1995) Epstein-Barr virus immortalizing genes. *Trends Microbiol.* **3,** 105–109.
2. Kieff, E. (1996) Epstein-Barr virus and its replication, in *Virology*, 3rd edition (Fields, B. N., Knipe, D. M., Howley, P. M., et al., eds.), Lippincott-Raven, Philadelphia, PA, pp. 2343–2396.
3. Kilger, E., Kieser, A., Baumann, M., and Hammerschmidt, W. (1998) Epstein-Barr virus-mediated B-cell proliferation is dependent upon latent membrane protein 1, which simulates an activated CD40 receptor. *EMBO J.* **17,** 1700–1709.
4. Farrell, P. J. (1998) Signal transduction from the Epstein-Barr virus LMP-1 transforming protein. *Trends Microbiol.* **6,** 175–178.
5. Wang, D., Liebowitz, D., and Kieff, E. (1985) An EBV membrane protein expressed in immortalized lymphocytes transforms established rodent cells. *Cell* **43,** 831–840.
6. Baichwal, V. R. and Sugden, B. (1988) Transformation of Balb 3T3 cells by the BNLF-1 gene of Epstein-Barr virus. *Oncogene* **2,** 461–467.
7. Gires, O., Zimber-Strobl, U., Gonnella, R., Ueffing, M., Marschall, G., Zeidler, R., et al. (1997) Latent membrane protein 1 of Epstein-Barr virus mimics a constitutively active receptor molecule. *EMBO J.* **16,** 6131–6140.
8. Liebowitz, D., Wang, D., and Kieff, E. (1986) Orientation and patching of the latent infection membrane protein encoded by Epstein-Barr virus. *J. Virol.* **58,** 233–237.

9. Henderson, S., Rowe, M., Gregory, C., Croom, C. D., Wang, F., and Longnecker, R. (1991) Induction of bcl-2 expression by Epstein-Barr virus latent membrane protein 1 protects infected B cells from programmed cell death. *Cell* **65,** 1107–1115.
10. Laherty, C. D., Hu, H. M., Opipari, A. W., Wang, F., and Dixit, V. M. (1992) The Epstein-Barr virus LMP1 gene product induces A20 zinc finger protein expression by activating nuclear factor kappa B. *J. Biol. Chem.* **267,** 24157–24160.
11. Huen, D. S., Henderson, S. A., Croom-Carter, D., and Rowe, M. (1995) The Epstein-Barr virus latent membrane protein-1 (LMP1) mediates activation of NF-κB and cell surface phenotype via two effector regions in its carboxy-terminal cytoplasmic domain. *Oncogene* **10,** 549–560.
12. Mitchell, T. and Sugden, B. (1995) Stimulation of NF-κB-mediated transcription by mutant derivatives of the latent membrane protein of Epstein-Barr virus. *J. Virol.* **69,** 2968–2976.
13. Devergne, O., Hatzivassiliou, E., Izumi, K. M., Kaye, K. M., Kleijnen, M. F., Kieff, E., and Mosialos, G. (1996) Association of TRAF1, TRAF2, and TRAF3 with an Epstein-Barr virus LMP1 domain important for B-lymphocyte transformation: role in NF-κB activation. *Mol. Cell. Biol.* **16,** 7098–7108.
14. Floettmann, J. E., and Rowe, M. (1997) Epstein-Barr virus latent membrane protein-1 (LMP1) C-terminus activation region 2 (CTAR2) maps to the far C-terminus and requires oligomerisation for NF-κB activation. *Oncogene* **15,** 1851–1858.
15. Sandberg, M., Hammerschmidt, W., and Sugden, B. (1997) Characterization of LMP-1's association with TRAF1, TRAF2, and TRAF3. *J. Virol.* **71,** 4649–4656.
16. Mosialos, G., Birkenbach, M., Yalamanchili, R., VanArsdale, T., Ware, C., and Kieff, E. (1995) The Epstein-Barr virus transforming protein LMP1 engages signaling proteins for the tumor necrosis factor receptor family. *Cell* **80,** 389–399.
17. Izumi, K. M. and Kieff, E. D. (1997) The Epstein-Barr virus oncogene product latent membrane protein 1 engages the tumor necrosis factor receptor-associated death domain protein to mediate B lymphocyte growth transformation and activate NF-κB. *Proc. Natl. Acad. Sci. USA* **94,** 12,592–12,597.
18. Kaye, K. M., Devergne, O., Harada, J. N., Izumi, K. M., Yalamanchili, R., Kieff, E., and Mosialos, G. (1996) Tumor necrosis factor receptor associated factor 2 is a mediator of NF- kappa B activation by latent infection membrane protein 1, the Epstein- Barr virus transforming protein. *Proc. Natl. Acad. Sci. USA* **93,** 11,085–11,090.
19. Kieser, A., Kilger, E., Gires, O., Ueffing, M., Kolch, W., and Hammerschmidt, W. (1997) Epstein-Barr virus latent membrane protein-1 triggers AP-1 activity via the c-Jun N-terminal kinase cascade. *EMBO J.* **16,** 6478–6485.
20. Karin, M., Liu, Z., and Zandi, E. (1997) AP-1 function and regulation. *Curr. Opin. Cell Biol.* **9,** 240–246.
21. Angel, P. and Karin, M. (1991) The role of Jun, Fos and the AP-1 complex in cell-proliferation and transformation. *Biochim. Biophys. Acta* **1072,** 129–157.
22. Hibi, M., Lin, A., Smeal, T., Minden, A., and Karin, M. (1993) Identification of an oncoprotein- and UV-responsive protein kinase that binds and potentiates the c-Jun activation domain. *Genes Dev.* **7,** 2135–2148.
23. Derijard, B., Hibi, M., Wu, I. H., Barrett, T., Su, B., Deng, T., et al. (1994) JNK1: a protein kinase stimulated by UV light and Ha-Ras that binds and phosphorylates the c-Jun activation domain. *Cell* **76,** 1025–1037.
24. Eliopoulos, A. G. and Young, L. S. (1998) Activation of the c-Jun N-terminal kinase (JNK) pathway by the Epstein-Barr virus-encoded latent membrane protein 1 (LMP1). *Oncogene* **16,** 1731–1742.

25. Kyriakis, J. M., Banerjee, P., Nikolakaki, E., Dai, T., Rubie, E. A., Ahmad, M. F., et al. (1994) The stress-activated protein kinase subfamily of c-Jun kinases. *Nature* **369,** 156–160.
26. Rosette, C. and Karin, M. (1996) Ultraviolet light and osmotic stress: activation of the JNK cascade through multiple growth factor and cytokine receptors. *Science* **274,** 1194–1197.
27. Ip, Y. T. and Davis, R. J. (1998) Signal transduction by the c-Jun N-terminal kinase (JNK) - from inflammation to development. *Curr. Opin. Cell Biol.* **10,** 205–219.
28. Sakata, N., Patel, H. R., Terada, N., Aruffo, A., Johnson, G. L., and Gelfand, E. W. (1995) Selective activation of c-Jun kinase mitogen-activated protein kinase by CD40 on human B cells. *J. Biol. Chem.* **270,** 30,823–30,828.
29. Berberich, I., Shu, G., Siebelt, F., Woodgett, J. R., Kyriakis, J. M., and Clark, E. A. (1996) Cross-linking CD40 on B cells preferentially induces stress-activated protein kinases rather than mitogen-activated protein kinases. *EMBO J.* **15,** 92–101.
30. Terada, K., Kaziro, Y., and Satoh, T. (1997) Ras-dependent activation of c-Jun N-terminal kinase/stress-activated protein kinase in response to interleukin-3 stimulation in hematopoietic BaF3 cells. *J. Biol. Chem.* **272,** 4544–4548.
31. Xia, Z., Dickens, M., Raingeaud, J., Davis, R. J., and Greenberg, M. E. (1995) Opposing effects of ERK and JNK-p38 MAP kinases on apoptosis. *Science* **270,** 1326–1331.
32. Kyriakis, J. M. and Avruch, J. (1996) Sounding the alarm: protein kinase cascades activated by stress and inflammation. *J. Biol. Chem.* **271,** 24,313–24,316.
33. Liu, Z. G., Hsu, H., Goeddel, D. V., and Karin, M. (1996) Dissection of TNF receptor 1 effector functions: JNK activation is not linked to apoptosis while NF-κB activation prevents cell death. *Cell* **87,** 565–576.
34. Natoli, G., Costanzo, A., Ianni, A., Templeton, D. J., Woodgett, J. R., Balsano, C., and Levrero, M. (1997) Activation of SAPK/JNK by TNF receptor 1 through a noncytotoxic TRAF2-dependent pathway. *Science* **275,** 200–203.
35. Smith, A., Ramos-Morales, F., Ashworth, A., and Collins, M. (1997) A role for JNK/SAPK in proliferation, but not apoptosis, of IL-3-dependent cells. *Curr. Biol.* **7,** 893–896.
36. Sanchez, I., Hughes, R. T., Mayer, B. J., Yee, K., Woodgett, J. R., Avruch, J., et al. (1994) Role of SAPK/ERK kinase-1 in the stress-activated pathway regulating transcription factor c-Jun. *Nature* **372,** 794–798.
37. Sambrook, J., Fritsch, E. F., and Maniatis, T. (1989) *Molecular Cloning: A Laboratory Manual,* 2nd ed., Cold Spring Harbor Laboratory Press, Cold Spring Harbor, NY.
38. Minden, A., Lin, A., McMahon, M., Lange-Carter, C., Derijard, B., Davis, R. J., et al. (1994) Differential activation of ERK and JNK mitogen-activated protein kinases by Raf-1 and MEKK. *Science* **266,** 1719–1723.
39. Chen, C. and Okayama, H. (1987) High-efficiency transformation of mammalian cells by plasmid DNA. *Mol. Cell. Biol.* **7,** 2745–2752.
40. Chen, C. A. and Okayama, H. (1988) Calcium phosphate-mediated gene transfer: a highly efficient transfection system for stably transforming cells with plasmid DNA. *Biotechniques* **6,** 632–638.

# 36

# In Vitro Assays for the Detection of Protein Tyrosine Phosphorylation and Protein Tyrosine Kinase Activities

**Sara Fruehling and Richard Longnecker**

## 1. Introduction

The ability of Epstein-Barr virus (EBV) to establish and maintain a latent infection, one of the defining characteristics of a herpesvirus infection, is a complex phenomenon. It requires viral control of the host-cell environment to maintain the latent viral genome indefinitely, even in the presence of cellular activating signals. The consistent detection of the latent membrane protein 2A (LMP2A) in EBV infection in vivo and the ability of LMP2A to downmodulate signals through the B-cell receptor (BCR) in vitro suggest a vital role of LMP2A in the maintenance of EBV latency. Studies of LMP2A have shown that specific sequences of the amino-terminal domain interact with multiple cellular proteins, downmodulate cellular protein tyrosine phosphorylation, and downmodulate cellular protein tyrosine kinase activities *(1–6)*. These LMP2A functional studies have involved in vitro assays to determine the phosphorylation patterns of both LMP2A and cellular signal transducers before and after BCR crosslinking. In addition, the kinase activities of protein tyrosine kinases potentially downmodulated by LMP2A have been investigated by in vitro auto kinase assays. The methodology for the detection of tyrosine phosphorylated cellular and viral proteins and the detection of the auto kinase activities of cellular protein tyrosine kinases by in vitro kinase assays are described in this chapter.

### *1.1. Immunoprecipitation of Tyrosine Phosphorylated Proteins*

The detection of tyrosine phosphorylated cellular and viral proteins is performed by various combinations of immunoprecipitation-immunoblot experiments using antibodies specific to phosphotyrosine (APT). For a general survey of all tyrosine phosphorylated proteins within a cell, an APT immunoprecipitation followed by an APT Western blot will detect all viral and cellular proteins that are tyrosine phosphorylated in the cellular preparation. The generation of cellular protein lysates before and after a defined stimulus provides a method of studying the changes that occur in protein

From: *Methods in Molecular Biology, Vol. 174: Epstein-Barr Virus Protocols*
Edited by: J. B. Wilson and G. H. W. May © Humana Press Inc., Totowa, NJ

tyrosine phosphorylation in response to the stimulus. Stimulation of the BCR in B lymphocytes leads to a well defined signal cascade involving the activation of many cellular proteins by tyrosine phosphorylation *(7–11)*. Stimulation of the BCR in vitro is achieved by the addition of anti-immunoglobulin crosslinking antibodies and the phosphorylation of downstream proteins occurs immediately upon addition of crosslinking antibodies. For specific phosphorylation analysis of a known cellular or viral protein, "LMP2A" or "Syk" for example, an LMP2A or Syk immunoprecipitation followed by an APT Western blot will determine whether LMP2A or Syk protein is tyrosine phosphorylated. The use of lysates made from unstimulated cell preparations vs cells stimulated through the BCR at various time-points reveals any changes in tyrosine phosphorylation after BCR crosslinking. Reversing the order of the experiment, an APT immunoprecipitation followed by a LMP2A or Syk Western blot, will give similar results. Both will determine whether or not LMP2A or Syk protein is tyrosine phosphorylated. However, this reversal tends to be less sensitive, owing to the less specific immunoprecipitation step. In this method, all phosphorylated proteins in the lysate will be immunoprecipitated with the APT antibody and therefore the amount of LMP2 or Syk in each immunoprecipitation is quantitatively less than if LMP2A or Syk were specifically immunoprecipitated from the lysate as a first step.

Quality APT antibodies are available commercially that can be used in both immunoprecipitation and immunoblot protocols. Two widely used APT antibodies are P420 and 4G10 that are available from Santa Cruz Biotechnology (Santa Cruz, CA) and Upstate Biotechnology Inc. (Lake Placid, NY), respectively. Antibodies against proteins involved in cellular signaling pathways are also commercially available. Companies such as Santa Cruz Biotechnology, Transduction Laboratories (Lexington, KY), and Upstate Biotechnology Inc. have a wide selection of antibodies (both monoclonal and polyclonal) available for use. Antisera against LMP2A are not available commercially but monoclonal antibodies (MAbs) have been made successfully *(2)*. Enzyme-conjugated secondary antibodies are readily available from many companies, including Amersham Life Sciences (Arlington Heights, IL), Jackson ImmunoResearch Laboratories (West Grove, PA), Pierce (Rockford, IL), and Transduction Laboratories.

### 1.2. Detection of Auto Kinase Activities by In Vitro Kinase Assays

An in vitro kinase assay determines whether or not enzyme activity is present in a given sample. The detection of kinase activity is based on the transfer of radiolabeled phosphate from ATP to a target substrate by the phosphotransferase activity of the kinase. The technique uses antibodies specific to the kinase to immunoprecipitate the kinase and then uses that partially purified kinase preparation as a source of enzyme activity. The in vitro auto kinase assay protocol requires γ-[$^{32}$P]ATP as the labeled donor substrate and the kinase itself as the target (acceptor) substrate. The addition of an exogenous substrate can also be used to assay the phosphotransferase activity of the kinase with an exogenous target substrate (*see* Chapter 35). Enolase is frequently used as a target protein for the assay of protein tyrosine kinases. Conditions such as the pH, salt concentration, concentrations of

$Mg^{2+}$ and $Mn^{2+}$, and temperature all have the potential to effect enzymatic activity and should be optimized for each assay.

## 2. Materials

### *2.1. Cellular Activation and Lysis*

1. RPMI: serum free RPMI-1640 medium.
2. Supplemented RPMI: RPMI-1640 medium containing 10% inactivated fetal bovine serum (FBS), 1000 U/mL of penicillin, and 1000 μg/mL of streptomycin for maintaining B-cell lines at 37°C in 5% $CO_2$ incubator.
3. 1% Triton-X Lysis buffer: 1% Triton X-100, 50 m*M* Tris-HCl, pH 7.4, 150 m*M* NaCl, 2 m*M* EDTA, 10 μg/mL (each) pepstatin and leupeptin, 1 m*M* sodium orthovanadate, and 0.5 m*M* phenylmethylsulfonyl fluoride (PMSF), use ice-cold (*see* **Note 1**).
4. Anti-immunoglobulin $F(ab')_2$ antibody (*see* **Note 2**).

### *2.2. Immunoprecipitation*

1. Protein A or G Sepharose, 50% slurry in lysis buffer (*see* **Note 3**).
2. Immunoprecipitating antibodies: anti-phosphotyrosine (APT) antibody, anti-LMP2A antibody, and antibodies against specific cellular signal transducers.
3. 1% Triton X-100 lysis buffer as wash buffer (as in **Subheading 2.1.**).
4. 2X sodium dodecyl sulfate (SDS) sample buffer: 50 m*M* Tris-HCl, pH 6.8, 2% SDS, 100 m*M* β-mercaptoethanol, 0.1% bromophenol blue, 10% glycerol.
5. Heat-block or water bath (70–95°C).

### *2.3. Western Blot (see also Chapter 26)*

1. SDS-polyacrylamide gel (6–10% acrylamide).
2. SDS-polyacrylamide gel electrophoresis (PAGE) apparatus.
3. 5X SDS electrophoresis buffer: 25 m*M* Tris-HCl, 250 m*M* glycine, pH 8.3, 0.1% SDS.
4. Protein standards.
5. Transfer apparatus.
6. PVDF membrane (i.e., Immobilon-P, Millipore, Bedford, MA) and filter papers.
7. Transfer buffer: 20 m*M* Tris-HCl, pH 8.3, 192 m*M* glycine, 10% methanol.
8. Tris-buffered saline-Tween (TBST): 10 m*M* Tris-HCl, pH 7.4, 150 m*M* NaCl, and 0.05–0.2% Tween. Buffer used for the dilution of antibody solutions and for washing and blocking the membranes.
9. Membrane blocking buffer. 3–5% nonfat dried milk or bovine serum albumin (BSA, fraction V) diluted in TBST.
10. Primary and horseradish peroxidase-conjugated secondary antibodies, diluted in TBST.
11. Enhanced chemiluminescence (ECL) chemicals for development.
12. Plastic sheet protectors.
13. Cassettes and film.

### *2.4. In Vitro Auto Kinase Assay*

1. Kinase buffer: 50 m*M* Tris-HCl, pH 7.4, 10 m*M* $MgCl_2$, 10 m*M* $MnCl_2$.
2. Kinase reaction mix: 10 μCi per 25 μL γ-[$^{32}$P]-ATP in kinase buffer.
3. Materials for SDS-PAGE (*see* **Subheadings 2.2.** and **2.3.**).
4. Gel dryer.
5. Cassettes and film.

## 3. Methods

### 3.1. Cellular Preparation

1. Remove the desired number of cells from cell culture and pellet cells gently (400*g* for 10 min).
2. Resuspend pelleted cells in 5–10 mL of RPMI and wash three times to remove extra serum proteins and other soluble factors (400*g* for 10 min).
3. Equilibrate washed cells in RPMI for 15 min at 37°C (*see* **Note 4**). This resting period in the absence of serum is essential for the detection of serum responsive proteins in an inactivated state. After incubation, the cells are ready for lysis and/or stimulation.

### 3.2. Cellular Activation and Preparation of Lysates

1. Remove cells from incubator.
2. Before BCR stimulation, remove 1 mL of cells for an unstimulated time-point(s) (*see* **Note 4**) and transfer cells into a micro-centrifuge tube containing 300 µL of ice-cold 1% Triton X lysis buffer.
3. Vortex the lysate and place on ice for 15 min to insure complete cell lysis.
4. Stimulate the remaining cells with 25 µg of anti-Immunoglobulin antibodies per mL and quickly remove 1 mL of stimulated cells (*see* **Note 4**) at each time-point into a micro-centrifuge tube that contains 300 µL of ice-cold 1% Triton X lysis buffer (*see* **Note 5**).
5. Immediately vortex each lysate and place on ice for 15 min.
6. Remove insoluble material by centrifugation at 4°C (10,000*g* for 15 min), repeat if necessary. The cleared supernatants are now ready for immunoprecipitation.

### 3.3. Immunoprecipitation

1. Incubate the prepared cell lysates with 25–40 µL of protein A or G Sepharose (50% slurry) for 1 h at 4°C to preclear each lysate of proteins that bind nonspecifically to the Sepharose.
2. Remove Sepharose beads by centrifugation (10,000*g* for 15 min). Save supernatants and transfer to new micro-centrifuge tubes.
3. Incubate cleared lysates with the appropriate antisera for 1 h at 4°C. Use 1–3 µg of antibody per immunoprecipitation (*see* **Note 6**).
4. Capture immune complexes with 25-40 µL of protein A- or G-Sepharose (50% slurry) for 1 h at 4°C (*see* **Note 3**).
5. Remove supernatant by centrifugation (1,000*g* for 10 min).
6. Wash precipitated immune complexes (beads) four times with cold 1% Triton X lysis buffer.
7. Remove wash buffer from the bead pellet and resuspend beads in 2X SDS sample buffer.
8. Denature samples at 70–95°C for 10 min (*see* **Note 7**).
9. Separate immunoprecipitated proteins by SDS-PAGE (*see* Chapter 26).

### 3.4. Immunoblotting (see also *Chapter 26*)

1. Transfer separated proteins to Immobilon membrane.
2. Block the membrane in membrane blocking buffer for 1 h at room temperature (*see* **Note 8**).
3. Incubate membrane in primary antibody for 1 h at room temperature (*see* **Note 9**).
4. Wash membrane three times in TBST.
5. Incubate membrane with a horseradish peroxidase-conjugated secondary antibody for 30 min at room temperature.
6. Wash membrane an additional four times in TBST.
7. Detect proteins by enhanced chemiluminescence (ECL): Combine equal volumes of ECL

solutions A and B, cover membrane entirely with solution, and expose to mixed ECL solution for 1 min.

8. Remove membrane from ECL solution and place wet membrane in plastic sheet protector and expose to film. Time of exposure will vary from seconds to minutes depending upon the strength of the signal.

### 3.5. *In Vitro* Kinase Assays

1. Wash immune complexes four times with cold 1% Triton-X lysis buffer as performed in the standard immunoprecipitation protocol (*see* **Subheading 3.3., step 6**).
2. Wash immune complexes an additional two times with kinase buffer. This step removes the detergent from the immune complexes and provides the necessary $Mn^{2+}$ and $Mg^{2+}$ ions needed for kinase activity.
3. Remove kinase wash buffer and resuspend immune complexes in 25 µL of kinase buffer containing 10 µCi of γ-[$^{32}$P]-ATP per sample.
4. Incubate at room temperature for 20 min (*see* **Note 10**).
5. Stop reactions with the addition of 2X SDS sample buffer.
6. Denature samples at 70–95°C for 10 min and load onto a SDS-polyacrylamide gel.
7. After electrophoresis (*see* **Note 11**), remove the bottom of the gel with a razorblade just above the dye front. This will remove the nonincorporated [$^{32}$P] ATP and will eliminate the overexposure of the film at the bottom of the gel which might interfere with the detection of specific protein bands near the dye front.
8. Use a gel dryer apparatus to dry the gel. Two h at 80°C is adequate to dry a large gel (15 × 15 cm, 1.5-mm thickness) and the time can be shortened for smaller or thinner gels. Place the gel on 2 pieces of filter paper and cover top with plastic wrap to avoid $^{32}$P contamination of gel dryer.
9. Place dried gel (on filter paper, covered with plastic wrap) in a film cassette and expose to film. (The $^{32}$P signal will penetrate through the plastic wrap.) The use of an intensifying screen will enhance the sharpness of the image and exposure of the film at a lower temperature (–70°C) will help to stabilize the film image and often requires a shorter exposure time.

## 4. Notes

1. This lysis buffer contains a cocktail of chelating agents and phosphatase and protease inhibitors to inhibit most metallo-, serine-, and thiol-proteases. PMSF is the least stable of the included inhibitors and has a half-life of 35 min to 3 h depending on the temperature and pH of the solution. Therefore, it is recommended to add PMSF at each step of the protocol.
2. Use a F(ab')$_2$ fragment anti-immunoglobulin antibody instead of a whole Ig antibody for anti-Ig stimulation to eliminate cellular activation through the membrane Fc receptors.
3. The antibody class, subclass, and species may effect the binding affinity of the Fc portion of the antibody for either protein A or G Sepharose. Most antibodies work efficiently with protein A, but refer to an antibody reference to choose the apropriate Sepharose for a specific antibody ***(12)***.
4. For equilibration, place cells in a final volume of RPMI convenient for cell lysis. For example, if cells have been prepared for an experiment involving 3 activation time-points resuspend and equilibrate the cells in 3 mL of medium so that 1 mL of cells can be used for each time-point and the volume is convenient for lysis in a 1.5-mL micro-centrifuge tube.

5. For relatively long time-points (e.g., 5–10 min), place stimulated cells back in the 37°C incubator to maintain ambient growth conditions before cell lysis.
6. Dilute the antibody in lysis buffer or PBS and aliquot a larger volume of the diluted antibody into each immunoprecipitation for greater accuracy in dispensing 1–3 μg antibody per sample.
7. Standard denaturation by heating is generally done at 95°C, however, highly hydrophobic proteins (e.g., LMP2A) form high molecular weight aggregates at exposure to such high temperatures and do not effectively migrate in SDS-polyacrylamide gels. Denaturation of hydrophobic proteins at 70°C eliminates this problem.
8. The use of milk as a blocking buffer is usually the best option because it is cheap and provides a clean background. However, milk contains many phosphoproteins that will be detected by antibodies specific for anti-phosphotyrosine. This nonspecific reactivity will interfere with the experimental results. The use of BSA (fraction V) will alleviate this problem.
9. Dilute antibodies in blocking buffer or TBST at a concentration recommended by the manufacturer (if known) or perform trial experiments with various dilutions of primary antibody. Most MAbs work well in a 1:200 to 1:2000 dilution.
10. Use standard lab protocols for the handling of radio-isotopes. Wear apropriate protective clothing, use blocking tube racks for samples, and perform experiments behind a thick Plexiglas shield. The use of screw-capped, micro-centrifuge tubes will prevent dispersal of $^{32}$P-labeled liquids and contamination of centrifuges.
11. Stop electrophoresis of the gel when the dye front is still present in the gel (2–3 cm from the bottom of the gel) so that the nonincorporated [$^{32}$P] ATP will remain in the gel and not contaminate the buffer reservoir.

## References


1. Burkhardt, A. L., Brunswick, M., Bolen, J. B., and Mond, J. J. (1991) Anti-immunoglobulin stimulation of B lymphocytes activates src-related protein-tyrosine kinases. *Proc. Natl. Acad. Sci. USA* **88,** 7410–7414.
2. Fruehling, S., Lee, S., Herrold, R., Frech, B., Laux, G., Kremmer, E., et al. (1996) Identification of latent membrane protein 2A (LMP2A) domains essential for the LMP2A dominant-negative effect on B-lymphocyte surface immunoglobulin signal transduction. *J. Virology* **70,** 6216–6226.
3. Fruehling, S. and Longnecker, R. (1997) The immunoreceptor tyrosine-based activation motif of Epstein-Barr virus LMP2A is essential for blocking BCR-mediated signal transduction. *Virol.* **235,** 241–251.
4. Fruehling, S., Swart, R., Dolwick, K. M., Kremmer, E., and Longnecker, R. (1998) Tyrosine 112 of latent membrane protein 2A is essential for protein tyrosine kinase loading and regulation of Epstein-Barr virus latency. *J. Virol.* **72,** 7796–7806.
5. Miller, C. L., Burkhardt, A. L., Lee, J. H., Stealey, B., Longnecker, R., Bolen, J. B., and Kieff, E. (1995) Integral membrane protein 2 of Epstein-Barr virus regulates reactivation from latency through dominant negative effects on protein-tyrosine kinases. *Immunity* **2,** 155–166.
6. Panousis, C. G. and Rowe, D. T. (1997) Epstein-barr virus latent membrane protein 2 associates with and is a substrate for mitogen-activated protein kinase. *J. Virol.* **71,** 4752–4760.
7. Bolen, J. B. (1993) Nonreceptor tyrosine protein kinases. *Oncogene* **8,** 2025–2031.
8. Cambier, J. C., Pleiman, C. M., and Clark, M. R. (1994) Signal transduction by the B cell antigen receptor and its coreceptors. *Annu. Rev. Immunol.* **12,** 457–486.

9. DeFranco, A. L. (1995) Transmembrane signaling by antigen receptors of B and T lymphocytes. *Curr. Opin. Cell Biol.* **7,** 163–175.
10. Gold, M. R. and Matsuuchi, L. (1995) Signal transduction by the antigen receptors of B and T lymphocytes. *Int. Rev. Cytol.* **157,** 181–276.
11. Weiss, A. and Littman, D. R. (1994) Signal transduction by lymphocyte antigen receptors. *Cell* **76,** 263–274.
12. Harlow, E. and Lane, D. (1988) *Antibodies: A Laboratory Manual.* Cold Spring Harbor Laboratory Press, Cold Spring Harbor, NY, pp. 618.

# VIII

## Tissue and In Vivo Protocols

# 37

## Analysis of Apoptosis in Tissue Sections

**Vicki Save, Philip J. Coates, and Peter A. Hall**

### 1. Introduction

The recognition over the past decade that apoptosis represents a critical element in cell-number control in physiological and pathological situations has been well-reviewed *(1–4)*. In addition there is increasing recognition that many of the effects of chemo- and radio- therapeutic agents are mediated by apoptosis *(5–7)*. The seminal work of Kerr, Wyllie, and Currie *(8)*, building upon the earlier observations of Glucksmann *(9)* and Saunders *(10)*, should be read by those interested in assaying apoptosis because of the excellent photomicrographs that document the morphological features of the process. This is important because despite considerable progress in the understanding of the mechanistic basis of apoptosis, morphological analysis remains unquestionably the "gold-standard" for its assessment and quantitation.

Apoptosis is a regulated and active process. Although a diverse range of insults and physiological events can lead to apoptosis the process is remarkably stereotyped, with a program of activities leading to the final morphological events that are similar throughout phylogeny and may be recapitulated in most (if not all) cell types. Mounting data indicate that much of the machinery for the implementation of the apoptotic response is "hard-wired" in cells, being present all the time but kept in an "off" state: rapidly recruited into an "on" state if needed. Consequently, and despite much effort, there remain few biochemical markers of the apoptotic process that are specific for this complex regulated process. Similarly, although many potential regulators of apoptosis are described, critical examination of the available data indicates that there is little consensus on their value as markers of apoptosis.

A critical point for the quantitation of apoptosis is that, irrespective of the initiating insult, the time-course of apoptosis is very fast *(11,12)*. Moreover, the clearance of the resultant debris (either by professional phagocytes or bystander [amateur] phagocytes) is rapid. Coles et al. *(13)* suggested that clearance times of less than 1 h were typical. The rapid nature of apoptosis means that in any static analysis, a very small number of apoptotic cells observed at a given instant might, in fact, reflect a very considerable

From: *Methods in Molecular Biology, Vol. 174: Epstein-Barr Virus Protocols*
Edited by: J. B. Wilson and G. H. W. May © Humana Press Inc., Totowa, NJ

contribution to cell turnover. Dramatic evidence for this came from studies of the physiological contribution of apoptosis in renal development *(13)* and in the steady-state regulation of intestinal epithelial populations *(14)*. Although the process of apoptosis and its clearance is (as far as we can tell) always rapid, there may be some variation between cell types or in relation to different insults. This has important implications for the quantitation of apoptosis, as highlighted by Potten *(15)*.

Given its contribution to cell turnover in physiological, pathological, and toxicological situations, it is important to be able to identify and quantitate the process of apoptosis in cells and in tissues. Ideally, one would like a technique that is sensitive and highly selective for apoptosis, and it should also be easily applicable to routinely prepared tissue sections. Here we will review the various options that can be used to identify and quantitate apoptosis, concentrating on those methods applicable to tissues sections. A method for the identification of apoptosis using in situ end-labeling of DNA fragments (ISEL/TUNEL) is given.

### 1.1. Demonstration of Apoptosis: Comparison of Methods

#### 1.1.1. Morphology

The phenomenon of apoptosis is defined by a series of morphological changes *(8,16,17)*. The classical features are best seen by electron microscopy but can be observed at the light microscopic level using nucleic acid-binding dyes, such as hematoxylin, acridine orange, or propidium iodide (PI) *(8,13,16,18)*. The first signs of apoptotic cell death are a condensation of the nuclear material, with a marked accumulation of densely stained chromatin, typically at the edge of the nucleus. This is accompanied by cell shrinkage. Cytoplasmic blebs appear on the cell surface, best seen by time-lapse video-microscopy *(19)*, and the cell detaches from its neighbors. The nuclear outline often becomes highly folded and the nucleus breaks up, with discrete fragments dispersing throughout the cytoplasm. Eventually, the cells themselves fragment, with the formation of a number of membrane bounded apoptotic bodies. Apoptotic bodies are generally phagocytosed by surrounding cells, which are not necessarily derived from the mononuclear phagocytic system. Therefore, the most common sign of apoptosis in a tissue section is the presence of apoptotic bodies, which may be seen as extracellular bodies, or, after phagocytosis, inside other cells. Apoptotic bodies have a diverse appearance, particularly in regard to their size. They are generally oval or round in shape, and are most easily recognized when they contain large amounts of homogeneous, condensed chromatin. The morphological features of apoptosis have been extensively reviewed, and plentiful illustrations of both the light and electron microscopic appearances are provided in these publications *(8,16,17,20,21)*.

#### 1.1.2. DNA Laddering (see also *Chapter 20*)

A characteristic feature of apoptosis is DNA fragmentation. Wyllie *(22)* described in association with apoptosis nucleosomal fragmentation, which can be seen by agarose electrophoresis with a ladder of DNA bands representing multiples of 180–200 base pairs. This DNA "ladder" correlates with the early morphological signs of apoptosis *(23)* and so this technique has been widely used as a distinctive marker of the process *(24–28)*. DNA laddering is not seen in cells that have undergone necrosis, which rather show a random fragmentation pattern, leading to smears on agarose electrophoresis *(22)*. However, the method is not easily quantified and cannot be applied (in this form) to tissue sections. Moreover, although it is clear that DNA degradation is a common feature of apoptosis, it is also evident that not all cells that undergo apoptosis show the formation of a nucleosomal-sized ladder of DNA. In some cases, DNA fragmentation appears to be delayed *(29)*, whereas others have reported a complete lack of DNA laddering *(30)*. It has recently been shown that cells undergoing apoptosis may show only very limited DNA degradation, with the formation of 300 or 50 kilobase fragments *(31)*. These fragments are thought to represent the release of loops of chromatin from their attachment points on the nuclear scaffold. These changes cannot be seen on conventional electrophoresis, but require the use of pulsed-field gel electrophoresis (PFGE) to allow the separation of large DNA fragments.

#### *1.1.3. ISEL or TUNEL*

The property of DNA fragmentation in apoptosis can be utilized to identify cells undergoing this process *(32–36)* since certain enzymes can add labeled nucleotides to the DNA ends. The labeled nucleotides can then be identified by immunological methods akin to immunohistochemistry. Such methods were originally termed TUNEL (terminal deoxynucleotidyl transferase mediated UTP nick-end labeling) but are also referred to as ISEL (*In Situ* End-Labeling techniques). Strictly, the different names relate to the different enzymes employed and although there are theoretical and some practical differences, the similarity of technique and result make the names essentially interchangeable. A comparison of the methodologies employing TdT (TUNEL) and Klenow fragment of DNA polymerase (ISEL) was reported by Mundle et al. *(37)*, who demonstrated that TUNEL appeared more sensitive than ISEL. This is because TdT can label 3' recessed, 5' recessed or blunt ends of DNA, whereas ISEL labels only those with 3' recessed ends. All three types of DNA end are seen in apoptosis and thus in principle TdT-based methods should be more sensitive than Klenow polymerase methods. Despite this, in practice ISEL and TUNEL appear functionally interchangeable.

Irrespective of the enzyme employed a variety of labels could be used, including radioactive nucleotide triphosphates. However, methods based on the use of nonisotopic labels have been developed and are superior for a variety of reasons, including ease of use, stability, simplicity, and speed of detection, and the increased resolution obtained. Using this approach, it has been clearly shown that the amount and distribution of labeled cells is closely correlated with the amount and distribution of cells known to be undergoing apoptosis using other methods *(33–36)*. The method can be modified for fluorescence detection *in situ* or by flow cytometry or detection at the light or ultrastructural levels *(36,38)*. In addition, the use of immunocytochemistry for cell-surface antigens in combination with TUNEL/ISEL allows the identification of the particular cell types undergoing apoptosis, and could also be used to measure phenotypic changes in apoptotic cells *(36,39)* and with *in situ* hybridization methods *(40)*.

The protocol for TUNEL/ISEL is given later, based on our experience (***14,35,41,42***, and *see* **Note 1**). A number of variables must be considered when performing the technique. The staining results depend on a variety of factors, including the rapidity and extent of fixation, the extent and nature of proteolytic digestion, the specificity of the DNA polymerase, the extent of incorporation of labeled nucleotide triphosphate and the sensitivity of detection of the label.

### 1.1.4. Immunohistochemical Methods

In recent years, a large number of antibodies have been marketed for apoptosis research. The vast majority of these recognize proteins that can influence apoptosis in certain instances, but are neither universal nor specific. Indeed, because apoptosis is a consequence of the activation of pre-existing mechanisms within a cell, there has been relatively little progress in the identification and use of antigens whose expression is correlated with this form of cell death. Immunohistological detection of the expression of regulatory proteins (e.g., Bcl-2 or BAX) has been reported, but the utility of this approach as a marker of apoptosis is unsubstantiated. Moreover, there have been significant problems with the specificity of some reagents purported to be apoptosis specific and the authors urge extreme caution (*see,* for example, the caveat on BAX staining in **ref.** ***[45]***). A novel approach recently reported is the detection of Annexin V expression in apopotic cells as a consequence of membrane changes ***(46,47)***. Unfortunately this method requires the use of unfixed cells and cannot be applied (at present) to histological material. The use of antibodies to clusterin (also known as TRPM-2, or SGP-2) has also been correlated with apoptosis in certain situations, although this protein is not a universal marker, nor is it specific for apoptosis ***(48)***. Perhaps the most widely used immunhistochemical marker of apoptosis is the identification of tissue transglutaminase (tTG) ***(49,50)***, although even here recent data suggests that transglutaminase is not always induced during apoptosis ***(51)*** Finally, apoptosis can also be demonstrated by *in situ* hybridization ***(52)***, although the utility of this method also remains to be established.

### 1.1.5. Flow Cytometry

The detection of fragmented nuclei by flow cytometry is now a widely used and accepted method for the detection and quantitation of apoptosis ***(28,53)***. The methods rely upon the use of DNA binding dye (usually PI), which intercalates stoichiometrically with DNA and allows the quantitation of DNA content. A sub-G1 peak is reliably found to be indicative of apoptosis (because of the DNA fragmentation) and the peak size reflects the amount of apoptosis in the sample. The method is easily applied to cell suspensions and can also be applied to material derived from histological samples, although this is associated with higher "background levels" and of course results in the loss of potentially important spatial and micro-anatomical information. The appearance of phosphatidylserine on the cell surface can also be measured by FACS, through binding of FITC-tagged annexin V. Simultaneous staining with propidium iodide aids with the identification of the apoptotic cell population.

### 1.1.6. ELISA-Based Methods

A variety of enzyme-linked immunosorbent assay (ELISA)-based methods for the quantitation of apoptosis that are limited to cell culture systems have recently been developed and marketed (Boehringer Mannheim; Calbiochem, for example). These assays utilize the release of usually insoluble nuclear molecules into the cytoplasm of dying cells, and kits are available for the measurement of nucleosomes or nuclear matrix proteins. In addition, a Western blot method has also been proposed, based on the cleavage of the 113 kDa poly(ADP-ribose)polymerase into 89 kDa and 24 kDa fragments by members of the ICE-like proteases, which are activated during apoptosis ***(54)***.

#### *1.1.7. Conclusion*

Although we have a burgeoning knowledge of the mechanistic basis of apoptosis and an increasing recognition of its contribution to both physiological and pathological processes, the ability to objectively quantitate this process remains poorly developed. It is the view of these authors that if apoptosis is to be assessed in histological material, then there is no escape from meticulous and painstaking microscopy coupled with rigorous and meticulous quantitation. Whether it is the quantitation of morphologically defined events ("the gold standard") or of TUNEL/ISEL-defined events is in our view a relatively unimportant issue—they will correlate very well—and both have inherent problems. Arguably the morphological approach is perhaps more satisfactory, but curiously the additional complexity of TUNEL/ISEL attracts some workers! In the end, the choice of method will depend on the experience of the researcher in histological analysis and microscopy.

## 2. Materials

### *2.1. Materials in Common to ISEL and TUNEL*

1. Tissues and cells: *In situ* end-labeling techniques can be applied to cells grown in culture, to frozen tissue section, or to formalin-fixed, paraffin-embedded material, such as that found in surgical pathology archives.
2. Methanol/Acetone fix: 50% methanol, 50% acetone.
3. 4% paraformaldehyde: dissolve 4 g of paraformaldehye in 80 mL of water with gentle heating and addition of 1 *M* NaOH until the powder dissolves. Make up to 90 mL with distilled water and add 10 mL of 10X PBS.
4. 10X Phosphate-buffered saline (PBS): 1 L consists of 80 g NaCl, 2 g KCl, 14 g $Na_2HPO_4$ and 2 g $KH_2PO_4$. Adjust pH to 7.4 with HCl. Filter-sterilize through a 0.2-µm filter and store at 4°C.
5. Silane solution: 5 mL of 3-aminopropyltriethoxysilane (Sigma) in 250 mL of acetone.
6. Glass slides.
7. Ethanol: 100, 95, 90, and 70% with distilled water.
8. Methanol.
9. Proteinase K: A stock solution of proteinase K (Sigma; P2308) is prepared by dissolving 10 mg of enzyme in 1 mL of water, to give a 10 mg/mL concentration. The enzyme is aliquoted and stored frozen. The aliquots should not be thawed and re-frozen more than twice. For use, 5 mL of the stock solution is diluted into 5 mL of sterile 50 m*M* Tris/HCl, pH 8.0, 1 m*M* ethylenediammetetraacetic acid (EDTA).
10. Horseradish peroxidase-conjugated avidin (Dako Ltd.; P364) is made freshly by diluting 5 mL into 1 mL of PBS containing 1% bovine serum albumin (BSA) (Sigma; A9647).
11. Methanol with 0.5% or 3% $H_2O_2$.
12. Mayer's hematoxylin.

### 2.2. ISEL

1. *In Situ* end-labeling buffer: 0.01 m$M$ of each of biotin-dATP, dCTP, dGTP, and dTTP, in 50 m$M$ Tris-HCl, pH 7.5, 5 m$M$ $MgCl_2$, 10 m$M$ 2-Mercaptoethanol, 0.005% BSA (Molecular Biology grade, e.g., Sigma; B2518), and 5 U/mL Klenow fragment of DNA polymerase I. The labeling solution without polymerase can be prepared in bulk and stored frozen in aliquots, but the DNA polymerase must be added immediately prior to use. The biotinylated nucleotide can be obtained from Life Technologies Ltd. (cat. # 19534-016). Deoxynucleotide triphosphates can be purchased as a set from Boehringer Mannheim (cat. # 1277 049).
2. Diaminobenzidine-$H_2O_2$.

### 2.3. TUNEL

1. TdT buffer: 30 m$M$ TRIZMA base, pH 7.2, 140 m$M$ sodium Cacodylate, 1 m$M$ $CoCl_2$.
2. Terminal deoxynucleotidyl transferase (TdT) enzyme (Boehringer Mannheim).
3. dUTP biotin (Boehringer Mannheim).
4. AEC: 3-amino-9-ethyl-carbazole (AEC peroxidase substrate kit; Vector Lab.).

## 3. Methods

### 3.1. Fixation

Frozen material or tissue culture cells may be fixed by immersion for 10 min in Methanol/Acetone fix at –20°C, followed by air drying. Alternatively, a 4% solution of paraformaldehyde can be used. For the latter, fix sections for 10 min at 4°C, and then rinse slides in PBS. Tissues or cells which are to be used for TUNEL/ISEL should be fixed as quickly as possible, because delay causes significant artifacts.

Importantly, it has been shown that TUNEL/ISEL can be performed on sections of archival tissues after formalin fixation and storage as wax blocks. When using tissue sections that have been fixed in formaldehyde, it is necessary to use a protease in order to break some of the crosslinks formed between proteins, and thereby allow access of the reagents to the degraded DNA. Either pepsin or proteinase K can be used for this step, and the extent of digestion varies with the extent of fixation. In general, too much digestion leads to some nonspecific staining, whilst too little digestion results in a decrease in the intensity of staining of apoptotic cells. Proteolytic digestion is not required when using frozen cells or tissue sections fixed in acetone/methanol.

### 3.2. In Situ *End Labeling (ISEL, see Notes 1 and 2)*

1. To aid tissue adherance, silane-coat glass slides by soaking them for 60 min in silane solution.
2. Wash slides twice with distilled water for 10 min each wash.
3. Dry slides overnight at 60°C. Slides can be stored for several months under dry and dust-free conditions.
4. Cut 3–4-µm sections and mount on silane coated glass slides.
5. Paraffin embedded sections must be dewaxed, for nonembedded samples proceed to on to **step 8**. To dewax sections, dry mounted sections on the slides overnight at 40°C.
6. Place slides in fresh xylene for 10 min and repeat for a further 10 min in fresh xylene.
7. Rinse sections twice for 1 min in 100% ethanol, followed by 2 min in methanol and air-dry.

8. For formaldehyde-fixed samples: Digest with 100 μL/section of proteinase K for 30 min at 37°C (*see* **Notes 3** and **4**).
9. Wash sections in sterile distilled water three times, rinse in 70, 90, and 95% ethanol and air-dry.
10. Prepare 40–60 μL *in situ* end-labeling buffer for each section and keep on ice (*see* **Notes 5–7**).
11. Carefully pipet the mixture over the tissue section, and place a clean glass coverslip over the section to prevent evaporation.
12. Incubate at 37°C for 1 h in a moist chamber.
13. Terminate the reaction by washing sections in distilled water three times, being careful not to scratch the tissue surface when removing the coverslip.
14. Block endogenous peroxidase activity with methanol containing 0.5% $H_2O_2$ (100 vol) for 30 min (*see* **Note 8**). Wash three times in distilled water and rinse in PBS.
15. Incubate with diluted horseradish peroxidase-conjugated avidin (*see* **Notes 6** and **8**).
16. Wash in PBS three times (5 minutes each) and develop in diaminobenzidine-$H_2O_2$. Lightly counterstain with hematoxylin and mount in resin.
17. View under a light microscope, where apoptotic nuclei are stained brown and non-apoptotic cell nuclei appear blue (*see* **Notes 9–11**).

### 3.3. Terminal Deoxynucleotidyl Transferase Mediated UTP Nick-End Labeling (TUNEL) In Situ (see Note 1)

1. Dewax 1–2 μm paraffin sections of formalin-fixed samples as described in **Subheading 3.2., steps 1–6** (*see* **Note 12**).
2. Rinse sections twice for 1 min in ethanol, once for 2 min in methanol followed by a rinse in water.
3. Pre-treat sections with 100 μL/section of 10 mg/mL proteinase K for 20 min at room temperature (*see* **Notes 3** and **4**).
4. Wash sections four times for 1 min each in PBS.
5. To block endogenous peroxidase activity, place sections in a solution of 3% (v/v) $H_2O_2$ in methanol for 5 min at room temperature (*see* **Note 8**).
6. Wash in PBS four times for 1 minute each and finally wash in TdT buffer.
7. Incubate sections in 100 μL/section of a solution of 0.25 U/mL TdT and 1 nmol dUTP-biotin in TdT buffer at 37°C for 60 min in a humid environment (*see* **Notes 13** and **14**).
8. Incubate sections in 100 mL of horseradish peroxidase streptavidin (Dako) for 1 h at room temperature (*see* **Note 14**).
9. Incubate sections in AEC according to kit instructions.
10. Red-stained apoptotic nuclei can be visualized by light microscopy after approx 15 min.
11. Counterstain with Mayer's hematoxylin.

### 3.4. Quantitation

This is a real problem. Much of the currently available literature on apoptosis is problematic because of inadequate quantitation procedures. The application of stereological and morphometric principles to quantitation in histology is difficult: many authors get round this problem by ignoring it. Moreover, many texts on the subject are at best impenetrable. The use of flow cytometric methods does lend to the problem the advantages of objective assessment of large numbers of events (>$10^4$ typically): those wishing to use *in situ* techniques will not be easily able to match that, but will obtain valuable information relating to micro-anatomical variation, which may be of fundamental biological importance. It is worth restating that not only is the ability of cells to proliferate and differentiate regulated by position (anatomical and within cellular hierarchies) but so too is apoptosis ***(15)***. The critical issues are simply stated:

1. The confidence that can be placed upon the data depends on the effort and rigor invested in its generation;
2. Where the levels of apoptosis are low (the usual state of affairs), very large numbers of events must be quantitated for accuracy; and
3. Methods based on semi-quantitative approaches, the use of high-power fields as denominator, the failure to define reproducibility of assessment and methods that do not consider the heterogeneity implicit in biological samples are to be deprecated.

Given this what can be done?

### *3.4.1. What to Count?*

ISEL- or TUNEL-stained samples will make the microscopic assessment easier and perhaps more objective, particularly if the observer is not an experienced microscopist. On the other hand these methods *may* underestimate the true number of apoptotic bodies and may be influenced by artefacts (owing to fixation ***[14]*** or non-apoptotic processes ***[35,44]***). The former may not matter as the "error" will be systematic and the same in all samples. The latter is significant but can be minimized by careful control of sample handling. In the hands of an experienced microscopist then, fluorescent dye based assays ***(13)*** or even simple hematoxylin will be useful ***(14)***. Double-labeling may be useful in very specialized circumstances ***(14)*** and ISEL methods can be combined with both immunocytochemical techniques (*see* for example, **ref. *39***) and with *in situ* hybridization methods (*see* for example, **ref. *40***) to good effect.

### *3.4.2. How Many Events to Count?*

Pragmatism must be the key word, and there must be a compromise between the quality of the data, the time taken to generate that data, and the importance of the question. Although statistical approaches can be employed to determine how many events must be assessed (*see* **ref. *55*** for a discussion), the authors favor an experimental approach based on the generation of a "wandering mean" in a small number of representative examples from the population of cases to be studied. To generate this data, the following procedure should be undertaken.

Count the number of events (TUNEL/ISEL positive or apoptotic bodies) and total number of relevant cells in the first microscopic field. This will give the first score (A1 based on N1 cells). In the second field, the process is repeated and running scores recorded to give a running mean (A2 based on N2 cells). This process is repeated to give multiple running averages (A3, N3 . . . . . . An, Nn). If these are plotted, the mean will be seen to wander and eventually oscillate about a mean value and as N increases this will become less. This procedure can then define experimentally the number of events to be assessed to produce a given quality of data.

## 4. Notes

1. Specificity: TUNEL/ISEL can by no means be said to be specific for apoptosis. Fortunately, the discrimination between large numbers of stained cells in an area of necrosis,

and the presence of scattered cells undergoing apoptosis, should not pose a great problem to a trained histologist. However, of course, the effects of speed of fixation, and the penetration rates of fixative may also influence the staining characteristics of the tissue. For instance, if a large piece of tissue is immersed in fixative, there will be a significant delay before cells in the center of the tissue are fixed, with the possible result of autolysis. For most purposes, the TUNEL/ISEL technique can be considered a selective (rather than a specific) technique for the identification of apoptosis in histological material. The technique assists with the identification and quantitation of apoptosis, but must be employed in conjunction with simple morphological examination in order to exclude artefactual staining caused by technical aspects, and staining as a result of demonstrating DNA strand breaks resulting from other physiological or pathological processes.

2. A number of kits are available and work very well and have good documentation. For example, the ApopTag Plus Kit marketed by Oncor (Appligene), the *in situ* cell death detection kits (Boehringer Mannheim), or the FragEL kits (Calbiochem/Oncogene Research). However, these kits can be expensive and there is no reason why the component parts cannot be purchased from other competitive suppliers and incorporated into the methods. The ability to undertake these methods is critically based on having good basic histological and immunohistological skills.
3. Proteinase K should not be used if preparations have been fixed in methanol/acetone.
4. The conditions for proteolytic digestion may need to be varied, and it is advisable in the first instance to perform a series of digestions, varying the concentration of proteinase K from 1–20 mg/mL or digesting at room temperature or varying digestion time. Thinner sections will need less digestion. In principle, any enzyme with proteolytic activity can be used, but remember that enzyme preparations may be contaminated with nuclease activities, which could give false-positive results. For this reason, pepsin or proteinase K are good choices because the former is used at low pH, where nucleases would not be active, whereas the latter is supplied in a highly purified form and is effectively free of nuclease activity.
5. To avoid contamination by DNases, it is advisable to sterilize the solutions used in the TUNEL/ISEL procedure, particularly the labeling buffer, and to use sterile pipet tips and microcentrifuge tubes.
6. Digoxigenin-11-dUTP (Boehringer Mannheim) can be substituted for the biotinylated dATP at the same concentration (but note that the unlabeled nucleotides should then be dATP, dCTP, and dGTP). In this case, the reaction is detected by incubation with anti-digoxigenin antibodies (e.g., peroxidase conjugated anti-digoxigenin, cat. 1,207,733, diluted 1:200). Nucleotide triphosphates labeled with fluorescent markers are also available.
7. A variety of enzymes can be used for incorporation of the label. Klenow fragment of DNA polymerase I is preferable to the DNA polymerase I holoenzyme because it has the identical polymerase activity, but lacks the exonuclease activity which could cause artifactual labeling ***(43)***. Alternatively, one can use terminal deoxynucleotidyl transferase (TdT) ***(33)***, which adds on long tails of nucleotides to the 3' hydroxyl ends of DNA without the need for a template strand ***(43)***. It is extremely important to use the correct concentration of enzyme, as increased amounts will lead to nonspecific staining of morphologically normal nuclei ***(34,35)***. Obviously, insufficient enzyme will lead to a reduction in the staining of apoptotic nuclei.
8. This method uses detection of biotinylated sites with peroxidase and is highly suited for assessment of paraffin sections. The protocol should be amended if a different label has been used, or if a different detection system is preferred (e.g., fluorescent detection).

9. Modifications of the basic method are well-documented for flow cytometry *(36)*, and kits are also sold by Oncor, Appligene, and Boehringer Mannheim.
10. Controls. As with any technique, it is essential to perform a number of controls. A positive control section should be included with each batch, to test for variations in the intensity of staining from day to day. For each test section, an appropriate immunohistocemical control should be performed to test for the presence of endogenous enzyme activities and/or nonspecific binding of the detection reagents. This is most easily achieved by the exclusion of the enzyme or the labeled nucleotide from the TUNEL/ISEL reaction mixture.
11. Staining patterns and their interpretation. Irrespective of the enzyme or label employed, not all apoptotic bodies are intensely stained, and in particular, it is not uncommon to see that the extremely condensed nuclei are relatively unstained. This may be owing to problems with penetration of the reagents into these nuclei. The nuclei of non-apoptotic cells should be unstained by the technique, if the enzyme digestion has been performed correctly. A generalized staining of all or many apparently normal nuclei suggests that proteolytic digestion has been too harsh—a similar effect is seen if a DNAase treatment is used a positive control *(34,35)*. Necrotic cells are also stained by the method *(41)* and there are a number of situations in which staining can be seen in morphologically normal nuclei, for example in spermatogonia *(35)* and after exposure to some DNA damaging agents *(44)*. DNA breaks could be present as the result of fixation and processing procedures, which result in the accumulation of lower molecular weight DNA. In addition, the action of section cutting and various pretreatments, such as exposure to hydrogen peroxide to block endogenous peroxidase activity, might also cause DNA breaks in cells. In practice, this means that a range of concentrations of enzyme may need to be tested, particularly when using the technique for the first time.
12. An alternative to using xylene is to treat the sections for 5 min with Histoclear.
13. Incubate control slides without TdT enzyme.
14. Incubations must be done in a humid environment, such as a sealed box with wet paper towels, to avoid evaporation of the small liquid volumes.

## References


1. Korsmeyer, S. J. (1995) Regulators of cell death. *Trends Genet.* **11,** 101–105.
2. Wyllie, A. H. (1995) The genetic regulation of apoptosis. *Curr. Opin. Gen. Dev.* **5,** 97–104.
3. White, E. (1996) Life, death and the pursuit of apoptosis. *Genes Dev.* **10,** 1–15.
4. Kroemer, G. (1997) The proto-oncogene Bcl-2 and its role in regulating apoptosis. *Nature Med.* **3,** 614–620.
5. Eastman, A. (1990) Activation of programmed cell death by anti-cancer agents: cisplatin as a model system. *Cancer Cells* **2,** 275–280.
6. Dive, C. and Hickman, J. A. (1991) Drug-target interactions: only the first step in the commitment to a programmed cell death? *Br. J. Cancer* **64,** 192–196
7. Hickman, J. A. (1992) Apoptosis induced by anticancer drugs. *Cancer Metastasis Rev.* **11,** 121–139.
8. Kerr, J. F. R., Wyllie, A. H., and Currie, A. R. (1972) Apoptosis: A basic biological phenomenon with wide ranging implications in tissue kinetics. *Br. J. Cancer* **26,** 239–257.
9. Glucksman, A. (1951) Cell deaths in normal vertebrate ontogeny. *Biol. Rev.* **26,** 59–86.
10. Saunders, J. W. (1966) Death in embryonic systems. *Science* **154,** 604–612.
11. Sanderson, C. J. (1976) The mechanism of T-cell mediated cytotoxicity II. Morphological studies of cell death by time-lapse microcinematography. *Proc. Roy. Soc. Lond. B.* **192,** 241–255.

12. Matter, A. (1979) Microcinematographic and electron microscopic analysis of target cell lysis induced by cytotoxic T lymphocytes. *Immunology* **36,** 179–190.
13. Coles, H. S. R., Burne, J. F., and Raff, M. C. (1993) Large-scale normal cell death in the developing rat kidney and its reduction by epidermal growth factor. *Development* **118,** 777–784.
14. Hall, P. A., Coates, P. J., Ansari, B., and Hopwood, D. (1994) Regulation of cell number in the mammalian gastrointestinal tract: the importance of apoptosis. *J. Cell Sci.* **107,** 3569–3577.
15. Potten, C. S. (1996) What is an apoptotic index measuring? A commentary. *Br. J. Cancer* **74,** 1743–1748.
16. Wyllie, A. H., Kerr, J. F. R., and Currie, A. R. (1980) Cell death: The significance of apoptosis. *Int. Rev. Cytol.* **68,** 251–306.
17. Kerr, J. F. R., Searle, J., Harmon, B. V., and Bishop, C. J. (1987) Apoptosis, in: *Perspectives on Mammalian Cell Death* (Potten, C. S., ed.), Oxford Science Publications, Oxford, UK, pp. 93–128.
18. Gregory, C. D., Dive, C., Henderson, S., Smith, C. Williams, G. T., Gordon, J., and Rickinson, A. B. (1991) Activation of Epstein-Barr virus latent genes protects human B cells from death by apoptosis. *Nature* **349,** 612–614.
19. Evan, G. I., Wyllie, A. H., Gilbert, C. S., Littlewood, T. D., Land, H., Brooks, M., et al. (1992) Induction of apoptosis in fibroblasts by c-myc protein. *Cell* **69,** 119–128.
20. Ucker, D. S. (1991) Death by suicide: One way to go in mammalian cellular development? *New Biol.* **3,** 103–109.
21. Schwartz, L. M. and Osborne, B. A. (1993) Programmed cell death, apoptosis and killer genes. *Immunol. Today* **14,** 582–590.
22. Wyllie, A. H. (1980) Glucocorticoid-induced thymocyte apoptosis is associated with endogenous endonuclease activation. *Nature* **284,** 555–556.
23. Wyllie, A. H., Morris, R. G., Smith, A. L., and Dunlop, D. (1984) Chromatin cleavage in apoptosis: Association with condensed chromatin morphology and dependence on macromolecular synthesis. *J. Pathol.* **142,** 67–77.
24. Compton, M. M. and Cidlowski, J. A. (1986) Rapid *in vivo* effects of glucocorticoids on the integrity of rat genomic deoxyribonucleic acid. *Endocrinology* **118,** 38–45.
25. Cohen, J. J. and Duke, R. C. (1984) Glucocorticoid activation of a calcium dependent endonuclease in thymocyte nuclei leads to cell death. *J. Immunol.* **132,** 38–42.
26. McConkey, D. J., Hartzell, P., Duddy, S. K., Hakansson, H., and Orrenius, S. (1988) 2,3,7,8-Tetrachlordibenzo-p-dioxin kills immature thymocytes by $Ca^{2+}$-mediated endonuclease activation. *Science* **242,** 256–258.
27. Takano, Y. S., Harmon, B. V., and Kerr, J. F. R. (1991) Apoptosis induced by mild hyperthermia in human and murine cell lines: a study using electron microscopy and DNA gel electrophoresis. *J. Pathol.* **163,** 329–336.
28. Compton, M. M. (1992) A biochemical hallmark of apoptosis: Internucleosomal degradation of the genome. *Cancer Metastasis Rev.* **11,** 105–119.
29. Zakeri, Z. F., Quaglino, D., Latham, T., and Lockshin, R. A. (1993) Delayed internucleosomal DNA fragmentation in programmed cell death. *FASEB J.* **7,** 470–478.
30. Schwartz, L. M., Smith, S. W., Jones, M. E., and Osborne, B. A. (1993) Do all programmed cell deaths occur via apoptosis? *Proc. Natl. Acad. Sci. USA* **90,** 980–984.
31. Walker, P. R., Smith, C., Youdale, T., Leblanc, J., Whitfield, J. F., and Sikorska, M. (1991) Topoisomerase II-reactive chemotherapeutic drugs induce apoptosis in thymocytes. *Cancer Res.* **51,** 1078–1085.

32. Fehsel. K., Kolb-Bachofen, V., and Kolb, H. (1991) Analysis of TNF alpha-induced DNA strand breaks at the single cell level. *Am. J. Pathol.* **139,** 251–254.
33. Gavrieli, Y., Sherman, Y., and Ben-Sasson, S. A. (1992) Identification of programmed cell death in situ via specific labelling of nuclear DNA fragmentation. *J. Cell Biol.* **119,** 493–501.
34. Wijsman, J. H., Jonker, R. R., Keijzer, R., van de Velde, C. J. H., Cornelisse, C. J., and van Dierendonck, J. H. (1993) A new method to detect apoptosis in paraffin sections: in situ end-labelling of fragmented DNA. *J. Histochem. Cytochem.* **41,** 7–12.
35. Ansari, B., Coates, P. J., Greenstein, B. D., and Hall, P. A. (1993) In situ end-labelling detects DNA strand breaks in apoptosis and other physiological and pathological states. *J. Pathol.* **170,** 1–8.
36. Gold, R., Schmied, M., Rothe, G., Zischler, H., Breitschopf, H., Wekerle, H., and Laussmann, H. (1993) Detection of DNA fragmentation in apoptosis: application of in situ nick translation to cell culture systems and tissue sections. *J. Histochem. Cytochem.* **41,** 1023–1030.
37. Mundle, S. D., Gao, X. Z., Khan, S., Gregory, S. A., Preisler, H. D., and Raza, A. (1995) 2 in situ end labelling techniques reveal different paptterns of DNA fragmentation during spontaneous apoptosis in vivo and induced apoptosis in vitro. *Anticancer Res.* **15,** 1895–1904.
38. Migheli, A., Attanasio, A., and Schiffer, D. (1995) Ultrastructural detection of DNA strand breaks in apoptotic neural cells by in situ end-labelling techniques. *J. Pathol.* **176,** 27–35.
39. Kurrer, M. O., Pakala, S. V., Hanson, H. L., and Katz, J. D. (1997) Beta cell apoptosis in T cell-mediated autoimmune diabetes. *Proc. Natl. Acad. Sci. USA* **94,** 213–218.
40. Strater, J., Walczak, H., Krammer, P. H., and Moller, P. (1996) Simultaneous in situ detection of mRNA and apoptotic cells by combined hybridization and TUNEL. *J. Histochem. Cytochem.* **44,** 1497–1499.
41. Coates, P. J. (1994) Molecular methods for the identification of apoptosis in tissues. *J. °Histotechnol.* **17,** 261–267.
42. Coates, P. J., Hales, S. A., and Hall, P. A. (1996) The association between cell proliferation and apoptosis: studies using the cell cycle associated proteins Ki-67 and DNA polymerase alpha. *J. Pathol.* **178,** 71–77.
43. Sambrook, J., Fritsch, E. F., and Maniatis, T. (1989) M*olecular Cloning: A Laboratory Manual.* Cold Spring Harbor Laboratory Press, Cold Spring Harbor, NY.
44. Coates, P. J., Save, V., Ansari, B., and Hall, P. A. (1995) Demonstration of DNA damage/repair in individual cells using in situ end labelling: association of p53 with sites of DNA damage. *J. Pathol.* **176,** 19–26.
45. Coopersmith, C. M. and Gordon, J. I. (1997) gamma-Ray-induced apoptosis in transgenic mice with proliferative abnormalities in their intestinal epithelium: re-entry of villus enterocytes into the cell cycle does not affect their radioresistance but enhances the radiosensitivity of the crypt by inducing p53. *Oncogene* **15,** 131–141.
46. Martin, S. J. Reutelingsperger, C. P. M., McGahon, A. J., Rader, J. A., Vanschie, R. C. A., Laface, D. M., and Green, D. R. (1995) Early redistribution of plasma-membrane phosphatidylserine is a general feature of apoptosis regardless of the initiating stimulus: inhibition by overexpression of Bcl-2 and Abl. *J. Exp. Med.* **182,** 1545–1556.
47. Koopman, G, Reutlingsperger, C. P. M., Kuijten, G. A. M., Keehnen, R. M. J., Pals, S. T., and Vanders, M. H. J. (1994) Annexin-V for flow cytometric detection of phosphatidylserine expression on B cells undergoing apoptosis. *Blood* **84,** 1415–1420.

48. Garden, G. A., Bothwell, M., and Rubel, E. W. (1991) Lack of correspondence between mRNA expression for a putative cell death model (SGP-2) and neuronal cell death in the central nervous system. *J. Neurobiol.* **22,** 590–604.
49. Fesus, L., Thomazy, V., Autori, F., Ceru, M. P., Tarcsa, E., and Piacentini, M. (1989) Apoptotic hepatocytes become insoluble in detergents and chaotropic agents as a result of transglutaminase action. *FEBS Lett.* **245,** 150–154.
50. Cummings, M. (1996) Apoptosis of epithelial cells in vivo involves tissue transglutaminase upregulation. *J. Pathol.* **179,** 288–293
51. Szondy, Z., Molnar, P., Nemes, Z., Boyiadzis, M, Kedei, N., Toth, R., and Fesus, L. (1997) Differential expression of tissue transglutaminase during in vivo apoptosis of thymocytes induced via distinct signalling pathways. *FEBS Lett.* **404,** 307–313.
52. Hilton, D. A., Love, S., and Barber, R. (1997) Demonstration of apoptotic cells in tissue sections by in situ hybridization using digoxigenin-labelled poly(A) oligonucleotide probes to detect thymidine-rich DNA sequences. *J. Histochem. Cytochem.* **45,** 13–20.
53. Nicoletti, I., Migliorati, G., Pagliacci, M. C., Grignani, F., and Riccardi, C. (1991) A rapid and simple method for measuring thymocyte apoptosis by propidium iodide staining and flow cytometry. *J. Immunol. Meth.* **137,** 271–279.
54. Tewari, M., Quan, L. T., O'Rourke, K., Desnoyers, S., Zeng, Z., Beidler, D. R., et al. (1995) Yama/CPP32b, a mammalian homolog of CED-3, is a Crm-A inhibitable protease that cleaves the death substrate poly(ADP-ribose) polymerase. *Cell* **81,** 801–809.
55. Aherne, W. A. and Dunnill, M. S. (1982) Morphometry. Edward Arnold, London.

[illegible]

# 38

## Considerations in Generating Transgenic Mice

### *DNA, RNA, and Protein Extractions from Tissues— Rapid and Effective Blotting*

**Joanna B. Wilson and Mark E. Drotar**

### 1. Introduction

The mouse provides a powerful system to produce and study models of human disease. The ability to introduce, inactivate, or modify genes in mice has significantly advanced our understanding of molecular and cellular disease processes. New tools and novel applications of the classic techniques now permit spacial and temporal restrictions to be applied to in vivo gene expression. In this chapter, the expansive methods used to generate transgenic mice will not be presented as there are several comprehensive books on the topic, including one in this series *(1,2)*. In addition, the legislative requirements for working with animals will not be described here; suffice it to mention that transgenic animal production is a licensed procedure within the UK. Instead, considerations relating specifically to the application of transgenic techniques to studying Epstein-Barr virus (EBV)-associated diseases will be discussed.

#### *1.1. Transgene Expression*

The foremost consideration when generating a transgenic mouse by microinjection of zygotic nuclei is to design an appropriate expression vector. Expression of a viral gene in a tissue inappropriate to the disease states or at an undesirable developmental stage can lead to phenotypes that are difficult to interpret and to relate to the known diseases. With the EBV-associated diseases in mind, directing transgene expression to B-cells, T-cells, or epithelial cells are obvious targets (reviewed in **ref.** ***3***).

Expression in B-cells can be achieved using the enhancers of the immunoglobulin genes (heavy and light chain, both human and mouse). The most commonly used for a variety of transgenes has been the immunoglobulin heavy-chain intronic enhancer (upstream of the μ constant region) commonly referred to in the constructs as Eμ (examples of such can be found in **refs.** ***4–22***). This has been coupled to the gene

From: *Methods in Molecular Biology, Vol. 174: Epstein-Barr Virus Protocols*
Edited by: J. B. Wilson and G. H. W. May © Humana Press Inc., Totowa, NJ

under study either with the gene's own promoter *(4,19)*, or to a variety of heterologous promoters including the SV40 promoter *(7)*, Polyomavirus promoter *(9,13,18)* and an immunoglobulin promoter *(5,20)* amongst others. Using different promoters can lead to subtle, sometimes considerable, variations in gene expression patterns. For example, expression of Epstein-Barr viral nuclear antigen 1 (EBNA-1) from a transgene incorporating the Eμ enhancer and the Polyomavirus promoter is reasonably restricted to B-cells, possibly extending to T-cells in some lines *(18)*. However, expression of LMP1 from the same enhancer/promoter cassette, but in addition the transgene incorporating a partial LMP1 5' promoter along with the LMP1 gene internal promoters (ED-L1 and ED-L2) leads to widespread transgene expression in many tissues *(9)*. Indeed the EBV ED-L2 promoter alone proved to be effective in directing epithelial expression from a heterologous gene *(23)*.

Expression of several genes in T-cells has been achieved using a variety of promoters and enhancers, in particular the lck gene promoter has been frequently used (examples given by **refs.** ***24–30***). In addition, the promoters and/or enhancers for the interleukin 2 IL-2, IL-4, CD2, CD4, H-2K, perforin, MHC class II, T-cell receptor, and granzyme A and B genes, among others, have been used to direct expression to T-cells (examples given by **refs.** ***31–43***). In each case, whether expression is exclusive to T-cells, the T-cell subset targeted and the timing of expression is dependent on the combination of promoter, enhancer, and the gene to which it is juxtaposed.

Expression in epithelia can be directed by many enhancer/promoters and the first decision must be which tissue to target. For example, the mouse mammary tumor virus (MMTV) long terminal repeat has been frequently used to target expression to the mammary epithelium and a variety of cytokeratin promoters have been used to direct expression to particular epithelial layers, especially layers of the epidermis *(44)*. Human, murine, and bovine cytokeratin (K) promoters have been used where K5 and K14 promoters have been used to target basal-layer epidermal expression *(45–59)* and K1, K10, and involucrin promoters to target suprabasal transgene expression *(60–67)*. The K6 promoter has been used to target proliferative epidermal cells, particularly in the hair follicles *(68,69)*. We have used viral promoters, both the murine Polyoma virus early promoter and the EBV ED-L2 promoter to target epithelial expression, the latter being effective in certain mucosal epithelia as well as the epidermis *(9,23)*. Although the mouse skin may not be a tissue that is directly relevant to an EBV-associated disease state, the clear advantage of using this epithelium to model epithelial disorders (and the grounds why many other disease model studies have taken this approach) is the accessibility of the tissue. Phenotypes can be directly apparent and treatments can be applied topically. Moreover, for cancer studies, chemical carcinogenesis of the skin is a very well-studied approach, where several of the genetic changes relevant to tumorigenic progression have been defined.

Recent advances in conditional gene expression are now being successfully transferred to transgenic studies. The use of the tetracycline responsive binary system, derived from the *Escherichia coli* tetracycline-resistance operon *(70)* is one such. In this case, bitransgenic mice are generated where tetracycline or its derivatives (such as doxycyline) are used to control the activity of the Tet repressor protein (and recombinants thereof, which can be transcriptional activators), which binds to its cognate sequence, linked to the gene of interest *(71–77)*. Tetracycline can be simply supplied in the drinking water or administered in slow release pellets implanted subcutaneously *(74)*. When combined with the Cre-loxP site specific recombination system for inducing tissue-specific gene modifications (usually knockout) *(78–80)*, conditional, tissue-specific knock outs can be generated *(81)*. Localized induction of gene expression has been achieved by topical treatment with progesterone analogs *(82)*. Again in a binary system, a fusion of the truncated progesterone receptor and the yeast GAL4 DNA binding domain is targeted to express in the upper epidermal layers. Upon activation by topical antiprogestin treatment, focal induction of the second transgene linked to GAL4 binding sites is achieved. Use of a transient, conditional system can overcome problems previously encountered where embryonic or widespread transgene expression is toxic. In addition, such systems can come closer to modeling a disease resulting from infection, where only a small proportion of cells in a limited area express the heterologous protein and usually for a limited time.

### 1.2. Controls, Sampling, and Sample Preparation

The methods described in this chapter concern the preparation of samples for DNA, RNA, and protein analyses. In using a transgenic mouse system, the requirement for transgene genotyping is a constant feature. Where possible, transgenic mice can be bred to homozygosity for the transgene, obviating the need to transgene test at every generation, however, insertional disruption of a cellular gene leading to a recessive mutation, often precludes this option. Moreover, for any test of transgene effect, the best controls are transgene-negative siblings, where age, genotype, and environment are constant. Differences in mouse strain (the genetic background) can have a considerable effect on test parameters, particularly with regard to susceptibility to tumorigenesis and as such the use of syngeneic controls are imperative, often best provided by siblings. Similarly the environment, such as diet and pathogen status can influence the onset of tumorigenic disease and again, siblings provide the best control. Therefore, it is functional to maintain a transgenic line in the hemizygous state.

In examining the effects of transgene expression, the usual scenario is to compare a parameter with the wild-type, nontransgenic controls (preferably siblings as described earlier, or uninduced mice under inducible conditions). In order to investigate the differences between these two groups, sufficient animals need to be entered in to the study to be able to conduct a statistical analysis with the data to determine if the result is credible. It is important to bear in mind that in the living organism, data obtained between animals can vary considerably (even if they are genetically identical) and thus comparing one transgenic with one control is not a valid approach. In addition, subtle changes in cellular gene expression patterns as a response to transgene expression can have dramatic phenotypic consequences. The more subtle an induced change in the parameter being measured, the more samples must be entered into the study for statistical veracity.

Consequently, methods to optimize and speed the bulk preparation and analysis of genomic DNA samples are important. To date, we have not found a robotic method that yields genomic DNA of a comparable quality to the protocol described, but hopefully this is not too far off. The method described here allows for the production of DNAs of different purities, with stop-off points for rapid preparation simply for polymerase chain reaction (PCR) analyses and extended preparation steps for high quality and yield for more sensitive studies. The preparation of RNA and protein extracts from tissue samples differs only in the first steps to standard methods used for cultured cells.

### *1.3. Blotting and Hybridization*

In order to analyze transgene status, PCR is the most rapid detection method. However, although false-positives can be excluded with extensive care not to contaminate reagents and by always including the appropriate controls, it is difficult to eliminate false-negative results. If an animal is grouped in a negative batch in error, this could obviously have deleterious consequences on results where the group is used as a control. Blotting, although more time-consuming, is more reliable where this is critical. Slot blotting is considerably faster than Southern blotting and can be done in batches to be almost comparable in speed with PCR, whereas Southern blotting provides the additional information of transgene configuration (unique to each line), certainly useful in typing a line at the start of study. We have optimized both result detection and protocol speed for blotting. We routinely electroblot agarose gels (both DNA and RNA) ***(9,13,18)*** and use a simply made, but effective, prehybridization/hybridization buffer described by Church and Gilbert ***(83)***. In a direct comparison with capillary blotting and vacuum blotting, we have found the electroblotting method to give consistently better signal to background ratios than both other protocols and to be faster in its execution. This is true for Southerns and Northerns, with the only precaution that suitable cooling is required during blotting as described. In order to effectively compare transcript levels between several samples, the DNA slot-blot protocol has been modified for RNA slot blotting. Although all of these blotting protocols have been optimized for speed to deal with the many samples produced in transgenic mouse studies, no compromise in quality has been made, usually the reverse and as such the protocols are suitable for all blotting applications.

## 2. Materials

### *2.1. Genomic DNA Preparations from Tissues*

1. Tail solution: 50 m*M* Tris-HCl from a 1 *M* stock adjusted to pH 8.0 and autoclaved, 100 m*M* ethylenediaminetetraacetic acid (EDTA) from a 0.5 or 0.1 *M* stock adjusted to pH 8.0 and autoclaved, 100 m*M* NaCl from a 5 *M* autoclaved stock, 1% sodium dodecyl sulphate (SDS).
2. Proteinase K: make up to 10 mg/mL in distilled water and store at –20°C in aliquots.
3. Thermomixer: Eppendorf compact or equivalent.
4. Buffered phenol: Ultra-pure buffer saturated phenol (Gibco BRL or equivalent, *see* **Note 1**).
5. 2FC: 500 mL melted phenol, 500 mL chloroform, 10 mL isoamyl alcohol, 1 g 8-hydroxy quinoline; mix and saturate with TE, pH 8.0. Check that the pH of the aqueous layer lies between 7.0 and 8.0 (if not, replace buffer until it does). Store at room temperature in a glass bottle.
6. Chloroform-isoamyl alcohol: mix chloroform and isoamyl alcohol in a 24:1 ratio.

7. PLG tubes: phase-lock gel™ 1.5-mL tubes, heavy (for tail preps), light (for other tissues), spin for 20 s in a microcentrifuge at full speed (up to 16,000*g*) prior to use (Flowgen).
8. 10 *M* $NH_4$ acetate.
9. Ethanol: store aliquots at –20°C for efficient DNA precipitation.
10. 70% ethanol: ethanol in water.
11. TE, pH 8.0: 10 mM Tris-HCl, pH 8.0, 1 mM EDTA, pH 8.0. Autoclave.
12. Microcentrifuge and 1.5-mL tubes.

## 2.2. RNA and Protein Extraction

1. Homogenizer: Polytron (Kinematica AG) with PTA10s probe for use with 14-mL tubes and PTA7 probe for use with 5-mL tubes (or equivalent).
2. Phosphate-buffered saline (PBS): 2.7 m*M* KCl, 1.4 m*M* $KH_2PO_4$, 137 m*M* NaCl, 4.3 m*M* $Na_2PO_4$, pH adjusted to 7.3 with HCl.
3. RNA extraction buffer: any preferred RNA extraction buffer such as TRI-REAGENT (Sigma).
4. Protein extraction buffer: any preferred protein extraction buffer such as Rippa buffer: 150 m*M* NaCl, 0.5% Nonidet P40 (NP40) detergent, 0.5% sodium deoxycholate, 0.1% SDS, 5 m*M* EDTA, 20 m*M* Tris-HCl, pH 7.5. Freshly add protease inhibitors such as 1% Aprotinin (Sigma) and 1 m*M* PMSF (*see* **Note 2**).
5. Polypropylene round-bottom tubes: 14-mL 2059 tubes, 5-mL 2063 tubes, Falcon.
6. Stock SDS: 10% or 20% (w/v) SDS made up in distilled, autoclaved water.
7. Microcentrifuge and 1.5 mL tubes.

## 2.3. Southern and Northern Electroblotting

1. Denaturing solution: 0.4 *M* NaOH, 0.6 *M* NaCl.
2. Rocking platform: Hoeffer red rocker or equivalent.
3. 50X TAE: 242 g Tris base, 57.1 mL glacial acetic acid, 100 mL 0.5 *M* EDTA, pH 8.0. Make up to 1 L with $H_2O$.
4. Nylon membrane: Biodyne A or B (positively charged), 0.2- or 0.45-μm pore size, Pall biosupport membranes.
5. Whatman 3MM filter paper.
6. Transphor Tank: Hoefer Pharmacia Biotech Inc. TE62X with power lid (TE 50X, 100 V, 1.5 A constant current), or TE62 with separate power supply, cassettes, and sponges and cooling system, or similar electrophoretic tank system (*see* **Note 3**).

## 2.4. Slot Blotting

1. Slot blot apparatus: Schleicher and Schuell minifold 2 (or equivalent).
2. 1 *M* NaOH.
3. Nylon membrane: Biodyne A or B, (positively charged), 0.45 μm pore size, Pall biosupport membranes.
4. 3MM filter paper: Whatman.
5. 50X TAE: 242 g Tris base, 57.1 mL glacial acetic acid, 100 mL 0.5 M EDTA, pH 8.0. Make up to 1 L with $H_2O$.
6. Vacuum pump: Hoefer Red-Evac (PV.100) or equivalent.
7. Pasteur pipets.
8. TE, pH 8.0: 10 m*M* Tris-HCl, pH 8.0, 1 m*M* EDTA, pH 8.0. Autoclave.
9. Loading buffer (for RNA only): 17.8% (v/v) formaldehyde, 50% (v/v) pure, deionized formamide, 1X MOPS-E. For this, make up a stock of 10X MOPS-E: 10 m*M* EDTA, 200 m*M*

MOPS acid, 50 m*M* NaOAc, pH to 7.0 with NaOH. Upon autoclaving MOPS-E becomes discolored (yellow). Inhibit further buffer decomposition (and discoloration) by storing the buffer in a dark or foil-wrapped bottle at room temperature.
10. Heating block.
11. 20X SSC: 3 *M* NaCl, 0.3 *M* tri-sodium citrate, pH to 7.0 with 1 *M* NaOH.
12. Microcentrifuge and 1.5-mL tubes.

### 2.5. Membrane Hybridization, Washing, and Stripping

1. Church buffer: 1% (w/v) bovine serum albumin (BSA), 1 m*M* EDTA, 500 m*M* $NaPO_4$, 7% SDS, pH 7.2. To make up, prepare a 4X (1 *M*) stock solution of $Na_2HPO_4$ with 268 g $Na_2HPO_4 \cdot 7H_2O$, 8 mL $H_3PO_4$ made up to 1 L with water. For 200 mL Church buffer, use 50 mL of this 4X stock solution, 14 g SDS, 2 g BSA (RIA grade), 2 mL of 0.1 *M* EDTA, pH 8.0, made up to volume with water.
2. Roller tube oven: Hybaid midi oven and tubes, or equivalent.
3. 20X SSC: 3 *M* NaCl, 0.3 *M* tri-sodium citrate, adjust pH to 7.0 with 1 *M* NaOH.
4. Stock SDS: 10% or 20% (w/v) SDS made up in distilled, autoclaved water.
5. Formamide: pure grade, deionized.
6. Shaking platform water bath.
7. Plastic boxes with lids.
8. Plastic wrap.
9. X-ray film.

## 3. Methods

### 3.1 Genomic DNA Preparations from Tissues

1. This protocol can be used for many species and all tissue types, including tail, skin, internal organs, separated tissues or cell pellets. Prepare tissue directly after collection or snap-freeze in liquid nitrogen in 1.5-mL microtubes and store at –70°C. When preparing washed cell pellets, briefly vortex the cells in the residual liquid to loosen the pellet before DNA extraction or freezing (*see* **Note 4**).
2. The volumes given are appropriate for a piece of tissue of approx 5 $mm^3$, a tail segment of up to 1 cm or $10^8$ cell pellet. Scale up accordingly for larger samples. With each tissue in a 1.5-mL microtube, directly add 700 µL of tail solution.
3. Add 35 µL of proteinase K to each tube.
4. For tissues with a membranous capsule (such as the internal organs) and skin, mince the tissue finely with sharp scissors in the solution (*see* **Note 5**).
5. Incubate for 4 h to overnight at 55°C in a heating block, preferably with gentle mixing (*see* **Notes 6** and **7**).
6. Vigorously mix tube contents by hand (avoid vortexing) and centrifuge briefly (30 s) in a microcentrifuge at full speed (or approx 16,000g) to pellet cell debris (*see* **Notes 8** and **9**).
7. To extract proteins and peptides from the sample, transfer most of the sample (avoiding the debris) to PLG tubes (after briefly spinning the gel to the bottom of the tubes) (*see* **Note 10**). Add 500 µL of 2FC and mix thoroughly by tapping and inverting the tube. Do not vortex (*see* **Notes 11** and **12**).
8. Microcentrifuge at full speed, 16,000*g* for 5 min.
9. The PLG acts as a plug separating the organic and aqueous phases. Tip the top, aqueous layer containing the nucleic acids into a new 1.5-mL standard microtube. The lower phenol/chloroform layer will not be disturbed.

10. Add 100 µL of 10 *M* $NH_4$ acetate and mix.
11. Add approx 750 µL (to almost fill the tube) of ice-cold ethanol (*see* **Note 13**). Mix well to precipitate DNA (*see* **Note 14**).
12. Centrifuge in a microcentrifuge at 8,000*g* for 2 min (*see* **Note 15**) and decant ethanol, taking care not to discard DNA pellet.
13. Wash pellet with 1 mL of ice-cold 70% ethanol by gentle mixing and recentrifugation at 8,000*g* for 2 min and discarding ethanol.
14. Allow pellet to air-dry or vacuum dry (*see* **Note 16**).
15. Resuspend DNA in 215 µL of TE, pH 8.0 and incubate at 65°C for 15 min (up to 30 min if necessary) (*see* **Note 16**).
16. Use 15 µL (diluted 20-fold with water) to obtain an optical density reading ($OD_{260}$) for DNA concentration. For a 1 cm path length (quartz cuvet) the numerical value of the reading will equal the concentration in µg/µL for the sample. Store at 4°C indefinitely (*see* **Note 17**).

### 3.2. Total RNA and Protein Preparations

Total RNA or poly A selected RNA and proteins can be prepared from tissues using any of the commercially available kits and/or standard extraction solutions (*see* Chapters 5 and 26). Only the first step of tissue homogenization differs, as described here.

1. Collect or dissect tissue and snap-freeze in liquid nitrogen to avoid any RNA or protein degradation (*see* **Note 18**). Store at –70°C.
2. When preparing extracts, keep tissues on dry ice to avoid sample thawing while one sample at a time is homogenized.
3. Place a piece of tissue (up to approx 5 $mm^3$, scale up or down for larger or smaller pieces) directly into extraction solution of choice, in a round bottom polypropylene tube and homogenize immediately for at least 5 s, ensuring the tissue is thoroughly homogenized. For RNA extraction, use 3 mL of acidic phenol/guanidinium thiocyanate according to the method described by Chomczynski and Sacchi *(84)* and as fully detailed in Chapter 5. Alternatively, we routinely use TRI-REAGENT at 1 mL per 50–100 mg of tissue. For protein extraction use 1 mL of ice-cold extraction buffer including proteases. Reduce detergent concentration to minimize foaming of the sample (for example to 0.05% NP40 or 0.01% SDS, *see* **Note 2**).
4. After thorough homogenization of the sample, place it on ice while other samples are lysed. To avoid sample cross-contamination, thoroughly clean the probe of the homogenizer by running the homogenizer first in a solution of 1% SDS and then 3 changes of water, wiping the probe with sterile tissues between each run (*see* **Notes 19** and **20**).
5. For RNA extraction, proceed with the preparation as described in Chapter 5 or by the manufacturers instructions. For protein extraction, transfer the samples to microcentrifuge tubes on ice. Make up the detergent concentration to the required levels and vortex the samples to complete the extraction. Proceed as described in Chapter 26 for protein analysis (*see* **Note 21**).

### 3.3. Southern and Northern Electroblotting

Agarose gel electrophoresis of DNA and RNA is not described here as it is fully described in several other chapters in this volume. The protocol described here is applicable to any agarose gel system used (*see* **Note 22**) and parameters can be modified to be used with acrylamide gels.

1. For Southern (DNA) blotting, after taking the required gel image, denature the DNA in the gel by soaking the gel in enough denaturing solution to cover it in a dish (usually 200–300 mL), for 45 min, rocking gently.
2. Neutralize the gel by soaking, with rocking, 3 times for 15 min each in 0.5X TAE, using enough buffer to cover the gel (*see* **Notes 23** and **24**). Proceed to **step 4**.
3. For Northern (RNA) blotting, after gel electrophoresis, soak the gel (rocking) 3 times for 20 min each, in 1X TAE (*see* **Note 25**).
4. While gel is soaking, cut 1 piece of nylon membrane to size, 0.5 cm larger in both dimensions than the gel and pre-soak in 0.5X TAE for a Southern or 1X TAE for a Northern. Cut 2 pieces of 3MM filter paper to size, just larger than the nylon membrane. Fill the transphor tank with 0.5X TAE for a Southern or 1X TAE for a Northern (*see* **Note 26**).
5. Set up electroblot sandwich submerged in a large dish of 0.5 or 1X TAE (for Southern or Northern respectively) in the following order: plastic cassette (which will face positive electrode), foam sponge, one piece of wetted 3MM filter paper, pre-wet membrane, gel, one piece of wetted filter paper, foam sponge, plastic cassette. Ensure no air bubbles lie between the filter paper, membrane, and gel layers. Secure the cassette clips together still submerged (*see* **Notes 27** and **28**).
6. Holding the sandwich together, transfer it to the buffer-filled tank and slot into place (*see* **Note 29**). Gently agitate the loaded cassettes to dislodge any bubbles in the sponges resulting from transfer to the tank.
7. Transfer for a Southern (using 0.5X TAE) for 3 h at a constant 1.5 A (or just under, *see* **Note 3**) with cooling. The voltage should gradually drop from approx 60–45 V during the course of transfer. Transfer for a Northern (using 1X TAE) for 2.5–3 h at a constant 0.7 A (approx 40 V) with cooling (*see* **Note 30**).
8. Following transfer, fix or crosslink the nucleic acid to the membrane by baking at 80°C for 1 h and/or UV irradiation (*see* **Note 31**). Store membrane dry, wrapped in 3MM filter paper until hybridization.

### 3.4. DNA Slot Blotting

1. Use 5 µg of genomic DNA per slot. Aliquot the 5 µg DNA samples into microfuge tubes.
2. Make up to 120 µL with distilled water.
3. Add 40 µL of 1 *M* NaOH to denature DNA.
4. Vortex samples vigorously and incubate at room temperature for 10 min. During this time, cut 1 piece of nylon membrane and 2 pieces of 3MM filter paper to size (to fit the slot-blot apparatus). Soak the nylon membrane in 1X TAE for approximately 30 min at room temperature.
5. Add 160 µL of 10X TAE to samples.
6. Vortex samples, briefly spin to the bottom of the tube in a microfuge and put on ice.
7. Assemble slot blot apparatus with the 2 pieces of 3MM, briefly wetted in 1X TAE and with the soaked membrane on top, with the slotted manifold on top of this.
8. Attach to vacuum pump but do not turn the vacuum on yet.
9. Load all samples, including negative and positive controls (*see* **Note 32**).
10. Start vacuum. When all samples have passed through, without interrupting the vacuum, add 1 drop from a Pasteur pipet (approx 20 µL) of 5X TAE to each sample slot and let this be drawn through by the vacuum.
11. Disassemble apparatus, bake and/or UV-irradiate membrane to link the DNA (*see* **Note 31**). Store membrane dry, wrapped in 3MM filter paper until hybridization.

### 3.5. RNA Slot Blotting

1. Use 5 μg of total RNA per slot (*see* **Note 25**). Adjust aqueous RNA samples or resuspend precipitated RNA samples to 5 μg/10 μL in TE, pH 8.0, 0.1% SDS. Aliquot 5 μg samples into microfuge tubes.
2. Add 30 μL of loading buffer to each sample and vortex to mix. To denature secondary RNA structures, heat samples at 65°C for 10 min and then place tubes immediately on ice.
3. Add 10 μL of ice-cold 20X SSC to each sample.
4. Proceed with **steps 6–11** as for DNA slot blotting (*see* **Subheading 3.4.**)

### 3.6. Membrane Hybridization and Wash Conditions

The same conditions can be used for Southern, Northern and DNA and RNA slot-blots.

1. Pre-warm Church buffer to 68°C and ensure it is well-dissolved (the SDS can precipitate out under cool conditions). Prehybridize the membrane(s) in 8–10 mL of Church buffer in a roller tube for at least 1 h, but usually overnight, at 68°C rolling (*see* **Notes 33–35**).
2. Denature radiolabeled DNA probe (*see* **Note 36**) by heating it to 95°C (or boiling) and immediately transfer it to the 8 mL of prehybridization Church buffer within the roller tube. Swirl the tube to mix the probe in well and hybridize rolling overnight at 68°C (*see* **Note 34**).
3. Decant the hybridization solution into the appropriate radioactive waste container. Rinse the membrane in the rolling tube in 2X SSC, 0.1% SDS at room temperature (or perform this wash in a separate container). Decant the wash into radioactive waste.
4. Transfer the membrane to a plastic box and repeat the wash 3 more times using at least 200 mL, for 10 min at room temperature, shaking.
5. Finally, wash the membrane twice, under stringent conditions (*see* **Note 34**) using at least 200 mL of 0.1X SSC, 0.1% SDS at 68°C (pre-warm wash solution) for 30 min each, in a plastic box incubated in a shaking-platform water bath.
6. Blot excess liquid from membrane (but do not dry, *see* **Note 37**), plastic wrap, and expose to X-ray film as usual.
7. Store radiolabeled or stripped membranes in plastic wrap at –20°C. Membranes stored in this way can be effectively re-probed years after blotting.

### 3.7. Stripping Blots (*see* Note 38)

1. Place membrane in 200–300 mL of 0.5X SSC, 0.1% SDS with 50% formamide for DNA blots and 75% formamide for RNA blots (*see* **Note 39**), in a shaking water bath at 65°C for 45 min.
2. Wash membrane twice using 200–300 mL of 0.1X SSC, 0.1% SDS at 68°C (pre-warm wash solution) for 30 min each.
3. Expose membrane to X-ray film to ensure probe stripping is complete before prehybridizing and re-probing as described in **Subheading 3.6.**

## 4. Notes

1. To make your own, melt pure phenol (with care) in a 60°C water bath. Add an equal volume of 1 *M* Tris-HCl adjusted to pH 8.0, shake and store at 4°C overnight in a light protected (dark glass or covered) bottle. Replace the aqueous, upper, layer with TE, pH 8.0, shake well and leave overnight again at 4°C. Check the pH of the aqueous layer and continue to replace with TE, pH 8.0 until the phenol is buffered at pH 7.0–8.0. Store at 4°C.

2. Sample foaming upon homogenization can make it difficult to transfer the entire sample to new tubes resulting in sample loss. To reduce foaming when homogenizing, if necessary reduce detergent content of protein extraction buffer to 0.05% NP40, 0.01% SDS (or equivalent for other detergents). Make up to full detergent concentration following homogenization.
3. All the parameters for this protocol have been optimized with this electrophoretic transfer tank. We have found that this apparatus gives uniform transfer across a gel and the cooling system is very important. Optimal transfer of DNA is achieved at 1.5 A (or just below), as such, care should be taken when using the power lid not to exceed this as the fuse blows at 1.5 A. This problem is not incurred when using a separate power supply with a 2.0 A limit. It may be possible to use other electrophoretic transfer tanks, but the transfer parameters and timing may need to be altered for optimal conditions.
4. Hard-packed cells can be difficult to lyse, tending to remain in a clump if not loosened and reducing the subsequent DNA yield.
5. There is no need to mince tail; the fur and bones will remain following extraction.
6. The extraction proceeds more quickly if the tubes can be mixed gently during incubation (an Eppendorf thermomixer is ideal). This crude DNA extract can be stored indefinitely at 4°C without significant loss of DNA integrity.
7. An optional step if RNA contamination of the final sample is problematic is to treat at this stage with 20 µL of 10 mg/mL RNase A (DNase-free), by mixing and incubation at 37°C for 1–2 h.
8. For PCR analysis only, transfer the top two-thirds to a new tube and proceed to **step 10**, DNA precipitation; phenol extraction is not necessary.
9. This centrifugation step can be left out when doing more than one phenol or phenol/chloroform extraction.
10. Use of the phase-lock gel™ is not essential, but reduces protocol time by allowing the aqueous phase at **step 9** to be transferred to new tubes by tipping rather than pipetting. These tubes cannot be used effectively with buffered phenol alone, only with phenol chloroform mixtures or chloroform.
11. All steps requiring mixing should be done by vigorous tapping of the tube and not by vortexing, to minimize DNA shearing. If quality high molecular weight DNA is not necessary for the sample analysis, sample mixing can be done by gentle vortexing.
12. If a large tissue sample has been used or if purer DNA samples are required, use buffered phenol as a first extraction step before **step 7**. In this case, do not use PLG tubes (*see* **Note 9**). Then proceed on to **steps 7** and **18** with 2FC protein extraction, followed by chloroform-isoamylalcohol extraction, both with PLG tubes.
13. If some sample has been lost in the previous steps, do not add more than an equal volume of ethanol (except *see* **Note 14**) in order to preferentially precipitate high molecular weight genomic DNA and not low molecular weight, sheared DNA and RNA.
14. Ensure the DNA has come out of solution properly, visualized by a white feathery precipitate. If a large quantity of DNA has been extracted and is not precipitating properly (sometimes seen as a translucent blob in the solution), full precipitation may require further mixing by vigorously shaking the tube by hand, or the addition of a little more ethanol.
15. This slow, short spin is to preferentially pellet high molecular weight, genomic DNA. Longer or faster spins will also pellet any sheared DNA and RNA. Additional precipitation of RNA (visible following gel electrophoresis) will give misleading $OD_{260}$ values for the DNA concentration.

16. Avoid overdrying. If the pellet is absolutely desiccated, it will require a longer time at 65°C for resuspension. Leaving the sample overnight at 4°C will also aid suspension of large or too-dry pellets.
17. DNA prepared by this protocol can remain intact for many years stored at 4°C. Storage of high molecular weight aqueous DNA frozen may cause shearing. For long term, secure, storage, keep sample in ethanol as a precipitate (add 1/10 aqueous volume of 3 *M* NaOAc, plus 2 times aqueous volume of ethanol and mix) at –20°C.
18. To avoid contaminating signals from blood cells in certain tissues, such as the heart, rinse tissue in PBS, briefly blot off excess, and then snap-freeze.
19. A further precaution against cross-contamination of signals is to prepare any negative or control samples prior to positive samples. However, with thorough cleaning of the probe this should not be problematic.
20. To clean the probe after the final sample, finish up with a run in ethanol.
21. For protein concentration measurements we routinely use the Bradford assay with reagents from Bio-Rad.
22. For RNA gels we routinely use formaldehyde/formamide agarose gels electrophoresed in MOPS-E (*see* Chapter 5).
23. The use of TAE as the electrophoretic transfer buffer has been optimized with the use of Biodyne membranes.
24. There is no need to acid treat large DNA fragments as electrophoretic transfer is efficient for all DNA sizes using this protocol.
25. For RNA sample handling and electrophoresis, take all precautions against contamination with RNases. Treat glass and plastic ware (including gel boxes, gel combs, slot-blot manifold) by soaking for 10 min in 3% hydrogen peroxide at room temperature followed by thorough rinsing with DEPC water. DEPC-treat and autoclave non-Tris solutions and use DEPC treated water to make up TAE. A full description of precaution against RNases is given in Chapter 5.
26. Southern transfer is just as efficient using 1X TAE as with 0.5X TAE; the latter saves on reagent use. If Southerns are done frequently, buffer from gel electrophoresis (when using 1X TAE) can be diluted for use in the tank, buffer from the tank can be used for the next round of gel soaks. Keep Northern buffers separate and RNase-free.
27. To prevent bubbles from the sponges interfering with transfer, ensure these are thoroughly wetted in buffer before loading the gel sandwich by squeezing the sponges through several times under buffer.
28. The cassette sides are not identical and it is useful to routinely use one side as the base of the sandwich remembering this is the one which will face the positive electrode (to which the DNA will migrate).
29. The bottom cassette of the sandwich should face the positive electrode.
30. The cooling manifold with this system, using a constant flow of cold water, is sufficient to allow transfer without the problem of overheating. However, depending on the ambient temperature of the lab or the cooling water, if you find that the tank is overheating, pre-cooling the tank buffer in a cold room will help over come this or the entire apparatus can be located in a cold room.
31. We routinely bake the membrane for 1 h at 80°C for membrane uniformity before UV crosslinking the nucleic acid, either using an enclosed UV box such as a Stratalinker (Stratagene) or simply at a constant distance of 30 cm over a short-wave UV gel illuminator for 90 s (optimize according to the UV bulbs in your UV box).

32. Generate a record sheet to note the relative position/order of the samples at the start of the protocol and load the samples on the slot-blot apparatus according to the plan.
33. When using Church buffer, no denatured blocking DNA is required. Church buffer routinely gives clean backgrounds using Biodyne membranes when compared to other hybridization mixes based on Denhardt's solution and denatured DNA.
34. The temperature of hybridization and wash conditions depends on the stringency required. The conditions given are stringent, for an entirely homologous probe of sequence longer than 200 base pairs. For reduced homology or shorter probe fragments, the temperature of the hybridization and final washes should be reduced and the salt concentration of the washes increased.
35. Sealed plastic bags can be used instead of roller tubes, but containment of the liquid radioactivity is easier using tubes. Several membranes can be placed in a single tube if they are to be hybridized with the same probe. The volume of Church buffer used (8–10 mL) depends on the number of membranes in the tube and the size of the tubes. Membranes should be evenly wetted as the tube rotates.
36. DNA fragments can be radiolabeled by several methods, described in other chapters in this volume. We routinely use the random primer method with Klenow polymerase and $^{32}$P-dCTP (3,000 Ci/mmol), either preparing the individual constituents or using the Stratagene Prime-It II kit. For each hybridization, use 25 ng of DNA radiolabelled to a specific activity of at least $1 \times 10^9$ cpm. Probes must be purified away from unincorporated nucleotides, which would otherwise result in black background hybridization signals over the entire membrane. For this we use Stratagene NucTrap probe purification columns with the Push Column Beta Shield Device. All precautions for handling radioactive materials must be taken and local safety regulations concerning the use of radioisotopes must be adhered to.
37. Membranes that are fully dried after probing are difficult to strip effectively.
38. We have found that using this protocol, Southern, Northern, and slot blots can be effectively stripped and re-probed at least 5 times and up to 10 times.
39. RNA:DNA hybrids are more stable than DNA:DNA hybrids.

## References

1. Hogan, B., Constantini, F., and Lacy, E. (1986) *Manipulating the Mouse Embryo: A Laboratory Manual.* Cold Spring Harbor Laboratory, Cold Spring Harbor, NY.
2. Murphy, D. and Carter, D. A. (1993) *Transgenesis Techniques, Principles and Protocols,* Methods Mol Biol. vol. 18, Humana Press.
3. Wilson, J. B. (1997) Transgenic mouse models of disease and Epstein-Barr virus. *EBV Report* **4,** 63–72.
4. Adams, J. M., Harris, A. W., Pinkert, C. A., Corcoran, L. M., Alexander, W. S., Cory, S., et al. (1985) The c-myc oncogene driven by immunoglobulin enhancers induces lymphoid malignancy in transgenic mice. *Nature* **318,** 533–538.
5. Grosschedl, R. and Baltimore, D. (1985) Cell-type specificity of immunoglobulin gene expression is regulated by at least three DNA sequence elements. *Cell* **41,** 885–897.
6. Gerlinger, P., LeMeur, M., Irrmann, C., Renard, P., Wasylyk, C., and Wasylyk, B. (1986) B-lymphocyte targeting of gene expression in transgenic mice with the immunoglobulin heavy-chain enhancer. *Nucleic Acids Res.* **14,** 6565–6577.
7. Suda, Y., Aizawa, S., Hirai, S., Inoue, T., Furuta, Y., Suzuki, M., et al. (1987) Driven by the same Ig enhancer and SV40 T promoter ras induced lung adenomatous tumors, myc

induced pre-B cell lymphomas and SV40 large T gene a variety of tumors in transgenic mice. *EMBO J.* **6,** 4055–4065.

8. Schmidt, E. V., Pattengale, P. K., Weir, L., and Leder, P. (1988) Transgenic mice bearing the human c-myc gene activated by an immunoglobulin enhancer: a pre-B-cell lymphoma model. *Proc. Natl. Acad. Sci. USA* **85,** 6047–6051.
9. Wilson, J. B., Weinberg, W., Johnson, R., Yuspa, S., and Levine, A. J. (1990) Expression of the BNLF-1 oncogene of Epstein-Barr virus in the skin of transgenic mice induces hyperplasia and aberrant expression of keratin 6. *Cell* **61,** 1315–1327.
10. McDonnell, T. J., Nunez, G., Platt, F. M., Hockenberry, D., London, L., McKearn, J. P., and Korsmeyer, S. J. (1990) Deregulated Bcl-2-immunoglobulin transgene expands a resting but responsive immunoglobulin M and D-expressing B-cell population. *Mol. Cell Biol.* **10,** 1901–1907.
11. Iwamoto, T., Pu, M., Ito, M., Takahashi, M., Isobe, K., Nagase, F., et al. (1991) Preferential development of pre-B lymphomas with drastically down- regulated N-myc in the E mu-ret transgenic mice. *Eur. J. Immunol.* **21,** 1809–1814.
12. Akagi, K., Miyazaki, J., and Yamamura, K. (1992) Strain dependency of cell-type specificity and onset of lymphoma development in Emu-myc transgenic mice. *Jpn. J. Cancer Res..* **83,** 269–273.
13. Wilson, J. B. and Levine, A. J. (1992) The oncogenic potential of Epstein-Barr virus nuclear antigen 1 in transgenic mice. *Curr. Topics Microbiol. Immunol.* **182,** 375–384.
14. Haupt, Y., Bath, M. L., Harris, A. W., and Adams, J. M. (1993) bmi-1 transgene induces lymphomas and collaborates with myc in tumorigenesis. *Oncogene* **8,** 3161–3164.
15. Bodrug, S. E., Warner, B. J., Bath, M. L., Lindeman, G. J., Harris, A. W., and Adams, J. M. (1994) Cyclin D1 transgene impedes lymphocyte maturation and collaborates in lymphomagenesis with the myc gene. *EMBO J.* **13,** 2124–2130.
16. Lovec, H., Grzeschiczek, A., Kowalski, M. B., and Moroy, T. (1994) Cyclin D1/bcl-1 cooperates with myc genes in the generation of B-cell lymphoma in transgenic mice. *EMBO J.* **13,** 3487–3495.
17. Spanopoulou, E., Roman, C. A., Corcoran, L. M., Schlissel, M. S., Silver, D. P., Nemazee, D., et al. (1994) Functional immunoglobulin transgenes guide ordered B-cell differentiation in Rag-1-deficient mice. *Genes Dev.* **8,** 1030–1042.
18. Wilson, J. B., Bell, J. L., and Levine, A. J. (1996) Expression of Epstein-Barr virus nuclear antigen-1 induces B cell neoplasia in transgenic mice. *EMBO J.* **15,** 3117–3126.
19. Butzler, C., Zou, X., Popov, A. V., and Bruggemann, M. (1997) Rapid induction of B-cell lymphomas in mice carrying a human IgH/c-mycYAC. *Oncogene* **14,** 1383–1388.
20. Caldwell, R. G., Wilson, J. B., Anderson, S. J., and Longnecker, R. (1998) Epstein-Barr virus LMP2A drives B cell development and survival in the absence of normal B cell receptor signals. *Immunity* **9,** 405–411.
21. Ong, S. T., Hackbarth, M. L., Degenstein, L. C., Baunoch, D. A., Anastasi, J., and McKeithan, T. W. (1998) Lymphadenopathy, splenomegaly, and altered immunoglobulin production in BCL3 transgenic mice. *Oncogene* **16,** 2333–2343.
22. Wasserman, R., Zeng, X. X., and Hardy, R. R. (1998) The evolution of B precursor leukemia in the Eμ-ret mouse. *Blood* **92,** 273–282.
23. Nakagawa, H., Wang, T. C., Zukerberg, L., Odze, R., Togawa, K., May, G. H., et al. (1997) The targeting of the cyclin D1 oncogene by an Epstein-Barr virus promoter in transgenic mice causes dysplasia in the tongue, esophagus and forestomach. *Oncogene* **14,** 1185–1190.

24. Allen, J. M., Forbush, K. A., and Perlmutter, R. M. (1992) Functional dissection of the lck proximal promoter. *Mol. Cell Biol.* **12,** 2758–2768.
25. McGuire, E. A., Rintoul, C. E., Sclar, G. M., and Korsmeyer, S. J. (1992) Thymic overexpression of Ttg-1 in transgenic mice results in T-cell acute lymphoblastic leukemia/lymphoma. *Mol. Cell Biol.* **12,** 4186–4196.
26. Linette, G. P., Hess, J. L., Sentman, C. L., and Korsmeyer, S. J. (1995) Peripheral T-cell lymphoma in lckpr-bcl-2 transgenic mice. *Blood* **86,** 1255–1260.
27. Condorelli, G. L., Facchiano, F., Valtieri, M., Proietti, E., Vitelli, L., Lulli, V., et al. (1996) T-cell-directed TAL-1 expression induces T-cell malignancies in transgenic mice. *Cancer Res.* **56,** 5113–5119.
28. Carrasco, D., Rizzo, C. A., Dorfman, K., and Bravo, R. (1996) The v-rel oncogene promotes malignant T-cell leukemia/lymphoma in transgenic mice. *EMBO J.* **15,** 3640–3650.
29. Zornig, M., Hueber, A. O., and Evan, G. (1998) p53–dependent impairment of T-cell proliferation in FADD dominant-negative transgenic mice. *Curr. Biol.* **8,** 467–470.
30. Attar, R. M., Macdonald-Bravo, H., Raventos-Suarez, C., Durham, S. K., and Bravo, R. (1998) Expression of constitutively active IκB β in T cells of transgenic mice: persistent NF-κB activity is required for T-cell immune responses. *Mol. Cell Biol.* **18,** 477–487.
31. Zinkernagel, R. M., Pircher, H. P., Ohashi, P., Oehen, S., Odermatt, B., Mak, T., Arnheiter, H., Burki, K., and Hengartner, H. (1991) T and B cell tolerance and responses to viral antigens in transgenic mice: implications for the pathogenesis of autoimmune versus immunopathological disease. *Immunol. Rev.* **122,** 133–171.
32. Stewart, M., Cameron, E., Campbell, M., McFarlane, R., Toth, S., Lang, K., Onions, D., and Neil, J. C. (1993) Conditional expression and oncogenicity of c-myc linked to a CD2 gene dominant control region. *Int. J. Cancer* **53,** 1023–1030.
33. Hanna, Z., Simard, C., Laperriere, A., and Jolicoeur, P. (1994) Specific expression of the human CD4 gene in mature CD4+ CD8- and immature CD4+ CD8+ T cells and in macrophages of transgenic mice. *Mol. Cell Biol.* **14,** 1084–1094.
34. Brombacher, F., Schafer, T., Weissenstein, U., Tschopp, C., Andersen, E., Burki, K., and Baumann, G. (1994) IL-2 promoter-driven lacZ expression as a monitoring tool for IL-2 expression in primary T cells of transgenic mice. *Int. Immunol.* **6,** 189–197.
35. Grossman, W. J., Kimata, J. T., Wong, F. H., Zutter, M., Ley, T. J., and Ratner, L. (1995) Development of leukemia in mice transgenic for the tax gene of human T- cell leukemia virus type I. *Proc. Natl. Acad. Sci. USA* **92,** 1057–1061.
36. Lichtenheld, M. G., Podack, E. R., and Levy, R. B. (1995) Transgenic control of perforin gene expression. Functional evidence for two separate control regions. *J. Immunol.* **154,** 2153–2163.
37. Aguila, H. L., Hershberger, R. J., and Weissman, I. L. (1995) Transgenic mice carrying the diphtheria toxin A chain gene under the control of the granzyme A promoter: expected depletion of cytotoxic cells and unexpected depletion of CD8 T cells. *Proc. Natl. Acad. Sci. USA* **92,** 10,192–10,196.
38. Salmon, P., Boyer, O., Lores, P., Jami, J., and Klatzmann, D. (1996) Characterization of an intronless CD4 minigene expressed in mature CD4 and CD8 T cells, but not expressed in immature thymocytes. *J. Immunol.* **156,** 1873–1879.
39. Boyer, O., Zhao, J. C., Cohen, J. L., DePetris, D., Yagello, M., Lejeune, L., et al. (1997) Position-dependent variegation of a CD4 minigene with targeted expression to mature CD4+ T cells. *J. Immunol.* **159,** 3383–3390.
40. Lee, W. H., Park, Y. M., Kim, J. I., Park, W. Y., Kim, S. H., Jang, J. J., and Seo, J. S. (1998) Expression of heat shock protein 70 blocks thymic differentiation of T cells in transgenic mice. *Immunology* **95,** 559–565.

41. Rouleau, M., Cottrez, F., Bigler, M., Antonenko, S., Carballido, J. M., Zlotnik, A., et al. (1999) IL-10 transgenic mice present a defect in T cell development reminiscent of SCID patients. *J. Immunol.* **163,** 1420–1427.
42. Manjunath, N., Shankar, P., Stockton, B., Dubey, P. D., Lieberman, J., and von Andrian, U. H. (1999) A transgenic mouse model to analyze CD8(+) effector T cell differentiation in vivo. *Proc. Natl. Acad. Sci. USA* **96,** 13,932–13,937.
43. Na, S., Li, B., Grewal, I. S., Enslen, H., Davis, R. J., Hanke, J. H., and Flavell, R. A. (1999) Expression of activated CDC42 induces T cell apoptosis in thymus and peripheral lymph organs via different pathways. *Oncogene* **18,** 7966–7974.
44. Byrne, C., Tainsky, M., and Fuchs, E. (1994) Programming gene expression in developing epidermis. *Development* **120,** 2369–2383.
45. Vassar, R. and Fuchs, E. (1991) Transgenic mice provide new insights into the role of TGF-alpha during epidermal development and differentiation. *Genes Dev.* **5,** 714–727.
46. Guo, L., Yu, Q. C., and Fuchs, E. (1993) Targeting expression of keratinocyte growth factor to keratinocytes elicits striking changes in epithelial differentiation in transgenic mice. *EMBO J.* **12,** 973–986.
47. Missero, C., Serra, C., Stenn, K., and Dotto, G. P. (1993) Skin-specific expression of a truncated E1a oncoprotein binding to p105- Rb leads to abnormal hair follicle maturation without increased epidermal proliferation. *J. Cell Biol.* **121,** 1109–1120.
48. Williams, I. R. and Kupper, T. S. (1994) Epidermal expression of intercellular adhesion molecule 1 is not a primary inducer of cutaneous inflammation in transgenic mice. *Proc. Natl. Acad. Sci. USA* **91,** 9710–9714.
49. Williams, I. R., Ort, R. J., and Kupper, T. S. (1994) Keratinocyte expression of B7–1 in transgenic mice amplifies the primary immune response to cutaneous antigens. *Proc. Natl. Acad. Sci. USA* **91,** 12,780–12,784.
50. Arbeit, J. M., Munger, K., Howley, P. M., and Hanahan, D. (1994) Progressive squamous epithelial neoplasia in K14-human papillomavirus type 16 transgenic mice. *J. Virol.* **68,** 4358–4368.
51. Robles, A. I., Larcher, F., Whalin, R. B., Murillas, R., Richie, E., Gimenez-Conti, I. B., et al. (1996) Expression of cyclin D1 in epithelial tissues of transgenic mice results in epidermal hyperproliferation and severe thymic hyperplasia. *Proc. Natl. Acad. Sci. USA* **93,** 7634–7638.
52. Williams, I. R., Rawson, E. A., Manning, L., Karaoli, T., Rich, B. E., and Kupper, T. S. (1997) IL-7 overexpression in transgenic mouse keratinocytes causes a lymphoproliferative skin disease dominated by intermediate TCR cells: evidence for a hierarchy in IL-7 responsiveness among cutaneous T cells. *J. Immunol.* **159,** 3044–3056.
53. Gulliver, G. A., Herber, R. L., Liem, A., and Lambert, P. F. (1997) Both conserved region 1 (CR1) and CR2 of the human papillomavirus type 16 E7 oncogene are required for induction of epidermal hyperplasia and tumor formation in transgenic mice. *J. Virol.* **71,** 5905–5914.
54. Kaya, G., Rodriguez, I., Jorcano, J. L., Vassalli, P., and Stamenkovic, I. (1997) Selective suppression of CD44 in keratinocytes of mice bearing an antisense CD44 transgene driven by a tissue-specific promoter disrupts hyaluronate metabolism in the skin and impairs keratinocyte proliferation. *Genes Dev.* **11,** 996–1007.
55. Bol, D., Kiguchi, K., Beltran, L., Rupp, T., Moats, S., Gimenez-Conti, I., et al. (1998) Severe follicular hyperplasia and spontaneous papilloma formation in transgenic mice expressing the neu oncogene under the control of the bovine keratin 5 promoter. *Mol. Carcinog.* **21,** 2–12.

56. Brown, K., Strathdee, D., Bryson, S., Lambie, W. and Balmain, A. (1998) The malignant capacity of skin tumours induced by expression of a mutant H-ras transgene depends on the cell type targeted. *Curr. Biol.* **8,** 516–524.
57. Raife, T. J., Lager, D. J., Peterson, J. J., Erger, R. A., and Lentz, S. R. (1998) Keratinocyte-specific expression of human thrombomodulin in transgenic mice: effects on epidermal differentiation and cutaneous wound healing. *J. Investig. Med.* **46,** 127–133.
58. Xie, W., Wu, X., Chow, L. T., Chin, E., Paterson, A. J., and Kudlow, J. E. (1998) Targeted expression of activated erbB-2 to the epidermis of transgenic mice elicits striking developmental abnormalities in the epidermis and hair follicles. *Cell Growth Differ.* **9,** 313–325.
59. Pierce, A. M., Fisher, S. M., Conti, C. J., and Johnson, D. G. (1998) Deregulated expression of E2F1 induces hyperplasia and cooperates with ras in skin tumor development. *Oncogene* **16,** 1267–1276.
60. Greenhalgh, D. A., Quintanilla, M. I., Orengo, C. C., Barber, J. L., Eckhardt, J. N., Rothnagel, J. A., and Roop, D. R. (1993) Cooperation between v-fos and v-rasHA induces autonomous papillomas in transgenic epidermis but not malignant conversion. *Cancer Res.* **53,** 5071–5075.
61. Werner, S., Weinberg, W., Liao, X., Peters, K. G., Blessing, M., Yuspa, S. H., et al. (1993) Targeted expression of a dominant-negative FGF receptor mutant in the epidermis of transgenic mice reveals a role of FGF in keratinocyte organization and differentiation. *EMBO J.* **12,** 2635–2643.
62. Auewarakul, P., Gissmann, L., and Cid-Arregui, A. (1994) Targeted expression of the E6 and E7 oncogenes of human papillomavirus type 16 in the epidermis of transgenic mice elicits generalized epidermal hyperplasia involving autocrine factors. *Mol. Cell Biol.* **14,** 8250–8258.
63. Cui, W., Fowlis, D. J., Cousins, F. M., Duffie, E., Bryson, S., Balmain, A., and Akhurst, R. J. (1995) Concerted action of TGF-β 1 and its type II receptor in control of epidermal homeostasis in transgenic mice. *Genes Dev.* **9,** 945–955.
64. Carroll, J. M., Romero, M. R., and Watt, F. M. (1995) Suprabasal integrin expression in the epidermis of transgenic mice results in developmental defects and a phenotype resembling psoriasis. *Cell* **83,** 957–968.
65. Carroll, J. M., Crompton, T., Seery, J. P., and Watt, F. M. (1997) Transgenic mice expressing IFN-gamma in the epidermis have eczema, hair hypopigmentation, and hair loss. *J. Invest. Dermatol.* **108,** 412–422.
66. Feng, X., Peng, Z. H., Di, W., Li, X. Y., Rochette-Egly, C., Chambon, P., et al. (1997) Suprabasal expression of a dominant-negative RXR alpha mutant in transgenic mouse epidermis impairs regulation of gene transcription and basal keratinocyte proliferation by RAR-selective retinoids. *Genes Dev.* **11,** 59–71.
67. Wang, X. J., Greenhalgh, D. A., Jiang, A., He, D., Zhong, L., Medina, D., et al. (1998) Expression of a p53 mutant in the epidermis of transgenic mice accelerates chemical carcinogenesis. *Oncogene* **17,** 35–45.
68. Tinsley, J. M., Fisher, C., and Searle, P. F. (1992) Abnormalities of epidermal differentiation associated with expression of the human papillomavirus type 1 early region in transgenic mice. *J. Gen. Virol.* **73,** 1251–1260.
69. Fowlis, D. J., Cui, W., Johnson, S. A., Balmain, A., and Akhurst, R. J. (1996) Altered epidermal cell growth control in vivo by inducible expression of transforming growth factor β 1 in the skin of transgenic mice. *Cell Growth Differ.* **7,** 679–687.
70. Gossen, M. and Bujard, H. (1992) Tight control of gene expression in mammalian cells by tetracycline-responsive promoters. *Proc. Natl. Acad. Sci. USA* **89,** 5547–5551.

71. Furth, P. A., St. Onge, L., Boger, H., Gruss, P., Gossen, M., Kistner, A., et al. (1994) Temporal control of gene expression in transgenic mice by a tetracycline-responsive promoter. *Proc. Natl. Acad. Sci. USA* **91,** 9302–9306.
72. Passman, R. S. and Fishman, G. I. (1994) Regulated expression of foreign genes in vivo after germline transfer. *J. Clin. Invest.* **94,** 2421–2425.
73. Kistner, A., Gossen, M., Zimmermann, F., Jerecic, J., Ullmer, C., Lubbert, H., and Bujard, H. (1996) Doxycycline-mediated quantitative and tissue-specific control of gene expression in transgenic mice. *Proc. Natl. Acad. Sci. USA* **93,** 10,933–10,938.
74. Schultze, N., Burki, Y., Lang, Y., Certa, U., and Bluethmann, H. (1996) Efficient control of gene expression by single step integration of the tetracycline system in transgenic mice. *Nature Biotechnol.* **14,** 499–503.
75. Freundlieb, S., Schirra-Muller, C., and Bujard, H. (1999) A tetracycline controlled activation/repression system with increased potential for gene transfer into mammalian cells. *J. Gene Med.* **1,** 4–12.
76. Huang, C. J., Spinella, F., Nazarian, R., Lee, M. M., Dopp, J. M., and de Vellis, J. (1999) Expression of green fluorescent protein in oligodendrocytes in a time- and level-controllable fashion with a tetracycline-regulated system. *Mol. Med.* **5,** 129–137.
77. Xie, W., Chow, L. T., Paterson, A. J., Chin, E., and Kudlow, J. E. (1999) Conditional expression of the ErbB2 oncogene elicits reversible hyperplasia in stratified epithelia and up-regulation of TGFα expression in transgenic mice. *Oncogene* **18,** 3593–3607.
78. Gu, H., Zou, Y. R., and Rajewsky, K. (1993) Independent control of immunoglobulin switch recombination at individual switch regions evidenced through Cre-loxP-mediated gene targeting. *Cell* **73,** 1155–1164.
79. Gu, H., Marth, J. D., Orban, P. C., Mossmann, H., and Rajewsky, K. (1994) Deletion of a DNA polymerase β gene segment in T cells using cell type-specific gene targeting. *Science* **265,** 103–106.
80. Kuhn, R., Schwenk, F., Aguet, M., and Rajewsky, K. (1995) Inducible gene targeting in mice. *Science* **269,** 1427–1429.
81. St. Onge, L., Furth, P. A., and Gruss, P. (1996) Temporal control of the Cre recombinase in transgenic mice by a tetracycline responsive promoter. *Nucleic Acids Res.* **24,** 3875–3877.
82. Wang, X. J., Liefer, K. M., Tsai, S., O'Malley, B. W., and Roop, D. R. (1999) Development of gene-switch transgenic mice that inducibly express transforming growth factor β in the epidermis. *Proc. Natl. Acad. Sci. USA* **96,** 8483–8488.
83. Church, G. M. and Gilbert, W. (1984) Genomic sequencing. *Proc. Natl. Acad. Sci. USA* **81,** 1991–1995.
84. Chomczynski, P. and Sacchi, N. (1987) Single-step method of RNA isolation by acid guanidinium thiocyanate-phenol-chloroform extraction. *Anal. Biochem.* **162,** 156–159.

# 39

## In Vivo Assay of Cellular Proliferation

**John Curran**

### 1. Introduction

The use of bromodeoxyuridine (BrdU) incorporation into replicating DNA is a well-established and commonly used technique for identifying dividing cells in vivo and in cell culture. BrdU is a pyrimidine analog of thymidine that is incorporated into the DNA of cells in the S-phase of the cell cycle *(1–3)*. Intra-peritoneal injection of BrdU in mice results in nuclear incorporation only where DNA is being actively replicated. The loading time needed to label an S-phase cell to detectability is estimated at <0.2 h directly after injection of BrdU *(4)*. As the availability of BrdU decreases, the labeling time increases to about 0.65 h, 30 min after injection. Thereafter, cells that enter the S-phase continue to become detectably labeled for about 5–6 h. BrdU labeling therefore provides a method for rapidly detecting replicating DNA.

As well as an excellent diagnostic tool, BrdU has potential clinical applications. Phase 1 trials have been conducted to assess the effect of BrdU administration in conjunction with radiation therapy for the treatment of pancreatic cancer *(5)* and primary hepatobiliary cancers or colorectal liver metastases *(6)*. Radiation therapy is one of the most commonly used treatments for cancer. The use of high linear energy transfer (LET) radiation/densely ionizing radiation gives the highest likelihood of DNA damage within a tumor cell. Auger electrons are one such source of high LET and are 20 times more radiotoxic than low LET radiation such as X-rays or $\gamma$-rays. They are given off by a range of unstable radioactive nuclei, and are thought to be produced by these nuclei as a way of trying to form a new point of equilibrium. Essentially there is a rearrangement of outer and inner electrons resulting in a cascade of auger electrons. These act at short distances but are extremely damaging to DNA. In order to target this damage to the nucleus of tumor cells and increase the potency even further, BrdU is labeled with the auger electron emitting isotopes $^{77}$Br or $^{80}$Br. This targets the radiation directly to the DNA, killing the tumor cell. Iodo-deoxyuridine, another pyrimidine analog of thymidine that is incorporated into replicating DNA, can also be labeled with the auger electron emitting isotope $^{125}$I with the same effect. It is hoped that

From: *Methods in Molecular Biology, Vol. 174: Epstein-Barr Virus Protocols*
Edited by: J. B. Wilson and G. H. W. May © Humana Press Inc., Totowa, NJ

selective radiosensitization using BrdU may improve treatment for these types of cancer in the near future.

BrdU has also been used to identify the best method for anti-cancer drug administration in the treatment of liver metastases *(7,8)*. BrdU was administered to liver metastases via either the hepatic vein or the portal vein and the uptake of BrdU assessed. It was discovered that prophylactic treatment against liver metastases would be most effective when given via the hepatic artery as this route provided a much better distribution of drug.

Further clinical applications for BrdU include a potential role as an antiviral agent *(9–11)*. Using an in vitro model, BrdU has been shown to significantly inhibit human papillomavirus 11 (HPV-11) replication *(9)*. BrdU and its 5'-PAA and 5'-PFA phosphate esters have also been shown to have activity against herpes simplex virus (HSV), varicella-zoster virus (VZV), and human cytomegalovirus (HCMV) *(10)*. Finally, Epstein-Barr virus (EBV) thymidine kinase (TK) activity was significantly inhibited by BrdU, suggesting that BrdU or similar thymidine analogs may be the most suitable nucleoside antivirals to target TK activity *(11)*.

Other applications of BrdU include its use to analyze DNA structure *(12)*. Immunogold detection of BrdU as a marker of DNA synthesis was used to evaluate the three-dimensional chromatin arrangement during interphase and S-phase of the cell cycle. Scanning electron microscopy was used to conduct a detailed examination at the ultrastructural level.

It is the ability to detect BrdU and thus identify proliferating cells undergoing DNA replication which gives rise to its most common applications in research. There are two main types of experiment: 1) using BrdU to detect and measure DNA replication under different stimuli or 2) using BrdU as a marker of DNA replication in order to study cells that are actively proliferating. Some examples of the latter include the use of BrdU as a tool in measuring the degree of wound healing of partial-thickness wounds *(13)* and the use of BrdU to mark proliferating cells in order to study mRNA levels of specific genes during active DNA replication *(14)*. BrdU has also been used to track the fate of cells used in transplantation *(15–17)*. For example, sex-matched transfer of transgenic rat cells to a wild-type rat can be regarded as an autologous transplant because the only difference is the transgene itself. *In situ* hybridization (ISH) can be used to detect the transgene and then BrdU incorporation can be used to follow the survival of ISH positive cells. This method provides an excellent tool for studying autologous transplants.

The most common application of BrdU in research is as a tool to analyze the effects of stimuli or drugs on DNA replication. For example, the tissue specific effect of transgene expression on the proliferation rate of cells can be assayed using BrdU *(18–22)*. Transgenic mice can also be subjected to chemical stimuli or wounding and the effects on DNA replication assessed using BrdU *(23,24)*. BrdU labeling has been used to follow cell cycle regulation following activation via genotoxins *(25)* and to show that EBV latent infection suppresses a G2/M arrest. Thus, the in vivo techniques where BrdU has been associated and the uses to which this thymidine analog can be put, are many and varied. However, it is not the most commonly used technique to determine proliferation rates in vitro.

The most frequently used method of detecting levels of proliferation in vitro depends upon the uptake of tritiated thymidine ($^3H$) by cells *(26)*. Another commonly used technique to visualize proliferating cells is to use immunofluoresence where fluorescently tagged antibodies can detect dividing cells from culture or tissue section. Common targets are the proliferative cell nuclear antigen (PCNA) and the Ki67 antigen *(27)*. The latter technique can be carried out within one day but requires the use of expensive fluorescence microscopes to view results. The fluorescence is only temporary and long-term record storage requires images to be made. The former technique is also quite rapid but involves the use of a radio-isotope and therefore the need for specialized radio-isotope counters. The results from this are numerical and detailed investigation at the cellular level is not possible.

Although lengthier than the previous two techniques, BrdU incorporation studies can be carried out without the need for expensive equipment or radio-isotope dispensaries. BrdU is however a potent mutagen and carcinogen so all necessary caution should prevail when in use.

## 2. Materials

### 2.1. Preparation and Injection of BrdU

1. Bromodeoxyuridine (BrdU, Sigma B9285; *see* **Note 1**).
2. Saline: 0.85% in $H_2O$, sterilize by filter or autoclave.
3. Glass bijoux or equivalent vessels.
4. Syringes and needles (sterile).
5. Latex gloves.
6. Paper towels.
7. Cin-bin.
8. Shaver.
9. Electronic weighing scale.
10. 10% buffered neutral formalin fixative: 22.4 m*M* $NaH_2PO_4$, 45.8 m*M* $Na_2HPO_4$, 4% formaldehyde.

### 2.2. Fixing and Sectioning Samples

1. Phosphate-buffered saline (PBS): 58 m*M* $Na_2HPO_4$, 17 m*M* $NaH_2PO_4$, 68 m*M* NaCl.
2. Saline: 0.85% in $H_2O$, sterile.
3. Ethanol (EtOH) and 70% EtOH.
4. Frosted microscope slides.
5. 2% TESPA in acetone (3-aminopropyl triethoxysilane, Sigma A3648).
6. Acetone.
7. De-ionized water.
8. Slide rack and troughs.
9. Fine tweezers.
10. Baking oven with adjustable temperature setting.
11. Microtome.
12. Water bath.
13. Rocking/rolling platform.

### 2.3. BrdU Detection

1. Slide racks and troughs.
2. Histoclear (National diagnostics).
3. Ethanol (EtOH), 100, 90, 80, 70, and 30% in $H_2O$.
4. PBS: 58 m*M* $Na_2HPO_4$, 17 m*M* $NaH_2PO_4$, 68 m*M* NaCl.
5. Magnetic stirrer and stir-bar.
6. Hydrogen peroxide ($H_2O_2$): 30% stock solution and 1.3% solution: 4 mL of 30% stock solution, 96 mL methanol.
7. Trypsin solution: 0.1% trypsin and 0.1% $CaCl_2$, in 50 m*M* Tris, pH 8.0.
8. Vectastain *elite* ABC system (Vector Laboratories, PK6102).
9. Mouse $IgG_1$ anti-BrdU antibody, immunohistology grade (Sigma B2531).
10. Glass cover slips.
11. DAB tablets (3,3'-diaminobenzidine tetrahydrochloride, Sigma, D4418).
12. Bleach.
13. Harris Haematoxylin stain, freshly filtered (Sigma, HHS-16).
14. Scott's tap water: 81 m*M* $MgSO_4$ (20 g/L), 24 m*M* $NaHCO_3$ (2 g/L).
15. DPX mountant (Fluka, 44581).
16. Clear nail varnish.

## 3. Methods

### 3.1. Preparation of BrdU

1. As BrdU is a potent carcinogen, weigh out an amount by difference, that is transfer an amount to a glass bijoux and then weigh the difference in the closed solid container. Dissolve BrdU to a concentration of 125 mg/mL in water in the glass bijoux by heating the solution to 60°C . The bijoux should then be wrapped in tin foil and stored at 4°C as the stock solution (*see* **Note 1**).
2. Prepare a working solution of 25 mg/mL in sterile saline from the stock solution and store at 4°C wrapped in tin foil.
3. Each time the working solution is used it should first be heated to 60°C to dissolve any crystals that may have formed.

### 3.2. Injection of BrdU

Ensure that the legal requirements for animal work in your country are in place. All procedures involving the use of live mice in the UK must be conducted under Home Office licence and euthanasia according to a procedure listed in schedule 1.

1. If epidermal tissue is to be examined, mice should have their dorsal skin shaved 24 h prior to injection (*see* **Notes 2** and **3**).
2. Weigh each mouse on an electronic scale and record its weight.
3. Intraperitoneally (ip) inject each mouse (*see* **Notes 4** and **5**) with the equivalent of 2 μL of working BrdU solution per gram of mouse (*see* **Note 6**). Carry out all injections in a designated fume hood (*see* **Note 7**).
4. One hour postinjection the mouse should be euthanased according to accepted humane procedures in your country (*see* **Notes 8** and **9**).
5. Take the appropriate tissues into a clearly labeled bijoux containing 10% buffered neutral formalin fixative or snap-freeze according to the preferred method of analysis (*see* **Note 10**).

### 3.3. Fixing Tissue Samples

1. Leave the bijoux containing tissues from the BrdU-injected mice on a rolling platform at 4°C overnight in formalin fixative (*see* **Note 11**).
2. Wash the tissue as follows: 1 × 30 min in PBS, 1 × 30 min in saline, 2 × 15 min in saline:100% EtOH (1:1 ratio), and finally 2 × 15 min in 70% EtOH. Carry out all washes on a rolling platform at 4°C using sterile solutions.
3. Replace the final 70% EtOH wash with fresh 70% EtOH. Samples prior to paraffin embedding can be stored at 4°C.

### 3.4. Sectioning

1. To aid adherence of the tissue section to the slide, incubate frosted microscope slides in a rack (*see* **Note 12**) at room temperature (RT) for 50 s in 2% TESPA in a fume hood (*see* **Note 13**).
2. Transfer the slide rack immediately to acetone for 2 × 50 s washes.
3. Transfer the slide rack immediately to de-ionized water for 2 × 50 s washes.
4. Place slides face up on a paper towel-lined tray and bake dry at 42°C . Slides can now be stored in a slide box at RT until use.
5. Place the paraffin-embedded tissue block onto a microtome (*see* **Note 14**).
6. Cut 7 μm sections. Crank the microtome handle at a medium but constant pace for several turns. This produces a "ribbon" of sections.
7. Carefully pick up the sections using fine tweezers and place on a TESPA-coated slide. Clean the microtome blade with a fine brush after each tissue.
8. Carefully drop 30% EtOH over one edge of the section (*see* **Note 15**).
9. To smooth out the section, gently immerse the microscope slide in a small 37°C water bath filled with ultra pure water. The section will float off (*see* **Note 16**). Carefully place the same slide under the floating section and lift the slide such that the section adheres to the slide again (*see* **Note 17**).
10. Clearly label each slide with tissue details and then dry the slides with the section side facing up on a 42°C drying rack overnight. Slides can now be kept at RT in a slide box.

### 3.5. ABC Method for Detection of BrdU Incorporated Nuclei

1. Choose the slide samples which are to be BrdU stained (*see* **Note 18**).
2. Place the chosen slides in a slide rack and immerse the slides for 2 × 7 min in Histoclear (*see* **Notes 12** and **19**).
3. Immerse the slides through 2 × 100, 90, 80, and 70% EtOH concentrations respectively for 2 min each (*see* **Note 20**).
4. Wash the sections by immersing them for 3 × 30 min in PBS. Include a stir-bar to circulate the solution (*see* **Note 21**).
5. Immerse the sections in 1.3% $H_2O_2$ (in methanol) for 30 min (*see* **Notes 22** and **23**).
6. Wash the sections for 3 × 5 min in PBS with circulation (*see* **Note 21**).
7. Immerse the sections in warmed (37°C ) trypsin solution for 3 min (*see* **Notes 24** and **25**).
8. Wash the sections for 3 × 5 min in PBS with circulation (*see* **Note 21**).
9. Place the slides on paper towels with the section facing up. Add one drop (approx 50 μL) of 1% normal horse serum (supplied with Vectastain kit) directly onto each section and incubate at RT for 30 min (*see* **Note 26**).
10. Gently shake/dab off excess serum.
11. Add 10 μL of the undiluted primary anti-BrdU antibody to each section. Carefully place a glass coverslip over each section and incubate at RT for 1 h (*see* **Note 27**).

12. Wash the sections for 3 × 5 min in PBS with circulation. The coverslips will fall off during the washing and can be collected from the bottom of the trough.
13. Add 200 µL of the anti-mouse biotinylated IgG secondary antibody prepared as directed in the Vectastain Kit. Incubate at RT for 30 min (*see* **Note 28**).
14. Wash the sections for 3 × 5 min in PBS with circulation.
15. Prepare the ABC complex according to the Vectastain kit instructions and leave at RT for 30 min (*see* **Notes 29** and **30**).
16. Add one drop of the ABC complex to each section and incubate at RT for 1 h (*see* **Note 27**).
17. Wash the sections for 3 × 5 min in PBS with circulation.
18. Dissolve one 10 mg DAB tablet in 15 mL of PBS and 12 µL of 30% stock $H_2O_2$ (*see* **Notes 31** and **32**).
19. Place the slides on paper towels in the fume hood with sections face up and apply one drop of the DAB stain to each section individually. Leave for a maximum of 1 min (*see* **Note 33**). Quickly shake off excess DAB into bleach before placing the slide in a PBS wash trough to dilute the DAB and terminate the staining.
20. When all the sections have been DAB stained, immerse the slides in freshly filtered undiluted Harris's Haematoxylin for 10 s to counterstain the section (*see* **Note 34**).
21. Immediately but gently rinse all of the residual stain from the slides under running tap water.
22. Immerse the slides in Scott's tap water for 1 min (*see* **Note 35**).
23. Rinse the slides gently under running tap water for 1 min.
24. The sections are then dehydrated by immersing them through a series of ethanol baths of concentrations of 30, 50, 70, 90, and 100%. Each immersion is for 2 min (*see* **Note 20**).
25. Immerse the slides in 100% EtOH for 5 min.
26. Immerse the slides in histoclear for 2 min and then again in fresh histoclear for 7 min.
27. Mount the slides by adding a drop of DPX onto the section and placing a glass coverslip on top (*see* **Note 36**). Seal the edges with clear nail varnish. The slides can be stored indefinitely at RT.
28. View the sections through a suitably powerful light microscope. Nuclei that have incorporated the BrdU will be stained brown whereas those that have not will only show the blue counterstain.

### 3.6. Quantification

1. To obtain the BrdU count or a "mitotic index" for the tissue, sufficient samples and sections must be counted to yield results that are representative of the tissue. This is particularly important if results from two sample types (for example, where one is a control for a reagent under test) are to be compared. One method to obtain an index for a single section is to count labeled cells in a given area. For example, in obtaining the mitotic index for epidermal sections, the positively stained cells in interfolicular regions should be counted from one intact field of vision of the section where the magnification is 312.5 × (×25 lens and × 12.5 eyepiece; *see* **Note 37**). Where possible, all counts should be done "blind," that is without knowing whether the section is test or control, to avoid any possible count bias.
2. To obtain the mitotic index for the individual section, count at least 10 fields of vision and use the mean value as the index for the section (*see* **Note 37**).
3. To obtain a representative mitotic index for the tissue under the conditions applied (for example control or transgenic) sufficient samples must be taken from different mice (to ensure that any result is not owing to one aberrant mouse). Sufficiency will depend on the statistical test applied, but we usually aim for at least 5 mice in each test and control

category and 10 sections from each mouse tissue sample and apply the 2 sample *t*-test. It is important to ensure that controls are age and genotype matched and housed under the same conditions. Sibling controls are therefore usually the most appropriate.

## 4. Notes

1. Bromodeoxyuridine (BrdU) is a potent carcinogen. All procedures must be carried out in the fume hood. Contaminated plastics, needles, and mice must be kept separate from general waste and later incinerated. Gloves must be worn at all times and it is a sensible precaution to wear two layers of gloves in case one should inadvertently tear. Masks should be used when the BrdU powder is weighed out. Once in solution masks are not necessary.
2. There is suggestion that shaving, and evidence that accidental wounding caused by shaving, can result in increased cellular proliferation. Shaving 24 h prior to injection reduces this possibility.
3. Lift the mouse by the tail and allow it to grab onto the bars of the cage lid with its forepaws while gently pulling the mouse backwards. The mouse will continue to cling and resist your pressure thus remaining stretched. This makes shaving much easier.
4. To humanely pick up and hold a mouse securely, follow the procedure in **Note 3** such that the mouse is stretched. Using your forefinger and thumb, grasp the skin around the shoulder blades of the mouse such that its forepaws are slightly forced outwards. This should allow you to safely and securely pick up the mouse between your forefinger and thumb. Be careful of two things: 1) if your grip is loose the mouse could reach your finger with its teeth, and 2) they usually urinate, let it finish before turning it around to inject.
5. Having secured the mouse in one hand between finger and thumb, you can turn the mouse around to expose its stomach. This should allow simple ip injection.
6. It is also possible to BrdU label mouse pups. Here the working solution should be further diluted with sterile saline to 2.5 mg/mL so that each pup is injected with the equivalent of 20 μL of BrdU solution per gram of mouse.
7. Extreme care should be taken when injecting BrdU. Do so only in a designated fume hood, which must contain a sink for washing out after use. Dispose of all gloves, needles, syringes, paper towels, etc., in a designated and clearly labeled cin-bin.
8. Remember to wear gloves at all times when handling BrdU-injected mice. Larger time periods (up to 4 h) for incorporation of the BrdU pulse can be used, the optimal time will depend upon the tissue under study.
9. Ip injection provides a pulse of BrdU labeling. To track cells labeled in the pulse, mice can be euthanized and examined after the appropriate extended time delay. To continuously supply BrdU for an extended labeling period, BrdU can alternatively be administered in the drinking water, usually at a concentration of 0.8–1.0 mg/mL, changing the water every 2–3 d.
10. Cell suspensions, where appropriate, can also be obtained at this point and analyzed by flow cytometry.
11. Continual rotation ensures that the tissues are completely fixed.
12. The easiest way to coat multiple slides at once is to place them back to back in a slide rack. The rack can then be placed in its accompanying trough containing the liquid in use.
13. Plan how many different solutions and how many incubations are required to coat the slides. Have all the solutions prepared and ready in troughs, one trough for each incubation (6 troughs in total). This way the rack can be moved from trough to trough immediately each incubation period is over. Carry out all steps in a fume hood.

14. A cleaner cut section can be achieved if the paraffin embedded sample is kept in the fridge prior to sectioning.
15. The ribbon of sections will be wrinkly. Hold the slide at a 45° angle and drop 30% ethanol from the top of the slide. This will flatten out some of the creases.
16. Place the slide slowly into the water bath at a 45° angle. As soon as the section touches the water, it will come away from the slide and the rest of the section can then be eased off by further immersing the slide. This will completely flatten out the section and any remaining creases.
17. With practise and care, individual sections within a ribbon can be teased apart with fine tweezers to allow one single section per slide. This is difficult and it is generally easier to capture the entire ribbon and if desired, remove unwanted sections after the slide has dried.
18. Simple visual examination of each section on the microscope slide often reveals broken areas within the section or areas where the section has doubled over on itself slightly. Avoid using such sections.
19. Histoclear removes the paraffin from the sections while leaving the section untouched. Overnight incubation in xylene (or at least 2 h in fresh xylene) can also be used to dewax the sections. Always use xylene in a fume hood.
20. Passing the sections through ethanol of decreasing concentration hydrates the sections, just as increasing concentrations of ethanol dehydrates the samples. The simplest way of doing this is to have a series of troughs lined up, each containing the ethanol concentration to be used. This way the rack can be passed from trough to trough as previously indicated in **Note 13**.
21. Placing the trough plus stir-bar on a magnetic stirrer helps to circulate the solution and wash the sections.
22. The eventual detection of BrdU is facilitated by the Vectastain *elite* ABC kit (Vector laboratories), which is based on an immunoperoxidase detection system. For this reason it is necessary to block endogenous peroxidase activity using hydrogen peroxide.
23. Hydrogen peroxide is corrosive and causes burns. Skin and eye protection should be worn.
24. Make up the trypsin solution during the 30 min $H_2O_2$ incubation. Pour the liquid into a glass trough and place the trough in the 37°C waterbath. This allows the trypsin solution to equilibrate to the desired temperature for the incubation. A 15-min incubation at RT with Proteinase K (20 µg/mL in 50 m*M* Tris, pH 8.0) can be used as an alternative to trypsin.
25. Proteolytic cleavage is required for formalin-fixed, crosslinked samples. Digestion times will vary with the thickness of the section and the extent of fixation. Overdigestion will lead to nonspecific staining.
26. The 1% normal horse serum acts as a blocking agent to minimize background antibody signal. Horse serum is used because the secondary antibody in the BrdU detection step is raised in horse.
27. Covering the section with a glass coverslip reduces antibody evaporation. The coverslips can be cleaned and re-used.
28. The large volume of antibody means that no coverslips are necessary.
29. The two components of the ABC complex are Avidin and biotinylated horseradish peroxidase. Avidin has four binding sites for biotin and because of the dilutions used, at least one of these sites remains unbound and thus able to bind to biotin on the secondary antibody. During the ABC incubation the avidin:biotinylated HRP complex binds to the biotinylated secondary antibody through the biotin:avidin high-affinity binding site.
30. It is important to prepare the ABC complex 15 min into the secondary antibody step (**step 13**). The final 15 min of the secondary antibody step plus the $3 \times 5$ min PBS washes

allows the ABC complex to incubate at RT for 30 min and therefore be ready for use directly after the last PBS wash.

31. 3,3'-diaminobenzidine tetrahydrochloride (DAB) is a peroxidase substrate and is used to visualize individual BrdU-stained cells. Make up the DAB stain during the washes of **step 17**.
32. DAB is harmful and a possible carcinogen. It should always be handled with care in a fume hood. DAB can be deactivated with common bleach, and so this should always be available. It is also advisable to deactivate DAB with a little bleach prior to disposal into the drains.
33. Different lengths of exposure to DAB should be tested to optimize staining time. The longer the DAB is left the greater the orange background staining.
34. As with DAB exposure, the exposure time to Haematoxylin should be optimized. Any longer than 10 s and the background may become too blue.
35. This step is only necessary if the water quality in your area is hard. The Scott's tap water is designed to compensate for the hard water.
36. Gently drop the coverslip onto the drop of DPX and let the weight of the coverslip spread the DPX over the entire section. When the section is covered, the coverslip can be sealed in place by using clear nail varnish along the four edges.
37. A field of vision is defined as the visible area when examining a section at a particular magnification. When the count for one field of vision is complete, simply move the slide to another field of vision and so on.

## References


1. Gratzner, H. G. (1982) Monoclonal antibody to 5-Bromo- and 5-iododeoxyuridine: a new reagent for detection of DNA replication. *Science* **218,** 474–475.
2. Dolbeare, F., Gratzner, H., Pallavicini, M. G., and Gray, J. W. (1983) Flow cytometric measurement of total DNA content and incorporated bromodeoxyuridine. *Proc. Natl. Acad. Sci. USA* **80,** 5573–5577.
3. Morstyn, G., Hsu, S. M., Kinsella, T., Gratzner, H., Russo, A., and Mitchell, J. B. (1983) Bromodeoxyuridine in tumours and chromosomes detected with a monoclonal antibody. *J. Clin. Inv.* **72,** 1844–1850.
4. Hayes, N. L. and Nowakowski, R. S. (2000) Exploiting the dynamics of S-phase tracers in developing brain: Interkinetic nuclear migration for cells entering versus leaving the S-phase. *Dev. Neurosci.* **22,** 44–55.
5. Robertson, J. M., Ensminger, W. D., Walker, S., and Lawrence, T. S. (1997) A phase I trial of intravenous bromodeoxyuridine and radiation therapy for pancreatic cancer. *Intl. J. Radiat. Oncol. Biol. Physics* **37,** 331–335.
6. Robertson, J. M., McGinn, C. J., Walker, S., Marx, M. V., Kessler, M. L., Ensminger, W. D., and Lawrence, T. S. (1997) A phase I trial of hepatic arterial bromodeoxyuridine and conformal radiation therapy for patients with primary hepatobiliary cancers or colorectal liver metastases. *Intl. J. Radiat. Oncol. Biol. Physics* **39,** 1087–1092.
7. Ishida, H., Iwama, T., Yoshinaga, K., Gonda, T., and Idezuki, Y. (1998) Bromodeoxyuridine uptake by early liver metastases in rats: A comparison of the hepatic artery and portal vein infusion routes. *Surg. Today* **28,** 822–829.
8. Kuan, H-Y., Smith, D. E., Ensminger, W. D., Knol. J. A., DeRemer, S. J., Yang, Z., and Stetson, P. L. (1996) Regional pharmacokinetics of 5-bromo-2'-deoxyuridine and 5-fluorouracil in dogs: hepatic arterial versus portal venous infusions. *Cancer Res.* **56,** 4724–4727.

9. Clark, P. R., Roberts, M. L., and Cowsert, L. M. (1998) A novel drug screening assay for papillomavirus specific antiviral activity. *Antiviral Res.* **37,** 97–106.
10. Bird, R. M., Broadhurst, A. V., Duncan, I. B., Hall, M. J., Lambert, R. W., and Wong-Kai-In, P. (1986) Antiviral activity of 5'-PAA and 5'-PFA phosphate esters of 2'-deoxyuridines. *J. Antimicrob. Chemother.* **18,** 201–205.
11. Gustafson, E. A., Chillemi, A. C., Sage, D. R., and Fingeroth, J. D. (1998) The Epstein-Barr Virus thymidine kinase does not phosphorylate ganciclovir or acyclovir and demonstrates a narrow substrate specificity compared to the herpes simplex virus type 1 thymidine kinase. *Antimicrob. Agents Chemother.* **42,** 2923–2931.
12. Gobbi, P., Falconi, M., Vitale, M., Galanzi, A., Artico, M., Martelli, A. M., and Mazzotti, G. (1999) Scanning electron microscopic detection of nuclear structures involved in DNA replication. *Arch. Histol. Cytol.* **62,** 317–326.
13. Agren, M. S. (1999) Matrix metalloproteinases (MMPs) are required for re-epithelialization of cutaneous wounds. *Arch. Dermatol. Res.* **291,** 583–590.
14. Archer, C., Debiec-Rychter, M., Morse, P., Haas, G. P., and Wang, C. Y. (1999) Epithelial proliferation and expression of the aromatic amine activation enzyme N-acetyltransferase in the prostate of postnatal rat. *Anticancer Res.* **19,** 4013–4016.
15. Watanabe, N., Takai, S., Morita, N., Kawata, M., and Hirasawa, N. (1999) A method of tracking donor cells after simulated autologous transplantation: A study using synovial cells of transgenic rats. *Cell Tissue Res.* **298,** 519–525.
16. Seiler, M. J. and Aramant, R. B. (1995) Transplantation of embryonic retinal donor cells labelled with BrdU or carrying a genetic marker to adult retina. *Exp. Brain Res.* **105,** 59–66.
17. Aramant, R. B. and Seiler, M. J. (1992) Retina-to-Retina transplantation of embryonic donor cells, labelled with BrdU or carrying a genetic marker. *J. Neural Transplantation Plasticity* **3,** 283–284.
18. Sato, S., Kume, K., Ito, C., Ishii, S., and Shimizu, T. (1999) Accelerated proliferation of epidermal keratinocytes by the transgenic expression of the platelet-activating factor receptor. *Arch. Dermatol. Res.* **291,** 614–621.
19. Waikel, R. L., Wang, X-J., and Roop, D. R. (1999) Targeted expression of c-Myc in the epidermis alters normal proliferation, differentiation and UV-B induced apoptosis. *Oncogene* **18,** 4870–4878.
20. Snibson, K. J., Bhathal, P. S., Hardy, G. L., Brandon, M. R., and Adams, T. E. (1999) High, persistent hepatocellular proliferation and apoptosis precede hepatocarcinogenesis in growth hormone transgenic mice. *Liver* **19,** 242–252.
21. Machida, N., Brissie, N., Sreenan, C., and Bishop, S. P. (1997) Inhibition of cardiac myocyte division in c-myc transgenic mice. *J. Mol. Cell. Cardiol.* **29,** 1895–1902.
22. Wang, T. C., Koh, T. J., Varro, A., Cahill, R. J., Dangler, C. A., Fox, J. G., and Dockray, G. J. (1996) In vivo actions of insulin-like growth factor-I (IGF-I) on cerebellum development in transgenic mice: Evidence that IGF-I increases proliferation of granule cell progenitors. *Brain Res.* **95,** 44–54.
23. Ishikawa, T., Nakatsuru, Y., Zarkovic, M., and Shamsuddin, A. M. (1999) Inhibition of skin cancer by IP6 in vivo: Inhibition-promotion model. *Anticancer Res.* **19,** 3749–3752.
24. Wang, X-J., Greenhalgh, D. A., Jiang, A., He, D., Zhong, L., Medina, D., et al. (1998) Expression of a p53 mutant in the epidermis of transgenic mice accelerates chemical carcinogenisis. *Oncogene* **17,** 35–45.
25. Wade, M. and Allday, M. J. (2000) Epstein-Barr Virus suppresses a G2/M checkpoint activated by genotoxins. *Mol. Cell. Biol.* **20,** 1344–1360.

26. Roy, P., Paganelli, G. M., Faivre, J., Biasco, G., Scheppach, W., Saldanha, M. H., and Beckly, D. E. (1999) Pattern of epithelial cell proliferation in colorectal mucosa of patients with large bowel adenoma or cancer: An ECP case-control study. *Euro. J. Cancer Prevent.* **8,** 401–407.
27. Stavropoulos, N. E., Ioachim, E., Pappa, L., Hastazeris, K., and Agnantis, N. J. (1999) Antiproliferative activity of interferon gamma in superficial bladder cancer. *Anticancer Res.* **19,** 4529–4533.

# 40

# Topical Chemical Carcinogen Treatment in Mice

**John Curran**

## 1. Introduction

The mouse model of multi-step carcinogenesis has taken researchers a long way towards understanding the molecular events that underlie the transition from a normal cell to a transformed cell and neoplasia *(1)*. This model has been extended to transgenic mouse studies where one of the carcinogenic events (an activated oncogene or loss of a tumor-supressor gene) is supplied in transgenic form. This permits an examination of the consequences of the transgene expression (or loss of expression in the case of null mice) during the evolution of malignancy.

Many of the transgenic mice studied in this scenario have phenotypes reflecting early stages of carcinogenesis, but require further events to develop a malignancy *(2–10)*. Examples of epidermally expressed transgenic oncogenes that give rise to observable phenotypes include latent membrane protein 1 (LMP 1) *(2)*, Ha-*ras* *(3,4)*, transforming growth factor (TGF) $\beta_1$ *(5,6)*, TGF-$\alpha$ *(7–9)*, and v-*fos* *(10)*.

The chemical carcinogenesis protocol involves a single topical application of a mutagen to the dorsal skin of a susceptible strain of mouse (termed initiation), followed by repeated applications with a tumor promoter (promotion). This results in the formation of multiple discrete benign tumors called papillomas, 5–10% of which convert to carcinomas (malignant conversion). There is then the possibility of further conversion to a more aggressive tumor type and metastasis.

The first requirement is that the transgenic mouse must either be created in a strain of mice susceptible to tumor induction by chemical carcinogens or must be back-crossed to a susceptible strain. It has been well documented that there are marked strain differences in response to epidermal tumor promotion using chemical carcinogens *(11–13)*. This led to the identification of the following order of susceptibility to lesion formation: SENCAR> FVB> DBA/2> CD-1> C57Bl/6, where C57Bl/6 is the most resistant strain studied. In this respect, it is important to use an appropriate dose of carcinogen with respect to the strain of mice under study *(13)*. In the protocol described in this chapter, the dosage has been optimized for use with the FVB mouse strain.

From: *Methods in Molecular Biology, Vol. 174: Epstein-Barr Virus Protocols*
Edited by: J. B. Wilson and G. H. W. May © Humana Press Inc., Totowa, NJ

Initiation is achieved via a single topical application of a mutagen. One of the most frequently used mutagens for topical application is 7,12-Dimethylbenzanthracene (DMBA), a polycyclic aromatic hydrocarbon (PAH). PAHs are common environmental pollutants that have high carcinogenic properties ***(14)***. They are metabolically activated in cells by cytochrome p450 enzymes and/or peroxidases to DNA-damaging reactive intermediates. This damage is caused largely by the formation of stable DNA adducts ***(14)*** which result in transversion mutations (A to T). In over 90% of mouse skin tumors initiated with DMBA, the activating mutation has been identified as an A to T transversion at the second position of codon 61 of the Ha-*ras* gene ***(15–19)***. A smaller percentage display a mutation in codon 12 instead. Along with Ha-*ras* transgenic mouse studies ***(3,4)*** this is compelling evidence for the activation of the *ras* proto-oncogene as a principle event in initiation. Other carcinogens used as initiators include 3-Methylcholanthrene, N-Nitroso-N-ethylurea and N-Methyl-N'-nitro-N-nitrosoguanidine.

The promotion step in the mouse skin model consists of repeated treatment of initiated mouse skin with a tumor-promoting agent, a chemical carcinogen that is not necessarily a mutagen. This results in persistent general hyperplasia that is seen within 24 h, is maximal at 48–72 h, and can last for up 1 wk ***(20)***. There is a much wider choice of promoting agents available but the most potent promoters of mouse skin are phorbol esters such as 12-*O*-tetradecanoylphorbol-13-acetate (TPA). TPA has a wide variety of effects following topical application to mouse dorsal skin. For example, TGFβ1 mRNA and protein levels become elevated ***(21,22)***, TGFβ2 and TGFβ3 levels decrease ***(20)***, epidermal growth factor receptor (EGFR) ***(23,24)*** becomes activated, *erb* B2 and c-*src* ***(25)*** are also activated. These effects are mediated through TPA-responsive elements (TRE, an example of which is the Human collagenase TRE sequence TGAGTCA), which are located in the promoter regions of a number of different genes, modulating their expression ***(26)***. The AP-1 family of transcription factors bind to TRE sites and the composition of the AP-1 complex is dependent not only on the specific TRE but also on the adjacent sequence ***(27)***.

TPA binds to protein kinase C (PKC) and is thought to mimic the action of diacylglycerol (DAG) binding, to activate PKC ***(28,29)***. This activation of PKC by TPA is likely to be important in carcinogenesis because it leads to activation of several pathways including the mitogen-activated protein kinase kinase (MAPKK) ***(30)***. Because RAS is already activated by the application of DMBA in these chemical carcinogen studies, and RAS binds to RAF, targeting RAF to the membrane and activating it and the MAPKK pathway, this may amplify one of the PKC pathways further.

Thus, TPA promotion of susceptible mouse skin results in a plethora of events and the induction of a visible hyperplastic response. The events that occur after promotion are not clearly defined. One particular facet of phorbol ester treatment may be wholly responsible for papilloma formation, such as the induction of hyperplasia, or many of the resultant events may be required in tandem. Certainly the activation of PKC and the subsequent signal transduction pathways that will be stimulated may be important.

Other commonly used promoters include Phorbol-12-retinoate-13-acetate (RPA), chryserobin and ethyl phenylpropiolate. A tumor promoter is defined as any substance or event that results in the formation of pre-cancerous lesions on initiated skin. Therefore, other methods of tumor promotion include full-thickness skin wounding *(31,32)*.

Tumor promotion can be further divided depending on the type of promoter used. This led to the classification of stage 1 promoters (also called full or conversion promoters) and stage 2 promoters (propagation promoters). TPA and wounding belong to stage 1 promoters, whereas chemicals such as mezerein or RPA function as stage 2 promoters. Stage 2 promoters have only moderate or weak promoting activities but can give rise to tumors following short treatment with a stage 1 promoter *(33)*.

Repeated applications of TPA to DMBA-initiated mouse skin results in the formation of multiple discrete benign tumors called papillomas. Papillomas are thought to be clonal, arising from a single initiated cell that has an increased rate of proliferation with a concomitant decrease in the rate of differentiation *(1)*. The malignant conversion of a benign papilloma to a carcinoma is a relatively rare event, with approx 5–10% of papillomas converting to carcinomas. A further conversion step occurs with the progression from a squamous-cell carcinoma to the more aggressive spindle-cell tumor in which all organization and markers of epithelial differentiation are completely lost. This conversion step is rare with only 0.07 spindle-cell carcinomas formed per mouse (of the SENCAR strain) following DMBA and TPA treatment *(34)*.

The genetics of tumor susceptibility and tumor progression and conversion is gradually being determined. As well as the mutational activation of H-ras and overexpression of the mutant form, alterations in genes such as *cyclin D1*, *p53*, and $p16^{INK4A}$ frequently define the carcinogenic steps in this model system *(35–37)*.

The duration of chemical carcinogen treatment and the observation period after treatment will depend on the requirements of the study. The protocol described here follows a standard procedure of a single DMBA application followed by 20 wk of tumor promotion. Shorter promotion periods can be used to examine the contribution of another parameter (such as transgene expression) to promotion and the initiation step can be omitted to examine this component. The observation period can be extended up to 1 yr beyond chemical treatment. During the post-treatment period, some papillomas may regress and disappear while others will convert to carcinoma. It should be borne in mind that these in vivo studies must be conducted under the appropriate legislation and with humane end points. The development of papillomas in mice under this regime does not unduly affect the animals' breeding capacity or health but some papillomas may form in areas of natural abrasion and irritation. It is expedient to apply a health-scoring system for carcinoma progression in order to define when an animal should be removed from the study. Guidelines are available concerning the welfare of animals in experimental neoplasia in the UK and similar documents are likely to be available in other countries.

## 2. Materials

### 2.1. Equipment

1. Fume hood designated for use in chemical carcinogenesis studies. The hood should contain a sink.
2. Cin-bin designated for chemical carcinogen waste, or other appropriate waste container.

3. Pipets and aerosol-resistant tips designated for use with chemical carcinogens (*see* **Note 1**). Once used in this study these items should not be removed from the hood unless thoroughly cleaned.
4. Latex gloves. Gloves should be worn whenever mice are handled and two pairs should be worn during treatment (*see* **Note 1**).
5. Fridge/freezer designated for storage of chemicals and tissues from treated mice (*see* **Note 2**).
6. Electric or battery-operated shaver.
7. Dissection kit for use with treated animals only.
8. Sample collection vessels.
9. Liquid nitrogen carrier.

### 2.2. Chemicals

1. Hair removing cream: any standard brand available at chemists/drugstore.
2. 7,12-dimethylbenzanthracene (DMBA, Sigma D3254): 100X stock solution (12.5 mg/mL) dissolved in acetone and stored at –20°C (*see* **Notes 2** and **3**). 1X DMBA: stock solution diluted to 0.125 mg/mL in acetone and stored at –20°C.
3. 12-*O*-tetradecanoylphorbol-13-acetate (TPA, Sigma P8139): A stock solution of $2 \times 10^{-3}$ *M* is prepared by dissolving 25 mg TPA in 20 mL of acetone. Store stock solution at –20°C (*see* **Note 2**). $5 \times 10^{-5}$ *M* working solution diluted in acetone and stored at –20°C (*see* **Note 3**).
4. 70% Ethanol in water.
5. 10% buffered neutral formalin fixative: 22.4 m*M* $NaH_2PO_4$, 45.8 m*M* $Na_2HPO_4$, 4% Formaldehyde.
6. Liquid nitrogen.

## 3. Methods

### 3.1. Treatment Protocols

Begin treatment on mice of a uniform age; 8 wk old is preferable. Ascertainment of transgenic status or other parameter under test is preferably carried out following the removal of the animal from study, thereby conducting the study blind (*see* **Notes 4** and **5**). To allow meaningful statistical analysis of the experimental results, sufficient mice must be entered into the study. At least 10 mice should be used for each test parameter, but we usually aim for 30 mice in each category (*see* **Note 5**).

1. Identify all mice entered into the study so that their phenotypes can be monitored individually (*see* **Note 6**).
2. Remove fur from dorsal area using a shaver and/or hair removing cream the day prior to the first treatment (*see* **Notes 7** and **8**).
3. Remove the mouse from its cage and hold it by the tail on the lid of a spare cage lined with paper towels in a fume hood (*see* **Note 8**).
4. Pipet 200 µL of 1X DMBA directly but slowly onto the exposed dorsal skin (*see* **Notes 1** and **9**).
5. Discard all paper towels, tips, and gloves into the carcinogen waste container in the hood. All cages, cagetops, bottles, and bedding must be treated as if contaminated by carcinogens by all ancillary workers (*see* **Note 1**). Keep treated mice in their cages in the hood for 30 min to allow complete evaporation of the acetone before returning the cages to racks.

6. Allow one complete week (7 d) before commencing promotion with TPA.
7. Pipet 200 µL of $5 \times 10^{-5}$ *M* TPA directly but slowly onto the exposed dorsal skin (*see* **Notes 1, 8**, and **9**).
8. Repeat TPA treatment twice weekly for 20 wk (*see* **Note 7**).
9. Score lesion formation once per week (*see* **Subheading 3.2.**).
10. Continue to observe mice for up to a further 40 wk after treatment termination (60 wk total experimental time) or until all mice have been removed from the study (according to local rules for humane end point, e.g., United Kingdom Co-ordinating Committee on Cancer Research Guidelines for the Welfare of Animals in Experimental Neoplasia).
11. Continue to remove the fur from the dorsal area regularly using either a small and maneuverable shaver or hair removing cream. Remove fur at least 1 d prior to treatment (*see* **Note 7**). Take great care when shaving to avoid nicking any lesions that have formed.

### 3.2. Scoring Protocol

1. Carefully monitor every mouse in the study each week. Note the first appearance of papillomas and then count the numbers that have formed on each mouse. Note the first conversion to carcinoma and then the accumulation of carcinomas (*see* **Note 10**). Total numbers of lesions can be scored but it is usually more informative if the lesions are graded by size. We have used an effective scoring system for papillomas, where:
   1 < 0.2 cm in diameter
   2 = 0.2–0.5 cm in diameter
   3 = 0.5–1 cm in diameter
   4 > 1 cm in diameter (*see* **Note 11**).
2. When an animal is removed from the study and euthanized (*see* **Note 11**), take samples of papillomas and carcinomas. Tissue and lesion samples (or parts thereof) can be snap-frozen in liquid nitrogen for further analysis, placed in fixative (such as buffered formalin) for histopathological analysis (*see* **Note 10**), or taken into culture for the generation of squamous-cell carcinoma cell lines.

### 3.3. Measurements and Statistical Analysis

It is important to have entered sufficient numbers of mice in each treatment regime to validate any observed differences in the parameters under test.

1. Different measures of carcinogenesis can be examined. One measure is to calculate the average (mean) number of papillomas and carcinomas for each study group (e.g., transgenic and wild-type) at each week of the study and plot a line graph of lesion load vs time for each group (*see* **Note 5**).
2. Owing to the nature of this experiment it is difficult to analyze the resulting graph as a whole. The best approach is to analyze each time point separately. This allows direct comparison of the two study groups at any given time point. Using the Minitab statistical analysis program or similar software, conduct a Rankits plot to determine if the data is normally distributed.
3. If the data is normally distributed, conduct a two sample *t*-test to determine if the two groups differ significantly, using 95% confidence limits.
4. A further measurement that can be examined is the percentage of mice free of carcinoma (or the rate of first carcinoma appearance). An alternative measure of conversion rates can be gleaned by examining the total number of carcinomas per mouse over the total number of papillomas. However, the total number of carcinomas will have an artificial

ceiling owing to the removal of mice from the study (*see* **Note 11**) and thus not accurately reflects conversion rates. Following histopathological analysis, the percentage of carcinomas that are of the aggressive, spindle-cell type will reflect late tumorigenic events. In this manner, factors that influence early (papilloma) and late (carcinoma and malignancy) events can be analyzed.

## 4. Notes

1. Wearing two pairs of latex gloves during treatment provides added protection. The outer pair should be removed in the fume hood and disposed in the designated cin-bin. The inner pair can be disposed of normally. Aerosol resistant pipet tips and paper towels should also be disposed of in the same cin-bin. Always follow Control of Substances Hazardous to Health (COSHH in the UK) rules or local rules on the handling and use of carcinogens and all potentially contaminated equipment, including the mouse caging.
2. As the chemicals used in this procedure are carcinogens they should be clearly labeled and stored in enclosed containers and clearly labeled within the fridge/freezer. All tissues/carcasses should also be clearly labeled and stored in this manner.
3. The concentrations of DMBA and TPA recommended here are effective in the FVB mouse strain. Different concentrations and/or dosing regimes may be required when using different strains of mice *(13)*.
4. Although the animal identification (ID) must be known for accurate record collection, knowledge of its transgenic status may prejudice scoring of lesions. Transgenic status should be evaluated from a tissue (usually tail) biopsy carried out after the removal of the animal from the study.
5. It is unlikely that 60 mice (with one test and one control category) of 8 wk old will be ready to start treatment at one time. Start treatment whenever mice of 8 wk old become available and keep accurate records of ID numbers and start dates. Calculations, such as the average number of papillomas or carcinomas at a particular time point (e.g., after 15 wk of treatment) can only be completed when all of the mice in the study have passed this time point.
6. Commonly used forms of ID include ear punching, toe clipping, or the more expensive electronic chipping.
7. Shaving on a Monday is preferable. This allows DMBA application on the following Tuesday and then evenly spaced TPA applications every Tuesday and Friday for 20 wk. Repetition of hair removal, when necessary, can then be done on Mondays or Thursdays. Once lesions have formed, using hair removal cream is safer than using a shaver, to avoid nicking.
8. Lift the mouse by the tail and allow it to grab onto the bars of the cage lid with its forepaws while gently pulling the mouse backwards. The mouse will continue to cling and resist your pressure thus remaining stretched. This aids the shaving or cream removal and also allows easy application of chemicals. The paper towels lining the cage are to catch any spillage (*see* **Note 1**).
9. The liquid should be released faster than dropwise but not ejected out such that splashes occur. The acetone will ensure rapid spread of the DMBA/TPA over the entire exposed area while ensuring quick evaporation and drying.
10. Conversion of a papilloma to a carcinoma is apparent when the lesion becomes more embedded within the skin. A trained eye is valuable here. Precise diagnosis can only be determined subsequently by histopathological analysis.

11. In accordance with UK guidelines for humane end point of this procedure, mice must be sacrificed when they reach a maximum acceptable papilloma or carcinoma load or when a carcinoma reaches 2 cm in diameter. The maximum papilloma or carcinoma load should be subjectively determined by experienced staff blind to the test or control status of the mice. Further occasions when it is necessary to remove an animal from the study include an adverse, generalized skin reaction to the chemicals, wounding owing to fighting and papillomas or carcinomas that inhibit movement or reduce the animal's quality of life.

## References

1. Brown, K. and Balmain, A. (1995) Transgenic mice and squamous multistage carcinogenesis. *Cancer Metastasis Rev.* **14,** 113–124.
2. Wilson, J. B., Weinberg, W., Johnson, R., Yuspa, S., and Levine, A. J. (1990) Expression of the BNLF-1 oncogene of Epstein-Barr Virus in the skin of transgenic mice induces hyperplasia and aberrant expression of keratin 6. *Cell* **61,** 1315–1327.
3. Bailleul, B., Sarani, M. A., White, S., Barton, S. C., Brown, K., Blessing, M., et al. (1990) Skin hyperkeratosis and papilloma formation in transgenic mice expressing a *ras* oncogene from a suprabasal keratin promoter. *Cell* **62,** 697–708.
4. Greenhalgh, D. A., Rothnagal, J. A., Quintanilla, M. I., Orengo, C. C., Gagne, T. A., Bundman, D. S., Longley, M. A., and Roop, D. R. (1993) Induction of epidermal hyperplasia, hyperkeratosis, and papillomas in transgenic mice by a targeted v-Ha-*ras* oncogene. *Mol. Carcinogen.* **7,** 99–110.
5. Cui, W., Fowlis, D. J., Bryson, S., Duffie, E., Ireland, H., Balmain, A., and Akhurst, R. J. (1996) TGFβ1 inhibits the formation of benign skin tumours, but enhances progression to invasive spindle carcinomas in transgenic mice. *Cell* **86,** 531–542.
6. Fowlis, D. J., Cui, W., Johnson, S. A., Balmain, A., and Akhurst, R. J. (1996) Altered epidermal cell growth control *in vivo* by inducible expression of TGFβ1 in the skin of transgenic mice. *Cell Growth Diff.* **7,** 679–687.
7. Wang, X. J., Greenhalgh, D. A., Eckhardt, J. N., Rothnagal, J. A., and Roop, D. R. (1994) Epidermal expression of transforming growth factor-α in transgenic mice: induction of spontaneous and 12-*O*-tetradecanoylphorbol-13-acetate induced papillomas via a mechanism independent of Ha-*ras* activation or overexpression. *Mol. Carcinogen.* **10,** 15–22.
8. Vassar, R., Hutton, M. E., and Fuchs, E. (1992) Transgenic overexpression of transforming growth factor α bypasses the need for c-Ha-*ras* mutations in mouse skin tumorigenesis. *Mol. Cell. Biol.* **12,** 4643–4653.
9. Dominey, A. M., Wang, X. J., King, L. E. Jr., Nanney, L. B., Gagne, T. A., Sellheyer, K., et al. (1993) Targeted overexpression of transforming growth factor α in the epidermis of transgenic mice elicits hyperplasia, hyperkeratosis, and spontaneous, squamous papillomas. *Cell Growth Differ.* **4,** 1071–1082.
10. Greenhalgh, D. A., Rothnagel, J. A., Wang, X. J., Quintanilla, M. I., Orengo, C. C., Bundman, D. S., et al. (1993) Hyperplasia, hyperkeratosis and benign tumor production in transgenic mice by a targeted v-*fos* oncogene suggests a role for *fos* in epidermal differentiation and neoplasia. *Oncogene* **8,** 2145–2157.
11. DiGiovanni, J. (1989) Genetics of susceptibility to mouse skin tumour promotion, in *The Pathology of Neoplasia* (Sirica, A. E., ed.), Plenum Press, NY, pp. 247–273.
12. DiGiovanni, J., Walker, S. E., Beltran, L. M., Naito, M., and Eastin, W. C. (1991) Evidence for a common genetic pathway controlling susceptibility to mouse skin tumour promotion by diverse classes of promoting agents. *Cancer Res.* **51,** 1398–1405.

13. DiGiovanni, J., Imamoto, A., Naito, M., Walker, S. E., Beltran, L., Chenicek, K. J., and Skow, L. (1992) Further genetic analyses of skin tumor promoter susceptibility using inbred and recombinant inbred mice. *Carcinogenesis* **13,** 525–531.
14. Melendez-Colon, V. J., Luch, A., Seidel, A., and Baird, W. M. (1999) Cancer initiation by polycyclic aromatic hydrocarbons results from formation of stable DNA adducts rather than apurinic sites. *Carcinogenesis* **20,** 1885–1891.
15. Sukumar, S. (1989) *ras* oncogenes in chemical carcinogenesis. *Current Top. Microbiol. Immunol.* **148,** 93–113.
16. Sukumar, S. (1990) An experimental analysis of cancer: Role of *ras* oncogenes in multistep carcinogenesis. *Cancer Cells* **2,** 199–204.
17. Balmain, A. and Brown, K. (1988) Oncogene activation in chemical carcinogenesis. *Adv. Cancer. Res.* **51,** 147–182.
18. Brown, K., Buchmann, A., and Balmain, A. (1990) Carcinogen-induced mutations in the mouse c-Ha-*ras* gene provide evidence of multiple pathways for tumor progression. *Proc. Natl. Acad. Sci. USA* **87,** 538–542.
19. Kemp, C. J., Burns, P. A., Brown, K., Nagase, H., and Balmain, A. (1994) Transgenic Approaches to the Analysis of *ras* and *p53* Function in Multistage Carcinogenesis. Cold Spring Harbor Symposia on Quantitative Biology, vol. LIX, Cold Spring Harbor Laboratory Press, Cold Spring Harbor, NY, pp. 427–434.
20. Esherick, J. S., DiCunto, F., Flanders, K. C., Missero, C., and Dotto, G. P. (1993) Transforming growth factor β1 induction is associated with transforming growth factors β2 and β3 down-modulation in 12-*O*-tetradecanoylphorbol-13-acetate induced skin hyperplasia. *Cancer Res.* **53,** 5517–5522.
21. Akhurst, R. J., Fee, F., and Balmain, A. (1988) Localized production of TGFβ1 mRNA in tumour promoter-stimulated mouse epidermis. *Nature* **331,** 363–365.
22. Fowlis, D. J., Flanders, K. C., Duffie, E., Balmain, A., and Akhurst, R. J. (1992) Discordant transforming growth factor β1 RNA and protein localization during chemical carcinogenesis of the skin. *Cell Growth Diff.* **3,** 81–91.
23. Rho, O., Beltran, L. M., Gimenez-Conti, I. B., and DiGiovanni, J. (1994) Altered expression of the epidermal growth factor receptor and transforming growth factor alpha during multistage skin carcinogenesis in SENCAR mice. *Mol. Carcin.* **11,** 19–28.
24. Xian, W., Kiguchi, K., Imamoto, A., Rupp, T., Zilberstein, A., and DiGiovanni, J. (1995) Activation of the epidermal growth factor receptor by skin tumor promoters and in skin tumors from SENCAR mice. *Cell Growth Diff.* **6,** 1447–1455.
25. Xian, W., Rosenberg, M. P., and DiGiovanni, J. (1997) Activation of *erb* B2 and c-*src* in phorbol ester-treated mouse epidermis: possible role in mouse skin tumour promotion. *Oncogene* **14,** 1435–1444.
26. Rosenberger, S. F., Gupta, A., and Bowden, G. T. (1999) Inhibition of p38 MAP kinase increases okadaic acid mediated AP-1 expression and DNA binding but has no effect on TRE dependent transcription. *Oncogene* **18,** 3626–3632.
27. Ryseck, R. P. and Bravo, R. (1991) c-JUN, JUN B, and JUN D differ in their binding affinities to AP-1 and CRE consensus sequences: Effect of FOS proteins. *Oncogene* **6,** 533–542.
28. Nishizuka, Y. (1984) The role of protein kinase C in cell surface signal transduction and tumour promotion. *Nature* **308,** 693–697.
29. Nishizuka, Y. (1986) Studies and perspectives of protein kinase C. *Science* **233,** 305–312.
30. Marquardt, B., Frith, D., and Stabel, S. (1994) Signalling from TPA to MAP kinase requires protein kinase C, raf and MEK: reconstitution of the signalling pathway *in vitro*. *Oncogene* **9,** 3213–3218.

31. Clark-Lewis I. and Murray A. W. (1978) Tumor promotion and the induction of epidermal ornithine decarboxylase activity in mechanically stimulated mouse skin. *Cancer Res* **38,** 494–497.
32. DiGiovanni, J., Bhatt, T. S., and Walker, S. E. (1993) C57Bl/6 mice are resistant to tumor promotion by full thickness skin wounding. *Carcinogenesis* **14,** 319–321.
33. Hennings, H. and Boutwell, R. K. (1970) Studies on the mechanisms of skin tumour promotion. *Cancer Res.* **30,** 312–320.
34. Klein-Szanto, A. J. P., Larcher, F., Bonfil, R. D., and Conti, C. J. (1989) Multistage chemical carcinogenesis protocols produce spindle cell carcinomas of the mouse skin. *Carcinogenesis* **10,** 2169–2172.
35. Nagase, H., Bryson, S., Cordell, H., Kemp, C. J., Fee, F., and Balmain, A. (1995) Distinct genetic loci control development of benign and malignant skin tumours in mice. *Nature Genet.* **10,** 424–429.
36. Nagase, H., Mao, J. H., and Balmain, A. (1999) A subset of skin tumor modifier loci determines survival time of tumor-bearing mice. *Proc. Natl. Acad. Sci. USA* **96,** 15,032–15,037.
37. Frame, S., Crombie, R., Liddell, J., Stuart, D., Linardopoulos, S., Nagase, H., et al. (1998) Epithelial carcinogenesis in the mouse: correlating the genetics and the biology. *Philos. Trans. R. Soc. Lond. B. Biol. Sci.* **353,** 839–845.

# 41

# Separation of Epidermal Tissue from Underlying Dermis and Primary Keratinocyte Culture

**Jennifer Macdiarmid and Joanna B. Wilson**

## 1. Introduction

The epidermis shares many structural similarities to other epithelia throughout the body. All epithelia function as a barrier protecting the internal organs. The epidermis of the skin protects the exterior of the body, whereas other forms of epithelia line the airways, blood vessels, and gastrointestinal, urinary, and reproductive tracts. Some glandular epithelia secret substances such as sweat, mucus, and hormones. All epithelia are avascular and consist of closely packed cells, which are tightly attached to one another via cell junctions. This tight structure allows all epithelia to closely regulate the movement of materials such as ions, nutrients, and secretory products *(1,2)*.

Epithelial cells form continuous sheets, "simple" epithelia are one cell thick, whereas "stratified" epithelia are multilayered. "Pseudo-stratified" epithelia appear to have many layers, but in fact have only one layer of cells. All epithelia are anchored to a basement membrane. There are a variety of epithelial cell types. "Squamous" epithelial cells have a flat, scale-like shape, whereas "cuboidal" cells are cube-shaped, and "columnar" cells appear as tall rectangles. "Transitional" cells come in a variety of shapes; they line parts of the urinary tract and allow the epithelium to stretch and expand when necessary. The epidermis of the skin consists of keratinized, stratified squamous epithelium, whereas nonkeratinized, stratified squamous epithelium lines the mouth, tongue, and esophagus. Indeed, it is this epithelium that is susceptible to the Epstein-Barr virus (EBV)-associated malignancy Nasopharyngeal Carcinoma (NPC).

The skin can be divided into three main functional compartments: the epidermis, the dermis, and the skin appendages. The underlying dermis is considerably thicker than the epidermis, and consists mainly of connective tissue, which is composed of elastic and collagenous fibers. The dermis has relatively few cells; these include fibroblasts, which produce collagen, and macrophages and mast cells, which are involved in immunity. Developmentally, the dermis is of mesodermal origin.

From: *Methods in Molecular Biology, Vol. 174: Epstein-Barr Virus Protocols*
Edited by: J. B. Wilson and G. H. W. May © Humana Press Inc., Totowa, NJ

The epidermis is structurally very different from the dermis. It is derived from the fetal ectoderm, and is composed of tightly packed cells that form the stratified squamous epithelium. In the human, the epidermis, which covers most of the body, is around 100-μm thick, approx one-fortieth of the total thickness of the skin. However, epidermal thickness varies depending on the body region; the palms and soles exhibit a much thicker epidermis with 20–30 keratinocyte layers, whereas the epidermis of the protected inner upper arm exhibits only 3–4 keratinocyte layers. The human epidermis is much thicker than that of mammals with a protective pelt, for example, the epidermis of the mouse has only 2–3 keratinocyte layers.

There are four cell types within the epidermis: keratinocytes, melanocytes, Langerhans cells, and Granstein cells. The keratinocyte is the main cell type; it produces keratin, which gives the skin its strength, and epidermal lipids, which help to waterproof the skin. The keratinocyte also participates in immunity; it has been shown to produce various immunological mediators, including epidermal thymus-activating factor (ETAF), a homolog of interleukin 1 (IL-1), which activates the synthesis of neutrophil chemotactic peptides, and intercellular adhesion molecule (ICAM), a lymphocyte adhesion molecule that is expressed on the surface of keratinocytes. The melanocyte produces pigment and absorbs UV light, whereas Langerhans and Granstein cells interact with T cells during the immune response.

The epidermis in stratified epithelia consists of four distinct layers. During keratinization, cells are generated in the basal layer and pushed up to the surface. The four layers are:

1. The *stratum basale*, or basal layer. This is the innermost layer of the epidermis, and the only layer in which keratinocyte cell division occurs in healthy epidermis. The keratinocyte stem cells are organized in a single layer; following cell division, one daughter cell migrates to the stratum spinosum, while the other cell remains in the basal layer. Melanocytes are also found in the basal layer.
2. The *stratum spinosum* or germinative layer. This layer contains the majority of the living keratinocytes, which are organized into 8–10 rows of polyhedral closely packed cells. Melanin is present in this layer.
3. The *statum granulosum*. This granular layer consists of 3–5 rows of flattened keratinocytes, whose nuclei are undergoing nuclear disintegration. Nuclear breakdown is accompanied by cell death. The visible granules within the cells contain keratohyalin, a precursor compound of keratin.
4. The *stratum corneum*. This outermost layer of the epidermis is made entirely of dead, anucleate cells, which are filled with keratin. There are 25–30 rows of cells within this layer, which are continually shed and replaced.

Within the epidermis, the 10 nm keratin filaments are composed of specific pairs of type I and type II keratin. Type I keratins are acidic ($pK_i = 4.5 - 5.5$) and are relatively small (40–56.5 kDa), whereas type II keratins are more basic ($pK_i = 5.5 - 7.5$) and are larger (53–67 kDa). Different keratin (K) pairs are expressed in the different epithelia and in the different layers of stratified squamous epithelia; for example, in the epidermis K5 and K14 are expressed in the basal replicative layer, whereas terminally differentiating cells downregulate K5 and K14 and produce the differentiation specific keratins, K1 and K10. Finally, the suprabasal corneal cells express K3 and K12. Keratin pairs are therefore very useful markers of epidermal differentiation *(3–5)*.

The dermis and epidermis are held together by the basement membrane (or basal lamina). This is a complex structure that is composed of extracellular matrix proteins, including type IV collagen, laminins 1, 5, and 6, nidogen, and heparan sulphate proteoglycan. The basal keratinocytes are firmly attached to the basement membrane by hemidesmosomes, whereas the basement membrane is in turn routed to the dermis via dermal anchoring fibrils. Although the basement membrane forms a strong cohesive bond between epidermis and dermis, it allows for the passage of signaling molecules between the two layers, for example TGF-α produced in the dermis may act on keratinocytes. Lymphocytes and Langerhans cells can also pass through the basement membrane into the epidermis.

In addition to the dermis and epidermis, the skin appendages perform various essential functions within the skin. These organs are derived from the embryonic epidermis, and include hair follicles, nails, sebaceous glands, and the apocrine and eccrine sweat glands. Hair and nails act to protect the skin, whereas the sweat glands are involved in the regulation of body temperature.

When analyzing signal transduction and gene expression in the epidermis, it is often essential to first separate it from the dermis. The fact that the epidermis is considerably thinner than the dermis means that any dermal contamination could significantly alter results.

The main obstacle in separating the dermis from the epidermis is the basement membrane, which forms a strongly cohesive bond between them. Any separation technique must therefore loosen this bond. A second obstacle is the presence of hair follicles, which extend through the basement membrane deep into the dermis. For this reason, it is recommended that hairless skin samples be used wherever possible. In the case of mice, it is therefore easiest to use skin samples taken from pups before the first hair-growth cycle (which occurs at ~ 5 d). Skin from adult mice can be separated, but the bond between the two layers is much harder to break because of the many hair follicles, and the skin must first be shaved and treated with depilatory cream. Human skin is relatively hairless, and can therefore be separated more readily.

This chapter describes two techniques for epidermal/dermal separation. The first technique involves heat-shocking the skin sample at 55°C, cooling it to 0–4°C, then simply pealing the dermis away from the epidermis *(6)*. This technique is simple and fast, allowing for a rapid ex vivo manipulation time. However, exposure of the skin to a high temperature may affect temperature-sensitive proteins, and influence protein activity. The heat-shock process separates the epidermis from the basement membrane through the basal-cell cytoplasm, so this method is not optimal if the single basal layer of keratinocytes is desired *(7,8)*. Furthermore, ease of separation varies considerably according to the exact temperature and duration of the heat-shock process.

The second method involves separating the skin by enzymatic cleavage. In this case the skin sample is floated dermis side down on a 5% dispase solution, and left overnight at 4°C. If the sample is required for RNA work, RNA inhibitors such as vanadate can be added to the dispase or trypsin solution (*see* **Fig. 1**) *(9)*. The jelly-like

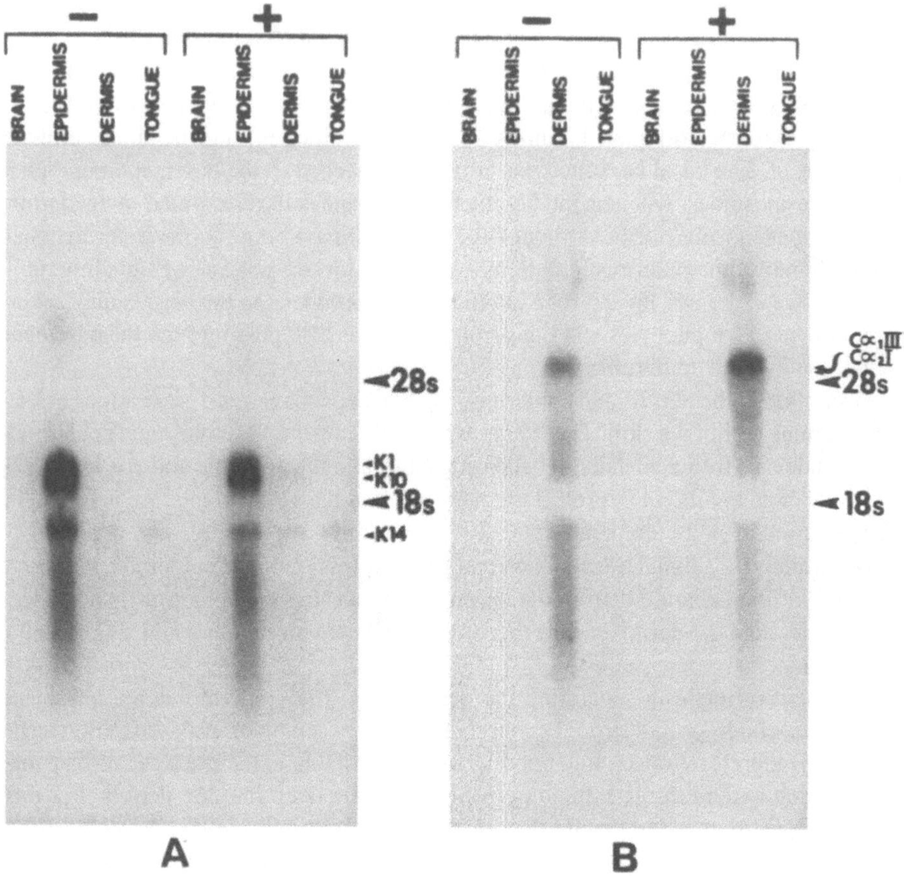


Fig. 1. Example of clean epidermal/dermal separation. Samples were separated using buffered trypsin with the inclusion of RVC as described, for RNA isolation. 20 μg samples of total RNA from a 1-d-old transgenic mouse carrying the PyLMP1 transgene (+) and a negative sibling (–) were Northern-blotted. **(A)** The Northern blot was probed with sequences for the murine K1, K10, and K14 genes, which are expressed in the epidermis. **(B)** The same blot was reprobed with sequences for the murine collagen α1(II) and α2(I) genes, which are expressed in the dermis.

dermis is then pealed off the intact epidermis. This protocol gives a consistently easy separation. The plane of separation by dispase is directly through the basement membrane; dispase acts as a type IV collagenase and effectively digests the bond between dermis and epidermis, leaving an intact epidermal sheet of live cells. As such, keratinocytes isolated in this manner can be cultured for further analyses. However, this technique involves considerably longer ex vivo manipulation time than the heat-shock method, which may influence the integrity or activation status of various proteins. The technique also utilizes dispase, a neutral protease that could potentially degrade proteins within the epidermal sample, and therefore affect results. For direct sample analyses after separation, it is recommended that both techniques are used in order to ascertain the optimal method for the particular application in hand.

## 2. Materials

### 2.1. Preparation of Murine Skin

1. 5-mL plastic bijouxs, and sealed small plastic bags.
2. Dissection tools including fine scissors and forceps.
3. 70% Ethanol: 70% ethanol (v/v) in distilled $H_2O$.
4. Antiseptic wash solution.
5. Phosphate-buffered saline (PBS): 170 m*M* NaCl, 3.35 m*M* KCl, 9.8 m*M* $Na_2HPO_4$, 1.83 m*M* $KH_2PO_4$. Autoclave. Store indefinitely at room temperature.
6. 5-cm (diameter) sterile plastic Petri dishes.

### 2.2. Epidermal-Dermal Separation by Heating

1. 50-mL sterile glass beaker.
2. 55°C water bath.
3. 25-mL universals.
4. Ice-cold PBS (*see* **Subheading 2.1.**).
5. 5-cm (diameter) sterile plastic Petri dishes.

### 2.3. Epidermal-Dermal Separation by Dispase

1. 5-cm (diameter) sterile plastic Petri dishes.
2. 0.5% dispase: 0.5% dispase (w/v) in distilled $H_2O$. Store for up to 1 mo at 4°C.
3. Sterile forceps.
4. Buffered trypsin: 5 m*M* KCl, 0.55 m*M* $KH_2PO_4$, 140 m*M* NaCl, 4 m*M* $NaHCO_3$, 5.5 m*M* D-glucose, 0.35 m*M* $Na_2HPO_4$, with 0.375% bovine pancreatic trypsin type III. Store for up to 1 mo at 4°C.
5. RNase-free buffered trypsin or dispase: prepare buffered trypsin or dispase as noted earlier, but include 45 m*M* ribonucleoside-vanadyl (RVC) complex, and use RNase-free $H_2O$. Store for up to 1 mo at 4°C. Before use, centrifuge the solution to pellet the RVC, transfer to a new container, and add fresh RVC.

### 2.4. Isolation of the Epidermis from the Dermis

1. 5-cm (diameter) plastic Petri dishes.
2. Sterile forceps.
3. Screw-top 2-mL tubes (Nunc).

### 2.5. Primary Keratinocyte Culture

1. PBS (*see* **Subheading 2.1.**).
2. Sterile scalpel.
3. Disposable cell scraper.
4. Trypsin/ethylenediaminetetraacetic acid (EDTA): 0.25% Trypsin, 1 m*M* EDTA (GibcoBRL, Life Technologies).
5. FCS: Fetal calf serum.
6. Sterile 25-mL plastic universals.
7. Keratinocyte culture medium: either KGM Bullet Kit, which contains Keratinocyte Basal Medium (KBM) and supplements, or KGM, which is complete Keratinocyte Growth Medium (Clonetics Corporation, San Diego, CA) (*see* **Note 1**).

8. Media supplements:
   a. If KBM is used, then the medium must be supplemented with insulin, hydrocortisone and EGF (supplied by Clonetics as part of the KGM BulletKit).
   b. If Dulbecco's Modified Eagle's Medium (DMEM) or MEM are used, then the medium must be supplemented with: 10% FCS, which has been chelated to remove calcium (*see* **Note 1**); 4 m*M* of Glutamine; 50 µg/mL of Penicillin and streptomycin.
   c. 1% fungizone to inhibit fungal growth from fresh tissue.
9. Gauze. Wrap pieces in foil and autoclave to sterilize.
10. Trypan blue solution: 0.4% trypan blue (Sigma), 0.8% NaCl, 0.6% $KH_2HPO_4$ in sterile $H_2O$. Use in a 4:1 ratio of trypan blue solution:cell suspension aliquot to count viable cells.
11. Hemocytometer.
12. Methyl cellulose (Aldrich Chemical Company).
13. PolyHEMA (Aldrich Chemical Company).

## 3. Methods

### *3.1. Preparation of Murine Skin*

1. Euthanase mouse according to the legally accepted procedure of your country (*see* **Notes 2** and **3**). Immediately place pup in a 5-mL sterile plastic Bijoux and place on ice. Adult mice can be placed in a sealed plastic bag and then kept briefly on ice.
2. If using mouse pups amputate limbs and tail (*see* **Note 4**).
3. Rinse the body in 70% Ethanol, and blot dry with a tissue. If the sample is to be used for subsequent primary cell culture, first wash the body once in antiseptic solution, then three times in 70% Ethanol, and finally rinse once in PBS.
4. Remove the skin with a dorsal longitudinal excision, endeavoring to obtain a single sheet (*see* **Note 5**).
5. Immediately place the skin dermis side down on a sterile plastic Petri dish. Use forceps to stretch the skin and flatten the edges down on the plastic (*see* **Note 6**). Proceed immediately onto the separation step (*see* **Note 7**).

### *3.2. Epidermal-Dermal Separation by Heating*

1. Preheat a 50-mL beaker of sterile $H_2O$ in a 55°C water bath (*see* **Note 8**). Prepare sterile 25-mL universals containing 10 mL of ice-cold PBS.
2. Take the flattened skin sample and place it in the beaker of 55°C water (*see* **Note 9**). Leave at 55°C for exactly 2 min (*see* **Note 10**).
3. Immediately immerse the skin in the ice cold PBS in a 25-mL universal. Leave on ice for exactly 3 min.
4. Remove the sample from PBS. Place on a sterile Petri dish and gently dab with clean tissue to remove the excess PBS (*see* **Note 11**).
5. Proceed immediately to **Subheading 3.4.**, the isolation of the epidermis from the dermis.

### *3.3. Epidermal-Dermal Separation by Dispase*

1. Pipet 5 mL of ice cold 0.5% dispase solution into a 5-cm Petri dish (*see* **Notes 12** and **13**).
2. Using two forceps, gently float the skin sample, dermal side down, on the dispase solution, taking care not to allow the sample to roll up (*see* **Note 14**). Place a lid on the Petri dish.
3. Incubate the samples at 4°C overnight (*see* **Note 15**).
4. Proceed immediately to **Subheading 3.4.**, the isolation of the epidermis from the dermis.

### 3.4. Isolation of the Epidermis from the Dermis

1. Place the sample on a dry, sterile Petri dish with the epidermal side down. Use forceps to flatten the sample, ensuring no edges are rolled up. The epidermis should adhere to the dry plastic (*see* **Note 16**).
2. Using two pairs of forceps and starting at one end of the sample, gently tease the jelly-like dermis away from the epidermis. The thick, pinky yellow dermis should come away easily, leaving the very thin, almost translucent white epidermis on the plastic (*see* **Note 17**).
3. If the samples have been separated using the dispase technique, they can be used immediately for primary cell culture (*see* **Subheading 3.5.**). Alternatively, for long-term storage, place the separate dermal and epidermal samples into screw top 2-mL tubes, snap-freeze them in liquid nitrogen, then store indefinitely at –70°C. These samples can be used for subsequent protein or RNA extraction (*see* **Note 13**) by standard protocols. Evidence of good separation can be obtained by analyzing the samples for dermal and epidermal specific markers such as collagens and keratins (*see* **Fig. 1**).

### 3.5. Primary Keratinocyte Culture

1. Place the freshly separated epidermis on a sterile Petri dish on ice, and use a sterile scalpel to chop the sample into fine segments. Use a disposable cell scraper and a little trypsin/EDTA solution to collect the tissue, and transfer the pieces into a sterile 25-mL universal.
2. Add 5 mL of trypsin/EDTA solution and digest the tissue pieces for 5 min at room temperature. Pipet the cells up and down to aid their separation (*see* **Notes 18** and **19**).
3. Filter the cells through gauze to obtain a single cell suspension (*see* **Note 20**). Deactivate the trypsin by adding FCS to 10% final volume. Pellet the cells by centrifugation for 5 min at 300*g*.
4. Resuspend the cell pellet in 5 mL of keratinocyte culture medium with the appropriate supplement (*see* **Note 1**). To quantitate the number of live cells in the sample, take an aliquot of cells and count live cells that do not take up trypan blue (trypan blue exclusion), using a hemocytometer and light microscopy (*see* **Note 21**).
5. To culture the cells, plate in the order of $2 \times 10^5$ cells onto a 5-cm tissue culture dish, using keratinocyte culture medium, a low calcium medium that contains supplements for proliferation (*see* **Notes 1** and **22**). Primary murine keratinocytes will survive at confluency but cannot be passaged, unlike human primary keratinocytes. If desired, a differentiation assay can be performed on the cells (*see* **Note 23**).

## 4. Notes

1. A variety of specialized primary keratinocyte growth media can be used depending on the assay. A commonly used medium is keratinocyte growth medium (KGM), from Clonetics Corporation, San Diego, CA. This medium can either be bought as a BulletKit, which contains keratinocyte basal medium and separate supplements, or as complete KGM. The KGM BulletKit allows supplement concentrations to be varied, whereas complete KGM requires less preparation. KGM is a serum-free medium. Other media such as DMEM and MEM may be used, but these media require serum, which must first be chelated in order to remove calcium. The calcium concentration of the culture medium is critical. 0.03 m*M* $Ca^{2+}$ will allow proliferation, limited by the capacity of the species type and the age of the donor. Higher calcium concentrations, such as 1.2 m*M* $Ca^{2+}$ will cause the cells to terminally differentiate ***(10,11)***.
2. The epidermal/dermal separation is easiest to perform on hairless skin, as hair follicles form a tight bond between the two layers. Optimally, murine skin samples should therefore be

taken from pups before the first hair emergence occurs (at ~5 d post partum). If adult skin must be used, the skin should be shaved and depilated, to remove as much hair as possible.

3. For this protocol, the legally accepted procedure for euthanazing mice in the UK is described under Home Office Schedule 1.
4. Tail can be stored indefinitely at –70°C for further DNA analysis. If required, brain and other tissues can also be stored at –70°C. DNA extracted from the brain yields large quantities of pure sample.
5. In the case of small mouse pups, it is optimal to remove the entire skin as a single sheet, which is easier to handle in further manipulations. Use forceps and scissors to gently tease the skin away from the dorsal incision, turn the torso over, and gradually loosen the skin over the anterior, snipping around the neck and tail region to free the skin. Finally turn the torso over again, and remove the skin from the body. For adult mice, it is not necessary to remove the entire skin; a square sheet of skin from the back should suffice.
6. This step is essential to prevent the skin from rolling up at the edges. The skin has a tendency to roll towards the dermis. It is particularly crucial that the skin does not roll up during the dispase separation, as the epidermis must not touch the dispase solution.
7. The skin sample can very quickly dry out and become brittle. Separation is impossible if this occurs. It is therefore recommended that each sample is dealt with individually at this stage, and that the procedure is performed as quickly as possible.
8. 55°C is the optimal heat-shock temperature for epidermal separation. However, for studies on sensitive proteins, the temperature can be lowered to retain the activity of the protein (for example, the sample can be heated to 52°C rather than 55°C) ***(12)***. In such cases, it is recommended that a range of temperatures is tried in order to optimize the results. It may be the case that the dispase separation protocol is a better method for such studies, as it does not involve exposing the proteins to high temperatures, so protein activity is more likely to be retained.
9. Curling of the skin sample will occur at this stage. This is unavoidable, and will be rectified later.
10. The heat-shock duration can be varied to achieve optimal results. We have found that 2 min at 55°C achieves excellent separation. Shorter heating times have resulted in a poorer epidermal separation, whereas longer times at 55°C may compromise the sample.
11. The sample is very fragile after heat-shock, and the epidermis is easily torn. Furthermore, the dermis easily sticks to the tissue. Caution must therefore be taken at this step not to rip the sample.
12. 0.375% buffered trypsin can be used in place of the 0.5% dispase solution. Exactly the same protocol applies for the two proteases, whereas the dispase is the "gentler" treatment.
13. If the epidermal sample is required for RNA work, then an RNase-free protease solution can be prepared that contains the RNase inhibitor ribonucleoside-vanadyl complex. Care should be taken thereafter to use sterile, RNase-free implements and solutions.
14. The skin sample should float on the dispase solution so that only the dermis is in contact with the protease. If the edges of the skin sample are allowed to roll, then the epidermis will touch the dispase, and proteolysis within the epidermis may occur.
15. Epidermal separation is possible once the samples have been incubated in dispase solution overnight, however, we have found that allowing the samples to incubate for 20 h in dispase solution at 4°C results in an excellent separation. Good separation using buffered trypsin can take as little as 5 h.
16. In order to allow the epidermis to adhere to the plastic, allow 10 s before removing the dermis. However, do not leave the sample for longer than this, because the skin can become dry and brittle, and the sample ruined.

17. Removal of the dermis from the epidermis should be performed with utmost care. The step is most easily performed when the sample is in a complete sheet, and the whole of the epidermis is anchored to the plastic. Ripping or fragmentation of the epidermis means that it is more likely to come off the plastic with the dermis. Care must therefore be taken to keep the epidermal sample intact.
18. A longer period of trypsin digestion with shaking may be required, depending on the sample type.
19. Passing the cell clumps through a syringe with a 18-guage needle will also help to disperse the cells.
20. Filtering may not be necessary if a single cell suspension, or obtaining an accurate cell count, is not required for the desired assay.
21. Dead cells take up trypan blue and can be distinguished from live cells by light microscopy. (*See* Chapter 42 for further details.)
22. Together, hydrocortisone, insulin, and EGF increase the growth rate and culture life span ***(13)***.
23. For a differentiation assay, resuspend the cells in DMEM with 1.44% methylcellulose, 10% FCS with 1.2 m*M* $Ca^{2+}$. Seed the cells at 1–4 × $10^5$/mL in this suspension medium, and use plastic dishes coated with polyHEMA (Aldrich Chemical Co.) to prevent cell adhesion. Differentiation can be assayed after 7–10 d incubation at 37°C, by examining the appearance of cornified envelopes ***(14)***.

## References


1. MacKie, R. (1991) *Clinical Dermatology*. Oxford University Press, Oxford, UK.
2. Harris, A. (editor) (1996) *Epithelial Cell Culture*. Cambridge University Press, Cambridge, UK.
3. Fuchs, E. (1988) Keratins as biochemical markers of epithelial differentiation. *Trends Genet.* **4,** 277–281.
4. Fuchs, E. (1993) Epidermal differentiation and keratin gene expression. *J. Cell Sci.* **17,** 197–208.
5. Fuchs, E. and Byrne, C. (1994) The epidermis: rising to the surface. *Curr. Opin. Genet. Dev.* **4,** 725–736.
6. Baumberger, J. P., Suntzeff, V., and Cowdry, E. V. (1942) Methods for the separation of dermis and some physiological and chemical properties of isolated epidermis. *J. Natl. Cancer Inst.* **2,** 413–423.
7. Marrs, J. M. and Voorhees, J. J. (1971) A method for the bioassay of an epidermal chalone-like inhibitor. *J. Invest. Dermatol.* **56,** 174–181.
8. Skerrow, C. J. and Skerrow, D. (1985) A survey of methods for the isolation and fractionation of epidermal tissue and cells, in *Methods in Skin Research* (Skerrow, D. and Skerrow, C. J., eds.), Wiley, New York, NY, pp. 609–650.
9. Wilson, J. B., Weinberg, W., Johnson, R., Yuspa, S., and Levine, A. (1990) Expression of the BNLF-1 oncogene of Epstein-Barr virus in the skin of transgenic mice induces hyperplasia and aberrant expression of Keratin 6. *Cell* **61,** 1315–1327.
10. Yuspa, S. H., Hawley-Nelson, P., Stanley, J. R., and Hennings, H. (1980) Epidermal cell culture. *Transplant.Proc.* **12,** 114–122
11. Hennings, H., Michael, D., Cheng, C., Steinert, P., Holbrook, K., and Yuspa, S. H. (1980) Calcium regulation of growth and differentiation of mouse epidermal cells in culture. *Cell* **19,** 245–254.
12. Slaga, T. J., Thomson, S., and Schwarz, J. A. (1977) Binding of dexamethasone by the subcellular fractions of mouse epidermis and dermis. *J. Invest. Dermatol.* **68,** 307–309.

13. Parkinson, E. K. and Yeudall, W. A. (1992) The epidermis, in *Culture of Epithelial Cells* (Freshney, R. I., ed.), Wiley-Liss, Inc., Chichester, NY, pp. 59–80.
14. Green, H. (1977) Terminal differentiation of cultured human epidermal cells. *Cell* **11,** 405–416.

# 42

# Selection and Enrichment of B Cells from Lymphoid Tissues

**Penelope Tsimbouri, Marie Anne O'Donnell, and Joanna B. Wilson**

## 1. Introduction

Transgenic mouse models that express Epstein-Barr virus (EBV) latent proteins in the B-cell compartment provide useful models to study the effects of these proteins at each stage of B-cell development and differentiation. In addition, many aspects of the murine immune system have been extensively studied and are similar to those of the human immune system.

The bone marrow is the source of hemopoietic stem cells which give rise to all blood cells. The progenitors of B cells develop into mature B cells within the specialized microenvironment of the bone marrow itself, whereas T-cell progenitors complete their development in the thymus. Mature B cells exit the bone marrow and migrate to the peripheral lymphoid organs via the blood.

The basic architecture of the peripheral lymph nodes (PLNs), spleen, and gut-associated lymphoid tissue (GALT) is similar. Each contains discrete areas where mature B cells recirculate and T cells are usually found in areas adjacent to these B-cell follicles. However, the peripheral lymphoid organs in the mouse differ from one another in the number of lymphocytes they contain and in the proportion of these cells that are B cells.

PLNs comprise a cortex, which contains mostly B cells organized into lymphoid follicles, and a paracortex region where most of the PLN T cells are located. The PLNs, though small, are numerous in the mouse body and if pooled together (not including the mesenteric lymph nodes, MLN) they can yield $5–10 \times 10^7$ lymphocytes, approx 25% of which are B cells. The spleen contains red pulp, which is the site of red blood cell destruction, and white pulp which contains lymphoid structures. Again, B cells are concentrated in discrete regions within the white pulp, the B-cell coronas, whereas T cells are mostly found in the adjacent periarteriolar sheath. The spleen

From: *Methods in Molecular Biology, Vol. 174: Epstein-Barr Virus Protocols*
Edited by: J. B. Wilson and G. H. W. May © Humana Press Inc., Totowa, NJ

provides the greatest source of B cells in the mouse with 50–60% of the 5–15 × $10^7$ splenocytes being of the B cell lineage. The GALT consists of large domed follicles of B cells; T cells are found between these follicles. A higher proportion of B cells than T cells is found in the GALT; typically 60–70% of the Peyer's Patch lymphocytes are B cells. The MLN can typically yield between $5 \times 10^6$ and $2 \times 10^7$ lymphocytes, approx 40% of which are B cells (numbers from our experience and reviewed in **ref. *1***).

There are several methods that can be used to purify B cells from mouse bone marrow and the peripheral lymphoid organs. These methods are equally applicable to isolating B cells from other species (including human) given the appropriate antibodies. The two techniques described in this chapter use magnetic beads to isolate different populations of cells based on their expression of different cell surface markers.

All B cells express a unique isoform of the CD45 cell surface molecule from an early stage in their development (B220). Mouse panB (B220) Dynabeads are iron particles coated with antibody that binds B220. B cells within a heterogeneous population can be labeled with the anti-B220 Dynabeads and the labeled B cells isolated from the other cell types by placing the sample within a magnet. The labeled B cells are positively selected and the unlabeled cells can be retained as the B cell depleted fraction.

Mature B cells from the spleen and peripheral lymph nodes can also be purified from other cell types by negative selection. Most of the other cell types in the spleen; T cells, immature B cells, macrophages, fibroblasts, etc., express the cell-surface marker CD43; however, mature B cells do not. Magnetic cell separation/sorting (MACS) Mouse CD43 microbeads are coated with antibody that binds CD43 and can be used to label the majority of cells in splenocyte samples that are not mature B cells. The labeled cells are then depleted from the heterogeneous population by passing the sample through a magnetic column; the cells labeled with CD43 microbeads remain in the column while the mature B cells are eluted. The labeled cells retained in the column can subsequently be eluted to provide the B-cell-depleted fraction.

The isolation of mouse B cells using positive selection with Mouse panB Dynabeads or by negative selection with CD43 MACS microbeads are both quite rapid, simple techniques that give high-purity B-cell fractions; typically the isolated B-cell fractions are 95% pure. Both techniques produce good recovery of B cells from the original cell sample and only a small fraction of B cells is lost. The techniques minimize potential damage to the cells, which is more likely with older techniques such as depletion of unwanted cell types by complement-mediated lysis *(2)*.

However, there are differences in the research applications for which the B cells isolated by positive selection (Mouse panB [B220] Dynabeads) and negative selection (Mouse CD43 MACS Microbeads) may be most suitable. Dynabeads are relatively large iron particles that remain bound to the B cells after isolation, which raises the possibility that the B cells can be activated through crosslinking of B220 molecules or other cell surface molecules adjacent to the B220 molecules. A protocol is given in this chapter for the detachment of the Dynabeads from the B cells, but this requires an overnight culture of the cells, during which the viability of primary cells may be greatly reduced. The positive selection of B cells using Dynabeads is probably more suited to isolation of B cells for subsequent purification of DNA, RNA, or protein from the purified B cells. However, if parameters are to be examined that may possibly be activated by B220 crosslinking, this should be taken into account. The CD43 MACS microbeads protocol described here is used to isolate B cells by negative selection, and the B cells obtained will not have been affected by the beads used for the labeling process. These bead-free B cells are therefore ideal for experiments involving culture, adoptive transfer, or *in vitro* activation of the primary B cells, as well as the extraction of DNA, RNA and protein. MACS also supply microbeads for the positive selection of mouse B cells and other cell types. MACS microbeads are extremely small iron oxide and polysaccharide particles and Miltenyi Biotec state that the labeled cells internalize and degrade the microbeads without the cells being activated, and so are suitable for the same applications as negatively selected cells. The MACS microbeads system is thus more flexible and a broader range of cell types can be isolated by positive selection. However, the Dynabeads method is slightly quicker to carry out and certainly less expensive.

## 2. Materials

### 2.1. General Materials

1. RPMI-P/S: RPMI-1640 medium (Gibco Life Technologies, cat. #31870-025) supplemented with 200 μg/mL Penicillin/Streptomycin (10,000 μg/mL, Gibco Life Technologies, cat. #15140-114).
2. Universal tubes: 25-mL plastic universal tubes (from any general equipment supplier).
3. Bijoux: 5-mL plastic (from any general equipment supplier).
4. 10X Phosphate-buffered saline (PBS): for 500 mL 50 g NaCl, 1.25 g KCl, 7 g $Na_2HPO_4$, 1.25 g $KH_2PO_4$, pH to 7.3 with HCl. Dilute 10X PBS prior to use to give 1X PBS (2.7 m*M* KCl, 1.4 m*M* $KH_2PO_4$, 137 m*M* NaCl, 4.3 m*M* $Na_2PO_4$) in sterile $H_2O$.
5. 15-mL tubes: 15-mL polypropylene centrifuge tubes (Corning Incorporated, cat. #430790).
6. Pastettes: 3 mL sterile Pasteur pipets (Jencons Scientific Limited, cat. #475-072).
7. Microfuge tubes: 1.5 mL (from any general equipment supplier).
8. FACS: Becton Dickinson with CellQuest software.
9. Primary cells from bone marrow, spleen or lymph nodes.
10. Fetal calf serum (FCS) (Gibco Life Technologies, cat #16010-076). Heat-inactivate for 30 min at 56°C and filter-sterilize before use.
11. Fine scissors.
12. Forceps.

### 2.2. Isolation and Preparation of Mouse Splenocytes and Bone Marrow Cells

1. Glass slides: Ground edges 90° twin-frost 76 × 26 × 1, 0–1, 2-mm (BDH, cat. #406/0184/04).
2. 5-cm Petri dishes.
3. 21G 1.5 needle and 2.5–5 mL syringe.
4. $NH_4Cl$ lysis buffer: Combine 9 volumes of 0.83% (w/v in $H_2O$) $NH_4Cl$ with 1 volume of 0.17 *M* Tris-HCl, pH 7.65, to give a final concentration of 0.75% $NH_4Cl$, 0.017 *M* Tris-HCl, pH 7.2. Check that the pH is pH 7.2, and filter-sterilize the buffer before use.
5. Trypan blue staining solution: trypan blue (0.4%) (Sigma), 0.8% NaCl, 0.06% $KH_2PO_4$.
6. Hemocytometer: Neubauer (**Fig. 1**).

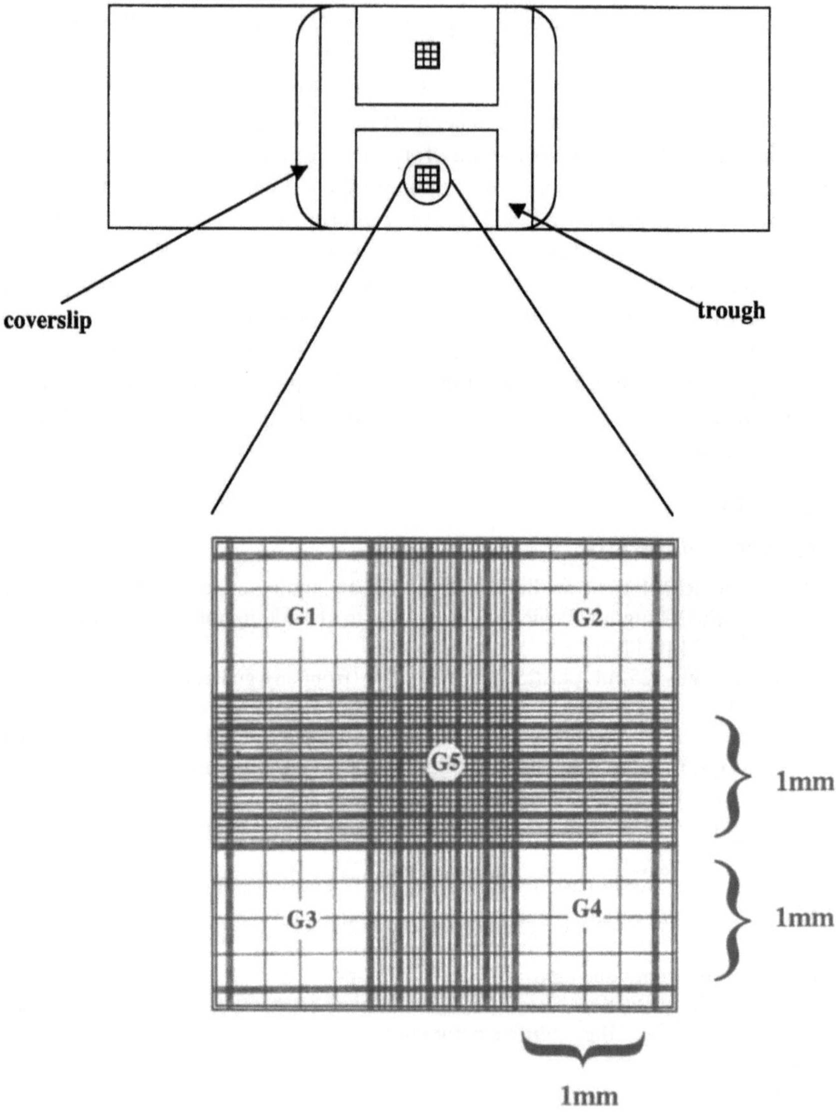


Fig 1. Standard hemocytometer ruling. Neubauer hemocytometer with a coverslip on top (top) and field of view seen typically under a 10× objective (below). Chamber depth is normally 0.1 mm.

### 2.3. Positive Selection of B220+ Mouse B Cells Using Dynabeads

1. B220 Dynabeads: DYNABEADS® Mouse panB *(220)* (Dynal, cat. #141.01).
2. PBS-1% FCS washing buffer: 1% FCS final concentration in PBS.
3. Dynal MPC Magnet (Dynal, cat. #120.02).
4. Rocking/rolling platform (from any general equipment supplier).

### *2.4. Isolation of Resting B Cells by Percoll Gradient*

1. Percoll: Percoll™ sterile (Amersham Pharmacia Biotech, cat. #17-0891-02).
2. Iso-osmotic Percoll: Mix 27 mL of Percoll with 3 mL of 10X PBS.
3. 70% Percoll: Mix 21 mL of iso-osmotic Percoll with 9 mL RPMI-P/S to give 70% Percoll.
4. 66% Percoll: Mix 9.43 mL of 70% Percoll with 0.57 mL RPMI-P/S.
5. 60% Percoll: Mix 8.58 mL of 70% Percoll with 1.42 mL RPMI-P/S.
6. 50% Percoll: Mix 7.14 mL of 70% Percoll with 2.86 mL RPMI-P/S.

### *2.5. Negative Selection of Mouse B Cells using MACS*

1. MACS buffer: PBS with 2 m*M* EDTA and 0.5% bovine serum albumin (BSA) R1A grade, Fraction V (Sigma, cat. #A-7888).
2. CD43 microbeads: (Miltenyi Biotec, cat. #498-01).
3. Octomacs magnet: (Miltenyi Biotec, cat. #421-09).
4. MS+ columns: (MS+ columns for Minimacs or Octomacs, Miltenyi Biotec, cat. #422-01).
5. MACS Multistand: (Miltenyi Biotec, cat. #423-03).
6. Pre-separation Filters: (30 μm, Miltenyi Biotec, cat. #414-07).

## 3. Methods

### *3.1. Isolation of Mouse Splenocytes and Lymph Node Cells*

1. Collect spleen(s) or LNs in approx 4 mL RPMI-P/S in a bijoux. The spleens or LNs can be stored briefly on ice until they are processed.
2. Place tissue in a Petri dish with the RPMI-P/S from the bijoux. Pulverize the tissue between the rough sides of two glass slides.
3. Transfer the cell suspension to a 15-mL tube using a pastette (*see* **Note 1**). Wash the Petri dish with approx 4 mL of RPMI-P/S and transfer the remaining cells to the 15 mL tube. Add more RPMI-P/S to the cells to make the total volume up to 14 mL.
4. Allow the larger chunks of debris to settle for approx 2–3 min. Transfer the supernatant to a new 15-mL tube using a pastette. Be careful to avoid transferring any debris.
5. Centrifuge the cells at 200*g* for 10 min at 4°C, discard the supernatant, and resuspend the cell pellet in 10 mL RPMI-P/S. To wash the cells, pellet by centrifugation again and discard the supernatant.
6. These cells are ready for red blood cell (RBC) lysis.

### *3.2. Bone-Marrow Cell Isolation*

1. Remove the femurs from the mouse using fine scissors. Place the femurs in a bijoux containing RPMI-P/S. The femurs can be stored briefly on ice until they are processed.
2. Remove any residual flesh from the bone and cut the epiphyses (the ends of the bones) using fine scissors.
3. Hold the bone with a pair of forceps and use a 2.5–5 mL syringe with a 21G 1.5 needle to force 2–3 mL RPMI-P/S through the shaft of the bone. The cells should come through very easily. This step can be repeated 2–3 times if required.
4. Resuspend the cells thoroughly using a pastette. Transfer the cell suspension to a 15-mL tube and wash the cells as described in **Subheading 3.1., step 5**.

### *3.3. RBC Lysis* (3)

1. Resuspend the cell pellet (bone marrow, spleen, or lymph node cells) at an approximate concentration of $3 \times 10^8$ cells/mL in $NH_4Cl$ lysis buffer (*see* **Note 2**). Splenocytes can be resuspended in approx 3 mL of $NH_4Cl$ lysis buffer per normal mouse spleen.

2. Incubate the cells at room temperature for 5 min, occasionally inverting the tube (*see* **Notes 3** and **4**).
3. Dilute the $NH_4Cl$ approx 5 fold by adding RPMI-P/S to the cells to make the final volume up to 14 mL. Invert the tube a few times to mix well.
4. Centrifuge the cells at 200*g* for 10 min at 4°C, discard the supernatant, and resuspend the pellet in 10 mL of RPMI P/S. To wash the cells, pellet by centrifugation again and discard the supernatant (*see* **Note 4**).
5. Resuspend the cell pellet in 10 mL of RPMI-P/S (*see* **Note 5**). Keep the cells on ice from this point onward. This cell suspension is ready for counting viable cells.

### 3.4. Viable Cell Counting: Trypan Blue Exclusion Method

1. Immediately before counting, ensure the cells are evenly distributed in the 10-mL suspension by gentle pipetting with a pastette.
2. Mix 100 µL of the cell suspension with 400 µL of trypan blue staining solution in a microfuge tube. Incubate the cells at room temperature for approx 5 min. Trypan blue will be taken up by the dead cells (*see* **Note 6**).
3. Count the cells using a hemocytometer (**Fig. 1**). Clean the surface of the hemocytometer using ethanol and clean tissue. Place the coverslip over the counting chamber.
4. Transfer 10 µL of stained cells to one half of the counting chamber. This volume should be sufficient to fill the semi-chamber area but not flood the surrounding trough (**Fig. 1**).
5. Count the cells in the four outer squares of the grid and the central square (G1–G5, large squares, **Fig. 1**) by light microscopy (40–100X magnification). Both live and dead cells can be scored as dead cells take up the dye and stain blue, while live cells exclude the dye and remain unstained (*see* **Note 6**).
6. Determine the average number of viable cells per large square (large squares are G1–G5 in **Fig. 1**, which are 1 $mm^2$ with a depth of 0.1 mm). To calculate the concentration of cells in your suspension, multiply the average count per large square by the dilution factor (5 in this case) and multiply by $10^4$ to give the number of viable cells/mL.
7. The total number of cells in the sample can be determined by multiplying the concentration of viable cells per mL by the total volume of cells (10 in this case).

### 3.5. Dynabeads Washing Procedure

Dynabeads mouse panB (B220) are supplied in a suspension containing $4 \times 10^8$ beads/mL in PBS containing 0.1% BSA and 0.02% $NaN_3$. Before use the beads need to be washed.

1. Resuspend the B220 Dynabeads thoroughly in the vial and transfer the desired amount to a microfuge tube.
2. Place the microfuge tube on a Dynal MPC magnetic device (or other appropriate magnetic device that will hold your tube in place) for 2 min and then pipet off the fluid. The fluid should be clear as the beads are drawn to the side of the tube next to the magnet.
3. Remove the tube from the magnet and add 1–2 mL of PBS-1% FCS washing buffer and resuspend the beads by inverting the tube 3–4 times.
4. Repeat **step 2** and resuspend the beads in the same volume of PBS-1% FCS washing buffer that was originally withdrawn from the vial.

### 3.6. Positive Selection of B220+ Mouse B Cells Using Dynabeads (see Note 7)

1. Prepare splenocytes, lymph node or bone marrow cells as described in **Subheading 3.1.** or **3.2.**, respectively. Lyse the RBCs and count the viable white blood cells (WBCs) as described in **Subheadings 3.3.** and **3.4.**
2. From the total count of WBCs make an estimate of the number of target cells in the sample (*see* Introduction). Centrifuge the cells at 200*g* for 5 min at 4°C and resuspend the cells in PBS-1% FCS washing buffer at a concentration of approx $1 \times 10^7$ target cells/mL. Transfer the cells to an appropriate-sized tube for the MPC magnetic device.
3. Pipet the required volume of B220 Dynabeads directly to the cell suspension to give a ratio of 4–10 beads per target cell (*see* **Note 8**).
4. Mix the cells and beads by vortexing for 1 s and incubate the cells for 20 min at 2–8°C on an apparatus that provides both gentle tilting and rotation (*see* **Notes 9** and **10**).
5. Place the tube in the magnetic device for 2 min at 4°C (*see* **Note 11**). The B cells labeled with the B220 Dynabeads should be drawn to the side of the tube. Pipet off the supernatant containing unlabeled cells (and keep if you wish to examine the B-cell-depleted cell pool; *see* **Note 12**).
6. Remove the tube from the magnet and resuspend the labeled cells in 1 mL of PBS-1% FCS washing buffer by gentle pipetting.
7. Repeat **steps 5** and **6** twice more and resuspend the selected B cells in the desired volume of medium or appropriate buffer. These cells can be counted and are ready for various research applications (*see* Introduction).

### 3.7. Detachment of B220 Dynabeads

The detachment of the B220 Dynabeads from the surface of the positively selected B cells may be required for some research applications *(4,5)*.

1. Incubate the labeled cell suspension from **Subheading 3.6.**, **step 7** in an incubator at 37°C, 5% $CO_2$ overnight in the appropriate culture medium.
2. After the overnight incubation, pipet the cells thoroughly but gently and transfer the cells to new tubes and place the tubes in the magnetic device. Leave the tubes in the magnet for 2 min to collect the detached B220 Dynabeads.
3. Transfer the supernatant containing the selected B cells to a fresh tube. These cells can be used for further experiments, although a significant loss of viability will result after this incubation when using normal, primary B cells.

### 3.8. Isolation of Resting Lymphocytes by Percoll Gradient

Activated lymphocytes are less dense than resting lymphocytes and they can be separated by Percoll gradient.

1. Prepare Percoll gradients in universal tubes. Hold the universal in one hand with the bottom of the tube resting on a flat surface to keep the tube steady. Tilt the tube so that it is at about 45° from horizontal. Pipet 2.5 mL of 70% Percoll into the bottom of the universal.
2. Overlay this 70% layer of Percoll with 2.5 mL of 66% Percoll. Hold the tip of the pipet against the lower side of the universal. Pipet the liquid out very slowly so that a very thin continuous trickle of Percoll travels down the side of the tube and lays over the 70% Percoll.
3. Repeat this technique to overlay the 66% Percoll layer with 2.5 mL of 60% Percoll and finish with a layer of 2.5 mL of 5 0% Percoll (*see* **Note 13**).

4. The universal can carefully be stood upright on a flat surface between adding each layer. At all times the tube should be handled carefully to keep the Percoll gradient steady (*see* **Note 14**).
5. Stand the Percoll gradient on ice for at least 15 min (*see* **Note 15**).
6. Prepare splenocytes, lymph node or bone marrow cells as described in **Subheadings 3.1.** or **3.2.**, respectively. Lyse the RBCs and count the viable WBCs as described in **Subheadings 3.3.** and **3.4.**
7. Resuspend the cells from 3–5 spleens (or the equivalent number of lymph node or bone marrow cells) in 2.5 mL of RPMI-P/S and then overlay them on the 50% Percoll layer using the same technique used when preparing the gradient. Overlay a further 2.5 mL of RPMI-P/S carefully on the cells to cushion the cells onto the surface of the Percoll gradient (*see* **Note 16**).
8. Centrifuge the Percoll gradient at 3000*g* for 15 min at 4°C with no brake.
9. There should be several interfaces in the Percoll gradient. Between the 60 and 50% layers, an interface of activated lymphocytes should be quite clear. Use a pastette to remove the medium on top of the gradient and discard it. The activated lymphocytes from the top interface can then be collected with a pastette and retained or discarded as required (*see* **Note 17**).
10. The resting lymphocyte layer should be between the 70–66% Percoll interface (*see* **Note 18**). Remove the Percoll layers above the resting lymphocytes and transfer the resting cells using a pastette to a new 15-mL tube (*see* **Note 19**).
11. To dilute the Percoll add RPMI-P/S to the cells to make the total volume up to 10 mL. Centrifuge at 200*g* for 10 min at 4°C and discard the supernatant. Resuspend the cells in 10 mL of RPMI-P/S and repeat this washing step twice more to remove all of the Percoll.
12. Resuspend the isolated resting cells in a suitable volume of RPMI-P/S for counting. These cells are ready for positive or negative selection.

### 3.9. Negative Selection of Mouse B Cells Using MACS (*see* Note 20)

1. Prepare splenocytes, lymph node or bone marrow cells as described in **Subheadings 3.1.** or **3.2.**, respectively. Lyse the RBCs and count the viable WBCs as described in **Subheadings 3.3.** and **3.4.** If resting B cells are required perform **Subheading 3.8.**
2. After counting the cells wash the cells once with 10 mL of MACS buffer as described in **Subheading 3.1., step 5.**
3. Resuspend the cells in MACS buffer to give a final concentration of $1.1 \times 10^8$ cells/mL (or $10^7$ cells in 90 µL) in a 15-mL tube. Add 10 µL of CD43 magnetic microbeads per 90 µL of cell suspension.
4. Mix the cells and microbeads well and incubate for 15 min in the fridge (6–12°C, *see* **Note 21**).
5. Add MACS buffer to the cells to make the total volume up to 10–20 times the labeling volume. Centrifuge the cells at 200*g* for 10 min at 4°C. Remove the supernatant, which contains excess beads, and discard.
6. Resuspend the labeled cells in 500 µL of MACS buffer per $10^8$ cells (*see* **Note 22**). If less than $10^8$ cells were used for labeling, then resuspend the cells in a minimum of 500 µL of MACS buffer. This labeled cell suspension is now ready for separation (step 9).
7. Place the columns to be used for separation in the appropriate-sized magnet (*see* **Note 23**). If using a minimacs or octomacs magnet pipet 500 µL of MACS buffer into the column and discard the flow-through.

8. Wet a pre-separation filter by passing 500 µL of MACS buffer through it and discard the flow-through. Place the wet pre-separation filter in the top of the column. Position a collection tube below the outlet of the column to collect the eluted cells.
9. Carefully pipet the cells from **step 6** onto the filter so that they pass through the filter into the column (*see* **Note 24**). The cells can then flow through the column and the unlabeled mature B cells should pass through while the labeled T cells and other CD43+ cell types should remain bound to the column. Wash the column three times with 500 µL of MACS buffer and collect the eluate with the eluted B cells (*see* **Note 25**).
10. The eluted cells can then be counted and used for further analyses.
11. A sample of the negatively selected B cells can be stained with anti-CD43 and anti-B220 and analyzed by FACS to establish the purity of the B-cell fraction isolated.
12. The CD43+ cells labeled with microbeads that were retained within the column can also be eluted. Remove the column from the magnet, pipet 1 mL of RPMI P/S onto the column and force the medium through with the syringe plunger supplied with the column. The CD43+ cells can then be counted and used for further analyses if required.

## 4. Notes

1. Three mL disposable wide-bore pastettes are very useful for resuspending and transferring cells in all the methods given here. Pastettes allow cell pellets to be thoroughly resuspended while minimizing the shear forces exerted on the cells.
2. With experience, it is desirable to estimate the volume of $NH_4Cl$ lysis buffer to use based on the size of the cell pellet rather than count the cells in each sample at this stage.
3. The samples in $NH_4Cl$ should be incubated at room temperature. Incubation of the cells at 37°C results in damage to the WBCs and at 4°C lysis is slower.
4. The 5-min incubation in $NH_4Cl$ should be enough to lyse the RBCs because of their permeability to ammonium ions. However, if cell lysis is not complete and RBCs are visible in the pellet at **step 4**, then **steps 1–4** should be repeated.
5. After RBC lysis, you may see debris floating in the sample. The debris is the cell membranes from lysed RBCs, which form aggregates. The debris can be removed using a pastette or the debris can be left to settle for 1–2 min and the supernatant containing the splenocytes transferred to a new tube.
6. Do not leave the cells in the staining solution for more than 30 min because the live cells will start to take up the dye and give false counts. If you have several samples, do only a few at a time.
7. This protocol can be applied to cells isolated from several different sources using the appropriate Dynabeads; for example, selection of human B cells using anti-human CD19 (Dynal M-450 CD19 Dynabeads #1111.03) Dynabeads.
8. It is important to keep the bead to target cell ratio between 4–10 beads per target cell. For example, 100 µL of the bead suspension will give $4 \times 10^7$ beads and the maximum number of target cells for this will be $1 \times 10^7$ target cells. If the bead/cell ratio is reduced below 4 then the yield will be affected.
9. The cells should be kept cold at 2–8°C and not at a lower or higher temperature because this may reduce the efficiency of attachment.
10. Avoid resuspending the cells using vigorous pipetting or vortexing as the shear forces exerted may damage the cells.
11. Perform all the subsequent steps at 4°C to reduce any nonspecific attachment of phagocytic cells to the dynabeads.

12. The supernatant containing the unlabeled cells can be retained. This supernatant comprises cells depleted of 95% of the B220+ B cells and will largely consist of T cells. This fraction can be used for further research applications.
13. It is a good idea to practice preparing the Percoll gradients before you use any tissue samples to ensure that you can maintain good control of the pipet and that a continuous trickle of Percoll is produced to form each layer of the gradient.
14. At this stage you cannot see any difference in the different layers of Percoll because they are all the same color and you cannot see the interfaces.
15. Before you place the universal tube containing the Percoll gradient into the ice, it is a good idea to make a hole the right size for the tube in the ice with either your finger or an empty universal. This minimizes the possibility of the Percoll gradient being disturbed.
16. At this stage you should be able to see the layer of cells resting on the surface of the top layer of the Percoll gradient and that there is a cushion of medium above the layer of cells.
17. The layers of cells at the interfaces below the activated cell layer at the 50–60% interface probably consist mostly of resting B cells. However, it is best to remove these to leave only the resting cells at the 70–66% layer to ensure that all activated cells have been excluded.
18. There may be a few unlysed RBCs visible at the bottom of the Percoll gradient, so when removing the resting cells you should try and avoid removing any RBCs as well.
19. A sample of the activated cells and resting cells can be stained for expression of CD23 (expressed on activated B cells) and FACS used to check that good separation of the activated cells in the Percoll gradient has been achieved.
20. This protocol can be applied to cells isolated from several sources using the appropriate MACS beads for selection, e.g., human B cells can be positively selected with CD19 Microbeads (Miltenyi Biotec, cat. #503-01) or negatively selected with B Cell Isolation Kit (Miltenyi Biotec, cat. #469-01).
21. The labeling of the cells should be carried out at 6–12°C. Incubation of the cells with the microbeads on ice results in less efficient labeling.
22. It is important to avoid producing air bubbles in the cells when resuspending them because the air bubbles can get trapped in the column and stop the flow of cells.
23. Different columns can be used for different sized magnets. If using cells from individual spleens MS+ columns and octo/minimacs are appropriate. If several spleens have been pooled, the midimacs system is more suitable with LD+ columns, which are specially designed for depletion. The different types of column retain different numbers of labeled cells and differ in the total number of cells that can be applied to the column. The number of cells to be retained from a sample can be estimated based on the proportion of B cells (*see* Introduction) expected for the lymphoid tissue used. The estimate of the number of retained cells can then be used to decide which column is appropriate.
24. It is important to filter the cells to ensure that a single cell suspension is applied to the column and that no clumps are present.
25. If the sample stops flowing through the column before all the sample has passed through then this is probably because an air bubble is trapped at the top of the column. A yellow (200 μL) pipet tip can be used to try and dislodge any air bubbles.

## References

1. Janeway, C. A. and Travers, P. (1994) *Immunobiology: The Immune System in Health and Disease.* Current Biology Series, Blackwell Scientific Publications, New York, London.

2. Klaus, G. G. B. (1987) *Lymphocytes: A Practical Approach.* Practical Approach Series, IRL Press, Oxford.
3. Boyle, W. (1968) An extension of the 51Cr-release assay for the estimation of mouse cytotoxins. *Transplantation* **6**,761–764.
4. Anderson, G., Jenkinson, E. J., Moore, N. C., and Owen, J. J. T. (1993) MHC class II-positive epithelium and mesenchyme cells are both required for T-cell development in the thymus. *Nature* **362,** 70–73.
5. Yang, J. C., Perry-Lalley, D. and Rosenberg, S. A. (1990) Tumour-infiltrating lymphocytes with in vivo antitumour activity. *J. Biol. Res. Mod.* **9,** 149–159.

# 43

## Detection of Immunoglobulin Gene Rearrangements

**Robert G. Caldwell and Richard Longnecker**

### 1. Introduction

Epstein-Barr virus (EBV) has been shown to effect immunoglobulin (Ig) gene rearrangement under certain experimental conditions. When used to establish primordial human B cell clones from bone marrow and liver samples, some clones exhibited abnormal Ig expression *(1–5)*. B cells from LMP2A transgenic mice can exit the bone marrow and colonize the spleen without surface Ig expression *(6)*. These transgenic B cells were less able to appropriately rearrange Ig heavy-chain (HC) genes, but correctly rearranged Ig light-chain (LC) genes. By contrast, latently infected B cells isolated from human peripheral blood have a memory B-cell phenotype, expressing both IgM and IgD *(7)*. This chapter details experiments that can be used to monitor Ig gene rearrangements in murine B-cell samples. However, these methods can be modified to monitor human B-cell Ig gene rearrangements as well as T-cell receptor gene rearrangements in lymphoid tissue types by designing specific primers as required. Immunoglobulin (Ig) HC and LC gene rearrangement in murine B cells occurs in a specifically coordinated manner. The genes encoding for the mature polypeptides must be assembled from several gene fragments spaced across several thousand kilobases of genomic DNA. For the Ig HC gene, one of 12 diversity ($D_H$) segments joins to one of four joining segments ($J_H$) to create a rearranged D-$J_H$ segment. One of several hundred variable ($V_H$) gene segments is then joined to the $DJ_H$ segment (**Fig. 1**). Once a HC protein is expressed from one allele, rearrangement of the remaining HC locus is allelically excluded *(8)*. Most of the Ig LC proteins are expressed from the kappa locus (κ), with only a small percentage being expressed from the lambda (λ) allele, approx 95 and 5%, respectively *(9)*. After the Ig HC has correctly rearranged, one of several hundred Ig LC variable segments (Vκ) joins to a joining segment (Jκ) allowing the expression of the LC protein. Again, expression at one of the LC alleles excludes the remaining allele *(8)*. If neither Vκ is utilized, the Vλ sequences are rearranged. These proteins form a tetrameric complex of two identical HC proteins with two identical LC proteins on the surface of immature B cells. The membrane bound Ig serves as the

From: *Methods in Molecular Biology, Vol. 174: Epstein-Barr Virus Protocols*
Edited by: J. B. Wilson and G. H. W. May © Humana Press Inc., Totowa, NJ

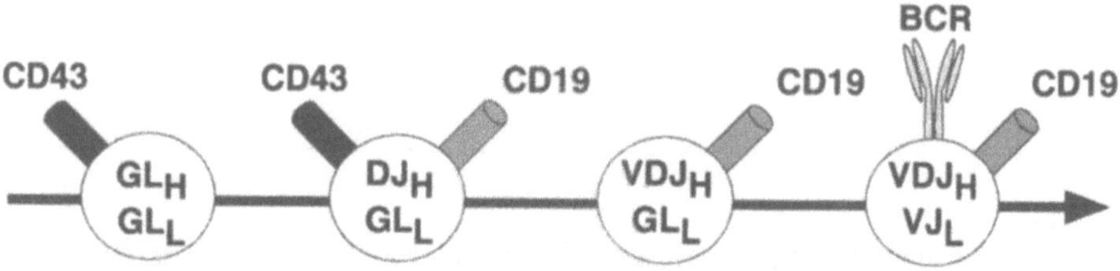


Fig. 1. Schematic of Ig HC gene rearrangements during B-cell development.

**Table 1**
**Primer Sets, Expected Size of Amplified PCR Products, and Oligoprobe Usage**

| Target | 5' Primer | Probe | 3' Primer | Expected size |
|---|---|---|---|---|
| $D_H$ to $J_H4$ | $D_HL$ | $J_H3$ | $J_H4$ | ~1033, ~716, ~333 bp |
| $V_H$ to $DJ_H4$ | $V_H558$ | $J_H3$ | $J_H4$ | ~1058, ~741, ~358 bp |
| $V_H$ to $DJ_H4$ | $V_H7183$ | $J_H3$ | $J_H4$ | ~1058, ~741, ~358 bp |
| $V_H$ to $DJ_H4$ | $V_HQ52$ | $J_H3$ | $J_H4$ | ~1058, ~741, ~358 bp |
| Vκ to Jκ | Vκ degenerate | OL110 | OL109 | ~647, ~311 |
| RAG gene (control) | OL106 | OL121 | OL107 | 560 bp |

antigen specific portion of the B-cell receptor (BCR). The same rearranged gene is alternatively spliced to allow expression and secretion of antigen-specific antibodies in activated plasma cells.

In order to detect Ig gene rearrangements in a pool of lymphoid cells, both degenerate and specific oligonucleotide primers are used to amplify the various possible Ig gene rearrangements. These polymerase chain reaction (PCR) products are separated by agarose gel electrophoresis, transferred to nylon membrane, and subsequently probed with oligonucleotide probes to the J segments of rearranged HC and LC genes (**Table 1, Fig. 2**). Changes in temperatures, times, pH, and other parameters in the protocol may be necessary depending on the equipment utilized and specific samples being examined in these experiments. The following procedures designed to examine murine bone marrow gene rearrangements can be modified to examine DNA rearrangements in splenic and peripheral B cells, as well as T-cell populations.

## 2. Materials

### *2.1. Isolation of Bone Marrow Cells*

1. Femurs and/or other long bones from mouse.
2. 26G1/2 needle and 10 mL syringe (e.g., Becton Dickenson can supply both).
3. PBS: To prepare 1 L, dissolve 8 g NaCl, 0.2 g KCl, 1.44 g $Na_2HPO_4$, 0.24 g $KH_2PO_4$ into 800 mL distilled water. Adjust pH to 7.4 with HCl. Adjust final vol to 1 L with distilled water. Sterilize by autoclaving. Store at 4°C.

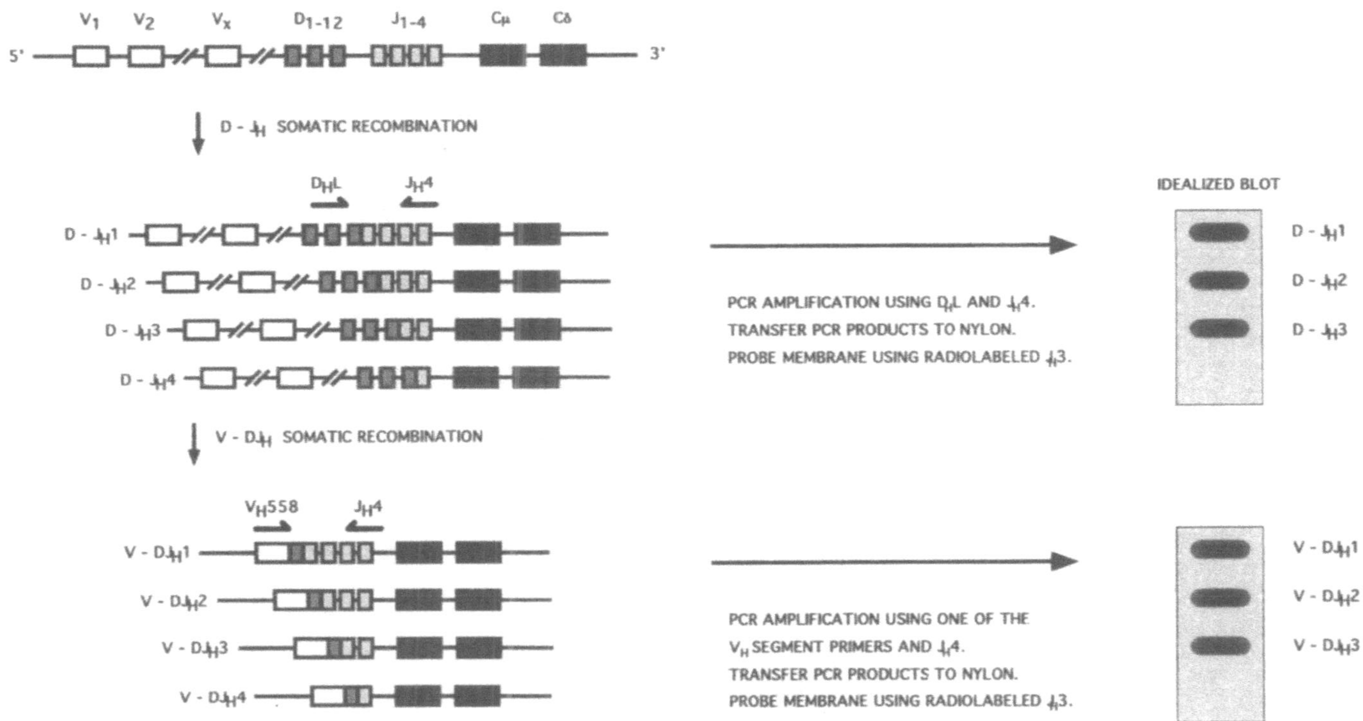


Fig. 2. Representation of PCR amplification and subsequent Southern hybridization detection of immunoglobulin gene rearrangements.

4. Nytex membrane (Tetko Inc., Depew, New York, Cat. #3-40/26), or other suitable material for filtering tissue debris from cell preparations.
5. Microscope and hemocytometer (VWR, Cat. #15170-168) with cover slips (VWR, Cat. #66198-002) or other method for cell counting.

### 2.2. Genomic DNA Purification

1. DNA Lysis Buffer: 100 m*M* Tris-HCl pH 7.5, 100 m*M* NaCl, and 10 m*M* EDTA.
2. 12 × 75 mm polypropylene tubes (Falcon Cat. #2063).
3. 10% sarkosyl.
4. 10 mg/mL proteinase K in water. Store aliquots at –20°C.
5. Incubating oven or water bath.
6. Buffer saturated phenol (GibcoBRL, Cat. #15513–039).
7. Tube rotator or other agitation device able to accept 12 × 75-mm tubes.
8. Chloroform.
9. Tabletop centrifuge with adapters able to accept 12 × 75-mm tubes.
10. Absolute ethanol.
11. TE Buffer: 10 m*M* Tris-HCl, pH 8.0, 1 m*M* EDTA.
12. Spectrophotometer or other DNA quantification methodology.

### 2.3. PCR Amplification

1. Taq DNA polymerase and manufacturer's 10X buffer (e.g., Pharmacia, Cat. #27-0799-01).
2. For analyzing mouse immunoglobulin gene rearrangements, utilize the following custom oligonucleotide sequences:

| | |
|---|---|
| $D_HL$ | GGAATTCGMTTTTTGTSAAGGGATCTACTACTGTG ***(11)*** |
| $V_H558$ | CGAGCTCTCCARCACAGCCTWCATGCARCTCARC ***(11)*** |
| $V_H7183$ | CGGTACCAAGAASAMCCTGTWCCTGCAAATGASC ***(11)*** |
| $V_HQ52$ | CGGTACCAGACTGARCATCASCAAGGACAAYTCC ***(11)*** |
| $J_H4$ | TCCCTCAAATGAGCCTCCAAAGTCC ***(11)*** |
| Vκ degenerate | GGCTGCAGSTTCAGTGGCAGTGGRTCWGGRAC ***(10)*** |
| OL106 | TACCCTGAGCTTCAGTTCTGCACC ***(6)*** |
| OL107 | TGACTGTGGGAACTGCTGAACTTT ***(6)*** |
| OL109 | TCCCTCCTTAACACCTGATCTGAG ***(6)*** |

M = A or C, R = A or G, S = G or C, W = T or A, Y = C or T

3. dATP, dGTP, dCTP, dTTP oligonucleotides (e.g., Pharmacia, Cat. #27-2050-01).
4. Programmable DNA thermocycler.

### 2.4. Agarose Gel Electrophoresis and Southern Blotting

1. Ethidium Bromide: 10 mg/mL solution (*see* **Note 1**).
2. 0.5 *M* EDTA, pH 8.0: To prepare 1 L, dissolve 186.1 g of disodium ethylenediaminetetraacetate · $2H_20$ into 800 mL distilled water. Adjust pH to 8.0 with several drops of 10 *N* NaOH. The EDTA will not go into solution until the pH nears 8.0. Adjust final volume to 1 L with distilled water. Sterilize by autoclaving.
3. 50X TAE Buffer: Dissolve 242 g of Tris base, 57.1 mL of glacial acetic acid, and 100 mL of 0.5 *M* EDTA, pH 8.0 into a final volume of 1 L with distilled water.
4. 1X TAE Running Buffer: Dilute 20 mL of 50X TAE Buffer and 12.5 µL of 10 mg/mL EtBr into a final volume of 1 L distilled water as needed.
5. 1.5% agarose: dissolve 1.5 g agarose into 100 mL of 1X TAE Running Buffer. Agarose will dissolve into solution upon heating in a microwave oven for 3–5 min at high heat.

Handle hot solution with gloved hands. Prepare solution in Erlenmeyer flask to reduce risk of boiling over. Add 2–3 µL of ethidium bromide solution before pouring the gel.

6. 6X xylene cyanol loading buffer: 30% glycerol, 0.25% xylene cyanol
7. Slab gel electrophoresis apparatus and power supply.
8. DNA standard markers (e.g., *Hae*III digested ϕX174 markers, Promega, Cat. #G1761). Dilute markers to a final volume of 1 µg/10 µL in 1X xylene cyanol buffer.
9. 0.8 *N* NaOH solution.
10. 0.25 *N* HCl solution.
11. 20X SSC: To prepare 1 L, dissolve 175.3 g NaCl and 8.2 g sodium citrate into 800 mL of distilled water. Adjust pH to 7.0 with several drops of 10 *N* NaOH. Adjust final volume to 1 L. Sterilize by autoclaving. Dilute to desired concentration as needed.
12. Nylon membrane (e.g., Genescreen Plus, NEN Dupont, Cat. #NEF988).
13. Filter paper (e.g., VWR, Cat. #28303).
14. Vacuum transfer apparatus. This protocol describes methods utilizing vacuum transfer, however other methods including capillary and electrophoretic transfer methodologies would also be appropriate.

### 2.5. Oligonucleotide Hybridization

1. Hybridization Solution: 6X SSC, 10 m*M* sodium pyrophosphate, 2 m*M* EDTA, 0.1% sodium dodecyl sulfate (SDS), 100 µg/mL denatured fish sperm DNA.
2. T4 polynucleotide kinase (T4 PNK), and manufacturer's 10X buffer (e.g., Pharmacia, Cat. #27-0736-01)
3. 10 µCi $\gamma^{32}$P ATP specific activity of 3000 Ci/mmol; 10 mCi/mL in aqueous solution (Amersham, Cat. #AA0068)
4. For analyzing mouse immunoglobulin gene rearrangements, utilize the following custom oligonucleotide sequences:

| | |
|---|---|
| $J_H3$ | GTCTAGATTCTCACAAGAGTCCGATAGACCCTGG *(11)* |
| OL110 | CGTTTTATTTCCAGCTTGGTCCCC *(6)* |
| OL121 | GAGTTTCAGTGCTCGTTGAGTCAG |

5. ProbeQuant G-50 Micro Columns (Pharmacia, Cat. #27-5335).
6. Geiger counter.
7. Heat sealable bags or incubating oven flasks for membrane incubation.
8. Incubating oven or water bath.

### 2.6. Membrane Washing

1. 20% SDS.
2. Wash Solution: 5X SSC, 0.1% SDS. To prepare 1 L, add 250 mL of 20X SSC and 5 mL of 20% SDS to 500 mL of distilled water. Bring final vol to 1 L with distilled water.
3. Appropriate vessel for washing membranes.
4. Incubating oven or water bath.
5. Geiger counter.
6. Autoradiographic film and film developing equipment.

## 3. Methods

### 3.1. Isolation of Bone Marrow Cells

1. Dissect femurs and/or other long bones from the mouse. Snip ends off of each bone (*see* **Notes 2** and **3**).

2. Flush bone marrow cells from dissected femurs using a 26G1/2 needle and syringe filled with 10 mL of ice-cold PBS. Maintain cells on ice (*see* **Notes 4** and **5**).
3. Pass cells through Nytex membrane thereby removing tissue debris.
4. Determine cell number and calculate cell concentration using a hemocytometer or other cell-counting methodology.

### 3.2. Genomic DNA Purification

1. Resuspend $5 \times 10^6$ cells in 950 µL of DNA Lysis Buffer, in a $12 \times 75$ mm polypropylene tube.
2. Add 50 µL of 10% sarkosyl, mix gently.
3. Add 10 µL of 10 mg/mL proteinase K, mix gently, and incubate 2 h (or overnight) at 55°C.
4. Add 1 mL of buffered phenol, rotate for 2 h (or overnight), room temperature.
5. Spin for 5 min at 600*g* and room temperature. Remove aqueous phase to new tube.
6. Add 0.5 mL of buffered phenol, 0.5 mL of chloroform, and rotate for 2 h (or overnight) at room temperature.
7. Spin for 5 min at 600*g* and room temperature. Remove aqueous phase to new tube.
8. Add 2.5 mL of absolute ethanol, invert tube gently. The DNA will precipitate in a visible flocculent form.
9. Spin for 5 min at 600*g* and room temperature. Pour off ethanol and aspirate residual ethanol droplets. Work quickly and do not allow genomic DNA to dry completely (*see* **Note 6**).
10. Resuspend the DNA in 500 µL of TE Buffer. Allow DNA to dissolve by incubating at 65°C for more than 30 min.
11. Quantitate 1:100 dilution of DNA by spectrophotometry and determine DNA concentration.
12. Prepare 100 µL of 25 ng/µL genomic DNA solution in TE Buffer to be used in PCR reactions.

### 3.3. PCR Reactions (*see* Note 7)

1. Prepare 25 µL, PCR reactions containing 250 ng of genomic DNA, 1X PCR buffer, 1 U of Taq, 1 µ*M* of each necessary oligonucleotide primers (*see* **Table 1** and **Note 8**), and 0.2 m*M* of each dNTP. Prepare a cocktail for multiple DNA samples as needed.
2. Preheat the thermocycler to 95°C. Place reaction tubes into thermocycler.
3. Perform the amplification cycles (15 s at 94°C, 30 s at 58°C, and 75 s at 72°C) 30 times followed by a single 15-min period at 72°C. A final step of 4°C can be added to maintain samples at 4°C until they can be removed from the thermocycler.

### 3.4. Southern Transfer (*see* Note 9)

1. Prepare an appropriately sized 1.5% agarose gel with ethidium bromide to contain all PCR samples and DNA standards. The gel should be as thin as possible for maximum DNA transfer. Submerge gel in electrophoresis apparatus containing 1X TAE Running Buffer with ethidium bromide.
2. Add 4 µL of 6X xylene cyanol loading buffer per PCR reaction and load onto the agarose gel. Load one lane with 10 µL of ϕX174 DNA markers beside PCR samples.
3. Perform electrophoresis for desired time utilizing sufficient electric current depending on the size of the gel and length of electrophoresis apparatus. Allowing the xylene cyanol dye front to progress approx 7–8 cm from the sample wells should be sufficient.

4. Cut nylon membrane to 1 cm wider than gel on each side.
5. Cut filter paper to 2 cm wider than gel on each side.
6. Soak the gel in 0.25 *N* HCl for 10 min to fragment large DNA molecules.
7. Soak the gel in 0.4 *N* NaOH for 30 min to denature the DNA.
8. Set up vacuum transfer layers in decreasing size from bottom to top: filter paper, then nylon membrane, then vacuum gel apron, then agarose gel. Perform the transfer for 1 h in 0.4 *N* NaOH. Exact times may vary depending upon the thickness of the gel.
9. Upon completion of transfer, denote PCR lanes by depressing a ball-point pen through sample wells in gel and marking individual lanes.
10. Disassemble transfer apparatus and rinse membrane in 2X SSC for 5 min to remove agarose debris.
11. PCR samples transferred to Genescreen nylon membrane need no further fixation and are ready to be probed using oligonucleotide hybridization. Other membranes need to be fixed by either UV irradiation or oven baking.

### 3.5. Oligonucleotide Hybridization (*see* Note 10)

1. Incubate membrane in 10 mL of Hybridization Solution for more than 30 min at 60°C in a sealed plastic bag, or incubation oven flask.
2. While preincubation is proceeding, prepare oligonucleotide probe by combining the following reagents at 37°C for 1 h: 25 µ*M* of the appropriate oligonucleotide, 10 µCi of $\gamma^{32}P$ ATP, 1X T4 polynucleotide kinase (PNK) buffer, 1 U of PNK in 25 µL final volume. $J_H3$ and OL110 will detect Ig HC and LC gene rearrangements, respectively. OL121 will detect the control amplification (*see* **Table 1** for oligoprobe usage.)
3. Prespin ProbeQuant G-50 columns for 1 min at 735*g*.
4. Remove unincorporated $\gamma^{32}P$ ATP from the oligonucleotide probe by spinning reaction through G-50 column at 735*g* for 2 min.
5. Incubate membrane with 10 mL of fresh Hybridization Solution containing the prepared oligonucleotide probe at 60°C overnight.

### 3.6. Wash Membrane

1. Rinse membrane briefly in 10 mL of Wash Solution, then gently agitate membrane in enough fresh Wash Solution to cover membrane for 15 min at room temperature (*see* **Note 11**).
2. Examine membrane for specific radiolabeled oligoprobe hybridization using Geiger counter (*see* **Note 12**).
3. Repeat **step 1**, as required. Two washes at room temperature are typically sufficient. However, one wash at 37°C may be necessary to remove significant amounts of nonspecific radiolabeled background.
4. Wrap damp membrane in plastic wrap and expose to autoradiography film for 3 h. Repeat exposure for optimum detection period as needed.

## 4. Notes

1. Extreme care should be used when preparing this solution because EtBr is a powerful mutagen. All electrophoresis equipment is dedicated for use with EtBr-containing solutions. EtBr is used in both the agarose solution and the 1X TAE running buffer.
2. When flushing cells from long bones, it is useful to remove as much muscle tissue as possible from the bone during dissection. This will allow visualization of the bone marrow as the cells are being flushed.

3. For preparation of cells from spleen and thymic tissues, crush dissected organs between the frosted ends of glass slides. Tissue debris will be filtered during **step 3**.
4. Use separate needles for each sample to reduce risk of contaminating samples from different animals. Precautions minimizing or eliminating sample contamination should be maintained during any experiment owing to the sensitivity of PCR amplification. It may be necessary to utilize barrier filtered micropipettor tips to eliminate DNA cross-contamination.
5. If red blood cells (RBCs) are contaminating the sample, they can be lysed by resuspending original lymphoid cell preparation (**step 2** in **Subheading 3.1.**) in 5 mL of RBC Lysis Buffer (Sigma, Cat. #R7757) for 5 minutes at room temperature. This solution should be removed from remaining cells by washing cells twice in cold PBS.
6. When resuspending DNA, it is critical that the genomic DNA does not dry completely. Dry genomic DNA does not dissolve well in TE Buffer. It is better to leave a few small droplets of ethanol with DNA than to allow the DNA to dry completely.
7. Variability between PCR machines, DNA quality, primer quality, reagent purity, Taq DNA polymerase manufacturers, PCR tube quality, and PCR cycle number can greatly affect the reproducibility of the PCR reactions. Optimization of each of these variables may be necessary for specific samples.
8. The $D_H$L primer is degenerate at two positions giving homology to 9 of the 10 murine D segment minigenes ***(11)***. The HC variable segment primers ($V_H$558, $V_H$7183, and $V_H$Q52) are degenerate primers representing sequences from the three respective murine V segment gene families (J558, 7138, and Q52) ***(11)***. These gene families are utilized in 62.5, 7 and 5% of Ig-positive splenic B cells in C57BL/6 mice, respectively ***(12)***. Therefore, depending on the murine species examined, PCR amplification efficiency will differ depending on which V segment primer set is used.
9. Depending on efficiencies of the PCR reaction, as well as membrane transfer and washing, it may be necessary to probe only a fraction of the total PCR reaction. The remainder of the reaction can be stored at 4°C for future analysis or reanalysis.
10. It is not necessary to probe the control PCR reactions, because the efficiency of this amplification is greater than the immunoglobulin amplifications. The RAG sequence is present in every cell of a pool, whereas the individual Ig rearrangements are represented in a fraction of total B cells (*see* **Note 8**). The readily amplified control PCR reactions can be visualizing by ethidium bromide staining of the agarose gel. However, if necessary, the control PCR reactions can be probed using radiolabeled OL121. This probe hybridization is very efficient and discrete visualization of bands may be enhanced by probing a fraction of the total PCR reaction. This blot may also need to be washed at 60°C to remove excess nonspecifically bound probe.
11. Because each radiolabeled oligoprobe will have a different annealing temperature, each blot utilizing a different probe should be washed separately.
12. Washing the radioactive membrane is a sensitive procedure. Because of their decreased annealing temperature, radiolabeled oligoprobes wash off the membrane much more rapidly than longer DNA probes. Between washes, monitor the membranes with a partially occluded Geiger detector field. This will allow for more precise monitoring of radiolabeled oligoprobe hybridization. If the edges of the membrane are relatively clean, but the center of the membrane is very radioactive, stop washing. It is always possible to continue washing a damp membrane if there is still too much background radiation after a short 1–2 h exposure to autoradiography film. If the membrane dries completely, the probe will be difficult to remove.

## References

1. Ernberg, I., Falk, K., and Hansson, M. (1987) Progenitor and pre-B lymphocytes transformed by Epstein-Barr virus. *Int. J. Cancer* **39,** 190–197.
2. Gregory, C. D., Kirchgens, C., Edwards, C. F., Young, L. S., Rowe, M., Forster, A., et al. (1987) Epstein-Barr virus-transformed human precursor B cell lines: altered growth phenotype of lines with germ-line or rearranged but nonexpressed HC genes. *Eur. J. Immun.* **17,** 1199–1207.
3. Katamine, S., Otsu, M., Tada, K., Tsuchiya, S., Sato, T., Ishida, N., Honjo, T., and Ono, Y. (1984) Epstein-Barr virus transforms precursor B cells even before immunoglobulin gene rearrangements. *Nature* **309,** 369–372.
4. Kubagawa, H., Burrows, P. D., Grossi, C. E., Mestecky, J., and Cooper, M. D. (1988) Precursor B cells transformed by Epstein-Barr virus undergo sterile plasma-cell differentiation: J-chain expression without immunoglobulin. *Proc. Natl. Acad. Sci. USA* **85,** 875–879.
5. Kubagawa, H., Cooper, M. D., Carroll, A. J., and Burrows, P. D. (1989) Light-chain gene expression before heavy-chain gene rearrangement in pre-B cells transformed by Epstein-Barr virus. *Proc. Natl. Acad. Sci. USA* **86,** 2356–2360.
6. Caldwell, R. G., Wilson, J. B., Anderson, S. J., and Longnecker, R. (1998) Epstein-Barr virus LMP2A drives B cell development and survival in the absence of normal B cell receptor signals. *Immunity* **9,** 405–411.
7. Babcock, G. J., Decker, L. L., Volk, M., and Thorley-Lawson, D. A. (1998) EBV persistence in memory B cells in vivo. *Immunity* **9,** 395–404.
8. Rajewsky, K. (1996) Clonal selection and learning in the antibody system. *Nature* **381,** 751–757.
9. Takemori, T. and Rajewsky, K. (1981) Lambda chain expression at different stages of ontogeny in C57BL/6, BALB/c and SJL mice. *Eur. J. Immun.* **11,** 618–625.
10. Schlissel, M. S. and Baltimore, D. (1989) Activation of immunoglobulin kappa gene rearrangement correlates with induction of germline kappa gene transcription. *Cell* **58,** 1001–1007.
11. Schlissel, M. S., Corcoran, L. M., and Baltimore, D. (1991) Virus-transformed pre-B cells show ordered activation but not inactivation of immunoglobulin gene rearrangement and transcription. *J. Exp. Med.* **173,** 711–720.
12. ten Boekel, E., Melchers, F., and Rolink, A. G. (1997) Changes in the V(H) gene repertoire of developing precursor B lymphocytes in mouse bone marrow mediated by the pre-B cell receptor. *Immunity* **7,** 357–368.

# Index

A

Apoptosis assays,
chromatin changes, 181–182
DNA fragmentation, 185, 189, 348
morphology, 347–348
TUNEL/ISEL, 181–182, 184–185, 347–348, 352–354
Allelic exchange, 27–29
Antibodies, 219, 222–223

B

B cells,
B220, 412
cell cycle distribution, 129
development, 423–424
enrichment, 411–421
expression in, 361
infection of,
with mini-EBV, 23, 31
Blotting,
Northern,
capillary, 48, 54
electroblotting, 55, 364, 367–368
hybridization, 56, 369
stripping, 369
Blotting *(cont.)*,
slot blot, 364
DNA, 368
RNA, 369
stripping, 369
Southern,
capillary, 107, 192
electroblotting, 364, 367–368
hybridization, 193, 369, 429
stripping, 369
vacuum, 428–429
Western, 219, 229–242, 340
chemiluminescence, 230, 236–237, 340
stripping, 237
Bone marrow, 412, 415, 427–428
BrdU,
applications, 379–381
preparation, 382
proliferation assays, *see* Proliferation

C

Carcinogenesis, 391–393
Carcinogens, chemical, 391–399
treatment protocol, 394–395
CAT assay, 259, 266–267

From: *Methods in Molecular Biology, Vol. 174, Epstein-Barr Virus Protocols*
Edited by: J.B Wilson and G. H. W. May © Humana Press Inc., Totowa, NJ

cDNA library,
construction, 37
plating, 40
screening, 40
Cell count (viable), 166
Alamar Blue, 169
Trypan Blue exclusion, 140, 167, 168, 416
Cell lines, *see also* EBV strains
BL2, 156
BL41, 156
C33A, 165
EJ, 165
EREB2–5, 316
HaCat, 165, 173
HEK293, 316, 331
Hela, 165
IARC171, 156
IB-4, 68
Jurkat, 156
L428, 156
Loukes, 149
Patas, 150
RHEK-1, 165
SCC12F, 165, 173
Chimeric receptors, 314
Complimentary strand transcripts (CTRs), 37–43
Conditional gene expression, 362
CsCl plasmid purification, 29
Cytotoxic T-cells, *see* T-cells

**D**

Disease models, 361–363, 391, 411
DNA,
blotting, *see* Blotting, Southern; Blotting, slot
DNA *(cont.)*,
coupling to magnetic beads, 274
CsCl purification, 29
electrophoresis,
field inversion, 189, 191
Gardella gel, 111, 113
gel/mobility shift assay, 273, 289–294
elution from gels, 115
extraction, 16
*in situ* hybridization, 79, 85–86, 93–94, 97
labelling,
end labelling, 18, 292, 429
nick translation, 72, 85, 282
random priming, 189, 192
strand breaks, 181–182, 184–185
preparation, genomic, 366, 428
primers, 18
transfection,
calcium phosphate mediated, 46, 53, 149–150, 265
DEAE method, 266
electroporation, 16, 137–140, 158, 320
lipofection, 319, 331, 333
Double-stranded RNA-activated protein kinase (PKR), 297, 300, 304
Dynabeads, *see* Magnetic-activated cell sorting; Magnetic DNA affinity purification

**E**

EBV genes,
BARF1, 147
BART (CST), 4, 37
BHLF1, 139

EBV genes *(cont.)*,
EBER, 4, 45, 80, 86, 297–310
EBNA-1, 4, 13, 219–220, 279
EBNA-2, 4, 23, 219–220, 232, 259–261, 271
EBNA-3A (3), 4, 23, 219–220
EBNA-3B (4), 4, 219–220
EBNA-3C (6), 4, 23, 219–220, 232
EBNA-LP (5), 4
LMP-1, 4, 23, 159–161, 219, 231, 232, 250, 391
chimeric and mutated variants, 313–323
kinases regulated by, 325–336
LMP-2 (A/B), 4, 219, 337–343, 423
nomenclature, 4
EBV strains/cell lines,
Akata, 119, 243
B95-8, 3, 119, 126
map, 5–11
Daudi,
deletion, 7
P3HR1, 23, 119
deletion, 7
Raji, 3, 119
deletion, 8, 9, 11
Electrophoresis, *see* DNA; RNA; Protein
Electroporation, *see also* DNA transfection, of *E. coli*, 256
Epithelial cells,
differentiation, 173
suspension culture, 174, 175
epidermis, 401–404
separation from dermis, 403–407
expression in, 362
Epithelial cells *(cont.)*,
growth, 165
primary culture, 407
raft culture, 174, 176–179
Epitope tag, 319, 327
Expression library, 279
screening of, 282–284

F

FACS, *see* Fluorescence-activated cell sorting
FISH, *see* Fluorescence *in situ* hybridization
Fluorescence-activated cell sorting, 103, 155, 159, 350
Fluorescence *in situ* hybridization, 67

G

GAL4 fusion proteins, 249, 259, 261, 363
Gardella gel, 111, 113
Glycoproteins,
biosynthetic radiolabeling, 243
GST fusion protein purification, 330

I

Immortalization assays, 147
Immunofluorescence, *see* Fluorescence-activated cell sorting
Immunoglobulin,
gene rearrangement, 423–431
heavy chain enhancer, 361
IgG subtypes, 334
Immunohistochemistry, 80, 87, 350
APAAP method, 95
Immunoprecipitation, *see* Protein

Interphase cells,
preparation of, 71
In vitro transcription, 297, 302
In vitro translation, 300, 304

**J**

JNK, 325–328

**K**

Kinase assays, 325, 331–333, 338, 341

**L**

Labelling, *see* DNA; RNA; Glycoproteins
Latent genes, *see* EBV genes
Latent infection, 79–81
LCLs, *see* Lymphoblastoid cell lines
Luciferase assay, 259, 266–267
Lymph nodes, 411, 415
Lymphoblastoid cell lines (LCLs), 23, 80, 139, 199, 203
cell cycle distribution, 129
generation of, 125
Lymphocytes, 411–421
Lytic cycle,
induction, 121
genes, 12

**M**

MACS, *see* Magnetic-activated cell sorting
Magnetic-activated cell sorting, 103, 106, 155, 158, 412–413, 416–419
Magnetic DNA affinity purification, 271, 273
Metaphase cells,
preparation of, 71
Mini-EBV plasmids, 23–36, 327
Mononuclear cells,
isolation of, 105

**N**

NFκB, 325–328
Nuclear extracts, preparation, 292

**O**

OriLyt, 23
OriP, 23
oriP-based plasmids, 13

**P**

PCR, *see* Polymerase chain reaction
Peripheral blood mononuclear cells (PBMCs), 105, 125, 199, 203, 205, 213, 214, 417
isolation of, 105
Percoll gradient, 417–418
Phage,
isolation, 41, 284
preparation of extracts from lysogens, 285
Plasmids,
mini-EBV plasmids, 23
Homologous recombination, 27
CsCl purification, 29
oriP-based plasmids, 13
tet shuttle plasmids, 26, 28
Polymerase chain reaction, 424, 428
EBV-specific, 107, 111–112
quantitative, competitive, 13, 17, 18

Probes, *see* DNA; RNA
Proliferation,
BrdU incorporation, 133, 382–384
$^{3}$H-thymidine incorporation, 133, 151, 166, 168
immortalization assays, 147
MTT assay, 166, 169
serum dependence, 152
soft agar assay, 151
Protein,
blotting, *see* Blotting, Western
Bradford assay, 57
electrophoresis,
SDS-PAGE, 229, 234–235
gel/mobility shift assay, 273, 289–294
extraction, 234–235, 319, 331–332, 340, 367
from bacteria, 330
immunoprecipitation, 319, 327, 331–332, 337, 340
inhibition of synthesis, 49, 57
*in situ* hybridization, 93, 95
protein-protein interaction, 249, 256, 259–262
purification by DNA affinity, 271, 274
$^{35}$S-methionine labelling, 57
synthesis measurement in vivo, 57
tyrosine phosphorylation, 337

**R**

Red blood cell (RBC) lysis, 415
Regression assay, 199
Reporter genes/plasmids, 259–264
Reticulocyte lysate, *see* In vitro translation
RNA,
*in situ* hybridization, 72–73, 93–94, 97
blotting, *see* Blotting, Northern; Blotting, slot
expression on heterologous cells, 45–66
gel electrophoresis, 48, 54, 55
labelling, 84, 298, 303
preparation, 47, 53, 54, 367
RNA-protein interactions, 297
filter binding, 299, 303
UV crosslinking, 298, 303

**S**

SDS-PAGE, *see* Protein, electrophoresis
Skin, *see* Epithelial cells, epidermis
Spleen/Splenocytes, 411, 415

**T**

T-cells,
cytotoxic T-cells (CTLs), 203, 205, 209
epitope mapping, 209, 210
limiting dilution assay, 213
expression in, 362
memory T-cells, 204
$^{3}$H-thymidine incorporation, *see* Proliferation
Tissue,
fixing, 95, 352, 383
sectioning, 83–84, 95, 352–353, 383
Transfection, *see* DNA, transfection
Transgenic mice, 361–364, 380, 391, 404, 411, 423
sample preparation, 363, 366–367

Tumorigenicity, 152

V

Viability, *see* Cell count
Virus,
  infection, detection of, 93–94, 103–104, 111–112
  isolation, 119–123

Y

Yeast,
  isolation of DNA, 255
  protein extracts, 253
  transactivation potential, 254
  transformation, 252–254
  two-hybrid assay, 249
    mammalian cell variation, 260

MIX
Papier aus verantwortungsvollen Quellen
Paper from responsible sources
FSC® C105338

If you have any concerns about our products,
you can contact us on
**ProductSafety@springernature.com**

In case Publisher is established outside the EU,
the EU authorized representative is:
**Springer Nature Customer Service Center GmbH**
**Europaplatz 3, 69115 Heidelberg, Germany**

Printed by Libri Plureos GmbH
in Hamburg, Germany